MUSCULAR DYSTROPHY

Edited by **Madhuri Hegde**
and **Arunkanth Ankala**

Muscular Dystrophy
Edited by Madhuri Hegde and Arunkanth Ankala

Published by InTech
Janeza Trdine 9, 51000 Rijeka, Croatia

Publishing Process Manager Jana Sertic

Technical Editor Teodora Smiljanic

Cover Designer InTech Design Team

Additional hard copies can be obtained from orders@intechopen.com

Muscular Dystrophy, Edited by Madhuri Hegde and Arunkanth Ankala
p. cm.
ISBN 978-953-51-0603-6

For EU product safety concerns:
IN TECH d.o.o., Prolaz Marije Krucifikse Kozulić 3, 51000 Rijeka, Croatia,
info@intechopen.com or visit our website at intechopen.com.

Meet the editors

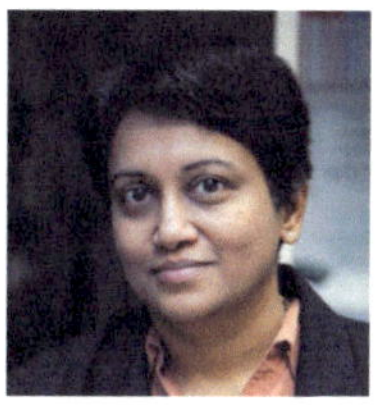

Dr Madhuri Hegde is an Associate Professor/Scientific Director at Emory Genetics Laboratory in the Department of Human Genetics. She received a BSc and an MSc from the University of Bombay, India, and a PhD from the University of Auckland, New Zealand. She performed post-doctoral studies at Baylor College of Medicine and is board certified in Clinical Molecular Genetics. The primary focus of her clinical work is the development of high-throughput sequencing strategies for rare disorders using sequence capture technologies, robotics, next generation sequencing, oligonucleotide array platforms, and predictive analysis tools. Her research is focused on functional analysis of sequence variants in disease-associated genes specifically for muscular dystrophies, with an ultimate goal of creating an algorithm for clinical interpretation of novel sequence variants. She is also involved in identifying novel disease genes using next-generation tools and a laboratory developed bridged whole exome sequencing approach.

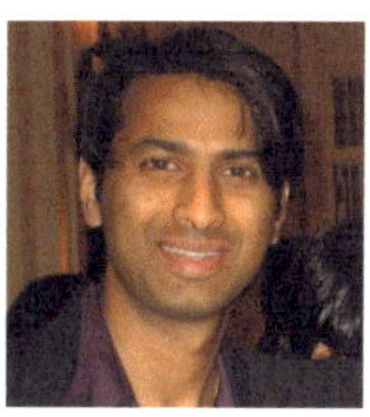

Dr Arunkanth Ankala is a Clinical Molecular Genetics Fellow at Emory Genetics Laboratory in the Department of Human Genetics. After receiving a Masters degree in Biochemistry from Bharatidasan University, India, he pursued his PhD at Mississippi State University in Molecular Biology. Later, he moved on to perform post-doctoral studies at Emory University School of Medicine in the department of Human Genetics. The primary focus of his clinical research work has been the understanding of the mechanisms underpinning the high frequency of intragenic deletions and duplications in human DMD gene causing Duchenne Muscular Dystrophy. His broader research interest has been the discovery of new disease causing genes associated with different muscular dystrophies especially congenital muscular dystrophies and limb-girdle muscular dystrophies. Using next generation sequencing technologies including targeted sequence capture technologies, whole exome sequencing and transcriptome analysis he has been actively involved in new gene discovery and diagnostic tool development for muscular dystrophies.

Contents

Preface

The journey of the development of an effective treatment for a disorder starts with the characterization of the clinical phenotype of an individual affected by the disorder. Genetic disorders run in families by autosomal recessive, dominant, X-linked or mitochondrial inheritance from either or both parents to child and within a few generations a group of individuals presenting a common phenotype are observed in the family. With the globalization of the scientific research, more and more such families are being identified and are being studied. Technological advancement in the field of clinical research has resulted in the rapid identification of novel disease-causing genes providing molecular diagnosis to the affected individuals. Identification of the causative gene initiates several studies to understand the pathophysiology of the disease, finally leading to the development of an effective therapy. This book provides a comprehensive overview of muscular dystrophy which is a group of inherited disorders characterized by muscle weakness and progressive muscle wasting. To date more than 30 different types and subtypes of muscular dystrophies have been identified, each of which is caused by mutations in a different gene. Therefore each subtype of muscular dystrophy needs to be studied individually. With an introduction to the different muscular dystrophies and the genes involved, the book comprises individual chapters contributed by different authors currently working in the field of muscular dystrophy.

This book aims to introduce the readers to the basic, clinical as well as translational research that is currently being carried on in various research laboratories around the globe. This includes wide aspects of the pathophysiology of the disorder, methods available for diagnosis of the disorder, therapeutic strategies being explored including those that are currently in the phase of clinical trials as well as tools and animal models available for further research.

The editors thank all the authors who have contributed to this book and hope the knowledge and ideas offered through this book provide the contemporary scientists with the right direction in which to further their interests in muscular dystrophy research.

Dr Arunkanth Ankala
Department of Human Genetics,
Emory University School of Medicine,
Atlanta,
USA

Dr Madhuri Hegde
Associate Professor,
Emory Genetics Lab Scientific Director,
Emory University School of Medicine, Atlanta,
USA

Section 1

Introduction to Muscular Dystrophies

1

Alpha-Dystroglycanopathy

Mieko Yoshioka
Department of Pediatric Neurology, Kobe City Pediatric and General Rehabilitation Center for the Challenged, Japan

1. Introduction

Alpha-dystroglycanopathies are a clinically and genetically heterogenous group of muscular dystrophies characterized by the reduced or absent glycosylation of alpha-dystroglycan (Muntoni et al., 2002). The hypoglycosylation of alpha-dystroglycan leads to decreased binding of its ligands, including laminin, agrin and perlecan in skeletal muscle and neurexin in the brain. The only known target for this type of glycosylation is alpha-dystroglycan, and together with other proteins of the dystrophin-glycoprotein complex it forms a link between extracellular matrix proteins and actin cytoskeleton. The clinical manifestations of alpha-dystroglycanopathies are extremely variable, leading to a broad spectrum of phenotypes with limb-girdle muscular dystrophy (LGMD) without mental retardation delineating the milder end, and Walker-Warburg syndrome (WWS), muscle-eye-brain disease (MEB) and Fukuyama type congenital muscular dystrophy (FCMD) the severe end (Muntoni & Voit, 2004) (Fig. 1). In most of the severe disorders, the eyes and the brain are affected in addition to congenital muscular dystrophy (CMD). Here, CMD is defined as onset of weakness prenatally or within the first 6 months of life, and LGMD is defined by later onset weakness, specifically after having acquired ambulation. The brain abnormalities are described as cobblestone lissencephaly; available pathological studies have demonstrated breeches of the glia limitans and over-migration of cortical neurons into the pial spaces. In WWS, the life-span of patients is severely reduced and brain and eye abnormalities extremely severe (Dobyns et al., 1989); MEB and FCMD patients generally survive beyond infancy, ocular manifestations are usually milder in FCMD than in MEB (Fukuyama et al., 1981, Santavuori et al., 1989). To date, mutations in six genes which encode putative or confirmed glycosyltransferases have been identified in these autosomal recessively inherited disorders: *Protein-O-mannosyl transferase 1* and *2* (*POMT1* and *POMT2*), *Protein-O-mannose 1,2-N-acetylglucosaminyltransferase 1* (*POMGnT1*), *Fukutin-related protein* (*FKRP*), *Fukutin* (*FKTN*), and *LARGE*. Initially, each gene was associated with one syndrome (original phenotype) : *POMT1* and *POMT2* mutations giving rise to WWS; *POMGnT1* mutations in patients with MEB; *FKRP* mutations in patients with congenital or late-onset muscular dystrophies (MDC1C and LGMD 2I); *FKTN* mutations in patients with FCMD; *LARGE* mutations in a patient with congenital muscular dystrophy type 1D (MDC 1D). Subsequently, mutation analysis in patients with milder or more severe syndromes within the dystroglycanopathy spectrum demonstrated allelic heterogeneity for different mutations in each of the dystroglycanopathy genes (Fig. 1). Null mutations in *POMT1, POMT2, POMGnT1, FKRP,*

FKTN and *LARGE* are associated with the most severe end of the clinical spectrum (WWS) of dystroglycanopathy, although not an absolute rule.

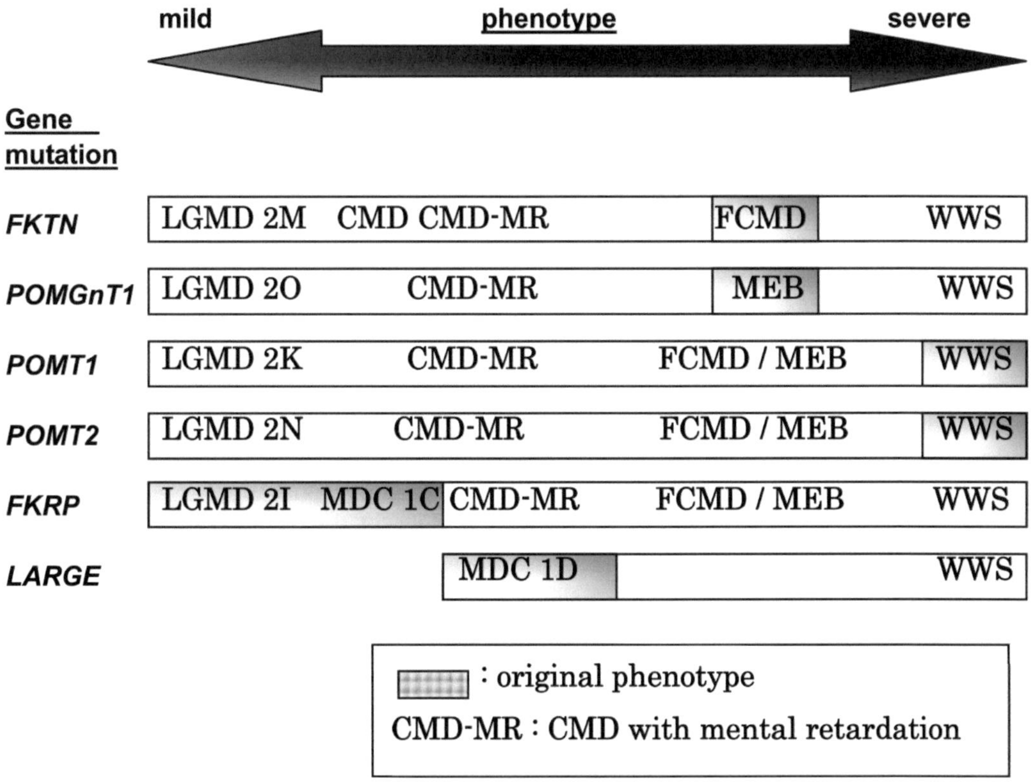

Fig. 1. Gene mutations and clinical phenotypes of alpha-dystroglycanopathy

2. Broader clinical spectrum and worldwide distribution of *FKTN* mutations

A wide clinical spectrum is also evident for the *FKTN* mutations that were first reported in patients with FCMD and later in patients with WWS and in patients with LGMD 2M without mental retardation. FCMD is the second most common form of muscular dystrophy in Japanese population after Duchenne muscular dystrophy, but is seen very rarely in other population. The incidence of FCMD is 3-10 per 100,000 or nearly half that of Duchenne muscular dystrophy in the Japanese population, with a carrier frequency of one in 80 and is one of the most common autosomal recessive disorder in Japan (Fukuyama & Ohsawa,1984). FCMD patients have muscular dystrophy with severe mental retardation and a neuronal migration abnormality. Epilepsy and eye abnormalities are also frequently associated with FCMD. Toda et al. (1993) localized the FCMD locus to chromosome 9q31-33 using genetic linkage analysis. They further defined the FCMD locus within a much smaller segment and also found evidence for strong linkage disequilibrium. Haplotype analysis using the markers D9S2105, 2107, and D9S172 indicated that most FCMD-bearing chromosomes in Japanese pedigrees were derived from a single ancestral founder (Toda et al., 1996). Most Japanese FCMD patients are homozygous for an ancestral founder mutation in FCMD gene, which arose from the insertion of a 3 kb retrotransposon element into the 3′ untranslated region (UTR). Some patients are compound heterozygous, carrying another mutation in addition to the founder insertion, and leading to a more severe FCMD variant (Kobayashi et al., 1998a). The absence of patients with two non-founder mutations in Japan led to the hypothesis that this may be lethal, however since 2003 compound heretozygosity for many different mutations have been described in non-Japanese populations, including homozygosity for nonsense mutations. To date, at least 24 different *FKTN* mutations have been described in non-Japanese patients and phenotypes of these patients cover the entire range of alpha-dystroglycanopathies (Yis et al., 2011).

We performed clinical studies in 41 families with FCMD examined between 1972 and 1992 (Yoshioka & Kuroki, 1994). These patients were diagnosed on the standard criteria of FCMD described by Fukuyama et al. (1960). After the discovery of FCMD gene, we investigated gene mutations of these FCMD families (Yoshioka et al., 2008). Here, we at first describe the clinical studies performed until 1992 and later analysis of the genotype-phenotype relationship in FCMD. We then present Japanese CMD patients with alpha-dystroglycanopathy with other gene mutations than *FKTN* and without any known gene mutation. In addition, we describe *FKTN* mutations outside Japan and compare them with Japanese FCMD patients.

2.1 Japanese FCMD patients diagnosed on standard criteria between 1972 and 1992

We performed clinical and genetic studies in 41 families with FCMD examined by us between 1972 and 1992 (Table 1) (Yoshioka & Kuroki, 1994). The diagnosis in these patients was established according to standard criteria described by Fukuyama et al. in 1960, which were, briefly, early onset hypotonia, joint contractures, severe mental retardation with occasional convulsions, and dystrophic abnormalities detected in the muscle biopsy specimen. Nine families (22%) had multiple affected children ("familial" FCMD). Unfortunately, two siblings in nine families had already died at the time of examination, and detailed clinical data other than their clinical diagnosis were therefore not available. The other 32 families had only one affected child ("sporadic" FCMD). Parental consanguinity was documented in 5 sporadic FCMD families and none of the familial cases. In total, 48 patients, including 7 sib pairs, were evaluated with regard to maximum motor ability, mental and convulsion states, cranial CT or MRI findings, and EEG and ophthalmological data.

	Total	Familial	Sporadic
Number of families	41	9	32
Consanguineous marriage	5	0	5
Number of patients	50	18	32
Male : female	22 : 28	5 : 13	17 : 15

Table 1. Patients with Fukuyama-type Congenital Muscular Dystrophy (FCMD) [diagnosed according to standard criteria between 1972 and 1992, reproduced from Yoshioka & Kuroki, 1994]

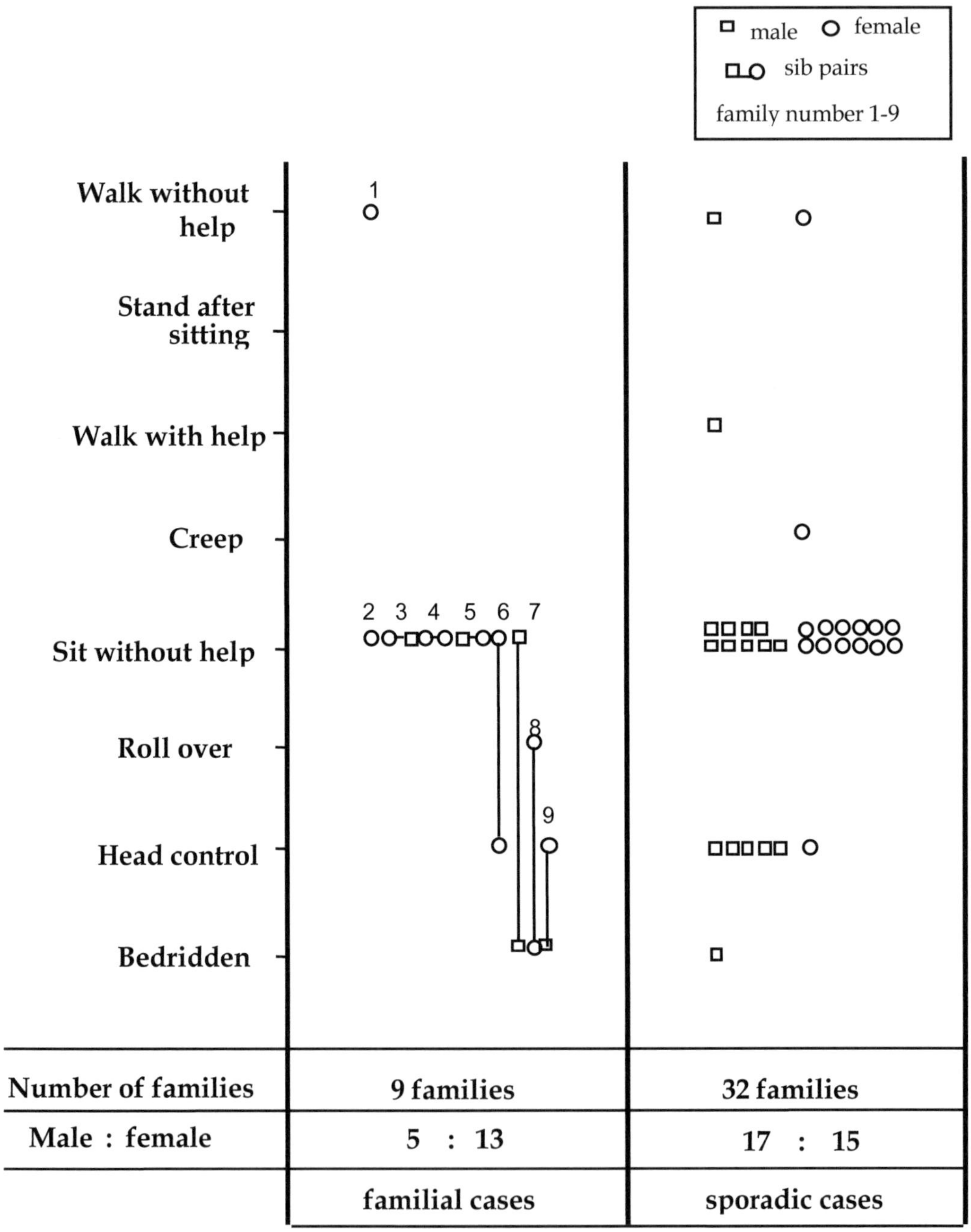

Fig. 2. Maximum motor ability in sib pairs and in familial and sporadic FCMD cases. The familial cases are numbered from 1 to 9. The members of each sib pair are connected by a line (Reproduced from Yoshioka & Kuroki, 1994).

Three patients in our familial group but only one in our sporadic group showed no head control ("bedridden"), whereas a few ambulatory patients were seen in both groups (Fig. 2).

The familial FCMD patients showed relatively more severe motor disability than that in the sporadic FCMD patients. The maximum motor ability in most patients in both groups consisted of sitting without help. Although the speech ability varied between sibs and between families (Fig. 3), all patients showed moderate to severe mental retardation. As for convulsion states, about half of the patients had febrile or afebrile convulsions in both familial and sporadic groups. The convulsion state in 7 sib pairs was the same; both sibs in 3 families had afebrile or febrile convulsions, while in 4 other families neither had convulsion. EEG showed paroxysmal discharges in three sibling pairs with convulsions, while in two of the other sibling pairs without convulsion a difference between siblings in EEG findings was apparent. Ophthalmologically, myopia, weakness of the orbicularis oculi, nystagmus, and optic nerve atrophy were common findings.

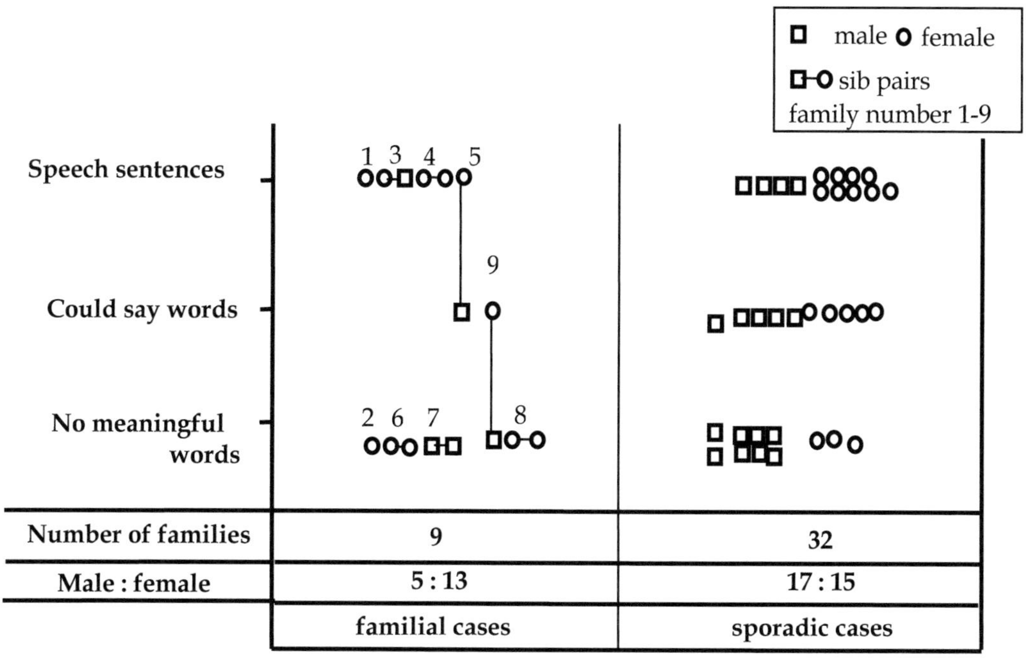

Fig. 3. Speech ability in sib pairs and in familial and sporadic FCMD cases. Familial cases are numbered from 1 to 9, and the members of each sib pair are connected by a line (Reproduced from Yoshioka & Kuroki, 1994).

Typical CT or MRI findings seen in FCMD were pachygyria or polymicrogyria of the fronto-temporo-occipital regions, moderate dilatation of the lateral ventricles, especially posteriorly (colpocephaly), the abnormal signal in the cerebral white matter, and cerebellar cysts closely related to polymicrogyria (Fig. 4). However, in one family (S-family), the elder brother had the typical CT findings of FCMD, while the younger brother had marked dilatation of the lateral ventricles and an occipital encephalocele (Fig. 5). In addition, retinal detachment was present in the younger brother at birth, whereas in the elder brother it developed at 3 years. Our study revealed that FCMD patients ranged from ambulatory to bedridden, and some were able to form sentences while others uttered no meaningful words. Convulsions were found in about half of the patients. Hydrocephalus, encephalocele and retinal detachment were rare but true findings in FCMD.

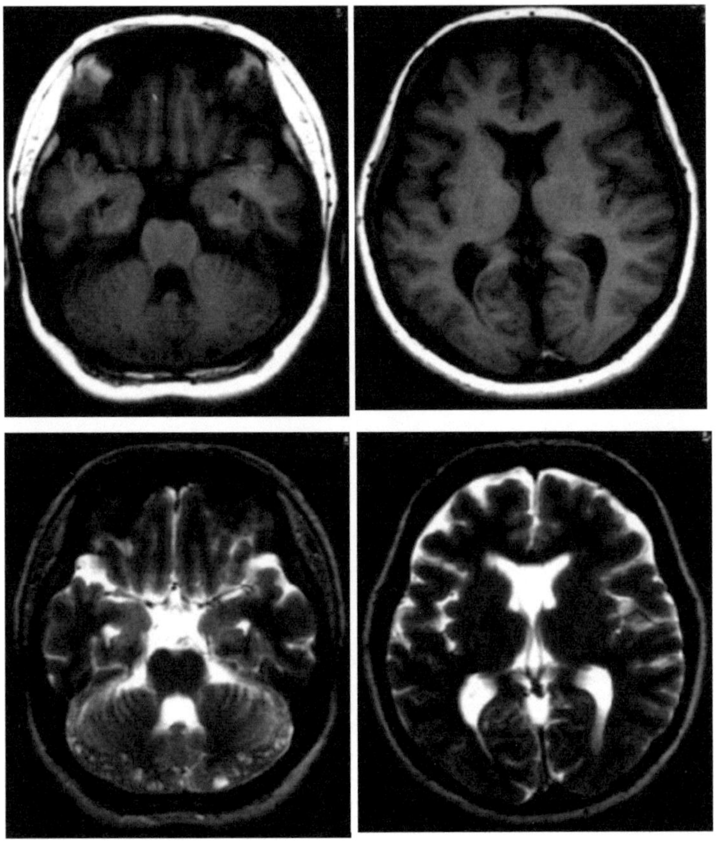

Fig. 4. Typical MR imaging in a FCMD patient aged 16 years. T1-(upper) and T2-(lower) weighted axial magnetic resonance images of the cerebellum (left) and cerebrum (right). Cerebral cortical dysplasia is mild, and numerous cysts closely related to polymicrogyria are seen in the cerebellum (Reproduced from Yoshioka et al., 2008).

Based on these observations, we considered the clinical spectrum of FCMD to be much broader than previously described and to overlap with that of "mild" WWS and of MEB.

2.2 Genetic study of S-family and further analyses of FCMD haplotype

The FCMD locus was initially localized to chromosome 9q31-33 by genetic linkage analysis and homozygosity mapping (Toda et al., 1993, 1994).

We analyzed one Japanese family (S-family) in which three siblings were affected with severe cerebral malformations in association with ocular anomalies and muscle disease (Yoshioka et al., 1992). Both parents were healthy and nonconsanguineous. The elder brother showed pachygyria on computed tomographic scan (Fig.5), retinal detachment in both eyes at the age of three years and dystrophic findings on a muscle biopsy. He was diagnosed clinically as having FCMD. The second pregnancy resulted in a male infant with anencephaly who survived for five minutes. Anencephaly was regarded as WWS with extreme brain abnormality. The third son exhibited at birth such characteristic features as pachygyria, encephalocele, hydrocephalus, retinal detachment in both eyes, elevated serum creatine kinase activity, and arthrogryposis multiplex congenita which were consistent with WWS (Fig.5).

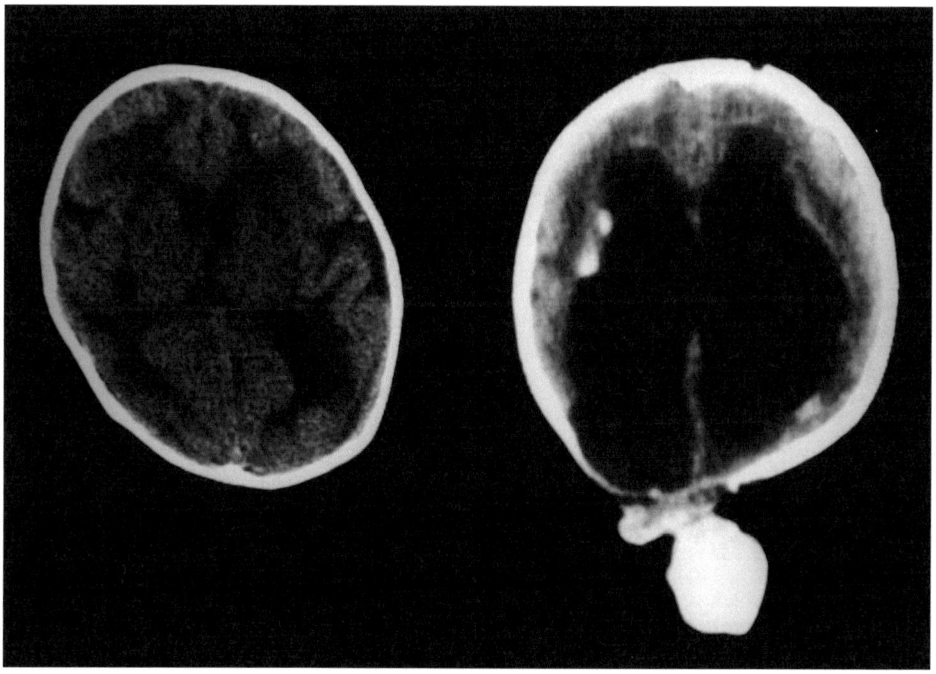

Fig. 5. Cranial computed tomographic scans of two siblings of S-family. Left: the first son at the age of 5 months. Moderate dilatation of the lateral ventricles, especially posteriorly (colpocephalic) and pachygyria in the temporo-parietal region are shown. The low density area in the white matter is apparent. Right: the third son at birth. Marked dilatation of lateral ventricles and occipital encephalocele are evident (Reproduced from Yoshioka & Kuroki, 1994).

Genetic analysis of this family was performed using polymorphic microsatellite markers flanking the FCMD locus (Toda et al., 1995). Genomic DNA was extracted from peripheral blood leukocytes of the parents, the first and the third siblings. Both patients (FCMD and WWS) shared exactly the same haplotype at seven marker loci spanning 16 cM and surrounding the FCMD locus. This suggests that both affected siblings should carry the same combination of FCMD alleles, each with a mutation. Since the patients of FCMD and WWS carry the identical combination of mutations on either allele of the FCMD locus, these clinical conditions are caused by the mutations in the same gene. The difference in clinical manifestations between FCMD and WWS may reflect the pleiotropy or variation of expressivity of the FCMD gene.

Later, it was found that one specific haplotype was shared by 82% of FCMD chromosomes (Kobayashi et al., 1998b). These data supported the hypothesis of a single founder of this disease in the Japanese population. Moreover, eight haplotypes different from the founder's were observed in FCMD chromosomes, indicating that eight different FCMD mutations in addition to the founder's have occurred in Japan. Thereafter, it was clarified that a retrotransposal insertion exists within this candidate-gene interval in all FCMD chromosomes carrying the founder haplotype. Two independent point mutations confirm that a mutation of this gene is responsible for the condition (Kobayashi et al., 1998a).

Using new polymorphic microsatellite markers, we genotyped five CMD patients from four families including the S-family who had severe eye and brain anomalies, such as retinal dysplasia and hydrocephalus (Yoshioka et al., 1999). All patients were heterozygous for the founder haplotype of the FCMD gene. In S-family, the Japanese founder haplotype of the FCMD gene was derived from the patients' mother and the haplotype, which cosegregate with nonsense mutation on exon 3 of the FCMD gene, was derived from their father (Fig. 6). Thus, two siblings were compound heterozygotes for FCMD. This showed severe eye anomalies such as retinal dysplasia or detachment and hydrocephalus could be included in the clinical spectrum of FCMD. The clinical spectrum of FCMD is much broader than previously presumed.

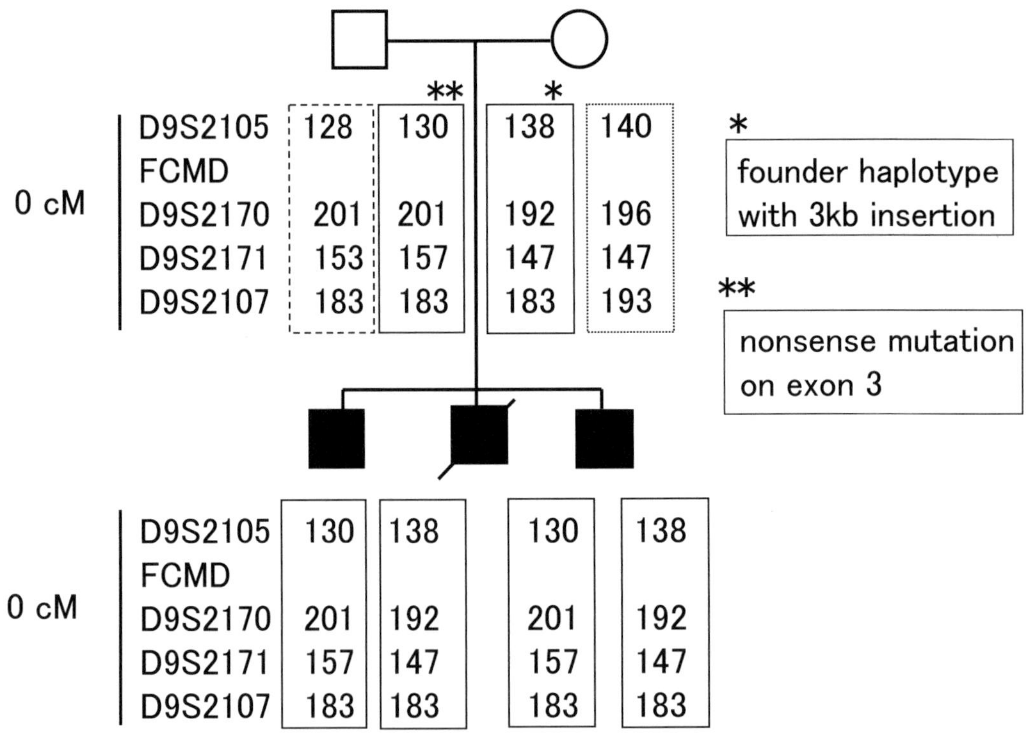

Fig. 6. Genotypes of S-family including two brothers at polymorphic microsatellite loci flanking the FCMD locus. This family is heterozygous for the founder insertion allele. The founder haplotype 138-192-147-183 for markers D9S2105-D9S2170-D9S2171-D9S2107 was derived from the patients' mother and the haplotype 130-201-157-183, which cosegregated with nonsense mutation on exon 3 of the FCMD gene, was derived from their father. Thus, two brothers are compound heterozygotes for the disease (Reproduced from Yoshioka et al., 1999).

To investigate the distribution and origin of the founder insertion of FCMD, Watanabe et al. (2005) screened a total of 4,718 control DNA samples from Japanese and other Northeast

Asian population. Fifteen founder chromosomes were detected among 2,814 Japanese individuals. Heterozygous carriers were found in various regions throughout Japan, with an averaged ratio of 1 in 188, although previous reports have estimated the carrier frequency to be as high as 1 in 80 and the incidence to be 3-10/100,000 births (Fukuyama & Ohsawa, 1984). In Korean populations, they detected one carrier in 935 individuals. However, they were unable to detect any heterozygous alleles in 203 Mongolians and 766 Mainland Chinese populations. These data largely rule out the possibility that a single ancestor bearing an insertion-chromosome immigrated to Japan from Korea or Mainland China and appear to confirm that FCMD carriers are rare outside of Japan.

2.3 Phenotype-genotype relationship in FCMD after discovery of FCMD gene, *FKTN*

Between 1994 and 2006, we diagnosed thirty-five patients with FCMD because they had the founder mutation homozygously or heterozygously, in Kobe City Pediatric and General Rehabilitation Center for the Challenged, Utano National Hospital, Shiga Medical Center for Children and Shizuoka Childrens's Hospital (Yoshioka et al., 2008). Among these 35 patients, we found 18 patients (eight boys and 10 girls) carrying a homozygous founder mutation (homozygous patients or homozygotes) and 17 patients (eight boys and nine girls) with a compound heterozygous mutation (heterozygous patients or heterozygotes). The range of follow-up was between one and 30 years (average 16.5 years) in homozygotes and between two and 19 years (average 12.8 years) in heterozygotes (Table 2).

	Homozygous patients	Heterozygous patients
Number of patients	18	17
Male : Female	8 : 10	8 : 9
Follow-up period : mean	16.5 years	12.8 years
Range : years : months	1 : 2~30 : 8	2 : 5~19 : 5
Maximum motor ability		
Bedridden	2	8
Head control	0	3
Sit without help	15	4
Walk without help	1	2
Mental status		
No meaningful words	2	11
Speak single words	5	5
Speak in sentences	11	1
Radiological findings		
Pachygyria/polymicrogyria	16	16
Hydrocephalus	0	2
Cephalocele	0	1
Ophthalmological findings		
Retinal dysplasia	0	7
Retinal detachment	0	5

Table 2. Clinical characteristics of FCMD patients diagnosed between 1994 and 2006 (Reproduced from Yoshioka et al., 2008)

Genomic DNA was extracted from patients' peripheral blood leukocytes. After digestion of genomic DNA with *Pvu*II, Southern hybridization was performed using fEco8-1 as a probe to detect the 3 kb founder insertion in the DNA. If a patient had only one founder insertion (compound heterozygotes), we then screened all exons and flanking introns of the *FKTN* gene by polymeraze chain reaction direct sequencing to detect nonsense or missense mutations. Some members had been genotyped with polymorphic microsatellite markers as described previously (Kobayashi et al., 1998b). Each chromosome containing the 3 kb retrotransposal insertion was concordant with the founder haplotype represented as 138-192-147-183 for markers D9S2105-D9S2170-D9S2171-D9S2107.

Clinical characteristics in both groups are summarized in Table 2. Most homozygotes could sit without help and speak in sentences, while half of the heterozygotes were bedridden and most spoke no meaningful words. Typical CT or MRI findings of FCMD were seen in almost all cases. These included polymicrogyria within the cerebral cortex that was primarily in the frontal lobes (Figs.4 and 5). In the cerebellum, numerous intraparenchymal cysts closely related to the polymicrogyria were seen at the hemispheres (Fig.4). More severe cortical dysplasia was usually found in heterozygotes than in homozygotes. Hydrocephalus and cephalocele were found only in heterozygotes. In particular, ophthalmological findings showed a clear difference between the two groups; retinal dysplasia and detachment were only found in heterozygotes.

In comparison with our study, systematic analysis of the FCMD gene in 107 unrelated patients by Kondo-Iida et al. (1999) revealed that 80 probands (75%) were homozygous for the 3 kb insertion, 25 (23%) were heterozygous, and two did not show the 3 kb insertion on either allele. In our study, however, the number of homozygotes and heterozygotes was almost the same. Although both groups included some sib pairs in our study, the number of probands was 16 for the homozygotes and 15 for the heterozygotes, which was also almost the same number. This result might be due to the small number of patients examined or a regional inclination in our study, as most of our patients lived in the western part (Kansai district) of Japan.

According to the report by Kondo-Iida et al. (1999), among patients homozygous for the founder mutation, 91.5% showed milder (stand or walk with or without support) or typical (able to sit unassisted or to slide on buttocks) phenotypes, and only 2.5% of cases were classified as severe (could sit only with support or had no head control), while among patients with heterozygous for the founder mutation, 92% showed severe phenotypes. This was true in our study, as most homozygotes could sit without help, while half of the heterozygotes were bedridden. It was speculated that because the 3'-UTR of a gene affects the stability of its mRNA, the 3 kb sequence inserted in that portion of the FCMD gene may alter the secondary structure of FCMD mRNA and render it unstable. This notion is supported by RT-PCR analysis that revealed low levels of the expected amplification product occurred in patients who were homozygous for the founder mutation and lower than normal in patients heterozygous for the insertion and another mutation. In other words, chromosomes carrying the 3 kb insertion may merely produce a lower level of mature fukutin than normal and generate a relatively mild phenotype. On the other hand, nonfounder mutations, which include nonsense and missense mutations within the coding region, cause major structural changes in the fukutin protein and thus are likely to produce severe effects.

2.4 Seizure-genotype relationship in FCMD patients diagnosed between 1994 and 2006

Mutational analysis of 35 patients with FCMD is shown in Table 3. Each chromosome containing the 3 kb retrotransposal insertion was concordant with the founder haplotype represented as 138-192-147-183 for markers D9S2105-D9S2170-D9S2171-D9S2107. Eighteen patients were homozygous for the 3 kb insertion and 17 were heterozygous. Mutations other than the 3 kb insertion were identified seven of the 12 heterozygous patients examined. These included five patients with a nonsense mutation in exon 3, one patient with a missense mutation in exon 5 and one patient with a nonsense mutation in exon 8. Among five patients with mutation in exon 3, afebrile seizures were found in three patients. One of them showed intractable seizures and the other developed infantile spasms at age six months. Two of five patients with a mutation in exon 3 had no seizures during follow-up as they died at ages 2 and 5 years, respectively, raising the possibility that seizures could

Haplotype	Location	Mutation	Type of mutation	No. of patients	Seizure status No. of patients
Homozygous for the founder haplotype (138-192-147-183)	3′ Untranslated region	3 Kb insertion	Instability of mRNA	18	Afebrile seizures : 8 Febrile seizures : 3 No seizure : 7
Heterozygous for the founder haplotype*				17	Afebrile seizures : 9 Febrile seizures : 5 No seizure : 3
130-201-157-183	Exon 3	R47X	Nonsense	5	Afebrile seizures : 3 (Intractable : 1, infantile spasms : 1) No seizure : 2 (died aged 2 and 5 years)
Not examined	Exon 5	M133T	Missense	1	Afebrile seizures : 1 (Intractable : 1)
Not examined	Exon 8	R307X	Nonsense	1	Febrile seizures : 1
139-201-155-183	Unknown**	Unknown	Unknown	4	Afebrile seizures : 3 (Intractable : 2) Febrile seizures : 1
148-196-153-183	Unknown	Unknown	Unknown	1	Febrile seizures : 1
128-199-155-183	Not done***	Not done	Not done	1	Afebrile seizures : 1
138-194-155-183	Not done	Not done	Not done	1	Febrile seizures : 1
138-199-147-191	Not done	Not done	Not done	1	No seizure : 1
138-196-147-191	Not done	Not done	Not done	1	Febrile seizures : 1
Not examined	Not done	Not done	Not done	1	Afebrile seizures : 1

* Haplotypes other than the founder's haplotype are shown below.
** Sequence analyzed, but no mutation found
*** Sequence analysis was not done yet.

Table 3. Relationship between genotypes and seizures in FCMD patients (Reproduced from Yoshioka et al., 2008).

develop later. All five patients also showed severe clinical manifestations suggestive of WWS. One patient with a missense mutation in exon 5 had intractable complex partial seizures and severe psychomotor retardation. However, one patient aged six years with a nonsense mutation in exon 8 developed a febrile seizure at the age of four years four months and he had no EEG paroxysmal discharges. On the other hand, five of twelve patients who underwent sequence analysis of chromosome without the 3 kb insertion revealed no mutation within the coding region of *FKTN*. It is probable that the mutations in these alleles lie in regulatory regions such as promoter sequences or intronic sequences critical for alternative splicing. Among them, four patients showed the same haplotype, 139-201-155-183, for markers D9S2105-D9S2170-D9S2171-D9S2107 and showed severe phenotypes. In addition, two of them had intractable seizures.

It is interesting that in this study seven of 18 (39%) homozygous and three of 17 (18%) heterozygous patients had no seizures during follow-up. Although two of our heterozygotes without seizures died at ages 2 and 5 years, respectively, all homozygotes without seizures were older than four years and two patients were over 30 years of age.

In addition, some had only febrile seizures throughout their life. Antiepileptic drugs were prescribed for half of the FCMD patients and no intractable seizures were observed in homozygotes. These facts showed that seizures occurring in FCMD patients were not always severe. Milder cortical dysplasia was suggested in FCMD, especially in homozygotes.

From these observations, it was concluded that mutational analysis of the FCMD gene could predict seizure prognosis. Heterozygotes usually developed seizures earlier than homozygotes and some heterozygotes showed intractable seizures. Special attention is necessary when treating epilepsy in heterozygotes. Mutational analysis other than the 3 kb insertion and haplotype analysis may also help to predict seizure prognosis.

2.5 Worldwide distribution of *Fukutin* mutation

A Turkish geneticist who had read our paper (Yoshioka et al., 1999) asked us to analyze her CMD patient. This Turkish boy had characteristics of WWS. Parents were first cousins, and their first son was unaffected. The infant was born by cesarean section and weighed 2,700 gm (25th percentile); his height was 50cm (50th percentile), and head circumference was 47 cm (>97th percentile). Physical examination showed respiratory difficulties, central cyanosis, generalized hypotonia, hydrocephaly, bilateral buphthalmus, and cataracts. Rieger's anomaly with iris atrophy and peripheral corneal adhesions was noticed. After cataract extraction of the right eye, ocular examination showed that the optic disc and the retina were hypoplastic. Cranial computed tomography showed hydrocephalus and cortical atrophy. After birth, this patient was supported by mechanical ventilation and died on the 10th day. Neuropathological examination showed agyric hemispheres with polymicrogyria in several cortical segments and severe cortical disorganization in other segments. The ventricles released 600ml of cerebrospinal fluid. CMD was also seen, with variation in fiber size, and fibrosis. Immunohistochemical analysis showed greatly reduced staining for alpha-dystroglycan, but normal immunoreactivity for beta-dystroglycan in the skeletal muscle membrane. Serum creatine kinase levels were greatly elevated.

Genetic analysis of this family was performed. As expected, the patient had no Japanese founder insertion. We then screened all exons and flanking introns of the fukutin gene in the patient by polymerase chain reaction direct sequencing. We detected a homozygous 1bp insertion mutation, nt504(insT), in exon 5 of *FKTN*. This mutation causes a frameshift, resulting in a premature termination at codon 157. Both parents and the brother were heterozygous for this mutation. This is the first case worldwide in which a *FKTN* mutation has been found outside the Japanese population (Silan et al., 2003).

Later, another Turkish boy with WWS phenotype was found to have a homozygous nonsense mutation in *FKTN* by the research group in the Netherlands (Beltran-Valero de Bernabe et al., 2003). The homozygous nonsense mutations within the coding region identified in two Turkish patients are predicted to cause a total loss of *FKTN* and are likely to produce a more severe phenotype which closely resembles WWS.

Manzini et al. (2008) assembled a large cohort of patients with typical WWS (43 affected individuals from 40 families), drawn from Middle Eastern consanguineous families (16 patients from 14 families) and from consanguineous and nonconsanguineous families from Europe and the Americas (27 cases). They found that 40% (16/40 families) of patients in their cohort carried mutations in the coding sequence of *POMT1, POMT2, FKRP* or *FKTN* with no *POMGnT1* or *LARGE* mutations detected. *FKTN* and *FKRP* mutations in particular were much more common than previously suggested and were mostly identified in non-consanguineous patients of European descent (6/27 cases). All Ashkenazi Jewish patients in their group shared an identical haplotype at the *FKTN* locus and the same homozygous mutation c.1167_1168insA in exon 9 suggesting a founder effect in this population. They identified the carrier frequency of this mutation to be 0.7% in the Ashkenazi population in Israel, which will be extremely informative for genetic testing. A striking difference was observed in the geographic distribution of mutations, as Middle East families were mostly carriers of *POMT1* mutations (35.7%, 5/14 families), while the most common cause of European/American cases was *FKTN* mutations (18.5%, 5/27 cases). An additional four USA Ashkenazi Jewish families with WWS were found to have a founder mutation in *FKTN* in this population (Chang et al., 2009).

The cohort consisted of 92 unrelated individuals who showed hypoglycosylation of alpha-dystroglycan at the sarcolemma by immunolabelling of skeletal muscle sections (80 patients) or had the clinical phenotype being highly suggestive of a alpha-dystroglycanopathy (12 patients) was analyzed the mutation of genes related to alpha-dystroglycanopathy (Godfrey et al., 2007). Homozygous and compound heterozygous mutations were detected in a total of 31 probands (34 individuals from 31 families). Mutations in *FKTN*, typically associated with FCMD in Japan were found in six patients, none of whom are of Japanese origin. Only two of these patients had structural brain involvement; one patient affected by WWS and one by a MEB-FCMD phenotype. The remaining patients had no structural brain involvement; one case had CMD-no mental retardation and never acquired the ability to walk but has normal IQ and five individuals from three families have entirely normal intellect and a mild LGMD phenotype (LGMD 2M). Interestingly in the latter two of these families, a dramatic response to steroid therapy was noted (Godfrey et al., 2006).

Vuillaumier-Barrot et al. (2009) reported four newly diagnosed Caucasian patients with *FKTN* mutations with a broad spectrum of phenotypes ranging from CMD associated with mental retardation to LGMD without central nervous system involvement. Two patients (two sisters) presented with CMD, mental retardation, and posterior fossa malformation including cysts, and brain atrophy at brain MRI. The other two patients had normal intelligence and brain MRI. Sequencing of the *FKTN* gene identified three previously described mutations and two novel misssense mutations.

In contrast to studies in Middle East families and European/American cases, a 10-year-old Korean boy with clinical features of FCMD was found to have homozygous Japanese insertion mutation (Lee et al., 2009). His parents were heterozygous carriers of the same mutation. He is the first genetically confirmed FCMD patient in Korea and the first non-Japanese patient carrying homozygous Japanese founder mutation. According to a large northeast Asian population study (Watanabe et al., 2005), the carrier frequency of 3-kb insertion mutation in Korean population is 1 in 935. Based on this observation, the incidence of FCMD by 3-kb insertion mutation is as low as 1 in 3,496,900 in Korea. On the other hand, the Japanese founder mutation was not detected in 766 mainland Chinese individuals (Watanabe et al., 2005). However, the first FCMD case was reported in the Chinese population with a Japanese founder 3-kb insertion and the other copy with a known c.139C>T mutation (Xiong et al., 2009). These Asian case reports emphasize the importance of considering the *FKTN* founder mutation for diagnostic purposes outside of Japan and suggest that segments of the Chinese, Korean and Japanese populations may have a recent common ancestor.

2.6 Milder phenotype of FCMD

The first indication that *FKTN* mutations may also cause a much less severe phenotype came from Murakami et al. (2006). They reported that six Japanese patients, all of whom were compound heterozygotes for *FKTN* founder mutation and a point mutation, had minimal muscle weakness, normal intellect and dilated cardiomyopathy. No mutation was found in the other responsible genes for alpha-dystroglycanopathy including *FKRP, POMGnT1, POMT1, POMT2,* and *LARGE* in these patients. Pathological findings in the biopsied skeletal muscles showed only minimal dystrophic changes, but have altered glycosylation of alpha-dystroglycan and reduced laminin binding ability. Cardiac involvement is the most remarkable finding in these patients. All the patients showed dilated cardiomyopathy, and two of them had life-threatening, rapidly progressive cardiac insufficiency. Cardiac involvement is rarely described in patients with alpha-dystroglycanopathy except for some patients with LGMD 2I.

Recently, milder cases of muscular dystrophy associated with *FKTN* mutations have also been reported in non-Japanese populations. Godfrey et al. (2006, 2007) reported on five non-Japanese children from three families with normal intelligence and limb-girdle phenotype, caused by heterozygous point mutations in the *FKTN* gene. Puckett et al. (2009) reported an additional two brothers with a LGMD phenotype due to compound heterozygous *FKTN* mutation. These two brothers had elevated CK, mild muscle weakness and normal cognition. They lack any cardiac or ocular abnormalities. In addition to their mild clinical presentation, patients were also unique from an ethnic and molecular standpoint. Their father was of European descent and their mother, Japanese. The children, however, did not possess the common Japanese founder mutation. Rather, the brothers had two *FKTN* missense mutations, one of which, c527T>C, had not been previously reported. This is significant, as the vast majority of patients reported have been either homozygous or heterozygous for the common retrotransposon insertion. Despite the milder skeletal muscle phenotype of these patients and those reported by Murakami et al. (2006), muscle biopsies show a reduction in fully glycosylated alpha-dystroglycan similar to severe forms of CMD, such as FCMD and MEB. This emphasizes that immunophenotype may correlate poorly with clinical severity.

3. Japanese patients with alpha-dystroglycanopthy with other gene mutations than *FKTN*

In Japan, FCMD is the most common form of CMD, whereas MEB, WWS, MDC1C and MDC1D were rarely seen. WWS has been observed in many population groups with a worldwide distribution (Dobyns et al., 1989). In contrast, both MEB and FCMD show striking founder effects. MEB was first described in Finland, where it is most prevalent, owing to a strong founder effect following by genetic drift (Santavuori et al., 1989, Haltia et al., 1997). Consequently, most MEB patients have come from a small, geographically isolated population in Finland, with few Caucasian exceptions. Taniguchi et al. (2003) examined 30 patients from various countries, including Japan and Korea, who were diagnosed as WWS, severe FCMD or MEB. Two Japanese patients were identified as compound heterozygotes of *POMGnT1* mutations. Severe hydrocephalus was observed prenatally by an ultrasonograph in both patients, and in one of them hydrocephalus required a ventriculo-peritoneal shunt at one year of age. Therefore, MEB patients may exist with a broader distribution than previously expected. Later, Matsumoto et al. (2005) performed detailed genetic and clinico-pathological analyses on 62 Japanese patients whose limb-muscle specimens showed altered glycosylation of alpha-dystroglycan. *FKTN* mutations were found in 54 patients (86%) examined, reflecting the most common form of CMD in Japan. In this study, the first patient with MDC1C (*FKRP* mutation) in oriental countries was found. Clinically, this patient showed severe muscle weakness from early infancy, marked elevation of serum CK level, calf hypertrophy, and normal intelligence; those are consistent with MDC1C. Further, the structural abnormality in the cerebellum was seen on brain MRI including disorganized folia and multiple cysts, those are commonly observed in FCMD/MEB. In addition, two MEB (*POMGnT1* mutations) and one WWS (*POMT1* mutation) were genetically confirmed. These studies show that patients with alpha-dystroglycanopathy in Japan have not only *FKTN* mutations but also have mutations of other genes such as *POMT1, POMT2, POMGnT1* and *FKRP*. Molecular genetic studies have been helpful in defining subgroups of CMD.

4. CMD patients without known gene mutations of alpha-dystroglycanopathy

We studied a Japanese CMD patient with brain abnormalities without *FKTN* mutation using immunohistochemical analysis of dystrophic muscle and full mutational analysis of *POMGnT1* and *FKRP* genes (Yoshioka et al., 2004).

Hypotonia and generalized muscle weakness became apparent during the first year of life. Consanguineous marriage was not noted. He obtained head control at 4 months, rolled over at 9 months, learned to sit unsupported at 12 months, crept at 19 months and stood with support at 26 months of age. At 4 years he could walk with the short leg braces using walker and speak two-word's sentences. Serum creatine kinase levels were markedly elevated (2,776 IU/L, normal range<130 IU/L). Brain MRI showed thick and bumpy cortices with shallow sulci and abnormal white matter changes (Fig. 7). Ophthalmologically, he had no abnormalities. Immunohistochemical analysis showed reduced staining of alpha-dystroglycan, while expression of merosin and beta-dystroglycan was normal (Fig. 8). Sequence analysis of *POMGnT1* and *FKRP* revealed no mutation.

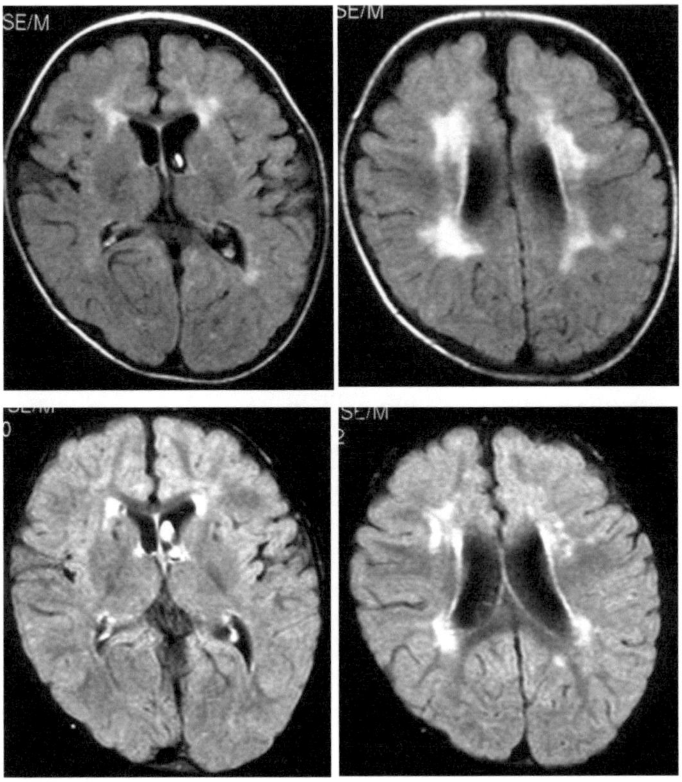

Fig. 7. MR imaging at 15 months of age (the upper line) and 26 months of age (the lower line) on T2-weighted sequences. The cerebral white matter shows symmetric high intensity, which decreases with age (Reproduced from Yoshioka et al. , 2004).

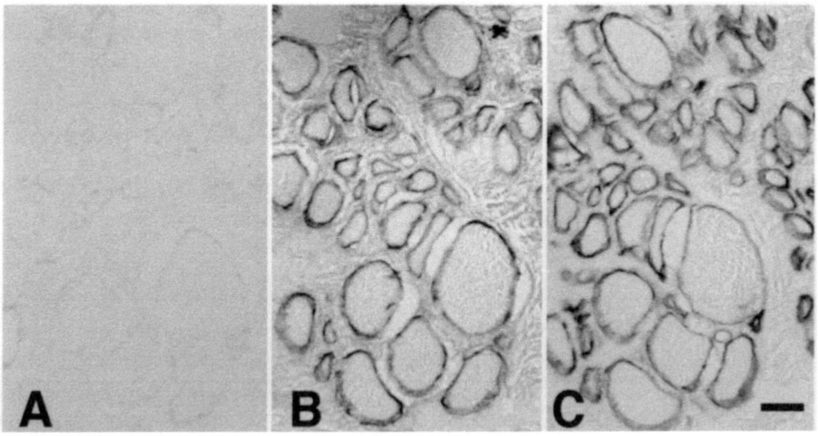

Fig. 8. Immunohistochemistry. Transverse serial frozen sections of skeletal muscle biopsies from the patient were immunostained with antibodies against alpha-dystroglycan (A), beta-dystroglycan (B), and laminin alpha-2 (merosin) (C). Note that beta-dystroglycan and laminin alpha-2 were present but alpha-dystroglycan was absent in sarcolemma of muscle fibers. Scale bar=20 micrometer (Reproduced from Yoshioka et al.,2004).

From these observations, this CMD patient seemed to belong to alpha-dystroglycanopathy. However, sequence analysis of *FKTN, POMGnT1 and FKRP* showed no mutations. Although analyses of *POMT1, POMT2* and *LARGE* are necessary, there seems to be still many CMDs whose causative genes are unknown. We previously reported these patients including this case as a variant of CMD (Yoshioka et al., 2002).

Among their 62 Japanese patients with alpha-dystroglycanopathy, Matsumoto et al. (2005) found four patients with no mutation in the known genes associated with glycosylation defects of alpha-dystroglycan. They were clinically diagnosed to have MEB or WWS. All four patients showed severe mental retardation, hypotonia from early infancy, and eye involvements. Brain MRI displayed type II lissencephaly, enlarged lateral ventricles, and hypoplastic brainstem and cerebellum. In the skeletal muscles, three patients who were clinically diagnosed as WWS showed severe dystrophic changes with marked fibrous tissue involvement. However, one patient who was clinically diagnosed as MEB showed only mild myopathic changes in his muscle.

It was true in non-Japanese patients with alpha-dystroglycanopathy. Although 31 among 92 probands (34%) with alpha-dystroglycanopathy had homozygous and compound heterozygous mutations in the known genes, a large number of remaining patients with clinico-pathological features indistinguishable from the ones with mutations were not found to have mutations in any of the genes studied (Godfrey et al., 2007). More, as yet undefined, genes are likely to be involved in the pathogenesis of the alpha-dystroglycanopathies. The identification of these genes may provide additional information on the pathway of glycosylation of alpha-dystroglycan.

5. Conclusion

Defects in genes responsible for altered glycosylation of alpha-dystroglycan cause a group of muscular dystrophies that are variably associated with central nervous and eye abnormalities, known as alpha-dystroglycanopathies. These comprise FCMD, MDC1C and 1D, WWS, and MEB. Mutations have been reported in six putative or demonstrated glycosyltransferases; *FKTN, FKRP, LARGE, POMT1, POMT2*, and *POMGnT1*. Although each disorder was initially associated with one gene, it has recently been shown that the spectrum of phenotypes is broader than previously thought, and all these syndromes can be associated with mutations in any of the six genes known to be involved in alpha-dystroglycan glycosylation (Fig. 1).

A wide clinical spectrum is also evident for the *FKTN* mutations that were first reported in patients with FCMD, and later also in patients with WWS, and in patients with LGMD. FCMD is most frequent in Japan, and relatively homogenous phenotype. The strikingly high prevalence of FMD among the Japanese appears to result from the initial founder effect, whose expansion occurred in relative isolation. Most FCMD-bearing chromosomes in Japan are derived from a single ancestral founder who lived a few thousands years ago. Seventy-five percent of Japanese patients are homozygous for the ancestral mutation and have a relatively milder phenotype than patients who are compound heterozygous for the ancestral mutation and another mutation. The Japanese founder 3′ insertion mutation is therefore regarded as a relatively mild mutation. The most common form of FCMD in Japan presents clinically with a combination of generalized muscle weakness, congenital structural brain malformations, seizures, decreased vision, and cardiomyopathy. Most patients are never able to walk independently and have moderate to severe cognitive delay. Japanese patients, who are compound heterozygous for the founder and another mutation, have much more severe WWS-like manifestations including hydrocephalus and microphthalmia.

However, an increasing number of *FKTN* mutations are being reported outside Japan. To date, at least 24 different *FKTN* mutations have been described in non-Japanese patients and phenotypes of these patients cover the entire range of alpha-dystroglycanopathies (Yis et al., 2011). Among 23 patients with CMD and mutations in the *FKTN* gene in non-Japanese populations, 10 patients had a WWS-like phenotype including severe brain and eye abnormalities, the remainder had a milder FCMD, MEB or LGMD phenotype. In addition to the Japanese founder mutation, the mutation c.1167insA in exon 9 has been found to be homozygous in seven non-consanguineous Ashkenazi Jewish families, with an estimated carrier frequency of the mutation of 0.7% in the Ashkenazi population in Israel. Affected patients in these Jewish families all had a severe WWS-like phenotype.

The WWS phenotype caused by *FKTN* mutations is associated with the presence of two loss-of-function mutations, although not an absolute rule. The relatively few reports of *FKTN* mutations in patients with mild phenotypes may be a result of ascertainment bias and the recent increase in the number of reports of such findings may result in increased mutation analysis in *FKTN* for such patients in the future.

In summary, these results confirm that outside Japan, muscular dystrophy due to *FKTN* mutations is not as rare as initially supposed, and could be associated with a large spectrum of phenotypes, compared to the relatively homogenous phenotype in the Japanese population.

Although alpha-dystroglycanopathy is still largely unknown, comprehensive mutation analysis in patients and genotype/phenotype correlation across the spectrum of disease caused by these genes may provide clues to gene function. Functional analysis in animal models will determine how these mutations affect the proteins.

6. References

Beltran-Valero de Bernabe D, van Bokhoven H, van Beusekom E, van den Akker W, Kant S, Dobyns WB, Cormand B, Currier S, Hamel B, Talim B, Topaloglu H & Brunner HG. (2003) A homozygous nonsense mutation in the fukutin gene causes a Walker-Warburg syndrome phenotype. *Journal of Medical Genetics* Vol.40, No.11, (November 2003), pp.845-848, ISSN 0022-2593

Chang W, Winder TI, LeDuc CA, Simpson LL, Millar WS, Dungan J, Ginsberg N, Plaga S, Moore SA & Chung WK. (2009) Founder *Fukutin* mutation causes Walker-Warburg syndrome in four Ashkenazi Jewish families. *Prenatal Diagnosis* Vol.29, No.6 (June 2009), pp.560-569, ISSN 0197-3851

Dobyns WB, Pagon RA, Armstrong D, Curry CJR, Greenberg F, Grix A, Holmes LB, Laxova R, Michels VV, Robinow M & Zimmerman RL. (1989) Diagnostic criteria for Walker-Warburg syndrome. *American Journal of Medical Genetics* Vol. 32, No. 2 (February 1989), pp.195-210, ISSN 0148-7299

Fukuyama Y, Kawazura M & Haruna H. (1960) A peculiar form of congenital progressive muscular dystrophy. Report of fifteen cases. *Paediatria Universitatis Tokyo* Vol. 4, No.4, (April 1960) pp.5-8, ISSN 0030-9303

Fukuyama Y, Osawa M & Suzuki H. (1981) Congenital progressive muscular dystrophy of the Fukuyama type --- clinical, genetic and pathological considerarions----. *Brain & Development* Vol.3, No.1, pp.1-29, ISSN 0387-7604

Fukuyama Y & Ohsawa M. (1984) A genetic study of the Fukuyama type congenital muscular dystrophy. *Brain&Development* Vol. 6, No. 4 , pp373-390, ISSN 0387-7604

Godfrey C, Escolar D, Brockington M, Clement EM, Mein R, Jimenez-Mallebrera C, Torelli S, Feng L, Brown SC, Sewry CA, Rutherford M, Shapira Y, Abbs S & Muntoni F. (2006) Fukutin gene mutations in steroid-responsive limb girdle muscular dystrophy. *Annals of Neurology* Vol. 60, No.5 (November 2006), pp.603-610, ISSN 0364-5134

Godfrey C, Clement E, Mein R, Brockington M, Smith J, Talim B, Straub V, Robb S, Quinlivan R, Feng L, Jimenez-Mallebrera C, Mercuri E, Manzur AY, Kinali M, Torelli S, Brown SC, Sewry CA, Bushby K, Topaloglu H, North K, Abbs S & Muntoni F. (2007) Refining genotype-phenotype correlations in muscular dystrophies with defective glycosylation of dystroglycan. *Brain* Vol. 130, No. 10, (October 2007), pp.2725-2735, ISSN 0006-8950

Haltia M, Leivo I, Somer H, Pihko H, Paetau A, Kivela T, Tarkkanen A, Tome F, EngvallE & Santavuori P. (1997) Muscle-eye-brain disease: A neuropathological study. *Annals of Neurology* Vol. 41, No. 2, (February 1997), pp.173-180, ISSN 0364-5134

Kobayashi K, Nakahori Y, Miyake M, Matsumura K, Kondo-Iida E, Nomura Y, Segawa M, Yoshioka M, Saito K, Osawa M, Hamano K, Sasakihara Y, Nonaka I, Nakagome Y, Kanazawa I, Nakamura Y, Tokunaga K & Toda T. (1998a) An ancient retrotransposal insertion causes Fukuyama-type congenital muscular dystrophy. *Nature* Vol. 394, No. 6691, (July 1998), pp. 388-392, ISSN 0028-0836

Kobayashi K, Nakahori Y, Mizuno K, Miyake M, Kumagai Y, Honma A, Nonaka I, Nakamura Y, Tokunaga K & Toda T. (1998b). Founder-haplotype analysis in Fukuyama-type congenital muscular dystrophy (FCMD). *Human Genetics* Vol. 103, No.3, (September 1998), pp. 323-327, ISSN 0340-6717

Kondo-Iida E, Kobayashi K, Watanabe M, Sasaki J, Kumagai T, Koide H, Saito K, Osawa M, Nakamura Y & Toda T. (1999) Novel mutations and genotype-phenotype relationships in 107 families with Fukuyama-type congenital muscular dystrophy (FCMD). *Human Molecular Genetics* Vol. 8, No. 12, (November 1999), pp.2303-2309, ISSN 0964-6906

Lee J, Lee BL, Lee M, Kim JH, Kim JW & Ki CS. Clinical and genetic analysis of a Korean patient with Fukuyama congenital muscular dystrophy. (2009) *Journal of the Neurological Sciences* Vol. 281, No. 1−2, (June 2009), pp. 122-124, ISSN 0022-510X

Manzini MC, Gleason D, Chang BS, Hill S, Barry BJ, Partlow JN, Poduri A, Currier S, Galvin-Parto P, Shapiro LR, Schmidt K, Davis JG, Basel-Vanagaite L, Seidahmed MZ, Salih MAM, Dobyns WB & Walsh CA. (2008) Ethnically diverse causes of Walker-Warburg syndrome (WWS): FCMD mutations are a more common cause of WWS outside of the Middle East. *Human Mutation* Vol. 29, No.11, (November 2008) E231-241, ISSN 1098-1004

Matsumoto H, Hayashi YK, Kim DS, Ogawa M, Murakami T, Noguchi S, Nonaka I, Nakazawa T, Matsuo T, Futagami S, Campbell KP & Nishino I. (2005) Congenital muscular dystrophy with glycosylation defects of alpha-dystroglycan in Japan. *Neuromuscular Disorders* Vol. 15, No. 5, (May 2005), pp.342-348, ISSN 0960-8966

Muntoni F, Brockington M, Blake DJ, Torelli S & Brown SC. (2002) Defective glycosylation in muscular dystrophy. *Lancet* Vol.360, No.9343, (November 2002), pp 1419-21, ISSN 0140-6736

Muntoni F & Voit T. (2004) The congenital muscular dystrophies in 2004: a century of exciting progress. *Neuromuscular Disorders* Vol. 14, No. 10, (October 2004), pp.635-649, ISSN 0960-8966

Murakami T, Hayashi YK, Noguchi S, Ogawa M, Nonaka I, Tanabe Y, Ogino M, Takada F, Eriguchi M, Kotooka N, Campbell KP, Osawa M & Nishino I. (2006) Fukutin gene mutations cause dilated cardiomyopathy with minimal muscle weakness. *Annals of Neurology* Vol. 60, No. 5, (November 2006), pp.597-602, ISSN 0364-5134

Puckett RL, Moore SA, Winder TL, Willer T, Romansky SG, Covault KK, Campbell KP & Abdenur JE. (2009) Further evidence of Fukutin mutations as a cause of childhood onset limb-girdle muscular dystrophy without mental retardation. *Neuromuscular Disorders* Vol. 19, No. 5, (May 2009), pp. 352-356, ISSN 0960-8966

Santavuori P, Somer H, Sainio K, Rapola J, Kruus S, Nikitin T, Ketonen L & Leisti J. (1989) Muscle-eye-brain disease (MEB). *Brain & Development* Vol. 11, No. 3, pp.147-153, ISSN 0387-7604

Silan F, Yoshioka M, Kobayashi K, Simsek E, Tunc M, Alper M, Cam M, Guven A, Fukuda Y, Kinoshita M, Kocabay K & Toda T. (2003) A new mutation of the fukutin gene in a non-Japanese patient. *Annals of Neurology* Vol. 53, No.3, (March 2003), pp.392-396, ISSN0364-5134

Taniguchi K, Kobayashi K, Saito K, Yamanouchi H, Ohnuma A, Hayashi YK, Manya H, Jin DK, Lee M, Parano E, Falsaperla R, Pavone P, Coster RV, Talim B, Steinbrecher A, Straub V, Nishino I, Topaloglu H, Voit T, Endo T & Toda T. (2003) Worldwide distribution and broader clinical spectrum of muscle-eye-brain disease. *Human Molecular Genetics* Vol.12, No.5, (March 2003), pp.527-534, ISSN 0964-6906

Toda T, Segawa M, Nomura Y, Nonaka I, Mastuda K, Ishihara T, Suzuki M, Tomita I, Origuchi Y, Ohno K, Sasaki Y, Takada K, Kawai M, Otani K, Murakami T, Saito K, Fukuyama Y, Shimizu T, Kanazawa I & Nakamura Y. (1993) Localization of a gene for Fukuyama type congenital muscular dystrophy to chromosome 9q31-33. *Nature Genetics* Vol. 5, No. 3, (November 1993) , pp 283-286, ISSN 1061-4036

Toda T, Ikegawa S, Okui K, Kondo E, Saito K, Fukuyama Y, Yoshioka M, Kumagai T, Kanazawa I & Nakamura Y. (1994) Refined mapping of a gene responsible for Fukuyama-type congenital muscular dystrophy: evidence for strong linkage disequilibrium. *American Journal of Human Genetics* Vol. 55, No.5, (November 1994), pp 946-950, ISSN 0002-9297

Toda T, Yoshioka M, Nakahori Y, Kanazawa I, Nakamura Y & Nakagome Y. (1995) Genetic identity of Fukuyama-type congenital muscular dystrophy and Walker-Warburg syndrome. *Annals Neurology* Vol. 37, No. 1, (January 1995), pp 99-101, ISSN 0364-5134

Toda T, Miyake M, Kobayashi K, Mizuno K, Saito K, Osawa M, Nakamura Y, Kanazawa I, Nakagome Y, Tokunaga K & Nakahori Y. (1996) Linkage-disequilibrium mapping narrows the Fukuyama-type congenital muscular dystrophy (FCMD) candidate region to <100 kb. *American Journal of Human Genetics* Vol. 59, No.6 , (December 1996), pp 1313-1320, ISSN 0002-9297

Vuillaumier-Barrot S, Quijano-Roy S, Bouchet-Seraphin C, Maugenre S, Peudenier S, Van den Bergh P, Marcorelles P, Avila-Smirnow D, Chelbi M, Romero NB, Carlier RY, Estournet B, Guicheney P & Seta N. (2009) Four Caucasian patients with mutations in the fukutin gene and variable clinical phenotype. *Neuromuscular Disorders* Vol. 19, No. 3, (March 2009), pp.182-188, ISSN 0960-8966

Watanabe M, Kobayashi K, Jin F, Park KS, Yamada T, Tokunaga K & Toda T. (2005) Founder SVA retrotransposal insertion in Fukuyama-type congenital muscular dystrophy and its origin in Japanese and northeast Asian populations. *American Journal of Medical Genetics* A Vol.138, No. 4, (November 2005), pp. 344-348, ISSN 0148-7299

Xiong H, Wang S, Kobayashi K, Jiang Y, Wang J, Chang X, Yuan Y, Liu J, Toda T, Fukuyama Y & Wu X. (2009) *Fukutin* gene retrotransposal insertion in a non-Japanese Fukuyama congenital muscular dystrophy [FCMD] patient. *American Journal of Medical Genetics Part A* Vol. 149A, No. 11, (November 2009), pp.2403-2408, ISSN 0148-7299

Yis U, Uyanik G, Heck PB, Smitka M, Nobel H, Ebinger F, Dirik E, Feng L, Kurul SH, Brocke K, Unalp A, Ozer E, Cakmakci H, Sewry K, Cirak S, Muntoni F, Hehr U & Morris-Rosendahl DJ. (2011) Fukutin mutations in non-Japanese patients with congenital muscular dystrophy: Less severe mutations predominate in patients with non-Walker-Warburg phenotype. *Neuromuscular Disorders* Vol. 21, No.1, (January 2011), pp.20-30, ISSN 0960-8966

Yoshioka M, Kuroki S, Nigami H, Kawai T & Nakamura H. (1992) Clinical variation within sibships in Fukuyama-type congenital muscular dystrophy. *Brain & Development* Vol. 14, No. 5 (September 1992), pp.334-337, ISSN 0387-7604

Yoshioka M & Kuroki S. (1994) Clinical spectrum and genetic studies of Fukuyama congenital muscular dystrophy. *American Journal of Medical Genetics* Vol. 53, No. 3, (November 1994), pp.245-250, ISSN 0148-7299

Yoshioka M, Toda T, Kuroki S & Hamano K. (1999) Broader clinical spectrum of Fukuyama-type congenital muscular dystrophy manifested by haplotype analysis. *Journal of Child Neurology* Vol. 14, No. 11, (November 1999), pp.711-715, ISSN 0883-0738

Yoshioka M, Kuroki K, Sasaki H & Baba T. (2002) A variant of congenital muscular dystrophy. (2002) *Brain & Development* Vol.24, No.1, (January 2002), pp.24-29, ISSN 0387-7604

Yoshioka M, Sugie K, Nishino I & Toda T. (2004) Immunohistochemical studies of a variant of congenital muscular dystrophy. *No to Hattatsu* (Japanese) Vol.36, No.1, (January 2004), pp.55-59, ISSN 0029-0831

Yoshioka M, Higuchi Y, Fujii T, Aiba H & Toda T. (2008) Seizure-genotype relationship in Fukuyama-type congenital muscular dystrophy. *Brain & Development* Vol. 30, No. 1 (January 2008), pp.59-67, ISSN 0387-7604

2

Nuclear Poly (A)-Binding Protein and Oculopharyngeal Muscular Dystrophy

Jnanankur Bag[*], Quishan Wang and Rumpa Biswas Bhattacharjee
University of Guelph, Department of Molecular and Cellular Biology, Guelph, Ontario, Canada

1. Introduction

Oculopharyngeal muscular dystrophy (OPMD) is an autosomal-dominant late-onset human genetic disease (Brais et. al, 1998). The symptoms usually appear around the age of fifty, and are characterized by drooping of the eyelid and swallowing difficulties. Both conditions may progress until the eyelid nearly or completely covers the eyeball (ptosis) and the ability to swallow is lost (dysphagia). In addition, patients suffer from proximal limb weakness; muscles of the shoulder and hip girdles may also gradually become weak. OPMD is highly prevalent amongst the French Canadian population of the Quebec province where almost one in every one thousand people is a carrier. In contrast only one in 100,000 people in Europe, including France is a carrier of OPMD. All cases of OPMD in Quebec could be traced to a single ancestor in the 15th century (Brunet et. al., 1990). OPMD is also more common amongst Bukhara Jews (Blumen et. al., 200). Possibly due to mass immigration during the 16th to 17th century, OPMD spread from Europe to many parts of the world (Hill et. al, 2001). OPMD patients have also been reported in Mexico, Thailand, Japan and China (Rivera et. al., 2008; Uyama et. al., 2000; Witoonpanich et.al., 2004; Ye et. al., 2011). A de novo germ line mutation has also been found in a Swiss OPMD patient (Gurtler et. al., 2006).

The mutation causing OPMD has been mapped to the gene encoding the nuclear poly (A) - binding protein PABPN1 at the short arm of chromosome 14 (14q11) of the human genome (Brais et. al., 1998). The human PABPN1 gene contains six GCG repeats following the AUG initiation codon. In OPMD patients expansion of the six GCG repeats to between 8-13 repeats have been found. A short poly alanines tract consisting of ten alanines is present at the N-terminal end of normal PABPN1. Six of these ten alanines are encoded by GCG while the last four alanines are coded by GCA. Compared to other trinucleotide expansion mutations such as the CAG expansion in Huntington's disease, the GCG expansion in OPMD is very modest and genetically stable. Mutations introducing two or more alanines are dominant whereas a single additional alanine expansion is recessive. Generally, the homozygous mutations exhibit more severe phenotypes than the heterozygotes. The severity of the disease increases with the increasing length of the GCG expansion, and also results in earlier onset of the disease (Messaed & Rouleau, 2009). The precise mechanism of trinucleotide repeat expansion in OPMD and other neurodegenerative diseases such as the

[*] Corresponding Author

Huntington is not clear. A slippage model, where the newly synthesized DNA strand dissociates and translocates to a new pairing position during DNA replication has been proposed. Perhaps this misalignment of the nascent strand in the repetitive tract results in the addition or deletion of repeats. Because of the stable nature of the GCG trinucleotide repeats of PABPN1 gene this model may not be applicable for the generation of mutation in OPMD patients. Unequal cross over during DNA replication may be the underlying mechanism for (GCG) repeat.

2. Structure and cellular function of PABPN1

Mammalian PABPN1 is a highly conserved nuclear RNA binding protein of 32.8 kDa with specificity for the poly (A) tract of eukaryotic mRNAs (Figure 1). It consists of one typical RRM domain with consensus RNP1 and RNP2 motifs in the central region of the polypeptide, separating the acidic glutamine rich N-terminal domain from the more basic arginine rich C- terminal domain (Kuhn et. al., 2003). The RNP domain and the C-terminal region of PABPN1 are required for binding to both RNA and its polypeptide partners. Interestingly the RNP domain of PABPN1 has no sequence similarity with the RNA binding domain of the cytoplasmic poly (A) - binding protein PABPC1 or other RNA binding proteins (Kuhn et. al., 2003). Recent crystal structure analyses of human PABPN1 suggest that PABPN1 RRM adopts a fold similar to canonical RRM structure consisting of a four stranded antiparallel β-sheet structure spatially arranged as β4β1β3β2. However, the fold of the third loop and dimerization of the crystal are distinct features of PABPN1 (Ge et. al., 2008).The nuclear localization signal is located between amino acids 289-306 and overlaps with the oligomerization domain (Abu-Baker et.al., 2005; Calado et.al., 2000). Due to the presence of the alanine tract PBPN1 is prone to aggregate formation. However, the polyalanine tract is not conserved, and is absent in Drosophila without any detectable loss of cellular function (Shinchuk et.al., 2005).

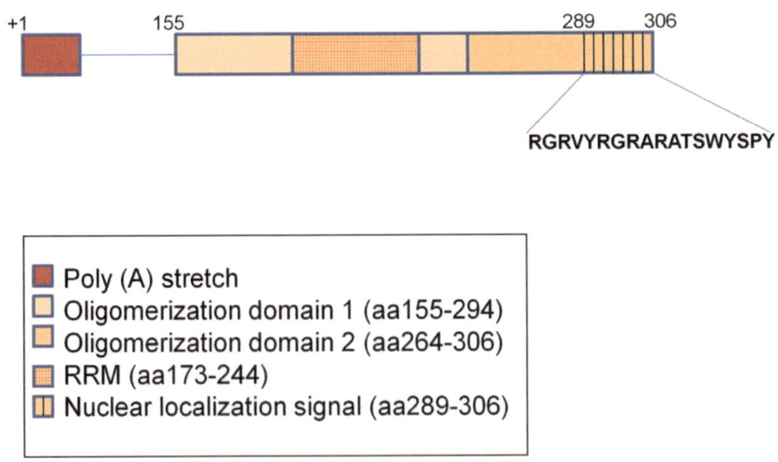

Fig. 1. Schematic diagram of various domains of PABPN1

The main cellular function of PABPN1 is to stimulate the elongation of poly (A) tract of eukaryotic mRNA, and at the same time control its length (Wahle, 1995). After the first ten adenine residues have been added PABPN1 binds to it as a monomer, and as the length of the poly (A) tract increases additional PABPN1 assembles on the tract at a packing density of 15 adenines per PABPN1 molecule (Bienroth et. al., 1993; Kuhn & Wahle, 2004; Wahle, 1995). Both cleavage and poly adenylation specific factor (CPSF) and PABPN1 stimulate the activity of poly (A) polymerase by mutually stabilizing their interaction with mRNA in a transient complex. Although both CPSF and PABPN1 alone can stimulate the polyadenylation by poly (A) polymerase but the extension of the 3` end is much faster when both are present. When the poly (A) tail length has reached 250-300 nucleotides, further extension of the poly (A) tract becomes very slow (Wahle, 1995). The oligomerization of PABPN1 is functionally important and may serve as a molecular ruler to determine the length of the poly (A) tract (Keller et. al., 2000). The wild type PABPN1 exists in equilibrium as monomers, dimmers and oligomers and filamentous complexes (Nemeth et. al., 1995). Expansion of the poly alanine tract in OPMD mutant PABPN1 enhances its aggregation property. However, no loss of cellular function due to this mutation has been detected (Messaed & Rouleau, 2009). In addition, PABPN1 can associate with RNA polymerase II along the chromatin axis before or shortly after the transcription initiation, and the assembly of PABPN1 on the poly (A) tract may be coupled to transcription (Bear et. al., 2003). Studies have shown that PABPN1 remains associated with the released mRNA-protein complex (mRNP) until it reaches the cytoplasmic side of the nuclear pore. Very little PABPN1 is present in the cytoplasmic side of the nuclear envelope suggesting perhaps during or shortly after passage through the nuclear pore PABPN1 is displaced by PABPC1 (Abu-Baker et. al., 2005; Afonia et. al, 1998; Calado et. al., 2000; Kraus et.al., 1994) . PABPN1 has also been shown to interact with the SKI-binding polypeptide (SKIP) transcription factor and stimulate myogenesis (Kip et. al., 2001). Depletion of PABPN1 in myoblasts prevents myogenesis and reduces the length of the poly (A) tract of mRNAs (Apponi et. al., 2010). Because, of the vital role of PABPN1 in mRNA metabolism it is not certain that whether the observed effect on myogenesis was related to a specific effect on myogenesis or due to impairment of global mRNA metabolism. The poly A extension mutant of PABPN1 appears to function normally in pol(A) tail elongation process. Since PABPN1 can interact with both RNA and polypeptide partners, like other RNA binding proteins additional interacting partners such as micro RNAs and signaling polypeptides may soon be detected to suggest additional cellular functions for PABPN1 .

3. Pathology of OPMD

The most distinctive feature of OPMD is the presence of intranuclear filamentous inclusions in skeletal muscle fibers. The inclusions are composed of aggregates of mutant PABPN1 and several additional proteins which will be discussed later. The filaments are less than 0.25 nm long tubular in structures with an average outer diameter of 8.5 nm and an inner diameter of 3 nm. Approximately 2-5% of nuclei of skeletal muscle cells of OPMD patients show the presence of nuclear inclusions (Tome et. al., 1997). The myo-pathological patterns of OPMD, which progress with age include variations in the diameter of muscle fibers; increase in the number of internal nuclei; and increased presence of endomysical connective tissues. Also, a variable number of typical rimmed vacuoles are found in OPMD muscle fibers (Uyama et. al., 2000). Recently, neuro-pathological abnormalities have also been described in some OPMD patients (Boukriche et. al., 2002). Recent studies using a transgenic mouse model of OPMD severe muscular atrophy of the fast glycolytic muscles were observed. Transcrsiptome analyses of the OPMD mouse muscle showed deregulation of a large number of genes by expression of OPMD mutant PABPN1 but not by the wild type PABPN1, and approximately one third of the affected genes were associated with muscle atrophy (Trollet et. al., 2010). There is a strong correlation between the presence of intra nuclear inclusions (INI) and the PABPN1 mutation. All patients whose muscle biopsy showed 8.5nm intranuclear filaments have expanded PABPN1 alleles (Bao et. al., 2002). This view was further supported by the formation of large mutant PABPN1 aggregates similar to the INI in cell culture models ectopically expressing human PABPN1. In cell culture models over expression of both wild type and mutant PABPN1 resulted in aggregate formation (Tavanez et. al., 2005). However, the wild type PABPN1 formed aggregates more slowly than what was observed with the poly alanine expanded mutant PABPN1 (Schinchuk et.al., 2005). More apoptotic cell death was also observed in cells with mutant PABPN1 aggregates (Bao et. al., 2002; Fan et. al., 2001; Tavanez et. al., 2005).

4. Misfolded protein aggregates

Misfolding of proteins may lead to formation of protein aggregates. This process could be triggered by many factors including oxidative and temperature stresses. In addition, point mutations and expansion of poly alanine or poly glutamine tracts may increase aggregation by favoring the assembly of the unfolded or partly folded monomers into the early pre-fibrillar species which can turn into aggregates with more distinctive morphologies called protofilaments or protofibrils. The protofibrils may act as seeds where other misfolded polypeptides are recruited to form insoluble fibrillar aggregates (Chiti et. al., 2003). For many years it was believed that the ability to form amyloid fibrils is limited to small number of proteins. However, more recent studies have uncovered that for some proteins the fibrillar aggregates represent a biochemically active form. For examples the aggregated fibers known as curli produced by *E. coli is* important for cell adhesion (Chapman et. al., 2002); yeast prion Sup35, a translation termination factor (eRF3) forms aggregates (Tuite et. al., 2011). Many studies support a role of Aβ amyloid aggregates in sealing capillaries following traumatic injuries (Atwood et. al., 2003). Studies have shown that *Aplysia* cytoplasmic poly adenylation element binding protein (CPEB) exists in two different structural isoforms, one being the soluble isoform and the other as a prion like protein aggregates, and interestingly the CPEB prion is involved in stimulating synaptic growth and long term memory (Si et. al., 2003). It is therefore, conceivable that the poly alanine expansion of PABPN1 results in a gain of function(s). Most RNA binding polypeptides, are capable of participating in a variety of cellular processes, thus it is likely that the OPMD mutation of PABPN1 results in the loss of some cellular functions while gaining one or more new biological activity. Future research needs to be directed towards unraveling additional cellular functions for both mutant and the wild type PABPN1.

Studies using synthetic peptides consisting of varying lengths of the homopolymeric alanines were used to determine the length of the alanines tract that leads to inclusions. Conformational transition to insoluble aggregates was found to depend on the length as well as concentration, temperature, and incubation time. No β sheet complex was detected with less than 8 alanines while ala 10- 15 showed significant conversion of monomeric peptides to β-sheet aggregates. Homopolymers of 15 or more alanines residues showed the highest conversion to aggregates under all conditions examined (Schinchuk et. al., 2005). These results agree with the in vivo observations that the OPMD mutant PABPN1 is more prone to form aggregates than the wild type PABPN1. *In vitro* studies also showed that fibril formation can be induced by low amounts of both mutant and wild type fibrils serving as seeds. Atomic force microscopy revealed morphlogic differences between wild type and mutant fibrils. In addition, the wild type fibrils were less resistant to solubilization by chaotropic agent guanidinium thiocyanate than what was observed for the mutant fibrils. Examination of the kinetics of fibril formation with PABPN1 fragments containing the polyalanine tract in real time using tryptophan fluorescence suggest that fibril formation coincides with the burial of the tryptophans in the fibrillar core. These studies did not detect any soluble pre-fibrillar intermediates suggesting that the unfolded soluble form directly converts into folded insoluble structure (Schinchuk et. al., 2005).

5. Cellular stress and PABPN1 aggregates

A variety of cellular stresses results in the formation of misfolded proteins, and in order to maintain cell viability and subsequent recovery when physiologically favorable conditions return most organisms produce a family of chaperones known as the heat shock proteins (HSPs) which helps the proper folding process (Daugaard et. al., 2007). It appears that the presence of mutant PABPN1 aggregates but not the wild type cohort in the nuclei produces a modest stress response resulting in the increase of HSP70 expression. Treatment of cells with indomethacin or $ZnS0_4$ augmented the stress response and further induction of HSP70 expression was observed (Figure 2). In addition, expression of HSP27, HSP40 and HSP105 also increased. Both ibuprofen and $ZnS0_4$ treated cells showed reduced level of protein aggregates and apoptotic cell death. Furthermore, in the drug treated cells all four HSPs were colocalized with the PABPN1 (Wang & Bag, 2008). These results suggest that HSPs interact with misfolded PABPN1 and are able to dissociate the aggregates by refolding it into its native form. Similar results were obtained by heat shock treatment of cells and over

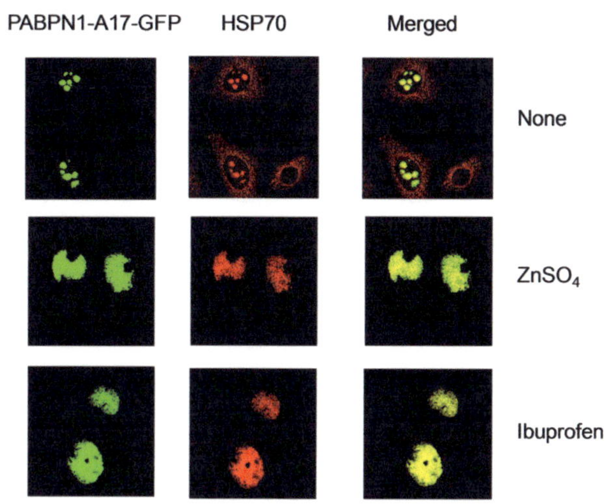

Fig. 2. Effect of different agents on aggregate formation by PABPN1-A17-GFP. HeLa cells were transfected with the PABPN1-A17-GFP expression vector and 48 hours after transfection, cells were treated with the indicated agents for 6 h and following a 24 h recovery period cells were examined for green fluorescence by confocal microscopy. HSP70 was detected by immunofluorescence with Texas red conjugated secondary antibody.

expression of HSP70 alone (Bao et. al., 2002' Wang et. al., 2005; Wang & Bag, 2008). Studies in our laboratory showed that deletion of the ATPase domain of HSP70, which is important for its chaperone function abolishes its ability to dissociate the mutant PABPN1 aggregates (unpublished).

6. Effect of PABPN1 on myogenesis

Despite the essential cellular function of PABPN1 in biogenesis of mRNA the pathologic symptoms are only seen in a restricted group of skeletal muscles such as the extraocular and pharyngeal muscles. Therefore, in addition to its role in mRNA biogenesis PABPN1 may be needed for proper differentiation of myogenic cells, which may be lost in mutant PABPN1 due to expansion of the poly alanine tract. Studies using a myoblast cell culture model showed that over expression of PABPN1 facilitates differentiation of myoblasts into myotubes (Kim et. al., 2001). PABPN1 has been shown to interact with SKIP which share significant homology to several transcriptional co activators such as Bx42 of *Drosophila melanogaster* (Wieland et. al., 1992), and mammalian NcoA-62 (Baudino et. al., 1998). SKIP appears to co-operate with PABPN1 in stimulating E box mediated tarnscription in presence of myoD by forming a hetero trimeric complex (Kim et. al., 2001. The N terminal domain of PABPN1 alone is necessary for interacting with SKIP. The C terminal domain including the RNA binding domains of PABPN1 are dispensable for its role in myogenesis (Kim et.al 2001). Although the poly alanine expanded PABPN1 also binds to SKIP *in vitro* (Tavanez et. al., 2009) it is not clear whether it can cooperate with MyoD to stimulate E box regulated transcription. However, this prospect is conceivable because of the location of poly alanines expansion is within the SKIP binding domain of PABPN1.

In addition to a loss of function in myogenesis the mutant PABPN1 may also gained a function albeit fortuitously, by trapping essential myogenic factors. Studies from our laboratory have indeed supports this hypothesis. We have shown that both myf 5 and Pax 3 co-localize with mutant PABPN1 aggregates but not with the wild type PABPN1 (Figure 3). Ectopic expression of wild type PABPN1 in C2C12 mouse myoblasts had a small beneficial effect on the expression level of various muscle specific proteins including myoD, myogenin, muscle creatine kinase, α-actin and slow troponin C. In contrast, expression of mutant PABPN1 reduced the abundance of those proteins (Figure 4) (Wang & Bag 2006).

The experimental results discussed above may explain why skeletal myogenesis could be affected but very little is known regarding specific targeting of the craniofacial muscles. To address this issue it has been proposed that continuous remodeling of the extraocular myofibers could result in selective loss of this muscle cells (Wirtschafter et. al., 2004). Since *in vivo* myonuclei of most skeletal muscles are post mitotic, therefore, continuous myofiber remodeling in extraocular muscle will require upregulation of genes in cell cycling and renewal of differentiated muscle cells (Wirtschafter et. al., 2004). The negative effect of mutant PABPN1 on myogenesis would show more pronounced effect on muscles that require more frequent rejuvenation than the other skeletal muscles over many years.

7. Protein aggregates and cell death

A direct connection between protein aggregation and cell death is controversial (Andrew et. al., 2000; Fan & Rouleau, 2003; Rubinsztein, 2002). Studies using live cell imaging have

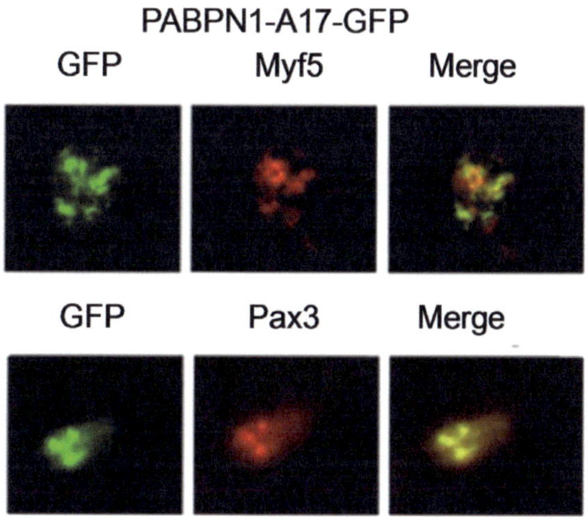

Fig. 3. Co-localization of Pax3/7 and Myf-5 in PABPN1-A17-GFP-transfected cells. Cells grown on coverslips were transfected and 48 h after transfection cells were fixed in methanol and incubated with the appropriate antibody. The green fluorescence of PABPN1-GFP and the red fluorescence of Texas red-conjugated secondary antibody were observed by fluorescence microscopy.

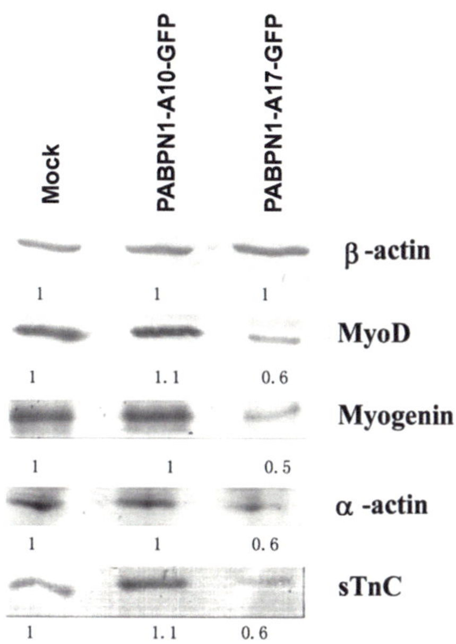

Fig. 4. Expression of muscle-specific proteins in PABPN1-A10 (or A17)-GFP-transfected cells. Cells were transfected with the appropriate Plasmid DNA after 2 days in the 2 days inthe differentiation medium, cells were lysed and the levels of various muscle proteins, were determined by Western blotting using jappropriate antibodies The Western blots were scanned and the levels of muscle proteins in transfected cells were determined and corrected for the difference in loading and transfection efficiency. The polypeptide levels in PABPN1-A17-GFP-transfected cells relative to that of the PABPN1-A10-GFP expressing cells are given at the bottom of each lane.

shown that cells expressing poly glutamine expanded huntingtin survives better than those without aggregates. It is believed that aggregation sequesters this protein and improves cell survival whereas the soluble oligomeric form of mutant huntingtin is more toxic to the cell (Arresate et. al., 2004). Whether the same is true for PABPN1 is not clear. The wild type PABPN1 naturally exists in a functional oligomeric form and is also present as aggregates in the speckles but these are not known to cause cell death. Two overlapping oligomerization domains are found within the C-terminal region of PABPN1. These domains are necessary for oligomerization and aggregation. Therefore, if the oligomeric form of mutant PABPN1 is toxic to the cell it must assume a different structure than that of the wild type protein. Indeed this may be the case since the sub nuclear location of wild type and mutant PABPN1 are different. The wild type PABPN1 was shown by immuno fluorescent microscopy to co-localize with the splicing factor SC35 and the nuclear matrix associated protein PML while the mutant PABPN1 did not (Messaed et. al., 2007; Tavanez et. al., 2005). However, this observation is paradoxical since both proteins seems to function normally in the poly adenylation process, and presence of wild type PABPN1 in the speckles is related to its role in transcription and splicing coupled polyadenylation. In contrast to the pro-apoptotic effect of mutant PABPN1 the wild type PABPN1 demonstrated anti-apoptotic function in mammalian cells. The wild type PABPN1 apparently up regulates the translation of anti apoptotic protein X-linked inhibitor of apoptosis (XIAP) which prevents activation of caspase 3 by inhibiting caspase 9 (Davies & Rubinsztein, 2011). Thus a loss of anti-apoptotic function of mutant PABPN1 may be responsible for cell death in OPMD muscles.

Several studies using cultured non-muscle cells as experimental models showed that strategies that reduced protein misfolding also decreased aggregate formation and cell death. Ectopic expression of the molecular chaperones HSP40 and HSP70 in cells transfected with the mutant PABPN1 reduce aggregate formation and cell death (Abu_Baker et. al., 2003; Bao et. al., 2002; 2004). Also anti-amyloid compounds such as Congo red and doxycyclin can reduce PABPN1 aggregate formation and cell death in a cell culture model (Bao et. al., 2004). We have shown that $ZnSO_4$, 8-hydroxyquinoline, indomethacin and ibuprofen induced HSP 70 expression, and nuclear localization of both HSP70 and the constitutive chaperone HSC 70 in mutant PABPN1 expressing HeLa cells, and reduced the formation of mutant PABPN1 aggregates and cell death (Wang et. al., 2005)

In several chronic neurodegenerative disorders including Alzheimer's, Huntington's, and Parkinson's, caused by the formation of protein aggregates, there is evidence that programmed cell death (apoptosis) may be involved (Desjardins & Ledoux, 1998). Apoptotic cell death has also been observed in cell models and transgenic mouse models of OPMD (Fan & Rouleau, 2003; Hino et. al., 2004; Dion et. al., 2005). However, the molecular mechanisms causing apoptosis remain elusive. Many studies suggest that in the aggregate containing cells, apoptosis proceeds through the up regulation of the tumor suppressor protein p53 (Bae et. al., 2005; Biswas et. al., 2005; Hooper et. al., 2007). Stabilization of p53 within the cell further leads to the activation of down stream proteins like PUMA (p53-upregulated modulator of apoptosis), Bax (Bcl-2-associated X protein) and Bad (Bcl-2-associated death promoter) that change the permeability of mitochondrial and endoplasmic reticulum membranes (Biswas et. al., 2005; Mattson, 2004). These events lead to the release of cytochrome C from mitochondria and calcium from the ER, which further activates the enzyme called caspase (Mattson, 2004). The cascades of proteolytic activities initiated by caspases are believed to trigger various morphological and biochemical aspects of the cell death process. Furthermore, in Huntington's disease, the GAPDH-Siah1 apoptotic pathway (Hara et. al., 2005) facilitates nuclear translocation of mHtt protein and the resultant neurotoxicity (Bae et. al., 2006). In addition to mitochondrial alterations, ER stress, due to the presence of misfolded polyglutamine has also been linked to the cell death in Huntington's and Alzheimer's disease models (Zhao & Ackerman, 2006).

We have demonstrated that although in OPMD cell death is restricted to a sub class of skeletal muscles, non muscle cells in culture also underwent apoptosis. This was not unexpected since PABPN1 is ubiquitously expressed. We found that in HeLa cells aggregation of the poly alanine expansion mutant PABPN1, favors apoptosis over necrosis or ER stress as cell death pathway. At the molecular level, cascades of biochemical events lead to apoptotic cell death due to the accumulation of mutant PABPN1 aggregates. Our results suggest that the apoptotic response to the accumulation of mutant PABPN1 aggregates was initiated by nuclear translocation of the glycolytic enzyme GAPDH. In the last decade several studies have shown that GAPDH is a multi-functional protein (Chuang et. al., 2005). This enzyme usually resides in the cytoplasm as a tetrameric active enzyme. As a response to cellular stress, the catalytic cysteine 150 of GAPDH is S-nitrosylated by nitric oxide, generated by the induction of inducible nitric oxide synthase (iNOS). It has been shown that Nitrosylated GAPDH binds to Siah1, an E3 ubiquitin ligase, and is transported to the nucleus as an inactive enzyme by piggy backing Siah1 (Hara et. al., 2005). The downstream target of GAPDH in the nucleus is p53 (Sen et. al., 2008). In our study, following ectopic expression of mutant PABPN1, we observed that the abundance of total as well as phosphorylated p53 was increased (Figure 5). p53 a tumor suppressor protein with wide ranging biological function including cell cycle arrest, apoptosis, and its abundance is known to increase in response to a variety of cellular damage (Green & Kroemer, 2009). In cells under stress, post translational modifications, especially phosphorylation and acetylation contribute to p53 stabilization and hence its activation (Sakaguchi et. al., 1998). It has been proposed that phosphorylation of p53 at ser 46 modulate the p53 gene promoter selection thereby dictating the fate of the cell to undergo p53 mediated apoptosis and/or growth arrest (Mayo et. al., 2005). The importance of phosphorylation in p53 mediated apoptosis was further underlined, by demonstrating that mutation of Ser46 to Ala decreases the ability of p53 to induce apoptosis (Oda et. al., 2000). It is known that p53 mediated apoptosis can be carried out by both transcription dependant and independent manner (Chuang et. al., 2005; Pietsch et. al., 2008). We found that in mutant PABPN1 cells, abundance of p53 and its phosphorylated isoform (p-p53) increases (Figure 5). Furthermore we also observed a redistribution of p53 in the nucleus and the mitochondria of mutant PABPN1 transfected cells (Figure 6). There was also a concomitant rise in the p53 transcription targeted pro apoptotic protein: Puma (Figure 5).

Thus, it appears that in mutant PABPN1 cells, activated p53 could be translocated to the nucleus and triggered the transcription dependant apoptosis (Wang et. al., 2007). This might be the reason why we did not observe acetylation of p53, since p53 acetylation occurs predominantly in transcription independent apoptosis (Yamaguchi et. al., 2009). However, both the transcription dependant and independent pathways are not necessarily mutually

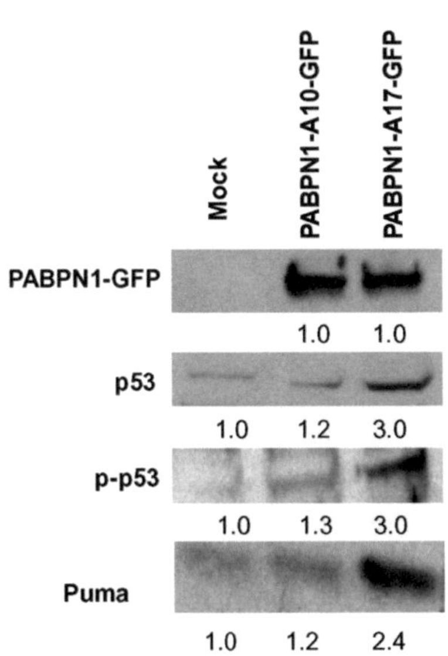

Fig. 5. PABPN1-A17 upregulates p53 and p53 mediated transcription: Following transfection, cells were harvested after 72 hours in SDS loading buffer. Whole cells extracts from PABPN1-A10, 17–GFP and mock-transfected HeLa cells were analyzed for apoptosis related proteins by western blotting. β-actin and GAPDH were used as loading controls.

exclusive. In fact, it has been suggested that the transcription dependent nuclear action of p53 cooperates with its transcription-independent, cytosolic/ mitochondrial action through activation of the *PUMA* gene (Chipuk et. al., 2005). Upon activation, Puma triggers apoptosis by releasing the p53 from its association with Bcl2 to activate Bax (Uo et. al., 2007;Wang et. al., 2007; Zhang et. al., 2009). Puma may also directly interact with Bax, promoting its mitochondrial translocation (Chipuk et. al., 2004; Zhang et. al., 2009). Puma may release p53 from its complex with Bcl2. The released p53 then could oligomerize the monomeric Bax in the cytosol causing the latter to induce mitochondrial outer membrane permeabilization (MOMP) (Dewson et. al., 2003; Jurgensmeier et. al., 1998). The activation of Bax by p53 is known to occur by a 'hit and run' style transient molecular associations (Chipuk et. al., 2004; Moll et. al., 2006; Green & Kroemer, 2009; Pietsch et. al., 2008).

It will be important to examine if a similar apoptotic signal contributes to cell death in muscle cells. In a recent study with the OPMD mouse model over-expression of Bcl2 rescued muscle weakness and apoptosis (Davies & Rubinsztein, 2011), therefore suggesting a similar Bax/Bcl2 pathway for apoptosis in both muscle and non-muscle cells. However, in the OPMD mouse the effect of Bcl2 on muscle weakness was transient, thus other cell death pathways may also contribute to cell death when Bax is inactivated by Bcl2. It is conceivable in the light of our observations in HeLa cells that increase in p53 level might eventually release Bax from Bcl2 mediated inactivation by sequestering Bcl2.

There are several pathways for apoptosis. The precise mechanism of apoptosis depends on developmental programs and the nature of the inducer (Green & Kroemer, 2009; Pietsch et. al., 2008). The Puma/Bax dependent pathway is usually triggered by a variety of cellular stress such as heat shock and oxygen stress (Uo et. al., 2007; Zhang et. al., 2009). The results of our study suggest that accumulation of misfolded protein aggregates also induces stress related apoptosis. In this context it is interesting to note that as discussed in a previous section a small but reproducible induction of a number of heat shock proteins including HSP70, HSP27, HSP40, and HSP105 was observed in mutant PABPN1 expressing cells (Wang & Bag 2008). Furthermore, all of these HSPs were found to be translocated to the cell nucleus and co-localize with the mutant PABPN1 aggregates. Further induction of HSPs using ibuprofen or indomethacin was shown to reduce the aggregate burden and apoptosis in mutant PABPN1 expressing cells (Wang & Bag 2008). HSP 70 has been shown to prevent heat stress induced apoptosis in cultured cells by preventing Bax translocation without directly interacting with Bax (Stankiewicz et. al., 2005). The mechanism how HSP70 induction with ibuprofen in mutant PABPN1 expressing cells prevents cell death will be of interest for further investigation.

The accumulated evidence supports a biochemical catastrophe model where loss of function combined with adventitious gain of function due to poly alanine expansion leads to cell death. The gain of function includes but not limited to increased aggregate formation, interaction with HSPs, trapping of various transcription factors and mRNAs. In studies using mtHtt aggregate formation in *C. elegans* it was shown that presence of mtHtt aggregates interferes with proper folding of normal cellular proteins and cell death could result from not only the aggregate burden of the mutant protein but also by the misfolding of many normal proteins which results in at the least reduction in the abundance of biologically active important cellular proteins (Gidalevitz et. al 2006). Since most studies measured protein abundance using western blotting techniques which does not measure the level of biological activity of the protein these changes has remained under explored.

The following hypotheses might explain the late onset and specificity of cellular targets *in vivo* of OPMD mutation: I) although aggregates can be cleared through proteasome degradation pathway, this pathway is not sufficient to completely prevent accumulation of aggregates; ii) aging is also associated with collapse of protein homeostasis resulting in accumulation of misfolded normal cellular proteins (Taylor & Dillin, 2011) and when this is combined with a mutation in an aggregate prone protein such as the PABPN1, it greatly increases accumulation of both mutant PABPN1 and many normal nuclear proteins in the intranuclear aggregates; iii) aging may also affect the ability to clear the aggregates through proteasome mediated decay; iv) although both muscle and non muscle cells undergo apoptosis, non-muscle cells are renewed through stem cells, in contrast since myogenesis is affected due to loss of function of mutant PABPN1, regeneration of differentiated muscle cells are affected; iv) skeletal muscles in adults are renewed only when injury occurs but in contrast the adult extraocular muscles undergo continuous remodeling (Wirtschafter et. al., 2004), therefore, extraocular muscles are more susceptible to the loss of myogenic role of mutant PABPN1.

8. Novel therapies for OPMD

Mouse and Drosophila models have been used to develop new therapies to treat OPMD. Administration of anti-amyloid agent doxycyclin to OPMD mice significantly reduced aggregate formation in muscle cells. In addition to its anti-amyloid properties doxycyclin also acts as an anti apoptotic agent to protect muscle cells (Davies et. al., 2006; 2008). In another study cystamine protected against the cytotoxicity of mutant PABPN1 in the OPMD mouse. Cysatmine inhibits transglutaminase 2 which is elevated in OPMD muscle cells (Davies et. al., 2010). Studies using the Drosophila model of OPMD single chain antibody against PABPN1 also produced nearly complete rescue of OPMD muscles and restored muscle gene expression (Chartier et. al., 2009). In a nematode model of OPMD the inhibitor of Sir2 sitinol also showed promising results in protecting muscle cells from apoptosis (Catoire et. al., 2008). Gene therapy approach using Bcl2 over expression also rescued OPMD mouse from muscle degeneration (Davies & Rubinsztein, 2011).

Several anti amyloid agents such as the disaccharide trehalose, and Congo red also worked in cell culture models of OPMD (Davies et. al., 2006). In our laboratory we have used ibuprofen, indomethacin, 8-hydroxy quinoline and $ZnSO_4$ to induce HSP 70 expression in HeLa cells. All of these agents significantly reduced the aggregate burden and cell death (Wang et.al., 2005). However these compounds have not been tested in an animal model yet. Ibuprofen's effectiveness was tested in a mouse model of Alzheimer disease without success. However, its conjugation with glutathione greatly improved its effectiveness in reducing aggregate formation and cell death in Alzheimer rats (Pinnen et. al., 2010). Zn^+ is an essential mineral nutrient and many people supplement their diet with it, as such, it is potentially a desirable treatment option. Similarly 8-hydroxy quinoline is also an approved agent used in animal feed as antimicrobial and antparasitic agent (Raether & Hanel, 2003). Its effective dose in the cultured cell is within the range of non-toxic dose. Various derivatives of this drug demonstrated their ability in reducing amyloid plaques in clinical trials on Alzheimer patients (Gouras & Beal 2001; Di Vaira et. al., 2004). In addition to the use of various pharmacological approaches in developing new therapies for OPMD, *in situ* myoblasts transfer by local administrations (Mouly et. al., 2006) or localized gene therapy of affected muscles using Bcl2 or HSP 70 gene expression should be considered.

9. References

Abu-Baker, A., Messaed, C., Laganiere, J., Gasper, C., Brais, B. & Rouleau, G. (2003). Involvement of the ubiquitin-proteasome pathway and molecular chaperones in oculopharyngeal muscular dystrophy. *Hum Mol Genet*, Vol. 12, No. 20, (October), pp. 2609–2623

Afonina, E., Stauber, R. & Pavlakis, G.N. (1998). The human poly(A)-binding protein 1 shuttles between the nucleus and the cytoplasm. *J Biol Chem, Vol.* 273, No. 21, (May), pp. 13015-21.

Andrew, P., Lieberman, M. & Fischbeck, KH. (2000). Triplet repeat expansion in neuromuscular disease. *Muscle Nerve*, Vol. 23, No. 6, (June). pp. 843–850

Apponi, LH., Leung, SW., Williams, KR., Valentini, SR., Corbett, AH. & Pavlath, GK. (2010). Loss of nuclear poly(A)-binding protein 1 causes defects in myogenesis and mRNA biogenesis. *Hum Mol Genet,* Vol. 19, No. 6, (December). pp. 1058-65

Arresate, M., Mitra, S., Schweitzer, E.S., Regal, M.R. & Finkbeiner, S. (2004). Inclusion body formation reduces levels of mutant Huntingtin and the risk of neuronal death. *Nature*, Vol. 431, No. 7010,(October), pp. 805–810

Atwood, CS., Bowen, RL., Smith, MA. & Perry, G. (2003). Cerebrovascular requirement for sealant, anti-coagulant and remodeling molecules that allow for the maintenance of vascular integrity and blood supply. *Brain Res Brain Res Rev,* Vol. 43, No. 1, (September), pp. 164-78

Bae, B-I., Xu, H., Igarashi, S., Fujimuro, M., Agrawal, N., Taya, Y., Hayward, S.D. & Sawa, A. (2005). p53 mediates cellular dysfunction and behavioral abnormalities in Huntington's disease. *Neuron,* Vol. 47, No.1, (July), pp. 29-41

Bao, Y., Cook, LJ., O'Donovan, D., Uyama, E. & Rubinsztein, DC. (2002). Mammalian, yeast, bacterial and chemical chaperones reduce aggregate formation and death in a cell model of oculopharyngeal muscular dystrophy. *J Biol Chem,* Vol. 277, No.14, (April), pp. 12263–12269

Bao, YP., Sarkar, S, Uyama, E. & Rubinsztein, DC. (2004). Congo red, doxycycline, and HSP70 over expression reduce aggregate formation and cell death in cell models of oculopharyngeal muscular dystrophy. *J Med Genet,* Vol. 41, No. 1, (January), pp. 47–51.

Bates, GP., Mangiarini, L., Mahal, A. & Davis, SW. (1997). Transgenic models of Huntington's disease. *Hum Mol Genet,* Vol. 6, No.10, (June), pp. 1633–1637.

Baudino, TA., Kraichely, DM., Jefcoat, SCJr., Winchester, SK., Partridge, NC. & MacDonald, PN. (1998). Isolation and characterization of a novel coactivator protein, NCoA-62, involved in vitamin D-mediated transcription. *J Biol Chem,* Vol. 273, No.26, (June), pp.16434-16441

Bear, DG., Fomproix, N., Soop, T., Björkroth, B., Masich, S. & Daneholt, B. (2003). Nuclear poly(A)-binding protein PABPN1 is associated with RNA polymerase II during transcription and accompanies the released transcript to the nuclear pore. *Exp Cell Res,* Vol. 286, No.2, (June), pp. 332–344

Behrouz, F., Enrique, P., Richard, AH. & Sylvie, E. (1995). Formation of an extremely stable polyalanine ß-sheet macromolecule. *Biochem Biophys Res Commun,* Vol. 211, No.1, (June), pp. 7–13

Bermano, G., Shepherd, RK., Zehner, ZE. & Hesketh, JE. (2001). Perinuclear mRNA localization by vimentin 3'-untranslated region requires a 100 nucleotide sequence and intermediate filaments. *FEBS Lett,* Vol. 497, No.2 ,(May), pp. 77–81

Bhushan, S., Malik, F., Kumar, A., Isher, HK., Kaur, IP., Taneja, SC. &. Singh, J. (2009). Activation of p53/p21/PUMA alliance and disruption of PI-3/Akt in multimodal targeting of apoptotic signaling cascades in cervical cancer cells by a pentacyclic triterpenediol from Boswellia serrata. *Mol Carcinog,* Vol.43, No.12, (December), pp.1093-108

Bienroth, S., Keller, W. & Wahle, E. (1993). Assembly of a processive messenger RNA polyadenylation complex. *EMBO J,* Vol. 12, No. 2, (February), pp. 585-594

Biswas, SC., Ryu, E., Park, C., Malagelada, C. & Greene, LA. (2005). Puma and p53 play required roles in death evoked in a cellular model of Parkinson disease. *Neurochem Res,* Vol. 30, No. 6-7, (June-July), pp. 839–845

Blasutig, IM., New, LA., Thanabalasuriar, A., Dayarathna, TK., Goudreault, M., Quaggin, SE., Li, SS-C., Gruenheid, S., Jones, N. & Pawson, T. (2008). Phosphorylated YDXV motifs and Nck SH2/SH3 adaptors act cooperatively to induce actin reorganization. *Mol Cell Biol,* Vol. 28, No.6, (January), pp.2035-2046

Blumen, SC., Nisipeanu, P., Sadeh, M., Asherov, A., Tome, FM. & Korczyn, AD. (1993). Clinical features of oculopharyngeal muscular dystrophy among Bukhara Jews. *Neuromuscul. Disord,* Vol. **3,** No. 5-6, (September-November), pp. 575–577

Boukriche Y, Maisonobe T. & Masson C. (2002) Neurogenic involvement in a case of oculopharyngeal muscular dystrophy. *Muscle Nerve,* Vol. 25, No.1, (January), pp. 98-101

Brais, B., Bouchard, JP., Xie, YG., Rochefort, DL., Chretien N., Tome, F.M., Lafrenier, R.G., Rommens, J.M., Uyama, E. & Nohira, O. (1998) Short GCT expansions in the PABPN1 gene cause oculopharyngeal muscular dystrophy. *Nat. Genet,* Vol. 18, No. 2, (February), pp. 164–166.

Brown, LY. & Brown, SA. (2004). Alanine tracts: the expanding story of human illness and trinucleotide repeats. *Trends Genet,* Vol. 20, No. 1, (January), pp.51-58

Brunet, G., Tome, FM., Samson, F., Robert, JM. & Fardeau, M. (1990). Oculopharyngeal muscular dystrophy: a census of French families and genealogic study. *Rev. Neurol,* Vol. 146, No.6-7,pp. 425–429

Burdon, RH. (1982). The human heat shock proteins: their induction and possible intracellular functions. In Schlesinger, M.J., Ashburner, M. and Tissieres, A. (eds), *Heat Shock from Bacteria to Man,* Cold Spring Harbor Laboratory, New York, USA

Calado, A., Tome, FMS., Brais, B., Rouleau, GA, Kuhn, U., Wahle, E. & Fonseca-Carmo, M. (2000). Nuclear inclusions in oculopharyngeal muscular dystrophy consist of poly(A) binding protein 2 aggregates which sequesters poly(A) RNA. *Hum Mol Genet,*Vol. 9, No. 15, (September), pp. 2321–2328

Carmichael, J., Chatellier, J., Woolfson, A., Milstein, C., Fersht, AR. & Rubinsztein, DC. (2000). Bacterial and yeast chaperones reduce both aggregate formation and cell death in mammalian cells models of Huntington's disease. *Proc Natl Acad Sci USA,*Vol. 97, No. 17, (August) pp.9701–9705

Catoire, H., Pasco, MY., Abu-Baker, A., Holbert, S., Tourette, C., Brais, B., Rouleau, GA., Parker, JA. & Néri, C. (2008). Sirtuin inhibition protects from the polyalanine muscular dystrophy protein PABPN1. *Hum Mol Genet,* Vol.17, Vol.14, (July), pp. 2108-2117

Chapman, MR., Robinson, LS., Pinkner, JS., Roth, R., Heuser, J., Hammar, M., Normark, S. & Hultgren, SJ. (2002). Role of Escherichia coli curli operons in directing amyloid fiber formation.*Science,* Vol.295, No.5556, (February), pp.851-855

Chartier, A., Raz, V., Sterrenburg, E., Verrips, CT., van der Maarel, SM. & Simonelig, M.(2009). Prevention of oculopharyngeal muscular dystrophy by muscular expression of Llama single-chain intrabodies in vivo. *Hum Mol Genet,*Vol. 18, No. 10, (May), pp. 1849-1859

Chen, S., Berthelier, V., Yang, W. & Wetzel, R. (2001). Polyglutamine aggregation behavior *in vitro* support a recruitment mechanism of cytotoxicity. *J Mol Biol,* Vol. 311, No. 1, (August) pp.173–182

Chen, Z., Li, Y. and Krug, R. (1999). Influenza A virus NS1 protein targets poly(A)-binding protein II of the cellular 3′ end processing machinery. *EMBO J,* Vol. 18, No.8, (April), pp. 2273–2283

Chipuk, JE., Kuwana, T., Bouchier-Hayes, L., Droin, NM., Newmeyer, DD., Schuler, M. & Green, DR. (2004). Direct activation of Bax by p53 mediates mitochondrial membrane permeabilization and apoptosis. *Science*, Vol. 303, No.5660, pp. 1010–1014

Chipuk, JE., Bouchier-Hayes, L., Kuwana, T., Newmeyer, DD. & Green, DR. (2005). PUMA couples the nuclear and cytoplasmic proapoptotic function of p53. *Science*, Vol. 309, No. 5741, (September), pp. 1732–1735

Chiti, F., Stefani, M., Taddei, N., Ramponi, G. & Dobson CM. (2003). Rationalization of the effects of mutations on peptide and protein aggregation rates.*Nature*, Vol.424, No.6950, (August), pp.805-808

Chuang, DM., Hough, C. & Senatorov, VV. (2005). Glyceraldehyde-3-phosphate dehydrogenase, apoptosis, and neurodegenerative diseases. *Annu Rev Pharmacol Toxicol*, Vol.45, pp.269-290

Corbeil-Girard, LP., Klein AF., Sasseville, AM., Lavoie, H., Dicaire, MJ., Saint-Denis A., Page, M., Duranceau, A., Codere, F., Bouchard, JP., Karpati, G., Rouleau, GA., Massie, B., Langelier, Y. and Brais, B. (2005). PABPN1 overexpression leads to upregulation of genes encoding nuclear proteins that are sequestered in oculopharyngeal muscular dystrophy nuclear inclusions. *Neurobiol Dis*, Vol. 18, No. 3 (April), pp. 551–567.

Cumming, CJ., Reinstein E., Sun Y., Antalify B., Jiang, Y., Ciechanovert, A., Orr, HT., Beaudet, AL. & Zoghbi, HY. (1999). Mutation of the E6-AP ubiquitin ligase reduces nuclear inclusion frequency while accelerating polyglutamine-induced pathology in SCAI mice. *Neuron*, Vol. 24, No. 4, (December), pp. 879–892

Daugaard, M., Rohde, M. & Jäättelä, M. (2007). The heat shock protein 70 family: Highly homologous proteins with overlapping and distinct functions. *FEBS Lett*, Vol. 581, No.19, (July), pp.3702-10.

Davies, JE., Wang, L., Garcia-Oroz, L., Cook, LJ., Vacher, C., O'Donovan, DG. & Rubinsztein, DC. (2005). Doxycycline attenuates and delays toxicity of the oculopharyngeal muscular dystrophy mutation in transgenic mice. *Nat Med*, Vol. 11, No.6, (June), pp. 672-677

Davies, JE. & Rubinsztein, DC. (2006). Polyalanine and polyserine frameshift products in Huntington's disease. *J Med Genet*, Vol.43, No.11, (June), pp.893-896

Davies, JE., Sarkar, S. & Rubinsztein, DC. (2008). Wild-type PABPN1 is anti-apoptotic and reduces toxicity of the oculopharyngeal muscular dystrophy mutation. *Hum Mol Genet*, Vol. 17, No. 8, (April), pp.1097-1108

Davies JE, Rose C, Sarkar S. & Rubinsztein DC. (2010). Cystamine suppresses polyalanine toxicity in a mouse model of oculopharyngeal muscular dystrophy. *Sci Transl Med*, Vol. 2, No. 34, (June), pp. 34ra40

Davies, JE. & Rubinsztein, DC. (2011). Over-expression of BCL2 rescues muscle weakness in a mouse model of oculopharyngeal muscular dystrophy. *Hum Mol Genet*, Vol. 20, No. 6, (March), pp.1154-1163

Desjardins, P. & Ledoux, S. (1998). The role of apoptosis in neurodegenerative diseases. *Metab Brain Dis*, Vol. 13, No. 2, ( ),pp. 79–96

Dewson, G., Snowden, RT., Almond, JB., Dyer, MJS. & Cohen, GM.(2003). Conformational change and mitochondrial translocation of Bax accompany proteosome inhibitor-induced apoptosis of chronic lymphocytic leukemic cells. *Oncogene*, Vol. 22, No.17, (May), pp. 2643-2654

Dhar, SK. & St Clair, DK. (2009). Nucleophosmin Blocks Mitochondrial Localization of p53 and Apoptosis. *J Biol Chem*, Vol. 284, No. 24, (June), pp. 16409–16418

Di Vaira, M., Bazzicalupi, C., Orioli, P., Messori, L., Bruni, B. & Zatta, P. (2004). Clioquinol, a drug for Alzheimer's disease specifically interfering with brain metal metabolism: structural characterization of its zinc(II) and copper(II) complexes. *Inorg Chem*, Vol. 43, No. 13, (May), pp. 3795–3797

Dion, P., Shanmugam, V., Gaspar, C., Messaed, C., Meijer, I., Toulouse, A., Laganiere, J., Roussel, J., Rochefort, D., Laganiere, S., Allen, C., Karpati, G., Bouchard, JP., Brais, B. & Rouleau, GA. (2005). Transgenic expression of an expanded (GCG) (13) repeat PABPN1 leads to weakness and coordination defects in mice. *Neurobiol. Dis*, Vol. 18, No.3, (April),pp. 528–536

Dreyfuss, G., Adams, S. & Choi, YF. (1984). Physical changes in cytoplasmic messenger ribonucleoproteins in cells treated with inhibitors of mRNA transcription. *Mol Cell Biol*, Vol. 4, No. 3,(March),pp. 415–423

Fan, X. & Rouleau, GA. (2003). Progress in understanding the pathogenesis of oculopharyngeal muscular dystrophy. *Can J Neurol Sci*, Vol. 30, No. (1), (February), pp. 8–14

Fan, XP., Dion, P., Laganiere, J., Brais, B. & Rouleau, GA. (2001). Oligomerization of polyalanine expanded PABPN1 facilitates nuclear protein aggregation that is associated with cell death. *Hum Mol Genet*, Vol. 10, No. 21, (October), pp. 2341–2351

Ge, H., Zhou, D., Tong, S., Gao, Y., Teng, M. & Niu, L. (2008). Crystal structure and possible dimerization of the single RRM of human PABPN1.Proteins, Vol. 71, No. 3, (May), pp.1539-1545

Gidalevitz, T., Ben-Zvi, A., Ho, KH. & Brignull, HR. (2006). Morimoto RI. Progressive disruption of cellular protein folding in models of polyglutamine diseases. *Science*, Vol. 311, No. 5766, (March) pp. 1471-1474

Gouras, GK. & Beal, MF. (2001). Metal chelator decreases Alzheimer ß-amyloid plaques. *Neuron*, Vol. 30, No.3, (June), pp. 641–642

Green, DR. & Kroemer, G. (2009). Cytoplasmic functions of the tumour suppressor p53. *Nature*, Vol. 458, No.7242, (April), pp. 1127-1130

Gürtler, N., Plasilova, M., Podvinec, M., Boesch, N., Müller, H. & Heinimann, K . (2006). A de novo PABPN1 germline mutation in a patient with oculopharyngeal muscular dystrophy. *Laryngoscope*, Vol.116, No.1, (January), pp.11-14

Hara, MR., Agrawal, N., Kim, SF., Cascio, MB., Fujimuro, M., Ozeki, Y., Takahashi, M., Cheah, JH., Tankou, SK., Hester, LD., Ferris, CD., Hayward, SD., Snyder, SH. & Sawa, A. (2005). S-nitrosylated GAPDH initiates apoptotic cell death by nuclear translocation following Siah1 binding. *Nat Cell Biol*, Vol. 7, No.7, (July), pp. 665–674

Heiser, V., Engemann, S., Brocker, W., Dunkel, I., Boeddrich, A., Waelter, S., Nordhoff, E., Lurz, R., Schugardt, N., Rautenberg, S. Herhaus, C., Barnickel, G., Böttcher, H., Lehrach, H. & Wanker, EE. (2002). Identification of benzothiazoles as potential polyglutamine aggregation inhibitors of Huntington's disease by using an automated filter retardation assay. *Proc Natl Acad Sci USA*, Vol.99, No.4, (December),pp. 16400–16406

Hill, ME., Creed, GA., McMullan, TF., Tyers, AG., Hilton-Jones, D., Robinson, DO. & Hammans, SR. (2001). Oculopharyngeal muscular dystrophy. Phenotypic and genotypic studies in a UK population. *Brain*, Vol. 124, No.3, (March), pp. 522-526

Hino, H., Araki, K., Uyama, E., Takeya, M., Araki, M., Yoshinobu, K., Mike, K., Kawazoe, Y., Maeda, Y., Uchino, M. & Yamamura, K. (2004). Myopathy phenotype in transgenic mice expressing mutated PABPN1 as a model of oculopharyngeal muscular dystrophy. *Hum Mol Genet*, Vol. 13, No. 2, (Jan), pp. 181-190

Hooper, C., Meimaridou, E., Tavassoli, M., Melino, G., Lovestone, S &, Killick, R. (2007). p53 is upregulated in Alzheimer's disease and induces tau phosphorylation in HEK293a cells. *Neuroscience Letters*, Vol. 418, No. 1, (May), pp. 34-37

Hyun, TH., Barreet-Connor, E. & Milne, DB. (2004). Zinc intakes and plasma concentrations in men with osteoporosis: The Rancho Bernardo study. *Am J Clin Nutr*, Vol. 80, No.3, (September), pp. 715-721

Jurgensmeier, JM., Xie, .Z, Deveraux, Q., Ellerby, L., Bredesen, D. & Reed, JC. (1998). Bax directly induces release of cytochrome *c* from isolated mitochondria. *Proc Natl Acad Sci USA*, Vol.95, No.9, (April), pp.4997-5002

Keller,RW., Kühn, U., Aragón, M., Bornikova, L., Wahle, E. & Bear, DG. (2000). The nuclear poly(A) binding protein, PABP2, forms an oligomeric particle covering the length of the poly(A) tail. *J Mol Biol*. Vol. 297, No.3, (March), pp. 569-583

Kelley, PM. & Schlesinger, M. (1978). The effect of amino acid analogues and heat shock on gene expression in chicken embryo fibroblasts. *Cell*, Vol. 15, No.4,(December), pp. 1277-1286.

Kerwitz, Y., Kuhn, U., Lilie, H., Knoth, A., Scheuermann, T., Friedrich, H., Schwarz, E. & Wahle, E. (2003). Stimulation of poly(A) polymerase through a direct interaction with the nuclear poly(A) binding protein allosterically regulated by RNA. *EMBO J*, Vol. 22, No.14, (July), pp. 3705-3714

Kim, YJ., Noguchi, S., Hayashi, YK., Tsukahara, T., Sahimizu, T. & Arahata, K. (2001). The product of an oculopharyngeal muscular dystrophy gene, poly(A)-binding protein 2, interacts with SKIP and stimulates muscle-specific gene expression. *Hum Mol Genet*, Vol. 10, No.11,(May), pp. 1129-1139.

Klein, AF., Ebihara, M., Alexander, C., Dicaire, MJ., Sasseville, AM., Langelier, Y., Rouleau, GA. & Brais B. (2008). PABPN1 polyalanine tract deletion and long expansions modify its aggregation pattern and expression. *Exp Cell Res*, Vol.314, No.8, (May), pp.1652-1666

Knights, CD., Catania, J., Giovanni, DD., Muratoglu, S., Perez, R., Swartzbeck, A., Quong, AA., Zhang, X., Beerman, T., Pestell, TR. & Avantaggiati, ML. (2006). Distinct p53 acetylation cassettes differentially influence gene-expression patterns and cell fate. *J Cell Biol*, Vol. 173, No.4, (May), pp.533-544

Krause, S., Fakan, S., Weis, K. & Wahle, E. (1994). Immunodetection of poly(A) binding protein II in the cell nucleus. *Exp Cell Res*, Vol.214, No.1, (September), pp.75-82

Kühn U, Nemeth A, Meyer S, Wahle E. (2003). The RNA binding domains of the nuclear poly(A)-binding protein. *J Biol Chem*, Vol. 278, No. 19, (May), pp. 16916-16925

Kühn, U. & Wahle, E. (2004). Structure and function of poly(A) binding proteins. *Biochim Biophys Acta*, Vol. 1678, No.2-3, (May), pp.67-84

Lagunas, L., Bradbury, CM., Laszlo, A., Hunt, CR. & Gius, D. (2004). Indomethacin and ibuprofen induce hsc70 nuclear localization and activation of the heat shock response in Hela cells. *Biochem Biophys Res Commun*, Vol. 313, No.4, (January), pp. 863-870.

Lee, BS., Chen, J., Angelidis, C., Jurivich, DA. & Morimoto, RI. (1995). Pharmacological modulation of heat shock factor 1 by antiinflammatory drugs resulted in protection against stress-induced cellular damage. *Proc Natl Acad Sci USA*, Vol. 92, No.16, (August), pp. 7207-7211.

Lenk, R., Ransom, L., Kaufmann, Y. & Penman, S. (1977). A cytoskeletal structure with associated polyribosomes from HeLa cells. *Cell*, Vol. 10, No.1, (January), pp.67–78

Li, P., Nijhawan, D., Budihardjo, I., Srinivasula, SM., Ahmad, M., Alnemri, ES. & Wang, X. (1997). Cytochrome C and dATP- dependant formation of Apaf-1/caspase-9 complex initiates an apoptotic protease cascade. *Cell*, Vol.91, No.14, (November), pp. 479-489

Mattson, MP. (2004). Pathways towards and away from Alzheirmer's disease. *Nature*, Vol.430, No.7000, (August), p.631-639

Mayo, LD., Seo, YR., Jackson, MW., Smith, ML., Rivera, GJ., Korgaonkar, CK. & Donner, DB. (2005). Phosphorylation of human p53 at serine 46 determines promoter selection and whether apoptosis is attenuated or amplified. *J Biol Chem*, Vol.280, No.28, (July), pp. 25953–25959

Messaed, C., Dion, PA., Abu-Baker, A., Rochefort, D., Laganiere, J., Brais, B. & Rouleau, GA. (2007). Soluble expanded PABPN1 promotes cell death in oculopharyngeal muscular dystrophy. *Neurobiol Dis*. Vol.26, No.3, (June), pp.546-57

Messaed, C. & Rouleau, GA. (2009). Molecular mechanisms underlying polyalanine diseases. *Neurobiol Dis*, Vol.34, No.3, (June), pp.397-405

Moll, UM., Marchenko, N. & Zhang, XK. (2006). p53 and Nur77/TR3-transcription factors that directly target mitochondria for cell death induction. *Oncogene*, Vol.25, No.34, (August), pp. 4725-4743

Mosser, DD., Caron, AW., Bourget, L., Denis-Larose, C. and Massie, B. (1997). Role of the human heat shock protein hsp70 in protection against stress-induced apoptosis. *Mol Cell Biol*, Vol.17, No.9, (September), pp.5317–5327

Mosser, DD. and Morimoto, RI. (2004). Molecular chaperones and the stress of oncogenesis. *Oncogene*, Vol.23, No.16, (April), pp. 2907–2918

Nakano, K. & Vousden, KH. (2001). PUMA, a novel proapoptotic gene, is induced by p53. *Mol Cell*, Vol. 7, No.3, (March), pp. 683-694

National Toxicology Program (1985) NTP toxicology and carcinogenesis studies of 8-hydroxyquinoline (CAS No: 1482-24-3) in F3441 N rats and B6C3F1 mice (feed studies). *Natl Toxicol., Program Tech. Rep. Ser*, Vol.276, (April) 1–170

Nemeth, A., Krause, S., Blank, D., Jenny, A., Jenö, P., Lustig, A. & Wahle, E. (1995). Isolation of genomic and cDNA clones encoding bovine poly(A) binding protein II. *Nucleic Acids Res*, Vol.23, No.20, (October), pp.4034-4041

Oda, E., Ohki, R., Murasawa, H., Nemoto, J., Shibue, T., Yamashita, T., Tokino, T., Taniguchi, T. & Tanaka, N. (2000). Noxa, a BH3-only member of the Bcl-2 family and candidate mediator of p53-induced apoptosis. *Science*, Vol.288, No.5468, (May), pp. 1053–1058

Oda, K., Arakawa, H., Tanaka, T., Matsuda, K., Tanikawa, C., Mori, T., Nishimori, H., Tamai, K., Tokino, T., Nakamura, Y. & Taya, Y. (2000). p53AIP1, a potential mediator of p53-dependent apoptosis, and its regulation by Ser-46-phosphorylated p53. *Cell*, Vol.102, No. 6, (September), pp. 849–862

Pallepati, P. & Averill-Bates, D. (2010). Mild thermotolerance induced at 40 degrees C increases antioxidants and protects HeLa cells against mitochondrial apoptosis induced by hydrogen peroxide: Role of p53. *Arch Biochem Biophys*, Vol.495, No.2, (March) pp.97-111

Pietsch, EC., Sykes, SM., McMahon, SB. & Murphy, ME. (2008). The p53 family and programmed cell death. *Oncogene*, Vol.27, No.50, (October), pp. 6507-6521

Pinnen, F., Sozio, P., Cacciatore, I., Cornacchia, C., Mollica, A., Iannitelli, A., D Aurizio, E., Cataldi, A., Zara, S., Nasuti, C. & Di Stefano A. (2011). Ibuprofen and Glutathione Conjugate as a Potential Therapeutic Agent for Treating Alzheimer's Disease. Arch Pharm (Weinheim). Vol.22, No. , *Arch Pharm Chem Life Sci*, Vol. 11, pp.139-148

Poirier, MA., Li, H., Macosko, J., Cai, S., Amzel, M. & Ross, CA. (2002). Huntingtin spheroids and protofibrils as precursors in polyglutamine fibrilization. *J Biol Chem*, Vol. 277, No.43, (October), pp. 41032-41037

Raether, W. & Hanel, H. (2003). Nitroheterocyslic drugs with broad spectrum activity. *Parasitol. Res*, Vol. 90, No.S1, (June) S19-S39

Rankin, J., Wyttenbach, A. & Rubinsztein, DC. (2000). Intracellular green fluorescent protein-polyalanine aggregates are associated with cell death. *Biochem J*, Vol.348, No.1, (May) 15-19.

Rivera, D., Mejia-Lopez, H., Pompa-Mera, EN., Villanueva-Mendoza, C., Nava-Castañeda, A., Garnica-Hayashi, L., Cuevas-Covarrubias, S. & Zenteno, JC. (2008). Two different PABPN1 expanded alleles in a Mexican population with oculopharyngeal muscular dystrophy arising from independent founder effects. *Br J Ophthalmol*, Vol. 92, No.7, (July), pp. 998-1002

Rubinsztein, DC. (2002) Lessons from animal models of Huntington's diseases. *Trends Genet*, Vol.18, No.4, (April),pp. 202-209

Sakaguchi, K., Herrera, JE., Saito, S., Miki, T., Bustin, M., Vassilev, A., Anderson, CW. & Appella, E. (1998). DNA damage activates p53 through a phosphorylation-acetylation cascade. *Genes Dev*. Vol.12, No. 18, (September),pp. 2831-2841

Sakahira, H., Breuer, P., Hayer-Hartl, MK. & Hartl, FU. (2002). Molecular chaperones as modulators of polyglutamine protein aggregation and toxicity. *Proc Natl Acad Sci USA*, Vol.99, No. Suppl 4, (June), pp.16412-16418

Saudou, F., Finkbeiner, S., Devys, D. & Greenberg, ME. (1998). Huntingtin acts in the nucleus to induce apoptosis but death does not correlate with the formation of intranuclear inclusions. *Cell*, Vol.95, No.1, (October), pp. 55-66

Schaffar, G., Breuer, P. & Botera, R. (2004). Cellular toxicity of polyglutamine expansion proteins: mechanism of transcription factor deactivation. *Mol Cell*, Vol.15, No.1, (July), pp.95-105

Scheffner, M., Huibregtse, JM., Vierstra, RD. & Howley, PM. (1993). The HPV-16 E6 and E6-AP complex functions as a ubiquitin-protein ligase in the ubiquitination of p53. *Cell*, Vol.75, No.3, (November) pp.495-505

Sen, N., Hara, MR., Kornberg, MD., Cascio, MM., Bae, B., Shahani, N., Thomas, B., Dawson, TM., Dawson, VL., Snyder, SH. & Akira, S. (2008). Nitric oxide-induced nuclear GAPDH activates p300/CBP and mediates apoptosis. *Nat Cell Biol*, Vol. 10, No. 7, (July), pp. 866-873

Shinchuk, LM., Sharma, D., Blondelle, SE., Reixach, N., Inouye, H. & Kirschner. DA. (2005). Poly-(L-alanine) expansions form core beta-sheets that nucleate amyloid assembly. *Proteins*, Vol. 61. No.3, (November), pp.579-589

Si, K., Giustetto, M., Etkin, A., Hsu, R., Janisiewicz, AM., Miniaci, MC., Kim, JH., Zhu, H. & Kandel, ER. (2003). A neuronal isoform of CPEB regulates local protein synthesis and stabilizes synapse-specific long-term facilitation in aplysia. *Cell*, Vol.115, No.7, (December), pp.893-904

Song, S. & Finkel, F. (2007). GAPDH and the search for alternative energy. *Nature Cell Biology*, Vol. 9, No. 8, (August) pp. 869 - 870

Stankiewicz, AR., Lachapelle, G., Foo, CP., Radicioni, SM. & Mosser, DD. (2005). Hsp70 inhibits heat-induced apoptosis upstream of mitochondria by preventing Bax translocation. *J Biol Chem*. Vol. 280, No.46, (November), pp. 38729-38739

Tavanez, JP., Calado, P., Braga, J., Lafarga, M. & Carmo-Fonseca, M. (2005). In vivo aggregation properties of the nuclear poly(A)-binding protein PABPN1. *RNA*, Vol.11, No.5, (May), pp.752-762

Tavanez, JP., Bengoechea, R., Berciano, MT., Lafarga, M., Carmo-Fonseca, M. & Enguita, FJ. (2009). Hsp70 chaperones and type I PRMTs are sequestered at intranuclear inclusions caused by polyalanine expansions in PABPN1. *PLoS One*, Vol. 4, No.7, (July), pp. e6418

Taylor, RC. & Dillin, A. (2011). Aging as an event of proteostasis collapse. *Cold Spring Harb Perspect Biol*. 2011 , Vol. 3, No.5, (May), pii: a004440. doi: 10.1101/cshperspect.a004440

Tomé, FM., Chateau, D., Helbling-Leclerc, A. & Fardeau M. (1997). Morphological changes in muscle fibers in oculopharyngeal muscular dystrophy. *Neuromuscul Disord*, Vol.7, No.Suppl 1, (October), pp.:S63-69.

Towbin, H. & Gordon, J. (1984). Immunoblotting and dot immunobinding: current status and outlook. *J Immunol Methods*, Vol.72, No. 2, (September), pp. 313–340

Trollet, C., Anvar, SY., Venema, A., Hargreaves, IP., Foster, K., Vignaud, A., Ferry, A., Negroni, E., Hourde, C., Baraibar. MA., 't Hoen, PA., Davies, JE., Rubinsztein, DC., Heales, SJ., Mouly, V., van der Maarel, SM., Butler-Browne, G., Raz, V. & Dickson, G. (2010). Molecular and phenotypic characterization of a mouse model of oculopharyngeal muscular dystrophy reveals severe muscular atrophy restricted to fast glycolytic fibres. *Hum Mol Genet*, Vol.19, Vol.11, (June), pp.2191-207

Trottier, Y., Devys, D., Imbert, G., Saudou, F., An, I., Lutz, Y., Weber, C., Agid, Y., Hirsch, EC. & Mandel, JL. (1995). Cellular localization of the Huntington's disease protein and discrimination of the normal and mutated form. *Nat Genet*, Vol.10, No1, (May), pp.104–110

Tuite, MF., Marchante, R. & Kushnirov, V. (2011). Fungal Prions: Structure, Function and Propagation. *Top Curr Chem*, Vol.30, (June) [Epub ahead of print]

Uyama, E., Tsukahara, T., Goto, K., Kurano, Y., Ogawa, M., Kim, YJ., Uchino, M. & Arahata, K. (2000). Nuclear accumulation of expanded PABP2 gene product in oculopharyngeal muscular dystrophy. *Muscle Nerve*, Vol. 23, No.10, (October), pp.1549-1554

van der Sluijs, BM., van Engelen, BG. & Hoefsloot, LH.(2003). Oculopharyngeal muscular dystrophy (OPMD) due to a small duplication in the PABPN1 gene. *Hum Mutat*, Vol. 21, No.5, (May), pp.553

Wahle, E. (1991) A novel poly(A)-binding protein acts as a specificity factor in the second phase of messenger RNA polyadenylation. *Cell*, Vol. 66, No.4, (August), pp. 759-768

Wahle, E., Listig, A., Jeno, P. & Maurer, P. (1993). Mammalian poly(A)-binding protein II. *J Biol Chem*, Vol. 268, No.4, (February), pp. 2937–2945

Wahle, E. (1995) Poly(A) tail length control is caused by termination of processive synthesis. *J Biol Chem*, Vol.270, No.6, (February), pp. 2800–2808

Wang, C. & Chen, J. (2003). Phosphorylation and hsp90 binding mediate heat shock stabilization of p53. *J Biol Chem*, Vol. 278, No.3, (January), pp. 2066–2071

Wang, P., Yu, J. & Zhang, L. (2007). The nuclear function of p53 is required for PUMA-mediated apoptosis induced by DNA damage. *Proc Natl Acad Sci USA*, Vol.104, No.10, (March), pp. 4054–4059

Wang, Q., Mosser, DD. & Bag, J. (2005). Induction of HSP70 expression and recruitment of HSC70 and HSP70 in the nucleus reduce aggregation of a polyalanine expansion mutant of PABPN1 in HeLa cells. *Hum Mol Genet*, Vol. 14, No.23, (October), pp. 3673-3684

Wang, Q. & Bag, J. (2006). Ectopic expression of a polyalanine expansion mutant of poly(A)-binding protein N1 in muscle cells in culture inhibits myogenesis. Vol. 340, No.3, (February), pp. 11-15

Wang, Q. & Bag, J. (2008). Induction of expression and co-localization of heat shock polypeptides with the polyalanine expansion mutant of poly(A)-binding protein N1 after chemical stress. *Biochem Biophysical Res Commun*, Vol. 370, No.1, (May), pp. 11-15

Wieland, C., Mann, S., von Besser, H. & Saumweber, H. (1992). The Drosophila nuclear protein Bx42, which is found in many puffs on polytene chromosomes, is highly charged. *Chromosoma*, Vol.101, No.8, (June), pp.517-525.

Wirtschafter, JD., Ferrington, DA. & McLoon, LK. (2004). Continuous remodeling of adult extraocular muscles as an explanation for selective craniofacial vulnerability in oculopharyngeal muscular dystrophy. *J Neuroophthalmol*, Vol.24, No.1, (March), pp.62-76

Witoonpanich, R., Phankhian, S., Sura, T., Lertrit, P., Phudhichareonrat, S. (2004). Oculopharyngodistal myopathy in a Thai family. *J Med Assoc Thai*, Vol. 87, No.12, (March), pp. 1518-21

Wolter, KG., Hsu, YT., Smith, CL., Nuchushtan, A., Xi, XG. & Youle, RJ. (1997) Movement of Bax from the cytosol to mitochondria during apoptosis. *J Cell Biol*, Vol. 139, No. 5, (December), pp. 1281-1292

Yamaguchi, H., Woods, NT., Piluso, LG., Lee, HH., Chen, J., Bhalla, KN., Monteiro, A., Liu, X., Hung, MC. & Wang, HG. (2009). p53 acetylation is crucial for its transcription-independent proapoptotic functions. *J Biol Chem*, Vol.284, No.17, (April), pp. 11171-11183

Ye, J., Zhang, H., Zhou, Y., Wu, H., Wang, C. & Shi, X. (2011). A GCG expansion $(GCG)_{11}$ in polyadenylate-binding protein nuclear 1 gene caused oculopharyngeal muscular dystrophy in a Chinese family. *Mol Vis*, Vol. 17, (May), pp.1350-1354

Zhang, Y., Xing, D. & Liu, L. (2009). PUMA promotes Bax translocation by both directly interacting with Bax and by competitive binding to Bcl-X L during UV-induced apoptosis. *Mol Biol Cell*, Vol.30, No. 13, (July), pp. 3077–3087

Zhao, L. & Ackerman, SL. (2006). Endoplasmic reticulum stress in health and disease. *Curr Opin Cell Biol*, Vol.18, No.4, (August), pp. 444–452

3

Myotonic Dystrophy Type 1 (DM1): From the Genetics to Molecular Mechanisms

Jonathan J. Magaña[1] and Bulmaro Cisneros[2]
[1]*Genetics Department, Genomic Medicine Laboratory, National Rehabilitation Institute;*
[2]*Genetics and Molecular Biology Department, CINVESTAV-IPN,*
Mexico

1. Introduction

For a long time, the human genome was considered an intrinsically stable entity; however, it is currently known that our human genome contains many unstable elements consisting of tandem repeat elements, mainly Short tandem repeats (STR), also known as microsatellites or Simple sequence repeats (SSR) (Ellegren, 2000). These sequences involve a repetitive unit of 1-6 bp, forming series with lengths from two to several thousand nucleotides. STR are widely found in pro- and eukaryotes, including humans. They appear scattered more or less evenly throughout the human genome, accounting for ca. 3% of the entire genome (Sharma et al., 2007). STR are polymorphic but stable in general population; however, repeats can become unstable during DNA replication, resulting in mitotic or meiotic contractions or expansions. STR instability is an important and unique form of mutation that is linked to >40 neurological, neurodegenerative, and neuromuscular disorders (Pearson et al., 2005). In particular, abnormal expansion of trinucleotide repeats (CTG)n, (CGG)n, (CCG)n, (GAA)n, and (CAG)n have been associated with different diseases such as fragile X syndrome, Huntington disease (HD), Dentatorubral-pallidoluysian atrophy (DRPLA), Friedreich ataxia (FA), diverse Spinocerebellar ataxias (SCA), and Myotonic dystrophy type 1 (DM1).

In 1909, Hans Gustav Wilhelm Steinert, as well as Frederick Eustace Batten and H.P. Gibb, described for the first time a muscular dystrophy characterized by progressive muscle weakness and myotonia (involuntary muscle contraction and delayed relaxation due to muscle hyperexcitability) denominated Myotonic dystrophy or Steinert disease (Schara and Schoser, 2006). Currently, two distinct mutations are known that lead to the clinical syndrome of DM: Myotonic dystrophy type 1 (DM1), caused by expansion of CTG repeats within the 3′ untranslated region of the Dystrophia myotonica-protein-kinase gene (*DMPK*) on chromosome 19 (Brook et al., 1992), and Myotonic dystrophy type 2, due to expansion of CCTG repeats in intron 1 of the Zinc finger protein gene (*ZNF9*) on chromosome 3 (Liquori et al., 2001). DM1 is an autosomal dominant inherited disease that represents the most common form of muscular dystrophy in adults with a prevalence of 1 in 8,000 individuals worldwide. In addition to muscular pathology, DM1 symptomatology includes cardiac conduction defects, insulin resistance, and cognitive alterations in the congenital form of the disease (Harper et al., 2002). For some time, it was difficult to decipher the manner in which a repeat expansion in the *DMPK* gene causes a multisystemic disease with dominant inheritance pattern. However, the fact that such a mutated region is transcribed but untranslated implies that mutant RNA might play a significant role in the disease process. Supporting this hypothesis, growing pieces of evidence obtained over the past 10 years have established that DM1- mutant RNA accumulates in the nuclei, disturbing RNA splicing and gene expression through sequestering of splicing and transcription factors, respectively (Day & Ranum, 2005; Ebralidze et al., 2004).

In this chapter, the clinical features of DM1 and the scientific pathway that allowed elucidation of the molecular basis of DM1 pathogenesis are described in detail. In addition, a discussion of recent developments in molecular therapy for fighting DM1 is provided.

2. Clinical aspects

DM1 is one of the most frequent genetic diseases and is also one of the most variable disorders. Symptoms and severity vary greatly among family members and between generations. Patients may even remain undiagnosed or be misdiagnosed for years, if not recognized as being a member of a family with DM1. However, within the broad spectrum of clinical symptoms, there are some distinct phenotypes according to age-of-onset and number of CTG repeats.

2.1 Multisystemic symptomatology

Clinical manifestations of DM1 involve a great number of organs and tissues and vary from the pre-/post-natal period to adulthood. Skeletal muscle pathology is the most characteristic feature of DM1. Impaired muscle relaxation from myotonia can lead to stiffness and cramping, especially in distal muscles of the hands, but it is rarely a significant complaint registered by patients. Muscle weakness and wasting start distally on distal limbs, neck, and face, and progress proximally over time, often leading to severe disability as the disease progresses (Schara and Schoser, 2006). Respiratory muscle involvement is common, and respiratory failure, either from the primary muscle process or from cardiopulmonary involvement, is a significant contributor to patient mortality (Machuca-Tzili L et al., 2005). A less well-defined but important disease feature is its effect on the Central nervous system (CNS) and cognition, which can be manifested by psychological dysfunction, mental retardation, excessive diurnal sleepiness, and neuropathological abnormalities (Rubinsztein et al., 1998; Laberge et al., 2009). Recent work has demonstrated global deficits with neuropsychological testing, as well as radiographic changes in the brains of affected individuals, including increased white matter lesion burden, decreased gray matter mass (especially in hippocampal and thalamic regions), and hypometabolism in frontal lobes (Di Constanzo et al., 2002a, 2008b; Ono et al., 2001). Alterations of personality associated with DM1 include avoidant personality, obsessive-compulsive, passive-aggressive, and schizotypic traits, whose occurrence is not attributable to the patients' disabling condition (Delaporte 1998; Winblad et al., 2005). Other studies have found severe impairment in all measurements of general intelligence and verbal fluency (Rubinsztein et al., 1997).

In addition to the effects on the CNS, 90% of patients with DM1 could develop cardiac abnormalities at some point of disease development. First-degree atrioventricular block and intraventricular conduction disorders are observed commonly in subjects with DM1, followed by lethal arrhythmias and occasional signs of cardiomyopathy. Echocardiograph findings include prolapsed mitral valve, depressed left ventricular systolic function, reductions in ejections fraction, fractional shortening, and reduced stroke volume (Melacini et al., 1995). In fact, sudden cardiac failure is one of the main causes of death in these patients and occurs with a high incidence of 30%. In the ocular system of these patients, the incidence of lens opacities is very high and manifests as posterior subcapsular, iridescent, multicolored cataracts. Moreover, changes in the Retinal pigment epithelium (RPE), known as Pigment pattern dystrophy (PPD), could be present in the peripheral retina or in macula, mimicking retinitis pigmentosa (Grover et al., 2002; Kim et al., 2009; Louprasong et al., 2010). The ocular muscles are also affected, resulting in external ophthalmoplegia, bilateral motility disturbance, obicularis oculi and levator muscle weakness, and ptosis. Other ocular defects include decreased vision and decreased intraocular pressure (Rosa et al., 2011). Patients with DM1 could also present endocrine defects including insulin resistance and gonadal atrophy (García de Andoin et al., 2005; Matsumura et al., 2009), as well as smooth muscle dysfunction, the clinical effects of which are observed mainly in the gastrointestinal tract and result in disordered esophageal and gastric peristalsis (Machuca-Tzili L et al., 2005).

2.2 Adult-onset and congenital myotonic dystrophy

Based on the clinical findings as well as age-at-onset and disease course, DM1 has been categorized into two main and somewhat overlapping phenotypes: adult-onset, and Congenital myotonic dystrophy (CDM). A rough correlation exists between CTG repeat tract size and these two main forms of DM1 (see Genetics of DM1 section).

Adult-onset presents the classical manifestations of DM1, including myotonia, muscle weakness, cardiac rhythm abnormalities, and endocrine and gonadal abnormalities. The disease progresses insidiously but can become debilitating in the fifth and sixth decades of life. Some authors have classified adult-onset in into two subtypes (mild and classic DM1) according to age-at-onset. Mild DM1 could be asymptomatic or may have only cataracts, mild myotonia, and/or diabetes mellitus. It usually begins in old age and patients may have fully active lives and normal or minimally shortened life span. Classic DM1 is the most common presentation of DM1. The predominant symptom is distal muscle weakness, leading to foot drop disturbance and difficulty with performing tasks requiring fine manual dexterity. Myotonia may interfere with daily activities and the typical face of the patients is principally caused by weakness of facial and levator palpebrae muscles; however, expressivity can be variable, and the presentation could include one or several DM1 features, including cardiac abnormalities, respiratory failure, endocrine abnormalities, smooth muscle dysfunction, cataracts, and hypersomnolence. Age-at-onset for classic DM1 is typically in the third of fourth decades of life, and presents uncommonly after 40 years of age. Nevertheless, in some cases, the pathology begins in the childhood stage (first decade of life), exhibiting evident facial weakness and myotonia, and more severe evolution characterized by low IQ, psychiatric alteration, and early cardiac abnormalities.

CDM is the most severe form of the disease and is usually inherited maternally (Harley et al., 1993). Prenatal stage is characterized by polyhydramnios and reduced fetal movement, all caused by muscle action failure. The main features of congenital DM1 include generalized hypotonia and weakness, pharyngeal weakness, and arthrogryposis, involving predominantly the lower limbs. Less constant features include facial diplegia, diaphragmatic paralysis, respiratory failure, decreased gastrointestinal-tract motility, congenital cataracts, and electrocardiographic abnormalities. Surviving infants exhibit delayed motor development and are often mentally retarded. Typically, affected infants have an inverted V-shaped upper lip, which is characteristic of significant bilateral facial weakness. It is noteworthy that myotonia is not observed in the first years of life (Schara and Schoser, 2006).

2.3 Prognosis and diagnosis of DM1

Life expectancy appears to be reduced in patients with DM1 and is variable depending on the clinical phenotype presented. Subjects with adult-onset DM1 have a nearly normal Quality of life (QOL) during childhood and early adulthood. Nevertheless, many patients become severely disabled by the fifth or sixth decades of life. Chest infections partly due to aspiration and diaphragm weakness are common and may precipitate respiratory failure. Sudden cardiac death is not uncommon, even in younger patients, but it may be preventable by cardiac pacemaker implantation (Machuca-Tzili L et al., 2005). In addition, treatment for diabetes mellitus including annual measurement of serum glucose and glycosylated hemoglobin concentration is indicated to improve the QOL of these patients. Approximate average age of death for patients with adult-onset disease is between 50 and 60 years, and when symptoms begin in the childhood stage, life expectancy is not necessarily reduced, but complications are more common.

In congenital DM1, stillbirths are seldom reported. In severe cases, mortality is high in the first hours and days of life, caused by respiratory insufficiency despite active resuscitation. After the neonatal period, prognosis is more favorable, and despite retarded motor development, all patients become able to walk independently at different ages. Death is frequent in these patients before the age of 30 years, which is caused suddenly by cardiomyopathy and cardiac arrhythmias (Harper, 2001). In the second decade of life, myotonia becomes a more prominent feature, in addition to classical symptoms observed in the adult-onset form, such as infertility and gastrointestinal problems.

An accurate diagnosis of DM1 is important, not only to enable a differential diagnosis among neurological diseases, but also to predict disease severity and to assist patients with appropriate medical monitoring and symptom management. For some time, clinical features were employed to establish the diagnosis of DM1; however, the disease's multisystemic and variable symptomatology caused misdiagnosis in some instances. For example, congenital DM1 could be clinically confused with several other congenital neuromuscular disorders, including myotonia congenita, congenital myopathies, spinal muscular atrophy type 1 or -2, congenital myasthenic syndromes, Möbius syndrome, Spinal muscular atrophy with respiratory distress (SMARD1), the congenital form of glycogenosis type 2, or anoxic brain damage (Harper, 2001; Harper & Monckton, 2004). In adults, Myotonic dystrophy type 2 (DM2) is the condition that is most similar to DM1; the symptoms are practically the same in both dystrophies. Other hereditary distal myopathies, such as hereditary myofibrillar myopathy, hereditary inclusion body myositis, distal muscular dystrophy (Miyoshi, Nonaka, Welander, Markesbery-Griggs), or limb-girdle muscular dystrophies could be confused (Bird, 2011). Currently, diagnosis of DM1 disease is based on DNA testing in individuals who are clinically suspected of having DM1. Patients may have had an electromyography and occasionally muscle biopsy and other tests prior to clinical suspicion of the diagnosis. Electromyography was the most helpful laboratory study prior to the availability of genetics. The combination of myotonic discharges and myopathic- appearing motor units, predominantly in distal muscles and the face, is highly suspicious of DM1. Because electrical myotonic discharges are not usually observed during infancy and many other disorders are associated with myotonia, including myotonia and congenital parmyotonia, this particular test should be taken only as a suggestive finding of DM1. Muscle biopsy is histologically grossly abnormal in clinically affected individuals. Features include variability in fiber size, fibrosis, rows of internal nuclei, sarcoplasmic masses, and an increased number of intrafusal muscle fibers. However, it should be emphasized that there is no clinical indication for performing a muscle biopsy to conducting the diagnosis of DM1 (The International Myotonic Dystrophy Consortium [IDMC], 2000). If clinical features suggest DM1 but DM1 genetic testing is negative, then DM2 testing should be performed. Finally, serum creatine kinase concentration may be mildly elevated in patients with DM1, but it is often normal in asymptomatic individuals.

The DNA test for DM1 is highly relevant because, it confirms the diagnosis in cases with clinically uncertain symptoms, eliminating the need for invasive muscle biopsy. Currently, molecular diagnosis identifies the DM1 mutations in 100% of affected subjects (IDMC, 2000). In addition, determination of insert sizes of CTG repeats aids relatively in predicting disease severity (see Table 1), which is especially useful in young asymptomatic subjects. Despite several advances in the field of DNA analytic techniques, identification of DM1 expanded alleles continues to represent a challenge because of the immense length and variability of expanded alleles and due to the extremely stable secondary structure formed by repetitive, CG-rich sequences. Mutation analysis is based on detection of expanded DMPK alleles, usually by Southern blot analysis. The use of Field-inversion gel electrophoresis (FIGE) and Pulsed-field gel electrophoresis (PFGE), as well as digoxigenin-labeled short CAG-repeat-specific, locked nucleic acid probes have increased the resolution of this technique (Jakubicza et al., 2004). However, Southern blot analysis is not suitable for routine clinical use because it is a time-consuming technique that requires large amounts of genomic DNA and the use in the majority of instances of radioactive probes. Moreover, Southern blot fails to detect premutated alleles and alleles with small expansions. PCR-based assays have been developed to replace Southern blot. PCR utilizing flanking primers allows for amplification up to approximately 100 CTG repeats, but it is unreliable above this size; thus, amplification of alleles with very large numbers of CTG repeats (>100) continue to require Southern blot analysis (Falk, 2006; Tishkoff, 1998; Warner, 1996). Certain improvements in amplification of alleles with large numbers of repeats have been obtained by adding highly stable Taq DNA polymerases, and PCR-enhancing agents, such as glycerol, betaine, and 7-deaza-dGTP to the master reaction (Cheng et al., 1996; Kakourou et al., 2010; Magaña et al., 2011a; Skrzypczak-Zielinska et al., 2009). Currently, identification of DM1 expanded alleles is performed through fluorescent PCR and capillary electrophoresis. The use of a fluorescently labeled primer permits detection of the amplified products by an Argon lasser, and its comparison with a molecular size marker allows sizing of alleles of <100 CTG repeats. Interestingly, a simple fluorescent PCR system that can rapidly identify the largest alleles for any disorder with CTG/CAG repeat expansion was developed (Warner et al., 1996). This method utilizes a fluorescently labeled locus-specific primer flanking the CTG repeat together with paired primers amplifying from multiple priming sites within the CTG repeat. Triplet repeat primed (TP-PCR) gives a characteristic ladder on the fluorescent trace, enabling rapid identification of large, pathological CTG repeats that cannot be amplified employing flanking primers. Although TP-PCR detects expanded alleles of all lengths, it does not allow for their sizing. In fact, samples with large CTG expansions identified by TP-PCR will require Southern blotting if accurate estimation of size is required (Magaña et al., 2011a). Therefore, there is no single method available yet that can reliably identify and size all ranges of expanded alleles in the DM1 locus.

3. Genetics of DM1

DM1 is the most common type of myotonic dystrophy in adults and it belongs to a growing group of genetic diseases caused by expansion of unstable microsatellite repeats. In 1992, DM1 was shown to be caused by an expanded CTG repeat in the 3'-Untranslated region (3'UTR) of the Dystrophy myotonic-protein kinase (*DMPK*) gene in chromosome 19q (Brook et al., 1992) (Figure 1). This gene is composed of 15 exons that encode several alternatively spliced isoforms of a serine/threonine protein kinase that range from 60-70 kDa. The number of CTG repeats in the *DMPK* gene is polymorphic. In unaffected individuals, length of the CTG expansion ranges from 5-34 repeats; this range of repeats is stably inherited and possesses a relatively low mutation rate. DM1 alleles present a range of intermediate alleles that is known as the "premutation range" and that includes between 35 and 49 CTG repeats (Table 1); this range is not clinically significant, but it is genetically unstable, which may cause the expansion of repeats in subsequent generations to reach the pathological range (IDMC, 2000), whereas affected individuals with as few as 50 repeats can exhibit symptoms of the disease in adulthood (Table 1).

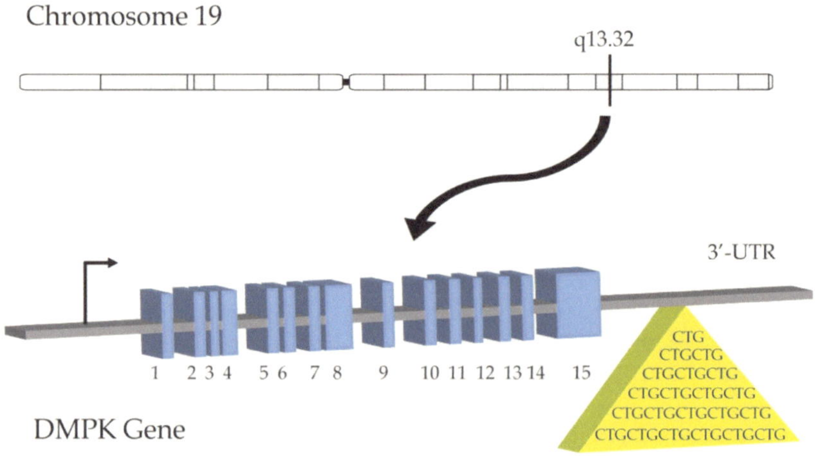

Fig. 1. *DMPK* gene. The *DMPK* gene is located in chromosome 19 at the q13.32 band. Blue rectangles indicate exons and the straight gray line, introns. The CTG repeat tract is located in the 3'unstranslated region of the gene.

In DM1, puzzling genetic phenomena, such as anticipation and the congenital form, which were difficult to explain by conventional Mendelian genetics, are largely attributable to the "dynamic" mutation. Expanded repeat size correlated inversely with age-at-onset, and repeat size increases in successive generations in DM1, providing the molecular basis for anticipation (Harper et al., 1992; Harley et al., 1992; Ashizawa et al., 1992). Paternal mutant alleles usually do not exceed 1,000 CTGs in offspring, whereas maternal transmission frequently gives rise to further expansions of mutant repeats beyond 1,000 CTGs in children with congenital myotonic dystrophy (Lavedan et al., 1993; Ashizawa et al., 1994). Premutation alleles tend to expand into the full-mutation range more frequently with paternal than with maternal transmission (Martorell et al., 2001; 2004). This accounts for the paternal origin of the *de novo* mutations of myotonic dystrophy. The terminal event of anticipation in DM1 is the congenital form, which accompanies severely compromised nuptial and reproductive capability. Consequently, anticipation is expected to deplete the population of patients with DM1 in gradual fashion. However, the prevalence of the disease has been relatively steady; in part, this can be explained by the considerable pool of normal individuals who have permutation alleles who can act as a reservoir for the future origin of new cases through genetic instability (Martorell et al., 2001).

Phenotype	CTG repeat size	Age-at-onset (years)
Normal	5-34	NA
Premutation	35-49	NA
Adult-onset (Mild)	50-150	60-70
Adult-onset (Classic)	100-1,000	10-30
Congenital	>1,000	From birth to 10

Table 1. Correlation between CTG repeat length and phenotype in DM1. NA, Not applicable.

3.1 Origin and distribution of the CTG repeat polymorphism

Myotonic dystrophy is one of the most common inherited neuromuscular disorders and has been described in global populations except for the majority of sub-Saharan ethnic populations (Krahe et al., 1995; Ashizawa & Epstein, 1991). Prevalence varies but generally ranges from 1/8,000-1/50,000 in European and Japanese populations (Harper et al., 2002). High prevalence has been reported in different regions of the world, such as Northeastern Quebec, Canada (Bouchard et al., 1989), and Istria, Croatia (Medica et al., 2004), with a founder effect. Based on the paucity of DM1 in sub-Saharan ethnic populations, it was postulated that the DM1 mutation occurred after human migration out of Africa (Ashizawa & Epstein, 1991). When the $(CTG)_n$ DM1 mutation was identified, it was found to be in complete linkage disequilibrium with the Alu 1-kb insertion (Alu^+) allele located 5 kb upstream of the $(CTG)_n$ repeat within the *DMPK* gene (Zerylnick et al., 1995). Since then, $(CTG)_n$ repeat expansion has always been found on the Alu^+ background in European and Asian populations (Krndija et al., 2005; Pan et al., 2001), with the exception of a Nigerian Yoruba family (Krahe et al., 1995). Subsequent analyses of $(CTG)_n$ and the $Alu^{+}/^{-}$ polymorphism in populations worldwide appears to point to the consensus that $(CTG)_5$ Alu^+ is the ancestral haplotype for all observed haplotypes and that $(CTG)_n$ expansion alleles have derived from this ancestral haplotype through expansion in successive generations of larger normal alleles with >18 CTG repeats (Tishkoff et al., 1998). Supporting this hypothesis, African-Negroid, African-American, and Taiwanese populations all exhibit low frequency of (CTG) >18 alleles and low DM1 prevalence (Acton et al., 2007; Goldman et al., 1994; Hsiao et al., 2003; Pan et al., 2001), whereas the relatively high frequency of (CTG) >18 alleles observed in Japanese, Yugoslav and European populations appears to be associated with moderate-to-high incidence of DM1 (Leifsdottir et al., 2005; Mladenovic et al., 2006). Thus, in the absence of epidemiological data for DM1, frequency estimation of $(CTG)_n$ alleles with >18 repeats in healthy population could be an indirect estimator of DM1 prevalence (Magaña et al., 2011).

Analysis of haplotypes of the DMPK region demonstrated that the majority of European and Asian DM1 $(CTG)_n$ expanded alleles are on one haploytpe (haplotype A) background, while the Nigerian DM1 mutation was found to be on a different haplotype background (Krahe, et al., 1995). Therefore, $(CTG)_5$ repeats in the *DMPK* gene is the most common allele in the majority of the populations; however, allelic distribution of other alleles is different among populations by means of the genetic drift effect on these populations or due to the genic flow caused by the emergence of new populations.

3.2 Expansion and Instability of CTG repeats

The molecular mechanism underlying repeat instability has yet to be completely elucidated. However, remarkable progress has been achieved through research done not only in patient-derived tissues and cells, but also in a variety of experimental systems, including *in vitro*, bacteria, yeast, and transgenic animal models. The use of these experimental models has recapitulated the expansion-prone instability of the expanded $(CTG)_n$ repeat, with degree of repeat instability in correlation with repeat size.

Age-dependent, tissue-specific somatic CTG repeat instability is observed in patients with DM1, with a strong bias toward expansions. The first wave of somatic instability has been suggested to occur between 13 and 16 weeks of gestation, and the second, which is less than the first, could continue throughout adulthood (Jansen et al., 1994). Likewise, a high degree of instability is detected in germ cells. In male gametes, smaller repeats are highly unstable, tending to enlarge significantly during spermatogenesis, while in female gametes, high instability is exhibited mainly in larger repeats (Martorell et al., 2004). It is thought that CTG repeats have already expanded in DM1-affected oocytes, leading to the conclusion that the initial CTG expansion occurs prior to completion of meiosis II of oogenesis (De Temmerman et al., 2004). In transgenic mice, the expanded $(CTG)_n$ repeat exhibits the majority of the characteristics of the expanded repeat in patients' tissues, including expansion bias, the parental gender effect, intergenerational instability, age-dependent increase, and inter-tissue variability of the repeat size (Fortune et al., 2000; Gourdon et al., 1997; Monckton et al., 1997; Seznec et al., 2000; 2001). Characterization of transgenic mice with expanded CTG-CAG repeats in the background of mismatch repair-gene deficiencies revealed that *Msh2*, *Msh3*, *Msh6*, and *Pms2* play important roles in repeat instability (Savouret et al., 2004; Van den Broek et al., 2002). Studies *in vitro* provide evidence that CTG-CAG repeats form non-B DNA structures during DNA replication (Wojciechowska et al., 2005); it is thought that the aberrant repair of these DNA intermediates is a source for development of the triplet repeat expansions. In *Escherichia coli*, CTG repeats are unstable by deletion prone, although expansions do occur depending on repeat length and direction of replication; the mechanism of instability includes slippage of the strands at the replication fork, gene conversion-like events, and recombination (Hashem et al., 2002). Analysis of CTG-CAG repeat instability in yeast has revealed the participation of molecules involved in DNA replication and repair (Shimizu et al., 2001). Although studies in bacteria and yeasts have provided insights into the mechanism of CTG repeat instability, their extrapolation to humans should be carefully considered due to obvious interspecies differences. Figure 2 depicts the major contributors to CTGG instability schematically. It is noteworthy that identification of the molecular mechanism causing expansion of CTG repeats might allow the design of therapeutic strategies against DM1, aimed at inducing deletions of the already expanded CTG repeats or preventing expansion from occurring.

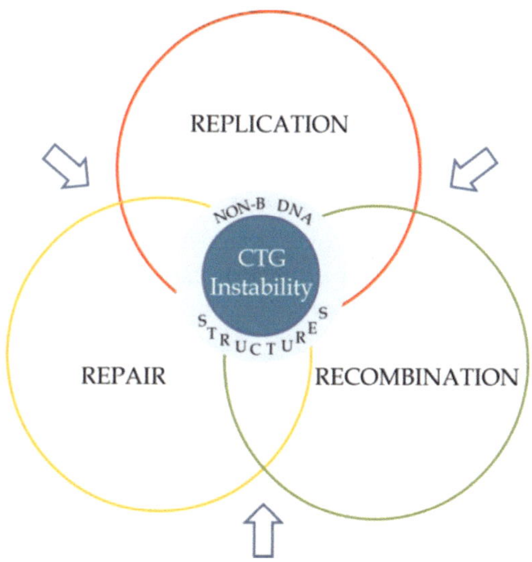

Fig. 2. Major contributors factor to CTG instability *in vivo*. Studies performed on cells and tissues from subjects with DM1, as well as on organism models including transgenic mice, bacteria, and yeast, have revealed that DNA segments containing expanded CTG repeats form unusual DNA structures that, in conjunction with alterations in the replication, recombination and repair processes, lead to CTG instability.

4. RNA-mediated mechanisms of pathogenesis

The mechanism by which the expanded CTG repeat leads to the multisystemic clinical phenotype of DM1 is not fully understood. Because of the location of $(CTG)_n$ in the 3' UTR, the gene's coding region remains intact in the mutant *DMPK* gene; however, the $(CTG)_n$ repeat is transcribed into the messenger RNA (mRNA) as a $(CUG)_n$ repeat. Recent studies have led to three major models of the disease mechanism for DM1 as follows: a) DMPK haploinsufficiency; b) loss-of-function of genes in the vicinity of the CTG repeat, and c) a toxic gain-of-function by the expanded CUG repeat in mutant *DMPK* mRNA.

a. Due to decreased levels of *DMPK* mRNA and protein in adult DM1 tissue (Fu et al., 1993), DMPK deficiency was proposed as the pathogenic mechanism of DM1 soon after identification of the DM1 mutation. The functional implications of a reduction in *DMPK* expression were genetically tested with the generation of knockout mice. *DMPK-/-* mice develop mild, late-onset, progressive skeletal myopathy, which suggested that DMPK might be necessary for the maintenance of skeletal muscle structure (Reddy et al., 1996). Subsequent divulged showed that DMPK-deficient mice also exhibited some cardiac-conduction abnormalities (Berul et al., 2000) and metabolic impairment such as abnormal glucose tolerance, reduced glucose uptake, and impaired insulin-dependent GLUT4 trafficking in muscle (Llagostera et al., 2007). However, the fact that *DMPK-/-* mice demonstrated solely a mild phenotype for only some DM symptoms and that no *DMPK* point mutations have been associated with a DM1 phenotype strongly suggested that the multi systemic features of DM1 were not caused by simply DMPK haploinsufficiency.

b. A second mechanism proposed to explain the pathogenesis of DM1 is based on the effect exerted by CTG expanded repeats on chromatin structure (Otten & Tapscott, 1995), which in turn might lead to partial silencing of neighboring *DMWD* (Dystrophia myotonica-containing WD repeat motif) and *SIX5* (Sine oculis homeobox homolog 5) genes (Alwazzan et al., 1999; Klesert et al., 1997; Sarkar et al., 2000). This hypothesis is supported by the fact that *DMWD* expression levels are reported as decreased in repeat expansion-bearing patients (Alwazzan et al., 1998; Gennarelli et al., 1999). Moreover, mutant analysis in *Drosophila* has shown that *D-Six4*, the closest *Six5* homolog in flies, is required for normal development of gonad muscle and mesodermal components. This suggested that human *Six5* could participate in muscle-wasting and testicular-atrophy phenotypes in DM1 (Kirby et al., 2001). However, *Six5* knockout mice only develop cataracts that lacked the distinctive iridescent opacities characteristic of cataracts of patients with DM1 (Klesert et al., 2000).

c. Data from patients as well as from transgenic mice and cell lines developed for DM1 modeling have offered compelling evidence in support of the third model, which proposes that CUG repeats in the pathogenic range fold into RNA hairpins that are not exported from the nucleus but that, instead, accumulate within ribonuclear foci, acquiring a new toxic function by trapping essential cellular RNA-binding proteins including alternative-splicing modulators and transcription factors, thus disturbing the gene-expression and alternative- splicing processes, respectively (Davis et al., 1997; Ebralidze et al., 2004; Ranum & Cooper 2006; Taneja et al., 1995).

4.1 Nuclear retention of mutant *DMPK* RNA

Preferential accumulation of mutant *DMPK* mRNA in nuclear foci has been observed by the Fluorescent *in situ* hybridization (FISH) technique in fibroblasts, myoblasts, and neurons from different nerve tissues (cerebral cortex, hippocampus, dentate gyrus, thalamus, substantia nigra, and brainstem) of subjects with DM1 (Davis et al., 1997; Day & Ranum, 2005; Machuca-Tzili et al., 2005). These findings have also been corroborated in muscle tissue of patients with DM1 by Northern blot analysis (Davis et al., 1997; Klesert et al., 2000; Wang et al., 1994). Furthermore, electron microscopy examination has revealed that the CUG-repeat RNA forms double-stranded RNA (Michalowski et al., 1999), which might impede its export to the cytoplasm. It has been demonstrated that nuclear accumulation of mutant transcripts increases in proportion to the number of CUG repeats, suggesting that the length of the (CUG)n tract strongly determines the formation of nuclear aggregates (Klesert et al., 2000). Furthermore, the number and morphology of ribonuclear foci in DM1 are also quite variable in different cell types and tissues; in proliferating DM1 cells in culture, these RNA-rich accumulations range from a few small foci in fibroblasts to dozens of larger foci in myoblasts. In contrast, only a few nuclear foci are observed in postmitotic cells, such as myofibers and cortical neurons.

Interestingly, mutant *DMPK* RNA is able to form ribonucleoprotein complexes by binding to certain RNA-binding proteins (Miller et al., 2000) including modulators of alternative-splicing and transcription factors, which are correspondingly depleted from their normal subcellular localizations (for review, see Llamusi & Artero, 2008). This aberrant event causes alteration in the normal expression of numerous muscular and neuronal proteins, supporting the multisystemic phenotype of the disease (see later). Given the fact that nuclear accumulation of mutant *DMPK* RNA is the basis for its toxic function, definition of the steps at which mutant mRNA transport is blocked would aid in improving the definition of the molecular basis of the pathology and eventually, in designing a therapeutic treatment (Mastroyiannopoulos et al., 2005).

4.2 Alternative-splicing misregulation

Accumulation of mutant *DMPK* mRNA in nuclei of muscle and nerve cells facilitates its aberrant union with proteins that participate in the regulation of nuclear processes, such as splicing modulators and transcription factors; thus, the normal function of a number of proteins might be impaired. Mutant mRNA of DM1 is able to interact and form aggregates with proteins that participate in the alternative splicing of pre-mRNAs, such as the Muscleblind-like family (MBNL1, MBNL2, and MBNL3), the CUG-binding protein 2 (ETR-3), the Protein kinase RNA-activated (Protein kinase R) PKR enzyme, and the heterogeneous nuclear ribonucleoprotein H (hnRNP H), which results in interference in developmentally regulated alternative splicing of defined pre-mRNAs (Fardaei et al., 2002; Jiang et al., 2004; Kanadia et al., 2003; Kuyumcu-Martínez & Cooper 2006; Mankodi et al., 2001; Miller et al., 2000). Furthermore, DM1 mutation cells activate CUG triplet repeat RNA-binding protein 1 (CUG-BP1), also denominated CUGBP1/Elav-like family member 1 (CELF1), through hyperphosphorylation and stabilization in the cell nucleus (Ho et al., 2005; Philips et al., 1998; Savkur et al., 2001; 2004; Timchenko et al., 2001). It is known that up to 74% of human genes undergo alternative splicing, during which exons or parts of exons can be skipped during pre-mRNA processing, resulting in the expression of multiple variant mRNAs; therefore, alternative-splicing misregulation could be the best explanation for the multisystemic characteristics of DM1 pathology. The function of these splicing regulators determines the tissue- and developmental phase- specific expression of certain protein isoforms (Taneja et al., 1995). Within this group of splicing regulators, CELF1 and MBNL are those that are best understood. CELF1 and MBNL1 play opposite roles in exon selection in several pre-mRNA transcripts; while MBNL1 promotes the transition of splicing from fetal to adult exons, CELF1 aids in retaining fetal exons. According to current evidence, the abnormal length of the (CUG)n segment determines the entrapment of muscle-bound MBNL proteins in ribonuclear aggregates and in the stabilized expression of CELF1, which in turn causes aberrant pre-mRNA splicing that results in abnormal expression of fetal splice isoforms in the tissues of adult subjects with DM1 (Figure 3).

To date, alterations in at least 14 pre-mRNA alternative-splicing events have been reported (Ranum & Day, 2006; Magaña et al., 2009), seven of which have been found in skeletal and cardiac muscle, affecting the following genes: *TNNT2* (cardiac Troponin T gene); *IR* (Insulin receptor gene); *MTMR1* (Myotubularin-related protein 1); *TNNT3* (skeletal muscle Troponin T gene); *RyR* (Ryanodine receptor gene); *SERCA2* (Sarco/endoplasmic reticulum calcium ATPase 2 gene), and *ClCN-1* (muscle-specific Chloride Channel) (Charlet et al., 2002; Ho et al., 2005; Kimura et al., 2005; Mankodi et al., 2002; Philips et al., 1998; Savkur et al., 2001). Moreover, alterations in the transcript processing of *Tau*, *NMDAR1* (N-methyl-D-aspartate receptor 1), and *APP* (Amyloid protein precursor) genes have been observed to occur in the brain of subjects with DM1 (De León & Cisneros, 2008; Jiang et al., 2004) (Figure 3).

It is noteworthy that utilization of transgenic mice and cellular models together with the information obtained in clinical trials has enabled correlation of alterations in transcript maturation with DM1 symptomatology. In subjects with DM1, the presence of an *IR* gene-derived mRNA that lacks exon 11 has been described, which results in the synthesis of an insulin-resistant receptor isoform (Savkur et al., 2001). This phenomenon could explain the development of diabetes in these individuals. Likewise, several studies have reported the expression of immature transcripts of *RyR* and *SERCA2* genes in skeletal muscle of patients with DM1; the products of these genes regulate calcium homeostasis during sarcolemma depolarization: at the beginning of muscle contraction, Ca^{2+} is released from the sarcoplasmic reticulum through ion channels formed by RyR, while SERCA2 pumps the former back to the lumen of the sarcoplasmatic reticulum to restore cytoplasmic Ca^{2+} levels, consequently inducing muscle relaxation. Thus, alterations in this process could be related with the muscle weakness observed in DM1. With respect to the employment of transgenic mice for studying DM1-associated mis-splicing, it has been reported that a transgenic mouse over-expressing CELF1 exhibits production of alternative TNNT2 gene mRNA with the inclusion of exon 5, which is exclusively observed in fetal tissues (Ho et al., 2005; Timichenko et al., 2001). Troponin T forms part of a protein complex that regulates actin-myosin interactions during muscle contraction. The fetal isoform is less sensitive to Ca^{2+}, resulting in a weaker cardiac-muscle contraction. Based on these observations, it has been proposed that aberrant processing of the Troponin T gene transcript might be the cause of the development of arrhythmia and the loss of myocardial function described in patients with DM1. Characterization of a second transgenic mouse that over-expressed CELF1 showed the presence of mRNA from the *ClCN-1* gene with inclusion of exon 7 in muscle tissue. The presence of exon 7 generates higher degradation of the transcript, with the consequent decrease in levels of the protein, a chloride-channel component (Charlet et al., 2002; Mankodi et al., 2002), which ultimately results in decreased transmembranal conductance of chloride ions in muscle fibers. This physiological alteration correlates with the classic clinical sign of DM1: myotonia. Supporting the crucial role of mis-splicing in the development of DM1, the knockout mouse for the *MBLN* gene (Mbln1 Δ^3/Δ^3) displayed alterations in the alternative splicing of *TNNT2, TNNT3,* and *ClCN-1* genes and consequently developed myotonia and cataracts. Comparison of two mouse models for DM1, one expressing the mutant *DMPK* RNA and the other *null* for the *Mbnl1*a gene, revealed that loss of MBNL1a explains only >80% of the splicing pathology due to expanded CUG RNA. Mbnl-independent mis-splicing effects were observed particularly on mRNAs for extracellular matrix proteins (Du et al., 2010).

Finally, the generation and characterization of cellular models for DM1 have additionally contributed to the identification of the molecular mechanism underling this pathology. A study on C2C12 cells, a mouse muscular-cell line, demonstrated that CELF1 sequestration by the mutant *DMPK* RNA impairs the translation of several myogenesis regulators, including MEF2A (myocyte-specific potentiator factor 2A), MyoD (Myogenin 2), and p21 (CdK 1A inhibitor), which ultimately cause impairment in the muscle differentiation program (Ho et al., 2005). Although the brain is considered the second most affected organ in DM1, the molecular basis of this pathology in the nervous system has not yet been elucidated. One of the most distinctive characteristics of brain damage in subjects with DM1 is the presence of hyperphosphorylated Tau aggregates in the neurocortex (Jiang et al., 2004). Tau is expressed abundantly in the peripheral and nervous systems and is especially enriched in the axons of mature and growing neurons, in which it is found associated with microtubules and on which it confers stability. Abnormal phosphorylation of Tau negatively affects its binding to microtubules, and ultimately its function, as has been described in Alzheimer disease. In the human brain, six Tau-protein isoforms are expressed as a result of the alternative splicing of exons 2, 3, and 10. Interestingly, expression of Tau isoforms, with the exclusion of exons 2/3 and 10, is favored in subjects with DM1 (Jiang et al., 2004; Wang et al., 2005). Exon 2 encodes for the N-terminal domain of Tau, which interacts with the axonal membrane, whereas exon 10 encodes for a microtubule-binding domain. Therefore, absence of these domains in the protein product might affect the function of Tau as a microtubule-stabilizer molecule, causing, at least in part, the neuronal damage observed in patients with DM1 (Wang et al., 2005). As mentioned previously, the brain of subjects with DM1 also exhibits alterations in *NMDAR1*-gene transcript maturation (Jiang et al., 2004), specifically in cortical and subcortical neurons. *NMDAR1* regulates synaptic transmission of excitation in the hippocampus, thus participating in the long-term potentiation and learning process (Tsien et al., 1996). Normally, the *NMDAR1* gene produces eight isoforms derived from alternative splicing of its premRNA; nevertheless, patients with DM1 preferentially produce an isoform with the inclusion of exon 5, which affects the affects the receptor's distribution and pharmacological properties. Hence, the presence of this abnormal isoform of NMDAR1 might be related with DM1-associated memory impairment (Cull-Candy et al., 2004; Winblad et al., 2006).

4.3 Leaching of transcription factors from chromatin

It has been recently observed that several transcription factors are sequestered by mutant *DMPK* RNA in muscle cells of subjects with DM1, including Sp1 (Specific protein 1), STAT1, and STAT3 (members of Signal transduction-family proteins and transcription activators), and the gamma subunit of the Retinoic acid receptor (RARγ) (Figure 3). This aberrant event removes the transcription factors from active chromatin, leading to disrupted gene-expression patterns. It is thought that the decreased *ClCN-1* gene expression observed in the muscle cells of patients with DM1 is due to the entrapment of Sp1 in nuclear foci containing mutant *DMPK* RNA, because Sp1 modulates the *ClCN-1* gene promoter positively. Supporting this idea, expression of the *ClCN-1* gene is restored in DM1 muscle cells by over-expression of Sp1 (Ebralidze et al., 2004). Further studies are required to fully understand the influence of mutant DMPK RNA on gene expression.

5. Perspectives of gene therapy

At present, treatment for DM1 is limited to symptomatic intervention and there is no therapeutic approach to prevent or reverse disease progression. However, elucidation of the molecular mechanisms underlying DM1 pathogenesis have allowed for the envisaging and developing of experimental approaches with therapeutic potential that are aimed at reversing DM1 symptomatology. Because the central core of DM1 pathogenesis is the gain-

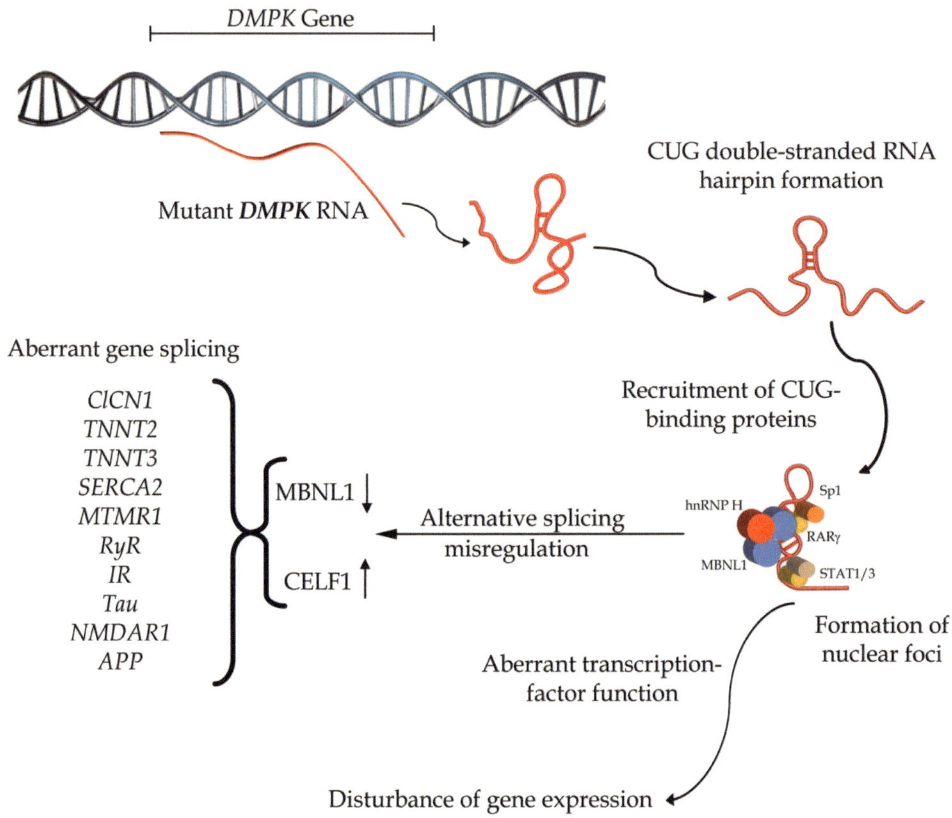

Fig. 3. RNA toxic gain-of-function model for DM1 pathogenesis. Mutant *DMPK* RNA accumulates in the nucleus of muscle and nerve cells, sequestering different regulatory proteins including splicing modulators MBNL1 and hnRNP H and transcription factors Sp1, STAT1, STAT3, and RARγ. Furthermore, expression of expanded CTG repeats causes, by means of an unknown mechanism, an increase in the activity of splicing modulator CELF1. The aberrant behavior of mutant *DMPK* RNA alters the activity of both splicing modulators and transcription factors, giving rise to impairment in the expression and function of a number of genes and ultimately, to the multisystemic DM1 phenotype.

of-function of mutant *DMPK* RNA, the majority of studies have been focused on targeting the mutant transcript to eliminate or ameliorate its toxic effects. However, alternative strategies centered on reversing DM1-associated spliceopathy without targeting the mutant *DMPK* RNA have remerged recently (Magaña & Cisneros, 2011; Mulders et al., 2010).

5.1 Degradation or neutralization of mutant *DMPK* RNA

Different approaches have been applied to target and cleave mutant *DMPK* RNA, including the use of antisense RNA, Antisense oligonucleotides (AONs), small interfering RNA (siRNA), and self-cleaving hammerhead ribozymes (Figure 4A). Antisense RNA complementary to (CUG)13 repeat-sequence AON was employed in human DM1 myoblasts carrying ~750 CTG repeats (Furling et al., 2003), resulting in preferential decay of mutant over wild-type *DMPK* transcripts and consequent normalization of myoblast fusion and glucose uptake via restoration of the expression and binding activity of *CELF1*. Further studies with a 2′-O-Methyl-phosphorothioate-modified AON (2′-MePS-AON) that targets CUG repeats were performed in immortal mouse myoblasts expressing the human *DMPK* gene with 500 CTG repeats (DM500 cell model) (Mulders et al., 2009) and in two following DM1 mouse models: the first carrying the Human skeletal alpha-actin (*HSA*) gene modified by the insertion of 250 CTG repeats in the 3′UTR (*HSA^LR^* mouse model) and the second, bearing the human *DM1* locus with 500 CTG repeats (DM500 mouse model) (Mankodi et al., 2000; Seznec et al., 2000). Promisingly, antisense treatment resulted in decreasing levels of mutant *DMPK*, reduction of ribonuclear foci, and correction of the DM1-associated, aberrant pre-mRNA splicing of several genes. Similar positive effects have been observed in DM1 myoblasts that have ~3,200 CTG repeats with the use of siRNAs (Langlois et al., 2005), and in DM1 myoblasts expressing approximately 750 CTG repeats with the employment of nuclear ribozymes that targeted and cleaved 3′UTR of *DMPK* mRNA (Langlois et al., 2003). However, the main limitation of these strategies lies in that all molecules recognize and cleave both mutant and wild-type *DMPK* mRNA with similar efficacy.

A more recent and attractive strategy against DM1 postulates that disruption of the aberrant RNA-protein interactions exerted by the *DMPK* mutant transcript with the alternative-splicing regulator MBNL1 would correct DM1-associated mis-splicing (Figure 4B). Supporting this hypothesis, a 25-nucleotide morpholino-type AON complementary to CUG-repeated RNA blocks the formation of the CUG-expanded MBNL1 complex in the HSA^{LR} transgenic mouse model, resulting in several beneficial effects, including decreased number of nuclear foci through MBNL1 protein redistribution in the nucleus, enhanced transport of CUG expanded-containing transcripts to the cytoplasm, alternative-splicing correction of MBNL1-dependent genes, normalization of transmembrane chloride-ion conductance, and reduction of myotonia (Wheeler et al., 2009). In this regard, identification of small molecules or multivalent modular compounds that specifically bind CUG repeats and that could competitively release sequestered MBNL1 would constitute a promising alternative strategy for neutralization of toxic RNA (Warf and Berglund, 2010; Warf et al., 2009).

5.2 Mis-splicing reversal

Sequestration of MBNL1 by mutant *DMPK* transcript in nuclear foci indicates that MBNL1 titration and loss-of-function is linked with the mis-splicing of particular genes. Furthermore, it was recently shown that activation of the PKC signaling pathway by CUG repeats leads to CELF1 hyperphosphorylation and stabilization, implicating this signaling event in DM1-associated mis-splicing (Philips et al., 1998; Savkur et al., 2001; Sergeant et al., 2001). Therefore, it has been hypothesized that modulation of the expression and/or activity of these two splicing factors would reverse DM1-associated spliceopathy (Figure 4C). Consistent with this idea, over-expression of *MBNL1* in a *Drosophila* model of DM1 expressing a non-coding mRNA containing 480 CUG repeats reduced the number of nuclear foci and suppressed the degenerative phenotypes caused by expanded repeats in muscle and eye tissue (de Haro et al., 2006). Moreover, over-expression of *MBNL1* mediated by an adeno-associated viral vector specifically corrected the mis-splicing of MBNL1-dependent genes including *Clcn1*, *Serca1*, and *Tnnt3* and reversed myotonia in the HSA^{LR} mouse model of DM1 (Kanadia et al., 2006). On the other hand, different mice models have been established to test the role of CELF1 activity in the development of muscle-wasting and cardiac disease in DM1 (Ho et al., 2005; Koshelev et al., 2010). Interestingly, specific blockage of PKC activity in an inducible mouse model for heart-specific expression of 960 CUG RNA repeats that developed cardiac arrhythmias, cardiomyopathy, and CELF1-associated spliceopathy (Wang et al. 2007) resulted in improved cardiac conduction and reduced misregulation of CELF1-mediated splicing events, which correlated with decreased phosphorylation and steady-state levels of CELF1 (Wang et al., 2009). Hence, the use of protein kinase C inhibitors to downregulate or to prevent upregulation of CELF1 activity would be an alternative therapeutic treatment for DM1. Finally, it is important to mention that correction of DM1 mis-splicing by modulation of *CELF1* and *MBNL1* expression should be considered with caution because artificial alteration of MBNL1 and/ CELF1 steady-state levels might alter the splicing pattern of a number of genes regulated by these proteins, with unknown consequences for muscle function.

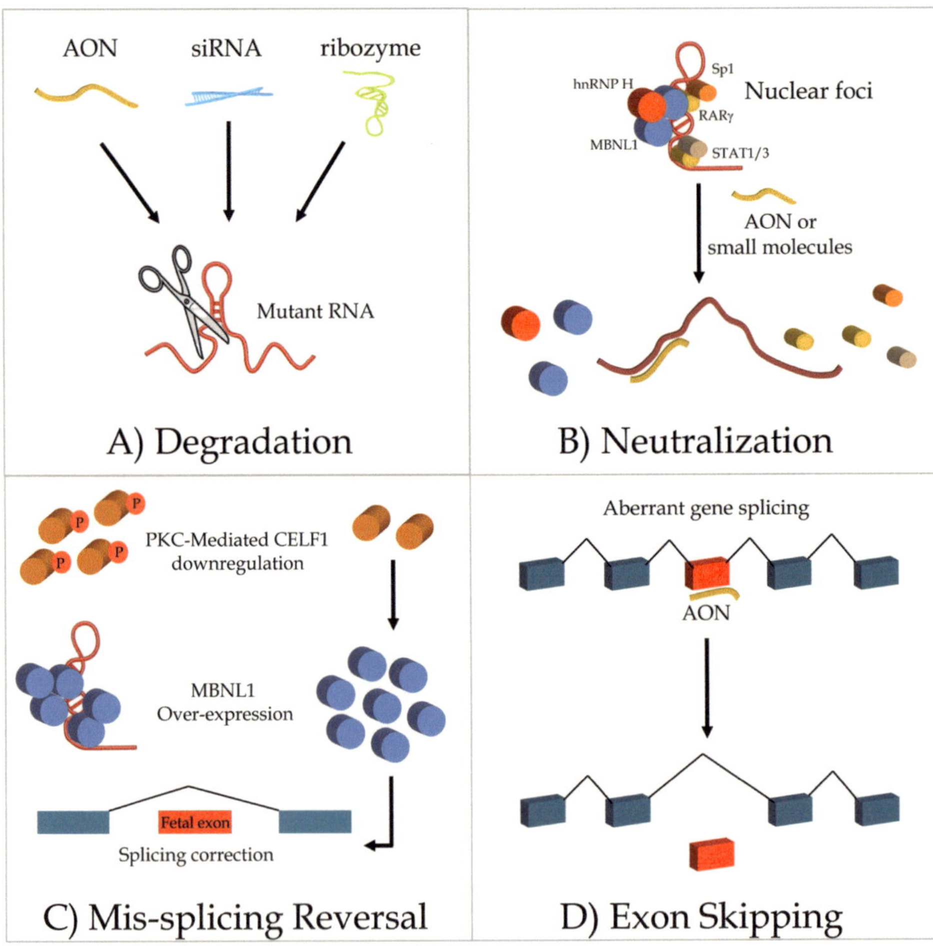

Fig. 4. Strategies for DM1 gene therapy. A) Degradation of mutant RNA by antisense oligonucleotides (AON), ribozyme, or siRNA. B) Neutralization of mutant RNA activity by blocking its interaction with the splicing regulator MBNL1 using AON or small chemical compounds. C) Mis-splicing reversal by ver-expression of MBNL1 or down-regulation of CELF activity. D) Exon skipping of mis-spliced genes (i.e. *CLCN1* gene) by splicing blockage with AON.

5.3 Exon skipping of mis-spliced genes

An alternative strategy to fight DM1 symptomatology is to correct aberrant splicing events by exon skipping of mis-spliced genes. The mechanism of exon skipping is based on the binding of AON to specific-target sense sequences of mis-spliced pre-mRNA genes to block the access of splicing machinery to splice sites, causing the elimination of specific exons(s) and their flanking regions, in order to restore an open-reading frame of the normal isoform (Alter et al., 2006; Lu et al., 2005) (Figure 4D). AON-mediated exon skipping appears to be a potent method for reversing DM1-associated myotonia caused by abnormal inclusion of exon 7a in *ClCN-1* mRNA. Normalization of *ClCN-1* current density, as well as elimination of myotonic discharges, were observed in two murine models (DM1 mouse model HSA^{LR}, and a transgenic mouse homozygous for *MBNL1*-gene disruption) after muscular injection of a morpholino-AON that targeted the 3' splice site of *ClCN-1* mRNA exon 7a and prevented inclusion of this exon in the mature transcript (Wheeler et al., 2007). Future exon-skipping strategies for DM1 should ensure muscle-specific uptake of therapeutic oligos after their systemic delivery, as well as the employment of a multiple AON cocktail designed to correct splicing at two or more transcripts involved in DM1 symptomatology.

6. Conclusions and future outlook

Conventional approaches to treatment of DM1 are supportative and have failed to slow or halt disease progression. Substantial progress has been made in understanding the disease-causing mechanisms of DM1, and now that it is clear that multisystemic phenotype of DM1 results directly from expression of a mutant expanded repeat RNA, the search for novel therapies is underway. Despite the tremendous progress obtained in several cell-based and animal models, in which degradation or neutralization of the mutant *DMPK* RNA results in reversal of mis-splicing and myotonia, there are a number of hurdles to overcome before implementation of RNA-based strategies in clinical trials, such as tissue-specific delivery, sustainability, and effectiveness of the therapeutic molecules.

7. Acknowledgments

This work was supported by the Science and Technology Institute of Mexico City (ICyTDF), Grant PIFUTP08-164.

8. References

Acton, R.T.; Rivers, C.A.; Watson, B.; & Oh S.J. (2007). DMPK-associated myotonic dystrophy and CTG repeats in Alabama African Americans. *Clinical Genetics,* Vol. 72, pp. 448-453, ISSN 0009-9163

Alter, J.; Lou, F.; Rabinowitz, A.; Yin, H.; Rosenfeld, J.; Wilton, S.D.; Partridge, T.A.; & Lu, Q.L. (2006). Systemic delivery of morpholino oligonucleotide restores dystrophin expression bodywide and improves dystrophic pathology. *Nature Medicine*. Vol.12, No.2, pp.175-177., ISSN 1078-8956

Alwazzan, M.; Hamshere, M.G.; Lennon, G.G.; & Brook, J.D. (1998). Six transcripts map within 200 kilobases of the myotonic dystrophy expanded repeat. *Mammalian Genome*. Vol.9, No.6, pp.485-487, ISSN 0938-8990

Alwazzan, M.; Newman, E.; Hamshere, M.G.; & Brook, J.D. (1999). Myotonic dystrophy is associated with a reduced level of RNA from DMWD allele adjacent to the expanded repeat. *Human Molecular Genetics*.Vol.8 pp.1491-1497, ISSN 0964-6906

Ashizawa, T.; & Epstein H.F. (1991). Ethnic distribution of myotonic dystrophy gene. *Lancet*. Vol 338 No. 8767, pp. 642-643. ISSN 0140-6736

Ashizawa, T.; Dunne, C.J.; Dubel, JR.; Perryman, M.B.; Epstein, H.F.; Boerwinkle, E.; & Hejtmancik, J.F.(1992). Anticipation in myotonic dystrophy. I. Statistical verification based on clinical and haplotype findings. *Neurology*. Vol 42, No. 10, pp. 1871-1877, ISSN 0028-3878

Ashizawa, T.; Dunne, P.W.; Ward, P.A.; Seltzer, W.K.; & Richards, CS. (1994). Effects of the sex of myotonic dystrophy patients on the unstable triplet repeat in their affected offspring. *Neurology*. Vol 44 No.1, pp. 120-122 , ISSN 0028-3878

Berul, C.I.; Maguire, C.T.; Gehrmann, J.; & Reddy, S. (2000).Progressive atrioventricular conduction block in a mouse myotonic dystrophy model. *Journal of Interventional Cardiac Electrophysiology*. Vol.4, No.2, pp.351-358 ISSN 1383-875X

Bouchard, G.; Roy, R.; Declos, M.; Mathieu, J.; & Kouladjian, K. (1989). Origin and diffusion of the myotonic dystrophy gene in the Saguenay region (Quebec). *The Canadian Journal of Neurological Sciences*. Vol 16, No.1 ,pp. 119-122 ISSN 0317-1671

Brook, J.D.; McCurrach, M.E.; Harley, H.G.; Buckler, A.J.; Church, D.; Aburatani, H.; Hunter, K.; Stanton, V.P.; Thirion, J.P.; & Hudson, T. (1992). Molecular basis of myotonic dystrophy: expansion of a trinucleotide (CTG) repeat at the 3' end of a transcript encoding a protein kinase family member. *Cell*, Vol 68, No.4, pp.799-808, ISSN 0092-8674.

Charlet, B.N.; Savkur, R.S.; Singh, G.; Philips, A.V.; Grice, E.A.; & Cooper, T.A. (2002). Loss of the muscle-specific chloride channel in type 1 myotonic dystrophy due to misregulated alternative splicing. *Molecular Cell* 2002; Vol. 10, pp.45-53, ISSSN 1097-2765

Cheng, S.; Barceló, J.M.; & Korneluk, RG. (1996). Characterization of large CTG repeat expansions in myotonic dystrophy alleles using PCR. *Human Mutation*, Vol. 7, No.4 , pp. 304-310, ISSN 1059-7794

Cull-Candy, S.G.; & Leszkiewicz, D.N.(2004). Role of distinct NMDA receptor subtypes at central synapses. *Science´s STKE: signal trasduction knowledge environment*. 2004; re16 ISSN 1525-8882

Davis, B.M.; McCurrach, M.E.; Taneja, K.L.; Singer, R.H.; & Housman, D.E. (1997). Expansion of a CUG trinucleotide repeat in the 3' untranslated region of myotonic dystrophy protein kinase transcripts results in nuclear retention of transcripts. *Proceedings National Academy Sciences of United States of America*, Vol.94, No.14, pp.7388-7393, ISSN 0027-8424

Day, J.W. & Ranum, L.P.; (2005). RNA pathogenesis of the myotonic dystrophies. *Neuromuscular Disorders*, Vol. 15, No.1, pp.5-16, ISSN 0960-8966

De Haro, M.; Al-Ramahi, I.; De Gouyon, B.; Ukani, L.; Rosa, A.; Faustino, N.A.; Ashizawa, T.; Cooper, T.A.; & Botas, J. (2006). MBNL1 and CUGBP1 modify expanded CUG-induced toxicity in a Drosophila model of myotonic dystrophy type 1. *Human Molecular Genetics*. Vol.15, No.13, pp.2138-2145, ISSN 0964-6906

De León, M. & Cisneros, B. (2008). Myotonic dystrophy 1 in the nervous system: From the clinic to molecular mechanisms. *Journal Neuroscience Reserch*, Vol. 86, No. 1, pp.18-26, ISSN 0360-4012

De Temmerman, N.; Sermon, K.; Seneca, S.; De Rycke, M.; Hilven, P.; Lissens, W.; Van Steirteghem, A.; & Liebaers, I. (2004). Intergenerational instability of the expanded CTG repeat in the DMPK gene: studies in human gametes and preimplantation embryos. *American Journal of Human Genetics* Vol.75, No.2, pp. 325-329, ISSN 0002-9297

Di Costanzo, A.; Di Salle, F.; Santero, L.; Tessitore, A.; Bonavita, V.; & Tedeschi, G. (2002) Pattern and significance of white matter abnormalities in myotonic dystrophy type 1: an MRI study. *Journal of Neurology*. Vol.249 , No.9, pp. 1175-82, ISSN 0340-5354

Di Costanzo, A.; Santoro, L.; de Cristofaro, M.; Manganelli, F.; Di Salle, F.; & Tedeschi, G. (2008). Familial aggregation of white matter lesions in myotonic dystrophy type 1. *Neuromuscular Disorders*. Vol.18, No.4, pp. 299-305, ISSN 0960-8966

Du, H.; Cline, M.S.; Osborne, R.J.; Tuttle, D.L.; Clark, T.A.; Donohue, J.P.; Hall, M.P.; Shiue, L.; Swanson, M.S.; Thornton, C.A.; & Ares, M. Jr. (2010) Aberrant alternative splicing and extracellular matrix gene expression in mouse models of myotonic dystrophy. *Nature structural & molecular biology*.2010 Feb;17(2):pp.187-93. ISSN 1545-9993

Ebralidze, A.; Wang, Y.; Petkova, V.; Ebralidse, K.; & Junghans, R.P. (2004). RNA leaching of transcription factors disrupts transcription in myotonic dystrophy. *Science*, Vol 303, No.5656, pp.383-387, ISSN 0036-8075.

Ellegren, H. (2000). Heterogeneous mutation processes in human microsatellite DNA sequences. *Nature Genetics*, Vol 24, No. 4, pp. 400-402, ISSN 1061-4036.

Falk, M.; Vojtiskova, M.; Lukas, Z.; Kroupová, I.; & Froster, U. (2006). Simple procedure for automatic detection of unstable alleles in the myotonic dystrophy and Huntington's disease loci. *Genetic Testing*, Vol. 10, No. 2, pp.85-97, ISSN 1090-6576

Fardaei, M.; Rogers, M.T.; Thorpe, H.M.; Larkin, K.; Hamshere, M.G.; Harper, P.S.; & Brook, J.D.(2002). Three proteins, MBNL, MBLL and MBXL, co-localize in vivo with nuclear foci of expanded-repeat transcripts in DM1 and DM2 cells. *Human Moecular Genetics*. Vol.11, No.7, pp.805-814, ISSN 0964-6906

Fortune, M.T.; Vassilopoulos, C.; Coolbaugh, M.I.; Siciliano, M.J.; & Monckton, D.G. (2000). Dramatic, expansion-biased, age-dependent, tissue-specific somatic mosaicism in a transgenic mouse model of triplet repeat instability. *Human Molecular Genetics*. Vol.9, No.3, pp. 439-445, ISSN 0964-6906

Fu, Y.H.; Friedman, D.L.; Richards, S.; Pearlman, J.A.; Gibbs, R.A.; & Pizzuti, A. (1993). Decreased expression of myotonin-protein kinase messenger RNA and protein in adult form of myotonic dystrophy. *Science* 1993; 36: 59-61 ISSN 0964-6906.

Furling, D.; Doucet, G.; Langlois, M.A.; Timchenko, L.; Belanger, E.; Cossette, L.; & Puymirat, J. (2003). Viral vector producing antisense RNA restores myotonic dystrophy myoblast functions. *Gene Therapy*.Vol.10, No.9, pp.795-802, ISSN 0969-7128

García de Andoin, N.; Echeverría, J.; Cobo, A.M.; Rey, A.; Paisán, L.; & López de Munain, A. (2005). A neonatal form of Steinert's myotonic dystrophy in twins after in vitro fertilization. *Fertility and Sterility*. Vol.84, No.3 pp. 756, ISSN 0015-0282

Gennarelli, M.; Pavón, M.; Amicucci, P.; Angelini, C.; Menegazzo, E.; Zelano, G.; Novelli, G.; & Dallapiccola, B. (1999). Reduction of the DM-associated homeo domain protein (DMAHP) mRNA in different brain areas of myotonic dystrophy patients. *Neuromuscular Disorders*. Vol.9, No.4, pp.215-219, ISSN 0960-8966

Goldman, A.; Ramsay, M.; & Jenkins, T. (1994). Absence of myotonic dystrophy in southern African Negroids is associated with a significantly lower number of CTG trinucleotide repeats. *Journal of Medical Genetics* . Vol.31, pp. 37-40, ISSN 002-2593

Gourdon, G.; Radvanyi, F.; Lia, AS.; Duros, C.; Blanche, M.; Abitbol, M.; Junien, C.; & Hofmann-Radvanyi, H. (1997). Moderate intergenerational and somatic instability of a 55-CTG repeat in transgenic mice. *Nature Genetics*. Vol.15, No.2, pp.190- 192, ISSN 1061-4036.

Grover, S.; Fishman, G.A.; & Stone, E.M. (2002). Atypical presentation of pattern dystrophy in two families with peripherin/RDS mutations. *Ophthalmology*. Vol.109, pp. 1110-1117, ISSN 0161-6420

Harley, H.G.; Rundle, S.A.; MacMillan, J.C.; Myring, J.; Brook, J.D.; Crow, S.; Reardon, W.; Fenton, I.; Shaw, DJ.; & Harper, P.S. (1993). Size of the unstable CTG repeat sequence in relation to phenotype and parental transmission in myotonic dystrophy. *American Journal of Human Genetics*. Vol.52, No.6, pp.1164-1174 ISSN 0002-9297

Harper, P.S. (2001). *Myotonic Dystrophy*. WB Saunders (3rd Ed), ISBN 0702021520, London

Harper, P.S.; van Engelen, B.G.; Eymard, B.; Rogers, M.; & Wilcox, D. (2002). 99th ENMC international workshop: myotonic dystrophy: present management, future therapy. 9-11 Naarden, The Netherlands. *Neuromuscular Disorders*, Vol.12, No.6, pp. 596-599, ISSN 0960-8966

Hashem, V.I.; Klysik, E.A.; Rosche, W.A.; & Sinden, R.R.; (2002). Instability of repeated DNAs during transformation in Escherichia coli. *Mutation Reserch*. Vol.502, No 1-2 , pp. 39-46,ISSN 0027-5107

Ho, T.H.; Bundman, D.; Armstrong, D.L.; & Cooper, T.A. (2005). Transgenic mice expressing CUG-BP1 reproduce splicing mis-regulation observed in myotonic dystrophy. *Human Molecular Genetics* Vol.14, No.11, pp.1539-1547, ISSN 0964-6906

Hsiao, K.M.; Chen, S.S.; Li, S.Y.; Chiang, S.Y.; Lin, H.M.; & Pan, H. (2003). Epidemiological and genetic studies of myotonic dystrophy type 1 in Taiwan. *Neuroepidemiology* .Vol.22, pp. 283-289, ISSN 0251-5350

Jakubiczka, S.; Vielhaber, S.; Kress, W.; Küpferling, P.; Reuner, U.; Kunath, B.; & Wieacker, P. (2004). Improvement of the diagnostic procedure in proximal myotonic myopathy/myotonic dystrophy type 2. *Neurogenetics*. Vol.5, No.1, pp. 55-59, ISSN 1364-6745

Jansen, G.; Willems, P.; Coerwinkel, M.; Nillesen, W.; Smeets, H.; Vits, L.; Howeler, C.; Brunner, H.; & Wieringa, B. (1994). Gonosomal mosaicism in myotonic dystrophy patients: involvement of mitotic events in (CTG)n repeat variation and selection against extreme expansion in sperm. *American Journal of Human Genetics* .Vol.54, No.4, pp. 575-585, ISSN 0002-9297

Jiang, H.; Mankodi, A.; Swanson, M.S.; Moxley, R.T.; & Thornton, C.A. (2004). Myotonic dystrophy type 1 is associated with nuclear foci of mutant RNA, sequestration of muscleblind proteins and deregulated alternative splicing in neurons. *Human Molecular Genetics* 2004; Vol,13, No. 24, pp.3079-3088, ISSN 0964-6906

Kakourou, G.; Dhanjal, S.; Mamas, T.; Serhal, P.; Delhanty, J.D.; & SenGupta, S.B. (2010). Modification of the triplet repeat primed polymerase chain reaction method for detection of the CTG repeat expansion in myotonic dystrophy type 1: application in preimplantation genetic diagnosis. *Fertility and Sterility*. Vol.94 , No.5, pp. 1674-1679, ISSN 0015-0282

Kanadia, R.N.; Johnstone, K.A.; Mankodi, A.; Lungu, C.; Thornton, C.A.; Esson, D.; Timmers, A.M.; Hauswirth, W.W.; & Swanson, M.S.(2003). A muscleblind knockout model for myotonic dystrophy. *Science*. Vol.302, No.5652, pp.1978-1980 ISSN 0036-8075

Kanadia, R.N.; Shin, J.; Yuan, Y.; Beattie, S.G.; Wheeler, T.M.; Thornton, C.A.; & Swanson, M.S. (2006). Reversal of RNA missplicing and myotonia after muscleblind overexpression in a mouse poly(CUG) model for myotonic dystrophy. *Proceedings of National Academy of Sciences of United States of America,* Vol.103, No.31, pp.11748-11753, ISSN 0027-8424

Kim, U.S.; Kim, J.S.; & Hwang, J.M. (2009). A Case of Myotonic Dystrophy With Pigmentary Retinal Changes. *Korean Journal of Ophthalmology* ,Vol.23, No.2, pp. 121-123, ISSN 1011-8942

Kimura, T.; Nakamori, M.; Lueck, J.D.; Pouliquin, Aoike F.; Fujimura, H.; Dirksen, R.T.; Takahashi M. P.; Dulhunty, A. F., & Sakoda, S. (2005). Altered mRNA splicing of the skeletal muscle ryanodine receptor and sarcoplasmic/endoplasmic reticulum Ca^{2+} -ATPase in myotonic dystrophy type 1. *Human Molecular Genetics* 2005, Vol.14, No. 15, pp.2189-2200, ISSN 0964-6906

Kirby, R.J.; Hamilton, G.M.; Finnegan, D.J.; Johnson, K.J.; & Jarman, A.P.(2001).Drosophila homolog of the myotonic dystrophy-associated gene, SIX5, is required for muscle and gonad development. *Current Biology.* Vol.10, No.13, pp. 1044-1049, ISSN 0960-9822

Klesert, T.R.; Otten, A.D.; Bird, T.D.; & Tapscott, S.J. (1997). Trinucleotide repeat expansion at the myotonic dystrophy locus reduces expression of DMAHP. *Nature Genetics.* Vol.16, No.4, pp. 402-406, ISSN 1061-4036

Klesert, T.R.; Cho, D.H.; Clark, J.I.; Maylie, J.; Adelman, J.; Snider, L.; Yuen, E.C.; Soriano, P.; & Tapscott S.J. (2000). Mice deficient in Six5 develop cataracts: implications for myotonic dystrophy. *Nature Genetics.* Vol.25, No.1, pp.105-109, ISSN 1061-4036

Koshelev, M.; Sarma, S.; Price, R.E.; Wehrens, X.H.; & Cooper, T.A. (2010). Heart-specific overexpression of CUGBP1 reproduces functional and molecular abnormalities of myotonic dystrophy type 1. *Human Molecular Genetics.* Vol.19, No.6, pp.1066-1075, ISSN 0964-6906

Krahe, R.; Eckhart, M.; Ogunniyi, A.O.; Osuntokun, B.O.; Siciliano, M.J.; & Ashizawa, T. (1995). De novo myotonic dystrophy mutation in a Nigerian kindred. *American Journal of Human Genetics.* Vol.56, No.5, pp.1067-1074, ISSN 0002-9297

Krndija, D.; Savić, D.; Mladenović, J.; Rakocević-Stojanović, V.; Apostolski, S.; Todorović, S.; & Romac, S. (2005). Haplotype analysis of the DM1 locus in the Serbian population. *Acta Neurologica Scandinavica.* Vol.111, No.4 , pp. 274-277, ISSN 0001-6314

krzypczak-Zielinska, M.; Sulek-Piatkowska, A.; Mierzejewski, M.; & Froster, U.G. (2009). New analysis method of myotonic dystrophy 1 based on quantitative fluorescent polymerase chain reaction. *Genetic Testing Molecular Biomarkers.* Vol.13, No.5, pp.651-655. ISSN 1945-0265

Kuyumcu-Martinez, NM; & Cooper, TA.(2006). Misregulation of alternative splicing causes pathogenesis in myotonic dystrophy. *Progress Moecularl Subcellular Biology,* Vol.44, pp. 133-159. ISSN 0079-6484

Laberge, L.; Bégin, P.; Dauvilliers, Y.; Beaudry, M.; Laforte, M.; Jean, S.; & Mathieu, J. (2009). A polysomnographic study of daytime sleepiness in myotonic dystrophy type 1. *Journal of neurology, neurosurgery, and psychiatry,* Vol.80, No.6, pp.642-646, ISSN 0022-3050

Langlois, M.A.; Lee, N.S.; Rossi, J.J.; & Puymirat, J.(2003). Hammerhead ribozyme-mediated destruction of nuclear foci in myotonic dystrophy myoblasts. *Molecular Therapy,* Vo. 7, No.5 Pt 1, pp 670-680, ISSN 1525-0016

Langlois, M.A.; Boniface, C.; Wang, G.; Alluin, J.; Salvaterra, P.M.; Puymirat, J.; Rossi, J.J.; & Lee, N.S. (2005). Cytoplasmic and nuclear retained DMPK mRNAs are targets for

RNA interference in myotonic dystrophy cells. *Journal of Biologial Chemistry* Vol.280, No.17, pp.16949-16954, ISSN 0021-9258

Lavedan, C.; Hofmann-Radvanyi, H.; Rabes, JP.; Roume, J.; & Junien, C. (1993). Different sex-dependent constraints in CTG length variation as explanation for congenital myotonic dystrophy. *Lancet.* Vol.341, No.8839, pp. 237. ISSN 0140-6736

Leifsdóttir, G.; Benedikz, J.E.; Jóhannesson, G.; Jónsson, J.J.; & Sveinbjörnsdóttir, S. (2005). Prevalence of myotonic dystrophy in Iceland. *Laeknabladid.* Vol.91, pp. 829-34, ISSN 0023-7213

Liquori, C.L.; Ricker, K.; Moseley, M.L.; Jacobsen, J.F.; Kress, W.; Naylor, S.L.; Day, J.W.; & Ranum, L.P. (2001). Myotonic dystrophy type 2 caused by a CCTG expansion in intron 1 of ZNF9. *Science*, Vol.293, No.5531, pp.864-867, ISSN 0036-8075.

Llagostera,E; Catalucci, D; Marti, L; Liesa, M; Camps, M; Ciaraldi, TP; Kondo, R; Reddy, S; Dillmann, WH; Palacin, M; Zorzano, A; Ruiz-Lozano, P; Gomis, R; & Kaliman, P. (2007).Role of myotonic dystrophy protein kinase (DMPK) in glucose homeostasis and muscle insulin action. *PLoS One,* Vol. 2, No.11, e1134. ISSN 1932-6203

Llamusi, B; & Artero, R. (2008). Molecular Effects of the CTG Repeats in Mutant Dystrophia Myotonica Protein Kinase Gene. *Current Genomics*. Vol.9, No.8, pp.509-516, ISSN 1389-2029

Louprasong, AC.; Light, DJ.; & Diller, RS. (2010). Spider dystrophy as an ocular manifestation of myotonic dystrophy. *Optometry* . Vol.81, pp. 188-193, ISSN 1529-1839

Lu, Q.L.; Rabinowitz, A.; Chen, Y.C.; Yokota, T.; Yin, H.; Alter, J.; Jadoon, A.; Bou-Gharios, G.; & Partridge, T. (2005). Systemic delivery of antisense oligoribonucleotide restores dystrophin expression in body-wide skeletal muscles. *Proceedings of National Academy of Sciences of United States of America,* Vol.102, No.1, pp.198-203, ISSN 0027-8424

Machuca-Tzili, L; Brook, D; & Hilton-Jones, D. (2005). Clinical and molecular aspects of the myotonic dystrophies: a review. *Muscle & Nerve* , Vol.32, No. 1, pp. 1-18, ISSN 0148-639X

Magaña, J.J.; Leyva-Garcia, N.; & Cisneros, B. (2009). [Pathogenesis of myotonic dystrophy type 1]. *Gaceta Medica de Mexico*, Vol.145, No.4, pp.331-337, ISSN 0016-3813

Magaña, J.J.; Cortés-Reynosa, P.; Escobar-Cedillo, R.; Gómez, R.; Leyva-García, N.; & Cisneros, B. (2011). Distribution of CTG repeats at the DMPK gene in myotonic dystrophy patients and healthy individuals from the Mexican population. *Molecular Biology Reports*. Vol.38, No.2, pp.1341-1346, ISSN 0301-4851

Magaña, J.J. & Cisneros, B. (2011). Perspectives on gene therapy in myotonic dystrophy type 1. *Journal of Neuroscience Research*, Vol.89, No.3, pp.275-285, ISSN 0360-4012

Mankodi, A.; Logigian, E.; Callahan, L.; McClain, C.; White, R.; Henderson, D.; Krym, M.; & Thornton, C.A. (2000). Myotonic dystrophy in transgenic mice expressing an expanded CUG repeat. *Science*. Vol.289, No.5485, pp.1769-1773, ISSN 0036-8075

Mankodi, A.; Urbinati, C.R.; Yuan, Q.P.; Moxley, R.T.; Sansone, V.; Krym, M.; Henderson, D.; Schalling, M.; Swanson M.S.; & Thornton, C. (2001) Muscleblind localizes to nuclear foci of aberrant RNA in myotonic dystrophy types 1 and 2. *Human Molecular Genetics,* Vol.10, No.19, pp. 2165-2170. ISSN 0964-6906

Mankodi, A.; Takahashi, M.P.; Jiang, H.; Beck, C.L.; Bowers, W.J.; Moxley, R.T. Cannon, S. C.; & Thornton C. A. (2002). Expanded CUG repeats trigger aberrant splicing of

CIC-1 chloride channel pre-mRNA and Hyperexcitability of skeletal muscle in myotonic dystrophy. *Molecular Cell*, Vol.10, No.1. pp.35-44, ISSN 1097-2765

Martorell, L.; Monckton, D.G.; Sanchez, A.; Lopez De Munain, A.; & Baiget, M. (2001). Frequency and stability of the myotonic dystrophy type 1 premutation. *Neurology*, Vol.56, No.3, pp. 328-335, ISSN 0028-3878

Martorell, L.; Gámez, J.; Cayuela, M.L.; Gould, F.K.; McAbney, J.P.; Ashizawa, T.; Monckton, D.G.; & Baiget, M. (2004). Germline mutational dynamics in myotonic dystrophy type 1 males: allele length and age effects. *Neurology*. Vol.62, No.2 pp.269-274, ISSN 0028-3878

Mastroyiannopoulos, NP; Feldman, ML; Uney, JB; Mahadevan, MS; & Phylactou, LA.(2005). Woodchuck post-transcriptional element induces nuclear export of myotonic dystrophy 3' untranslated region transcripts. *EMBO Reports*, Vol.6, No.5, pp.458-463, ISSN 1469-21X

Matsumura, T.; Iwahashi, H.; Funahashi, T.; Takahashi, M.P.; Saito, T.; Yasui, K.; Saito, T.; Iyama, A.; Toyooka, K.; Fujimura, H.; & Shinno, S. (2009). A cross-sectional study for glucose intolerance of myotonic dystrophy. *Journal of the Neurological Sciences*. Vol.276, No.1-2, pp. 60-65, INSS 0022-510X

Medica, I.; Logar, N.; Mileta, D.L.; & Peterlin, B. (2004). Genealogical study of myotonic dystrophy in Istria (Croatia). *Annales Genetique*. Vol.47, No.2, pp. 139-146, ISSN 0003-3995

Melacini, P.; Villanova, C.; Menegazzo, E.; Novelli, G.; Danieli, G.; Rizzoli, G.; Fasoli, G.; Angelini, C.; Buja, G.; Miorelli, M. et al. (1995). Correlation between cardiac involvement and CTG trinucleotide repeat length in myotonic dystrophy. *Journal of the American Collage of Cardiology*. Vol.25, No.1, pp.239- 245, ISSN 0735-1097

Michalowski, S.; Miller, J.W.; Urbinati, C.R.; Paliouras, M.; Swanson, M.S.; & Griffith, J.(1999). Visualization of double-stranded RNAs from the myotonic dystrophy protein kinase gene and interactions with CUG-binding protein. *Nucleic Acids Research*.Vol.27, No.17, pp.3534-3542, ISSN 0305-1048

Miller, J.W.; Urbinati, C.R.; Teng-Umnuay, P.; Stenberg, M.G.; Byrne, B.J.; Thornton, C.A.; & Swanson, M.S.(2000). Recruitment of human muscleblind proteins to (CUG)(n) expansions associated with myotonic dystrophy. The *EMBO Journal*.Vol. 19, No.17, pp.4439-4448, ISSN 0261-4189

Mladenovic, J.; Pekmezovic, T.; Todorovic, S.; Rakocevic-Stojanovic, V.; Savi, D. Romac, S; & Apostolski, S. (2006). Epidemiology of myotonic dystrophy type 1 (Steinert disease) in Belgrade (Serbia). *Clinical Neurology Neurosurgery*. Vol. 108, pp.757-760, ISSN 0303-8467

Monckton, D.G.; Coolbaugh, M.I.; Ashizawa, K.T.; Siciliano, M.J.; & Caskey, C.T. (1997) Hypermutable myotonic dystrophy CTG repeats in transgenic mice. *Nature Genetics*. Vol.15, No.2, pp.193-196. ISSN 1061-4036

Mulders, S.A.; Van den Broek, W.J.; Wheeler, T.M.; Croes, H.J.; Van Kuik-Romeijn, P.; De Kimpe, S.J.; Furling, D.; Platenburg, G.J.; Gourdon, G.; Thornton, C.A.; Wieringa, B.; & Wansink, D.G. (2009). Triplet-repeat oligonucleotide-mediated reversal of RNA toxicity in myotonic dystrophy. *Proceedings of National Academy of Sciences of United States of America*, Vol.106, No.33, pp.13915-13920, ISSN 0027-8424

Mulders, S.A.; Van Engelen, B.G.; Wieringa, B.; & Wansink, D.G.(2010). Molecular therapy in myotonic dystrophy: focus on RNA gain-of-function. *Human Molecular Genetics*, Vol.19, No.R1, pp.R90-97, ISSN 0964-6906

Myring, J.; Meredith, AL.; Harley, HG.; Kohn, G.; Norbury, G.; Harper, P.S.; & Shaw, D.J. (1992) Specific molecular prenatal diagnosis for the CTG mutation in myotonic dystrophy. *Journal of Medical Genetics.* Vol.29, No.11 pp. 785-788, ISSN 0022-2593

Ono, S.; Takahashi, K.; Kanda, F.; Jinnai, K.; Fukuoka, Y.; Mitake, S.; Inagaki, T.; Kurisaki, H.; Nagao, K.; & Shimizu, N. (2001). Decrease of neurons in the medullary arcuate nucleus in myotonic dystrophy.*Acta Neuropathologica.* Vol.102, No.1, pp.89-93, ISSN 0001-6322

Otten, A.D.; & Tapscott, S.J.(1995) Triplet repeat expansion in myotonic dystrophy alters the adjacent chromatin structure. *Proceedings of the National Academy of Sciences of the United States of America.*1995 Jun 6; Vol.92, No.12, pp.5465-546, ISSN 0027-8424

Pan, H.; Lin, H.M.; Ku, W.Y.; Li, T.C.; Li, S.Y.; Lin, C.C.; & Hsiao, K.M. (2001). Haplotype analysis of the myotonic dystrophy type 1 (DM1) locus in Taiwan: implications for low prevalence and founder mutations of Taiwanese myotonic dystrophy type 1. *European Journal of Human Genetics.* Vol.9, No.8, pp.638-641. ISSN 1018- 4813

Pearson, C.E; Nichol-Edamura, K.; & Cleary JD. (2005). Repeat instability: mechanisms of dynamic mutations. *Nature Review Genetics,* Vol.6, No10, pp.729-742 ISSN 1471-0056.

Philips, A.V.; Timchenko, L.T.; & Cooper, T.A.(1998). Disruption of splicing regulated by a CUG-binding protein in myotonic dystrophy. *Science.* Vol.280, No.5364, pp.737-741 ISSN 0036-8075

Ranum, LP; & Cooper, TA. (2006).RNA-Mediated Neuromuscular Disorders. *Annual Review of Neuroscience,* Vol. 29, pp. 259-277, ISSN 0147-006X

Reddy, S; Smith, DB; Rich, MM; Leferovich, JM; Reilly, P; Davis, BM; Tran, K; Rayburn, H; Bronson, R; Cros, D; Balice-Gordon, RJ; & Housman, D. (1996). Mice lacking the myotonic dystrophy protein kinase develop a late onset progressive myopathy. *Nature Genetics.* Vol.13, No.3, pp.325-335, ISSN 1061-4036

Rosa, N.; Lanza, M.; Borrelli, M.; De Bernardo, M.; Palladino, A.; Di Gregorio, M.G.; Pascotto, F.; & Politano, L. (2011). Low Intraocular Pressure Resulting from Ciliary Body Detachment in Patients with Myotonic Dystrophy. *Ophthalmology.* Vol.118, pp.260-264, ISSN 0161-6420

Rubinsztein, J.S.; Rubinsztein, D.C.; Goodburn, S.; & Holland, A.J. (1998). Apathy and hypersomnia are common features of myotonic dystrophy. *Journal of Neurology, Neurosurgery and Psychiatry.*Vol.64, No.4, pp.510-515, ISSN 0022-3050

Rubinsztein, J.S.; Rubinsztein, D.C.; McKenna, P.J.; Goodburn, S.; & Holland, A.J. (1997). Mild myotonic dystrophy is associated with memory impairment in the context of normal general intelligence. *Journal of Medical Genetics.* Vol.34, No.3 , pp.229-233, ISSN 0022-2593

Sarkar, P.S.; Appukuttan, B.; Han, J.; Ito, Y.; Ai, C.; Tsai, W.; Chai, Y.; Stout, J.T.; & Reddy, S. (2000). Heterozygous loss of Six5 in mice is sufficient to cause ocular cataracts. *Nature Genetics,* Vol. 25, No. 1, pp.110-114, ISSN 1061-4036

Savkur, R.S.; Philips, A.V.; & Cooper, T.A.(2001).Aberrant regulation of insulin receptor alternative splicing is associated with insulin resistance in myotonic dystrophy. *Nature Genetics* Vol.29, No.1, pp. 40-47, ISSN 1061-4036

Savkur, R.S.; Philips, A.V.; Cooper, T.A.; Dalton, J.C.; Moseley, M.L.; Ranum, L.P.; & Day, J.W.(2004). Insulin receptor splicing alteration in myotonic dystrophy type 2. *American Journal of Human Genetics.*Vol.74, No.6, pp.1309-1313, ISSN 0002-9297

Savouret, C.; Garcia-Cordier, C.; Megret, J.; te Riele, H.; Junien, C.; & Gourdon, G. (2004). MSH2-dependent germinal CTG repeat expansions are produced continuously in spermatogonia from DM1 transgenic mice. *Molecular Cell Biology*. Vol.24, No.2, pp. 629-637.ISSN 0270-7306

Schara, U.; & Schoser, B.G. (2006). Myotonic dystrophies type 1 and 2: a summary on current aspects. *Seminars in Pediatric Neurology*, Vol 13, No.2, pp 71-79, ISSN 1071-9091.

Sergeant, N.; Sablonniere, B.; Schraen-Maschke, S.; Ghestem, A.; Maurage, C.A.; Wattez, A.; Vermersch, P.; & Delacourte, A. (2001). Dysregulation of human brain microtubule-associated tau mRNA maturation in myotonic dystrophy type 1. *Human Molecular Genetics*. Vol.10, No.19, pp.2143-2155, ISSN 0964-6906

Seznec, H.; Lia-Baldini, A.S.; Duros, C.; Fouquet, C.; Lacroix, C.; Hofmann-Radvanyi, H.; Junien, C.; & Gourdon G.(2000). Transgenic mice carrying large human genomic sequences with expanded CTG repeat mimic closely the DM CTG repeat intergenerational and somatic instability. *Human Molecular Genetics* . Vol.9, No.8, pp.1185-1194, ISSN 0964-6906

Seznec, H.; Agbulut, O.; Sergeant, N.; Savouret, C.; Ghestem, A.; Tabti, N.; Willer, J.C.; Ourth, L.; Duros, C.; Brisson, E.; Fouquet, C.; Butler-Browne, G.; Delacourte, A.; Junien, C.; & Gourdon, G. (2002). Mice transgenic for the human myotonic dystrophy region with expanded CTG repeats display muscular and brain abnormalities. *Human Molecular Genetics*. Vol.10, No.23, pp.2717-26, ISSN 0964-6906

Sharma, P.C; Grover, A.; & Kahl, G.(2007). Mining microsatellites in eukaryotic genomes. *Trends in Biotechnology*, Vol.25, No. 11, pp. 490-498, ISSN 0167-7799.

Shimizu, M.; Fujita, R.; Tomita, N.; Shindo, H.; & Wells, R.D. (2001) Chromatin structure of yeast minichromosomes containing triplet repeat sequences associated with human hereditary neurological diseases. *Nucleic Acids Research Supplement*. No.1, pp.71-72, ISSN 0305-1048

Taneja, K.L.; McCurrach, M.; Schalling, M.; Housman, D.; & Singer, R.H. (1995). Foci of trinucleotide repeat transcripts in nuclei of myotonic dystrophy cells and tissues.*The Journal of Cell Biology*. Vol.128, No.6, pp.995-1002, ISSN 0021-9525

The International Myotonic Dystrophy Consortium (IDMC). (2000) New nomenclature and DNA testing guidelines for myotonic dystrophy type 1 (DM1). *Neurology*, Vol.54, No.6, pp.1218-1221, ISSN 0028-3878

Timchenko, N.A.; Cai, Z.J.; Welm, A.L.; Reddy, S.; Ashizawa, T.; & Timchenko, L.T.(2001).RNA CUG repeats sequester CUGBP1 and alter protein levels and activity of CUGBP1. *The Journal of Biological Chemistry*.Vol.276, No.11, pp.7820-7826, ISSN 0021-9258

Tishkoff, S.; Goldman, A.; Calafell, F.; Speed, W.C.; Deinard, A.S.; Bonne-Tamir, B.; Tishkoff, S.; Goldman, A.; Calafell, F.; Speed, W.C.; Deinard, A.S.; Bonne-Tamir, B.; Kidd, J.R,; Pakstis, A.J.; Jenkinns, T.; & Kidd, T.T. (1998). A global haplotype analysis of the myotonic dystrophy locus: implications for the evolution of modern humans and for the origin of myotonic dystrophy mutations. *American Journal of Human Genetics*, Vol.62, pp.1389-1402, ISSN 0002-9297

Tsien, J.Z.; Huerta, P.T.; & Tonegawa, S.(1996).The essential role of hippocampal CA1 NMDA receptor-dependent synaptic plasticity in spatial memory. *Cell* 1996; 87:pp.13271338, ISSN 0092-8674

Van den Broek, W.J.; Nelen, M.R.; Wansink, D.G.; Coerwinkel, M.M.; te Riele, H.; Groenen, P.J.; & Wieringa, B. (2002). Somatic expansion behaviour of the (CTG)n repeat in myotonic dystrophy knock-in mice is differentially affected by Msh3 and Msh6 mismatch-repair proteins. *Human Molecular Genetics*. Vol.11, No.2, pp .191-198, ISSN 0964-6906

Wang, G.S.; Kearney D.L.; De Biasi, M.; Taffet, G.; & Cooper, T.A. (2007). Elevation of RNA-binding protein CUGBP1 is an early event in an inducible heart-specific mouse model of myotonic dystrophy. *The Journal of Clinical Investigation*. Vol.117, No.10, pp.2802-2811, ISSN 0021-9738

Wang, G.S.; Kuyumcu-Martinez, M.N.; Sarma, S.; Mathur, N.; Wehrens, X.H.; & Cooper, T.A. (2009). PKC inhibition ameliorates the cardiac phenotype in a mouse model of myotonic dystrophy type 1. *Journal of Clinical Investigation*. Vol.119, No.12, pp.3797-3806, ISSN 0021-9738

Wang, Y.; Wang, J.; Gao, L.; Lafyatis, R.; Stamm, S.; & Andreadis, A.(2005). Tau exons 2 and 10, which are misregulated in neurodegenerative diseases, are partly regulated by silencers which bind a SRp30c.SRp55 complex that either recruits or antagonizes htra2beta1. *Journal of Biological Chemistry* 2005; 280: pp.14230-14239, ISSN 0021-9258

Wang, Y.H.; Amirhaeri, S.; Kang, S.; Wells, R.D.; & Griffith, J.D.(1994). Preferential nucleosome assembly at DNA triplet repeats from the myotonic dystrophy gene. *Science,* Vol. 265, No. 5172, pp.669-671, ISSN 0036-8075

Warf, M.B.; Nakamori, M.; Matthys, C.M.; Thornton, C.A.; & Berglund, J.A.; (2009). Pentamidine reverses the splicing defects associated with myotonic dystrophy. *Proceedings of National Academy of Sciences of United States of America,* Vol.106, No.44, pp.18551-18556, ISSN 0027-8424

Warf, M.B. & Berglund, J.A. (2010). Role of RNA structure in regulating pre-mRNA splicing. *Trends Biochemical Science*. Vol.35, No.3, pp.169-178, ISSN 0968-0004

Warner, J.P.; Barron, L.H.; Goudie, D.; Kelly, K.; Dow, D.; Fitzpatrick, D.R.; & Brock, D.J. (1996). A general method for the detection of large CAG repeat expansions by fluorescent PCR. *Journal of Medical Genetics,* Vol.33, pp.1022-1026 , ISSN 0022-2593

Wheeler, T.M.; Lueck, J.D., Swanson, M.S.; Dirksen, R.T.; & Thornton, C.A. (2007). Correction of ClC-1 splicing eliminates chloride channelopathy and myotonia in mouse models of myotonic dystrophy. *The Journal Clinical Investigation*. Vol.117, No.12, pp. 3952-3957, ISSN 0021-9738

Wheeler, T.M.; Sobczak K.; Lueck, J.D.; Osborne, R.; Lin, X.; Dirksen, R.T.; & Thornton, C.A. (2009). Reversal of RNA dominance by displacement of protein sequestered on triplet repeat RNA. Science 325(5938):336-339, ISSN 0036-8075

Winblad, S.; Lindberg, C.; & Hansen, S.(2006). Cognitive deficits and CTG repeat expansion size in classical myotonic dystrophy type 1 (DM1). *Behavioral and Brain Functions,* Vol. 2, pp.16. ISSN 1744-9081

Wojciechowska, M.; Bacolla, A.; Larson, J.E.; & Wells, R.D. (2005), The myotonic dystrophy type 1 triplet repeat sequence induces gross deletions and inversions. *Journal of Biological Chemistry*. Vol.280, No.2, pp.941-952, ISSN 0021-9258

Zerylnick, C.A.; Torroni, A.; Sherman, S.L.; & Warren, S.T.(1995). Normal variation at the myotonic dystrophy locus in global human populations. *American Journal of Human Genetics*. Vol.56, pp.123-130, ISSN 0002-9297

4

Possible Diverse Roles of Fukutin: More Than Basement Membrane Formation?

Tomoko Yamamoto[1], Atsuko Hiroi[1], Yoichiro Kato[1], Noriyuki Shibata[1], Makiko Osawa[2] and Makio Kobayashi[1]
[1]*Department of Pathology, Tokyo Women's Medical University,*
[2]*Department of Pediatrics, Tokyo Women's Medical University,*
Japan

1. Introduction

Fukutin is a gene responsible for Fukuyama-type congenital muscular dystrophy (FCMD) (Kobayashi et al. 1998). FCMD is associated with ocular and central nervous system (CNS) malformation characterized by cobblestone lissencephaly (Fukuyama et al. 1960; Osawa et al. 1997), and is included in α-dystroglycanopathy, one of the groups of muscular dystrophy. α-dystroglycan (α-DG) is one of the components of dystrophin-glycoprotein complex (DGC) linking extracellular and intracellular proteins (Fig. 1). *O*-linked glycosylation is a characteristic of α-DG, which is necessary for binding of extracellular matrix proteins to form the basement membrane. Causative genes of α-dystroglycanopathy are related to the glycosylation of α-DG, and hypoglycosylation of α-DG is involved in the pathogenesis of α-dystroglycanopathy (Martin 2005; Michele & Campbell 2003; Schessl et al. 2006).

The pathomechanism of muscular, ocular and CNS lesions of FCMD has gradually been elucidated, and the sequence of the *fukutin* gene is also known [GenBank: AB008226] (Kobayashi et al. 1998). Like other α-dystroglycanopathy diseases, reduced glycosylation of α-DG is observed at the cellular/basement membrane of the striated muscle, eye and CNS of FCMD patients (Hayashi et al. 2001; Yamamoto et al. 2010). Although fukutin is related to the glycosylation of α-DG, its actual role in the glycosylation is unknown. Moreover, post-transcriptional regulation of fukutin still remains to be elucidated. Interestingly, besides basement membrane formation, fukutin seems to have additional functions.

2. Diseases included in α-dystroglycanopathy

FCMD, muscle-eye-brain disease (MEB), Walker-Warburg syndrome (WWS), and some other types of muscular dystrophies such as MDC (congenital muscular dystrophy) 1C, MDC1D, limb girdle muscular dystrophy (LGMD) 2I and LGMD2K are in the disease category of α-dystroglycanopathy. FCMD is a congenital disease characterized by muscular dystrophy associated with CNS and ocular lesions. It is the second most common muscular dystrophy in Japan and was first described in 1960 by Fukuyama et al. (Fukuyama et al. 1960). MEB was initially reported in Finland, and ocular anomalies are especially conspicuous compared with FCMD (Pihko & Santavuori 1997). WWS is a severe disease and most of the patients die in infancy (Dobyns 1997). The CNS and eye are severely affected. The CNS lesions of FCMD, MEB and WWS are characterized by cobblestone lissencephaly, traditionally known as type II lissencephaly or polymicrogyria. Severe cases exhibit pachygyria. MDC1C (Brockington et al. 2001), MDC1D (Longman et al. 2003), LGMD2I (Brockington et al. 2001) and LGMD2K (Yis et al. 2011) are milder forms of α-dystroglycanopathy, in which CNS and eye lesions are less severe or absent. The clinical onset of LGMDs is late compared with that of congenital ones. Examples of animal models of α-dystroglycanopathy are fukutin chimeric mice (Chiyonobu et al. 2005; Masaki & Matsumura 2010), large^{myd} mice (Lee et al. 2005; Masaki & Matsumura 2010), large^{vls} mice (Lee et al. 2005; Masaki & Matsumura 2010), POMGnT1 knockout mice (Yang et al. 2007) and P0-DG null mice (Masaki & Matsumura 2010).

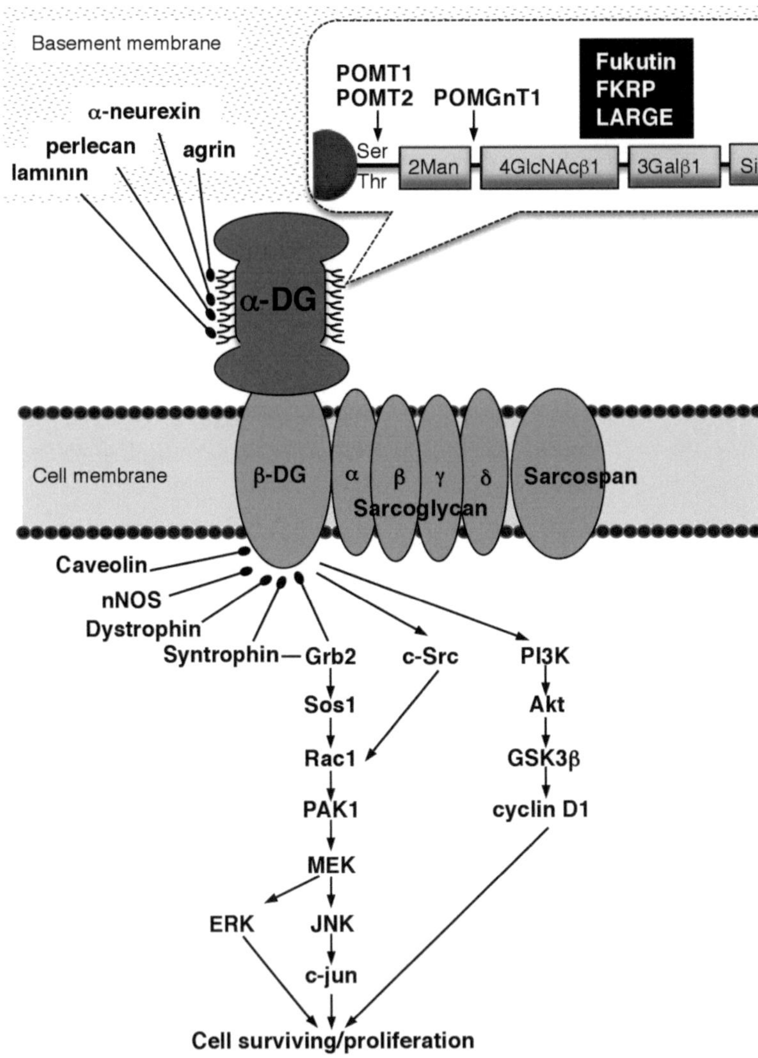

Fig. 1. A model of the dystrophin-glycoprotein complex in the skeletal muscle.

α-dystroglycanopathy shows the reduced glycosylation of α-DG at the cell/basement membrane. α-DG is a component of the DGC linking extracellular matrix and intracellular proteins (Fig. 1). It is a heavily glycosylated protein involved in the basement membrane formation by binding extracellular matrix proteins (Martin 2005; Michele & Campbell 2003; Schessl et al. 2006). Gene products involved in the glycosylation of α-DG include protein-*O*-mannosyltransferase 1 (POMT1), POMT2, *O*-linked mannose β1,2-*N*-acetylglucosaminyltransferase (POMGnT1), fukutin, fukutin-related protein (FKRP) and LARGE. α-dystroglycanopathy is caused by mutations of each gene. A wide spectrum of clinical disorders can be produced by mutations of one causative gene, especially *fukutin* and *FKRP* (Beltrán-Valero de Bernabé et al. 2003; Godfrey et al. 2007; Martin 2005; Schessl et al. 2006; Yis et al. 2011).

A common gene mutation of FCMD patients is homozygous founder mutation of *fukutin* (Kobayashi et al. 1998). However, a severe phenotype resembling WWS appears with heterozygous founder mutations and/or mutations that affect much of the coding protein (Beltrán-Valero de Bernabé et al. 2003; Cotarelo et al. 2008, Saito et al. 2000a), and milder phenotypes like LGMD have been reported (Godfrey et al. 2006; Godfrey et al. 2007; Murakami et al. 2006; Yis et al. 2011). *FKRP* mutations also produce clinical disorders over a wide spectrum covering most of the clinical phenotypes of α-dystroglycanopathy (Brockington et al. 2001; Martin 2005; Mercuri et al. 2006b; Schessl et al. 2006). *POMGnT1* is known as a gene responsible for MEB (Kano et al. 2002; Manya et al. 2003; Yoshida et al. 2001), but WWS is also associated with mutations of *POMGnT1* (Martin 2005; Schessl et al. 2006; Taniguchi et al. 2003). Major genes responsible for WWS are *POMT1* (Akasaka-Manya et al. 2004; Beltrán-Valero de Bernabé et al. 2002; Kim et al. 2004; Sabatelli et al. 2003) and *POMT2* (van Reeuwijk 2005), but milder phenotypes can occur as a result of their mutations (Balci et al. 2005; Biancheri et al. 2007; Mercuri et al. 2006a).

3. The glycosylation of α-DG for basement membrane formation, with regard to the pathogenesis of α-dystroglycanopathy

In striated muscle, glycosylated α-DG binds to several extracellular matrix proteins, such as laminin, agrin and neurexin, to form the basement membrane (Fig. 1) (Masaki & Matsumura 2010; Michele and Campbell 2003). After translation, DG is cleaved into α-and β-DG (Ibraghimov-Beskrovnaya et al. 1992; Michele and Campbell 2003). The C-terminal region of α-DG binds to the N-terminus of β-DG, a transmembrane protein. α-DG undergoes *N*-linked and *O*-linked glycosylation, and Sia-α-2,3-Gal-β-1,4-GlcNAc-β-1,2-Man-Ser/Thr in the mucin-like domain is involved in the interaction with laminin (Masaki & Matsumura 2010; Michele and Campbell 2003; Yoshida-Moriguchi et al. 2010). POMT1 together with POMT2 is required for the addition of mannose to a Ser/Thr residue (Manya et al. 2004), and POMGnT1 for the next step (Takahashi et al. 2001). These proteins possess glycosyltransferase activities (Manya et al. 2004; Takahashi et al. 2001). Although fukutin, FKRP and LARGE are related to the glycosylation of α-DG, it has not been fully elucidated how they work during the α-DG glycosylation (Martin 2005; Schessl et al. 2006). Recently, it has been clarified that phosphorylation on the *O*-linked mannose is required of α-DG for laminin binding, and this modification is mediated by LARGE (Yoshida-Moriguchi et al. 2010).

In α-dystroglycanopathy, epitopes recognized by monoclonal antibodies, IIH6 and VIA4-1 (Ervasti & Campbell 1993; Martin 2005; Michele and Campbell 2003), are reduced in the sarcolemma of the striated muscle, immunohistochemically. In western blotting, the hypoglycosylation is exhibited by a reduction of the molecular weight: a band of about 156 kDa in normal skeletal muscles shifts to a lower weight in muscles in cases of α-dystroglycanopathy. This hypoglycosylation is considered to cause a loss of α-DG function as a receptor for extracellular matrix proteins, which results in muscular dystrophy.

DGC similar to that of the skeletal muscle is observed in the peripheral and central nervous systems. In the CNS, the glia limitans is covered with the basement membrane where the glcosylated α-DG is observed. Morphological abnormalities of the basement membrane and the glia limitans have been reported in the CNS of FCMD (Fig. 2) (Nakano et al. 1996; Takada et al. 1987; Yamamoto et al. 1997; Yamamoto et al. 2010) and WWS (Beltrán-Valero de Bernabé 2002; Miller et al. 1991) patients and in mouse models of FCMD (Chiyonobu et al. 2005) and MEB (Yang et al. 2007). Fragile basement membrane caused by hypoglycosylation

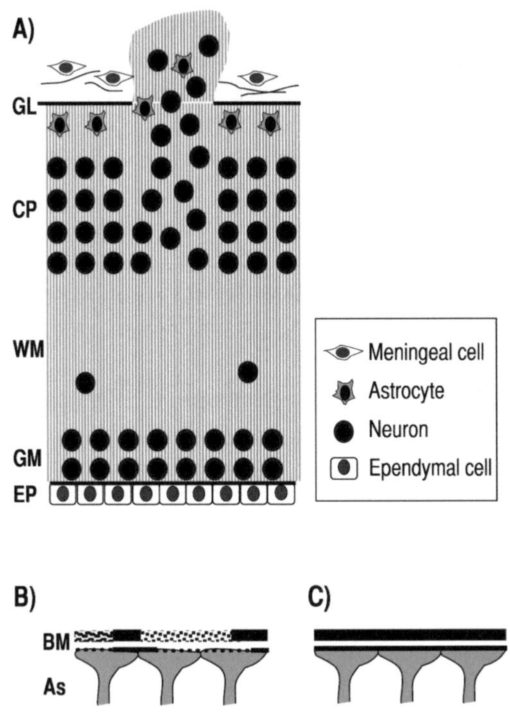

GL: glia limitans, CP: cortical plate, WM: white matter, GM: germinal matrix, EP: ependymal cells, BM: basement membrane, As: endfeet of astrocytes

Fig. 2. Schemas of the glia limitans of fetal FCMD cerebrum. A) Immature neurons and glia over-migrate into the leptomeninges through disruption of the glia limitans. B) The glia limitans is composed of astrocytic endfeet covered with the basement membrane. In the glia limitans of FCMD, both cell and basement membranes of astrocytes become ambiguous, even in the area without disruption, electron microscopically. Distribution of the abnormality is irregular. C) The cell and basement membranes are linear in controls.

of α-DG induces disruption of the glia limitans in the fetal period, which is considered to result in cobblestone lissencephaly. The glia limitans is formed by endfeet of astrocytes, and reduction of laminin binding has been observed in an astrocytoma cell line by knockdown of fukutin (data not shown). Astrocytes are considered to play an important role in the pathogenesis of the CNS lesion of α-dystroglycanopathy.

Thus, hypoglycosylation of α-DG at the basement membrane is involved in the pathogenesis of α-dystroglycanopathy. However, a wide clinical spectrum of disorders due to mutations of each causative gene might not be explained only by the abnormal basement membrane (Jiménez-Mallebrera et al. 2009).

4. Clinicopathological characteristics of FCMD

Generally, FCMD patients are found as a floppy infant, achieve peak motor function between 2 and 8 years, and die before 30 years old. They are mentally retarded, and more than 50% of patients have seizure. Abnormal eye movement and myopia are frequently seen, and cardiac symptoms may also be present (Fukuyama et al. 1960; Osawa et al. 1997). However, clinical manifestations of FCMD vary widely from mild to severe: patients of mild type can walk and talk meaningfully to some extent, while severe ones are very retarded and some cases may die *in utero*.

In the skeletal muscle, muscle fibers markedly decrease in number, which is associated with interstitial fibrosis and fatty infiltration. Myocardial fibrosis of varying degrees is observed in patients, particularly those more than 10 years old (Osawa et al. 1997). In eyes, retinal dysplasia with discontinuity of the inner limiting membrane is observed (Hino et al. 2001). In the cobblestone lissencephaly of post-natal patients, disorganization of cortical neurons, heterotopic glioneuronal tissues and surface fusions are seen, histologically (Kamoshita et al. 1976; Takada et al. 1984). Generally, the cerebral cortical lesion is extensive, but the cerebellum and brainstem are partially or mildly affected. Pachygyria and migration arrest are clear in severe cases mimicking WWS. On the other hand, a portion of the cerebral cortex shows an almost normal-looking appearance in mild cases. In fetal cases, the glia limitans formed by astrocytic endfeet in the CNS surface is disrupted, through which the glioneuronal tissues over-migrate into the leptomeninges (Fig. 2) (Nakano et al. 1996; Takada et al. 1987; Yamamoto et al. 1997; Yamamoto et al. 2010). Even in non-disrupted areas, both cell and basement membranes are abnormal, electron microscopically (Yamamoto et al. 1997; Yamamoto et al. 2010). The degree of disruption varies from case to case and even from area to area in a single patient (Takada et al. 1987; Yamamoto et al. 1997).

5. Functions of fukutin

5.1 *Fukutin* gene

Fukutin gene [GenBank, Accession AB038490] spans more than 100 kb of genomic DNA on chromosome 9q31 (Kobayashi et al. 1998; Toda et al. 1994). Fukutin mRNA composed of 10 exons is 7,349 bp with an open reading frame of 1,383 bp, beginning at base 112 (Kobayashi et al. 1998). Fukutin protein has 461 amino acids and the calculated molecular weight is 53.6 kDa, containing a hydrophobic signal sequence in the N-terminal (Kobayashi et al. 1998).

Retrotransposal 3-kb insertion of tandemly repeated sequences in the 3'-untranslated region is a common gene abnormality in FCMD patients and was determined as the ancestral founder haplotype (Kobayashi et al. 1998). Other mutations such as missense and nonsense mutations have been found (Beltrán-Valero de Bernabé 2003; Kobayashi et al. 1998). Japanese FCMD patients carry at least one copy of a founder mutation (Yoshioka 2009).

5.2 Functions of fukutin besides basement membrane formation in the nervous system

Fukutin is involved in basement membrane formation via the glycosylation of α-DG as described above. From the standpoint of CNS malformation, the most important component in the CNS is astrocytes that form the glia limitans. However, from the standpoint of total CNS function, the roles of fukutin in other components should be kept in mind during and after development (Fig. 3).

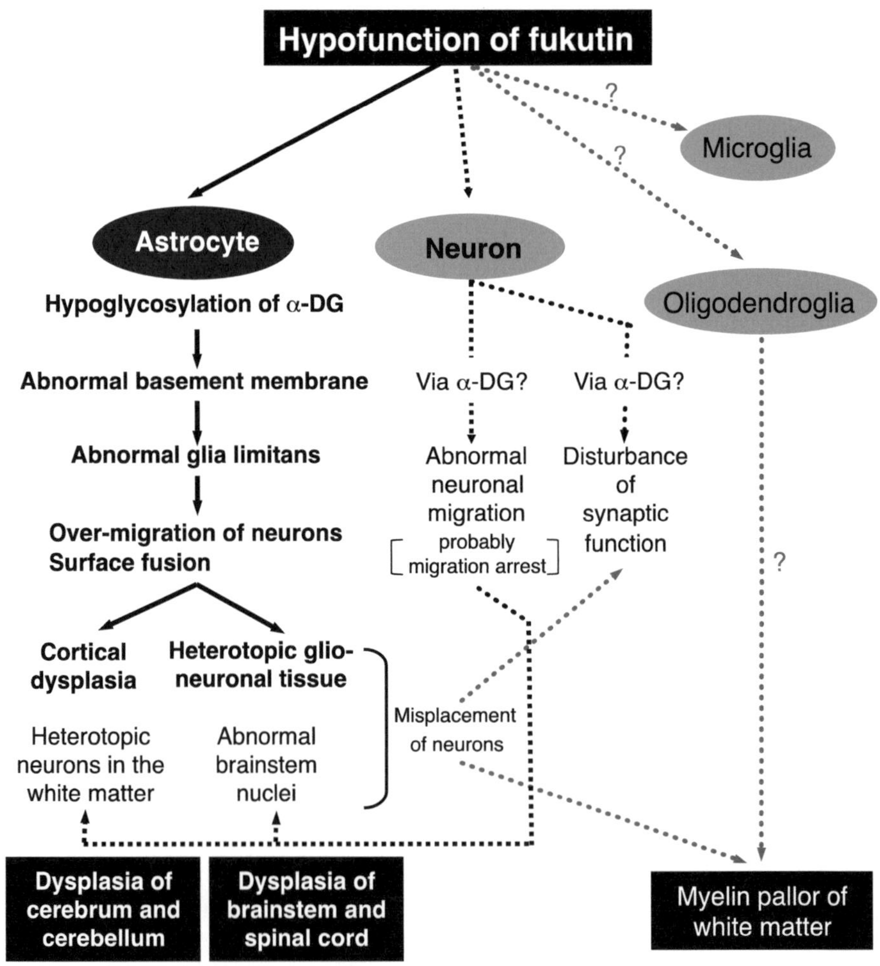

Fig. 3. Hypothesis for the CNS lesion of FCMD.

Fukutin is expressed in mature and immature neurons (Saito et al. 2000b; Sasaki et al. 2000; Yamamoto et al. 2002; Yamamoto et al. 2010). Mature neurons express α-DG detected by the antibody of VIA4-1, but not IIH6C4 (Hayashi et al. 2001; Hiroi et al. 2011; Saito et al. 2006). α-DG is considered to be involved in post-synaptic function (Moore et al. 2002; Satz et al. 2010). Since fukutin and the glycosylated α-DG are co-expressed in mature neurons, fukutin may be involved in synaptic function via the glycosylation of α-DG (Hiroi et al. 2011; Saito et al. 2006).

In the fetal cerebral and cerebellar cortex, fukutin and the glycosylated α-DG detected by VIA4-1 are co-expressed in immature neurons, especially in cells before and during migration (Hiroi et al. 2011). Fukutin may be involved in neuronal migration via the glycosylation of α-DG. However, this function appears to be minimal or immediately compensated for by other molecules because migration arrest in the FCMD brain is slight (Saito et al. 2003; Yamamoto et al. 2010), and forebrain histogenesis is preserved in mice with a neuron-specific deletion of DG (Satz et al. 2010).

The expression and function of fukutin in oligodendroglia and microglia are unclear. However, in the peripheral nerve, the DGC is found in Schwann cells, a counterpart of oligodendroglia, and is related to myelination and myelin maintenance (Masaki and Matsumura 2010). Fukutin-deficient chimeric mice exhibit a loss of myelination in the peripheral nerve (Masaki and Matsumura 2010; Saito et al. 2007), so that a function of oligodendroglia may be impaired.

Thus, fukutin is considered to have functions in neurons and glia, presumably mediated by the glycosylation of α-DG, which are not restricted to basement membrane formation. Interestingly, since neither mature nor immature neurons are positive for IIH6C4, the glycosylation of α-DG may be different between astrocytes and neurons (Hiroi et al. 2011). An experiment using mice genetically treated to lose DG in various patterns demonstrated a difference between glial and neuronal DG (Satz et al. 2010). Difference in DG glycosylation in different types of cells may be one of the reasons for the broad spectrum of CNS lesions of cobblestone lissencephaly (Satz et al. 2010).

5.3 Possible involvement of fukutin in neuroglial differentiation

The adult human cerebrum and cerebellum show less expression of fukutin than fetal ones, on immunohistochemistry and *in situ* hybridization (Saito et al. 2000b; Yamamoto et al. 2002). Fukutin expression is reduced after differentiation of cultured neuronal cells (Hiroi et al. 2011). Neuroblastoma cells extend neurites after knockdown of fukutin by RNAi (Fig. 4) (Hiroi et al. 2011). In an astrocytoma cell line, cells elongate cytoplasmic processes with increased expression of glial fibrillary acidic protein after knockdown of fukutin, and cells become epithelioid with an increase of Musashi-1 protein by transfection of fukutin (data not shown). Fukutin may be involved in neuroglial differentiation. In neurons, fukutin appears to prevent neuronal differentiation during migration. Although it is not clear whether this process is mediated by the glycosylation of α-DG, this seems very reasonable because immature neurons begin to differentiate after settlement in an appropriate site of the cortex.

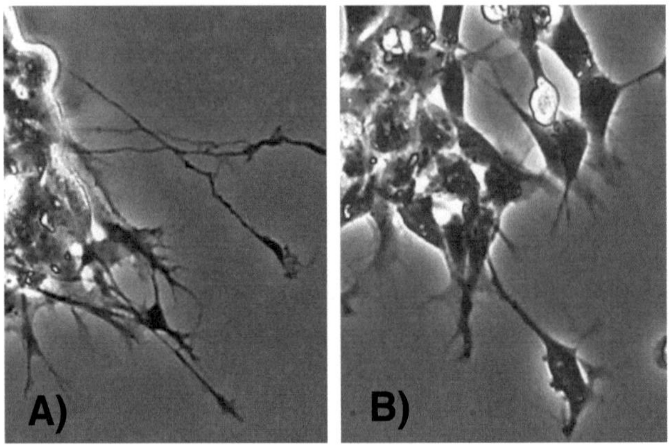

Fig. 4. RNAi in neuroblastoma cell line, IMR-32. After knockdown of fukutin, cells elongate neurites more (A) than in a control (B).

5.4 Functions of fukutin in somatic cells

Fukutin is expressed in various somatic organs (Kobayashi et al. 1998; Yamamoto et al. 2010). The DGC exists in epithelial cells, and DG plays a role in regulating cytoskeletal organization, cell polarization and cell growth in epithelial cells (Sgambato & Brancaccio 2005). Decrease of glycosylated α-DG has been reported in various cancers, and DG may act as a cancer suppressor (Sgambato & Brancaccio 2005). In a human non-tumorigenic mammary cell line, the percentage of cells in G_0/G_1 phase of the cell cycle is increased by DG overexpression (Sgambato et al. 2004). Since the DGC is linked to the cell signaling pathway (Oak et al. 2003) the glycosylation of α-DG can influence cell proliferation. At the C-terminus, β–DG binds to dystrophin and other intracellular proteins connecting to cell signaling pathways, such as growth factor receptor bound protein 2 (Grb2) involved in the MAPK/ERK cascade (Fig. 1) (Oak et al. 2003; Masaki and Matsumura 2010), with c-jun in the downstream region of the pathway (Oak et al. 2003). Tyrosine phosphorylation of the C-terminus of β-DG is dependent on c-src (Oak et al. 2003, Sotiga et al. 2001), and a signaling pathway is activated by laminin binding initiated by src family kinase (Zhou et al. 2007). The PI3K/AKT pathway is also involved (Langenbach et al. 2002).

Participating in the glycosylation of α-DG in epithelial cells as well (Yamamoto et al. 2008), fukutin may affect various epithelial cellular functions via the glycosylated α-DG. Fukutin may suppress cell proliferation/survival in epithelial cells because knockdown of fukutin in cancer cell lines made them proliferate more, at least in the short term (Yamamoto et al. 2008). There is a possibility of unknown functions of fukutin without intervention of the glycosylation of α-DG because nuclear localization of fukutin is suggested in cancer cell lines (Yamamoto et al. 2008). Involvement of fukutin in an immunological system is also supposed because fukutin is expressed in lymphoblast (Kobayashi et al. 1998).

The effects of fukutin might be different in different kinds of cells since cellular proliferation showed no change or rather a reduction after knockdown of fukutin in astrocytoma cells (data not shown). More experiments are required to clarify this point because there might have been some technical problems and alternative splicing has been reported in fukutin (Kobayashi et al. 2001).

5.5 Characteristics of fukutin mRNA with regard to neuroglial functions

In the CNS, synaptic plasticity is an important mechanism to adapt neurons to varying circumstances. Quick responses are needed at dendrites. Plasticity may also be required in astrocytes. Astrocytic endfeet are components of the blood-brain barrier (BBB), which maintains the CNS function by regulating transportation of water and various molecules. In the BBB, the basement membrane, positive for antibodies against glycosylated α-DG, VIA4-1 and IIH6C4, is formed between capillary and astrocytic endfeet. Moreover, the glycosylated α-DG is a receptor for some microorganisms (Cao et al. 1998; Kunz et al. 2005; Masaki and Matsumura 2010; Rambukkana et al. 1998). The glycosylation of α-DG should be prompt to adapt to varying circumstances at the most peripheral part of a cell.

There is a special type of mRNA called localized mRNA that is related to the maintenance of cell polarity, asymmetrical segregation and synaptic plasticity (López de Heredia and Jansen 2004; Ule and Darnell 2006). Localized mRNA has a binding site of an RNA-binding protein in the 3'-UTR region. A complex composed of mRNA and proteins is transported to peripheral areas of a cell such as dendrites, using a molecular motor like dynein and kinesin (López de Heredia and Jansen 2004). After reaching an appropriate site, the mRNA starts to be translated. mRNA of Arc, the immediate early gene product related to synaptic plasticity, is one of the localized mRNAs. A complex consisting of Arc mRNA and several proteins is transported along the microtubules and the mRNA undergoes local translation at a site of synaptic activity (Bramham et al. 2010). Kinesin is a motor of this complex. The transcription of Arc is regulated by cyclic AMP response element binding protein (CREB) (Bramham et al. 2010). A CRE-like sequence has been found in the fukutin gene promoter, and the transcription of fukutin may be regulated by CREB (Fang et al. 2005). Taking account of the possible functions of fukutin at the synapse and the BBB, it seems reasonable that fukutin mRNA is a localized mRNA. In the experiment using an astrocytoma cell line, Musashi-1 protein, one of the RNA-binding proteins, may bind to the 3'-UTR region of fukutin mRNA, suggesting that fukutin is a localized mRNA (data not shown).

6. Therapeutic strategies

From a therapeutic standpoint, many new strategies are underway for muscular dystrophy, particularly Duchenne muscular dystrophy (Collins & Bönnemann 2010; Cossu & Sampaolesi 2007; Muntoni et al. 2007; Odom et al. 2007). For α-dystroglycanopathy, full restoration of α-DG glycosylation might not be required (Kanagawa et al. 2009). Gene delivery using adeno-associated virus vectors may be applicable because causative genes of α-dystroglycanopathy are small enough to be packaged into this vector (Collins & Bönnemann 2010; Odom et al. 2007). Gene therapy using *LARGE* may be one of the candidates because gene transfer of *LARGE* restores α-DG receptor function not only in Large^{myd} mice but also in cultured cells from FCMD, MEB and WWS patients (Barresi et al. 2009). Transgenic overexpression of T-cell GalNAc transferase (*GALgt2*) in the skeletal muscle increases glycosylation of α-DG (Collins & Bönnemann 2010; Yoon et al. 2009). Transfer of *fukutin* restores glycosylation of α-DG in knock-in mice carrying the retrotransposal insertion in the mouse *fukutin* ortholog (Kanagawa et al. 2009).

However, there is a big underlying problem in patients with CNS malformation. Strategies might have to be different between muscle and CNS. The complicated structure of the CNS composed of several components should be noted. On FCMD, fukutin is expressed at least in astrocytes and neurons in the CNS. If the functions of fukutin in these cells are compensated for by other molecules after development, a therapy during the critical period *in utero* might be sufficient. In contrast, if fukutin continues to play important roles after development, lifelong therapy should be applied. In terms of future advances and applications of gene therapy for FCMD, it may be necessary to determine its precise roles to achieve an effective method while avoiding unprecedented side effects as much as possible. Since fukutin has several isoforms derived from alternative splicing (Kobayashi et al. 2001), investigations of each isoform may also be required.

7. Conclusion

Fukutin is related to the glycosylation of α-DG, which is involved in the pathogenesis of muscular dystrophy and ocular and CNS malformation of FCMD. Besides the basement membrane formation, fukutin has more diverse roles in other cells, including synaptic function and neuronal migration. Determination of the precise roles of fukutin seems to be important for further understanding of the disease and for future gene therapy.

8. Acknowledgement

The authors wish to thank Mr. Mizuho Karita, Mr. Hideyuki Takeiri, Mr. Fumiaki Muramatsu, Mrs. Noriko Sakayori and Mr. Shuichi Iwasaki for their excellent technical assistance and help in the preparation of this paper.

9. References

Akasaka-Manya, K.; Manya, H.; Endo T. (2004). Mutations of the *POMT1* gene found in patients with Walker-Warburg syndrome lead to a defect of protein O-mannosylation. *Biochem Biophys. Res. Commun*. 325, 75-79

Balci, B.; Uyanik, G.; Dincer, P.; Gross, C.; Willer, T.; Talim, B.; Haliloglu G.; Kale G.; Hehr U.; Winkler J.; Topaloglu H. (2005). An autosomal recessive limb girdle muscular dystrophy (LGMD2) with mild mental retardation is allelic to Walker-Warburg syndrome (WWS) caused by a mutation of the *POMT1* gene. *Neuromusc. Disord.* 15, 271-275

Barresi, R.; Michele, D.E.; Kanagawa, M.; Harper, H.A.; Dovico, S.A.; Satz, J.S.; Moore, S.A.; Zhang, W.; Schachter, H.; Dumanski, J.P.; Cohn, R.D.; Nishino I.; Campbell, K.P. (2004). LARGE can functionally bypass *a*-dystroglycan defects in distinct congenital muscular dystrophies. *Nat. Med.* 10, 696-703

Beltrán-Valero de Bernabé, D.; Currier, S.; Steinbrecher, A.; Celli, J.; van Beusekom, E.; van der Zwaag, B.; Kayserili, H.; Merlini, L.; Chitayat, D.; Dobyns, W.B.; Cormand, B.; Lehesjoki, A.-E.; Cruces, J.; Voit, T.; Walsh, C.A.; van Bokhoven, H.; Brunner, H.G. (2002). Mutations in the *O*-mannosyltransferase gene *POMT1* give rise to the severe neuronal migration disorder Walker-Warburg syndrome. *Am. J. Hum. Genet.* 71, 1033-1043

Beltrán-Valero de Bernabé, D., van Bokhoven H., van Beusekom E., van den Akker, W.; Kant, S.; Dobyns, W.B.; Cormand, B.; Currier, S.; Hamel, B.; Talim, B.; Topaloglu,

H.; Brunner, H.G. (2003). A homozygous nonsense mutation in the *fukutin* gene causes a Walker-Warburg syndrome phenotype. *J. Med. Genet.* 40, 845-848

Biancheri, R.; Falace, A.; Tessa, A.; Pedemonte, M.; Scapolan, S.; Cassandrini, D.; Aiello, C.; Rossi, A.; Broda, P.; Zara, F.; Santorelli, F.M.; Minetti, C.; Bruno, C. (2007). *POMT2* gene mutation in limb-girdle muscular dystrophy with inflammatory changes. *Biochem. Biophys. Res. Commun.* 363, 1033-1037

Bramham, C.R.; Alme, M.N.; Bittins, M.; Kuipers, S.D.; Nair, R.R.; Pai, B.; Panja, D.; Schubert, M.; Soule, J.; Tiron, A.; Wibrand, K. (2010). The Arc of synaptic memory. *Exp. Brain. Res.* 200, 125-140

Brockington, M.; Yuva, Y.; Prandini, P.; Brown, S.C.; Torelli, S.; Benson, M.A.; Herrmann, R.; Anderson, L.V.B.; Bashir, R.; Burgunder, J.-M.; Fallet, S.; Romero, N.; Fardeau, M.; Straub, V.; Storey, G.; Pillitt, C.; Richard, I.; Sewry, C.A.; Bushby, K.; Voit, T.; Blake, D.J.; Muntoni, F. (2001). Mutations in the fukutin-related protein gene (*FKRP*) identify limb girdle muscular dystrophy 2I as a milder allelic variant of congenital muscular dystrophy MDC1C. *Hum. Mol. Genet.* 10, 2851-2859

Cao, W.; Henry, M.D.; Borrow, P.; Yamada, H.; Elder, J.H.; Ravkov, E.V.; Nichol, S.T.; Compans, R.W.; Campbell, K.P.; Oldstone, M.B. (1998). Identification of alpha-dystroglycan as a receptor for lymphocytic choriomeningitis virus and Lassa fever virus. *Science* 282, 2079-2081

Chiyonobu, T.; Sasaki, J.; Nagai, Y.; Takeda, S.; Funakoshi, H.; Nakamura, T.; Sugimoto, T.; Toda, T. (2005). Effects of fukutin deficiency in the developing brain. *Neuromusc. Disord.* 15, 416-426

Collins, J.; Bönnemann, C.G. (2010). Congenital muscular dystrophies: toward molecular therapeutic interventions. *Curr. Neurol. Neurosci. Rep.* 10, 83-91

Cossu, G.; Sampaolesi, M. (2007). New therapies for Duchenne muscular dystrophy: challenges, prospects and clinical trials. *Trends Mol. Med.* 13, 520-526

Cotarelo, R.P.; Valero, M.C.; Prados, B.; Peña, A.; Rodríguez, L.; Fano, O.; Marco, J.J.; Martínez-Frías, M.L.; Cruces, J. (2008). Two new patients bearing mutations in the *fukutin* gene confirm the relevance of this gene in Walker-Warburg syndrome. *Clin. Genet.* 73, 139-145

Dobyns, W.B. (1997). Walker-Warburg and other cobblestone lissencephaly syndromes: 1995 update. In: *Congenital Muscular Dystrophies,* Fukuyama Y., Osawa M., Saito K. (eds), pp89-98, Elsevier, Amsterdam

Ervasti, J.M.; Campbell, K.P. (1993). A role for the dystrophin-glycoprotein complex as a transmembrane linkder between laminin and actin. *J. Cell Biol.* 122, 809-823

Fang, H.; Sodja, C.; Chartier, J.; Desbois, A.; Lei, J.; Walker, P.R.; Sikorska, M. (2005). Identification of a functional CRE in the promoter of Fukuyama congenital muscular dystrophy gene *fukutin*. *Mol. Brain Res.* 136, 1-11

Fukuyama, Y.; Kawazura, M.; Haruna, H. (1960). A peculiar form of congenital progressive muscular dystrophy. *Paediatr. Univ. Tokyo* 4, 5-8

Godfrey, C.; Escolar, D.; Brockington, M.; Clement, E.M.; Mein, R.; Jimenez-Mallebrera, C.; Torelli, S.; Feng, L.; Brown, S.C.; Swery, C.A.; Rutherford, M.; Shapira, Y.; Abbs, S.; Muntoni, F. (2006). *Fukutin* gene mutations in steroid-responsive limb girdle muscular dystrophy. *Ann. Neurol.* 60, 603-610

Godfrey, C.; Clement, E.; Mein, R.; Brockington, M.; Smith, J.; Talim, B.; Straub, V.; Robb, S.; Quinlivan, R.; Feng, L.; Jimenez-Mallebrera, C.; Mercuri, E.; Manzur, A.Y.; Kinali,

M.; Torelli, S.; Brown, S.C.; Swery, C.A.; Bushby, K.; Topaloglu, H.; North, K.; Abbs, S.; Muntoni, F. (2007). Refining genotypa-phenotype correlations in muscular dystrophies with defective glycosylation of dystroglycan. *Brain* 130, 2725-2735

Hayashi, Y.K.; Ogawa, M.; Tagawa, K.; Noguchi, S.; Ishihara, T.; Nonaka, I.; Arahata, K. (2001). Selective deficiency of α-dystroglycan in Fukuyama-type congenital muscular dystrophy. *Neurology* 57, 115-121

Hino, N.; Kobayashi, M.; Shibata, N.; Yamamoto, T.; Saito, K.; Osawa, M. (2001). Clinicopathological study on eyes from cases of Fukuyama type congenital muscular dystrophy. *Brain Dev.* 23 , 97-107

Hiroi, A.; Yamamoto, T.; Shibata, N.; Osawa, M.; Kobayashi, M. (2011). Roles of fukutin, the gene responsible for Fukuyama-type congenital muscular dystrophy, in neurons: possible involvement in synaptic function and neuronal migration. *Acta Histochem. Cytochem.* 44, 91-101

Ibraghimov-Beskrovnaya, O.; Ervasti, J.M.; Leveille, C.J; Slaughter, C.A.; Sernett, S.W.; Campbell, K.P. (1992). Primary structure of dystrophin-associated glycoproteins linking dystrophin to the extracellular matrix. *Nature* 355, 696-702

Jiménez-Mallebrera, C.; Torelli, S.; Feng, L.; Kim, J.; Godfrey, C.; Clement, E.; Mein, R.; Abbs, S.; Brown, S.C.; Campbell, K.P.; Kröger, S.; Talim, B.; Topaloglu, H.; Quinlivan, R.; Roper, H.; Childs, A.M.; Kinali, M.; Sewry, C.A.; Muntoni, F. (2009). A comparative study of α-dystroglycan glycosylation in dystroglycanopathies suggest that the hypoglycosylation of α-dystroglycan dose not consistently correlate with clinical severity. *Brain Pathol.* 19, 596-611

Kamoshita, S.; Konishi, Y.; Segawa, M.; Fukuyama Y. (1976). Congenital muscular dystrophy as a disease of the central nervous system. *Arch. Neurol.* 33, 513-516.

Kanagawa M.; Nishimoto A.; Chiyonobu T.; Takeda S.; Miyagoe-Suzuki Y.; Wang F.; Fujikake N; Taniguchi M.; Lu Z,; Tachikawa M.; Nagai Y.; Tashiro F.; Miyazaki J.; Tajima Y.; Takeda S.; Endo T.; Kobayashi K.; Campbell KP.; Toda T. (2009). Residual laminin-binding activity and enhanced dystroglycan glycosylation by LARGE in novel model mice to dystroglycanopathy. *Hum. Mol. Genet.* 18, 621-631

Kano, H.; Kobayashi, K.; Herrmann, R.; Tachikawa, M.; Manya, H.; Nishino, I.; Nonaka, I.; Straub, V.; Talim, B.; Voit, T.; Topaloglu, H.; Endo, T.; Yoshikawa, H.; Toda, T. (2002). Deficiency of α-dystroglycan in Muscle-Eye-Brain disease. *Biochem. Biophys. Res. Commun.* 291, 1283-1286

Kim, D.-S.; Hayashi, Y.K.; Matsumoto, H.; Ogawa, M.; Noguchi, S.; Murakami, N.; Sakuta, R.; Mochizuki, M., Michele, D.E.; Campbell, K.P.; Nonaka, I.; Nishino, I. (2004). *POMT1* mutation results in defective glycosylation and loss of laminin-binding activity in α-DG. *Neurology* 62, 1009-1011

Kobayashi, K.; Nakahori, Y.; Miyake, M.; Matsumura, K.; Kondo-Iida, E.; Nomura, Y.; Segawa, M.; Yoshioka, M.; Saito, K.; Osawa, M.; Hamano, K.; Sakakihara, Y.; Nonaka, I.; Nakagome, Y.; Kanazawa, I.; Nakamura, Y.; Tokunaga, K.; Toda, T. (1998). An ancient retrotransposal insertion causes Fukuyama-type congenital muscular dystrophy. *Nature* 394, 388-392

Kobayashi, K.; Sasaki, J.; Kondo-Iida, E.; Fukuda, Y.; Konoshita, M.; Sunada, Y.; Nakamura, Y.; Toda, T. (2001). Structural organization, complete genomic sequences and mutational analyses of the Fukuyama-type congenital muscular dystrophy gene, *fukutin*. *FEBS Lett* 489, 192-196

Kunz, S.; Rojek, J.M.; Kanagawa, M.; Spiropoulou, C.F.; Barresi, R.; Campbell, K.P.; Oldstone, M.B.A. (2005). Posttranslational modification of α-dystroglycan, the cellular receptor for arenaviruses, by the glycosyltransferase LARGE is critical for virus binding. *J. Virol.* 79, 14282-14296

Langenbach, K.J.; Rando, T.A. (2002). Inhibition of dystroglycan binding to laminin disrupts the PI3K/Akt pathway and survival signaling in muscle cells. *Muscle Nerve.* 26, 644-653

Lee, Y.; Kameya, S.; Cox ,G.A.; Hsu, J.; Hicks, W.; Maddatu, T.P.; Smith, R.S.; Naggert, J.K.; Peachey, N S.; Nishina, P.M. (2005). Ocular abnormalities in *Large*^{myd} and *Large*^{vls} mice, spontaneous models for muscle, eye and brain diseases. *Mol. Cell Neurosci.* 30, 160-172

Longman C.; Brockington, M.; Torelli, S.; Jimenez-Mallebrera, C.; Kennedy, C.; Khalil, N.; Feng, L.; Saran, R.K.; Voit, T.; Merlini, L.; Sewry, C.A., Brown, S.C., Muntoni, F. (2003). Mutations in the human LARGE gene cause MDC1D, a novel form of congenital muscular dystrophy with severe mental retardation and abnormal glycosylation of α-dystroglycan. *Hum Mol. Genet.* 12, 2853-2861

López de Heredia, M.; Jansen R.-P. (2004). mRNA localization and the cytoskeleton. *Curr. Opin. Cell Biol.* 16, 80-85

Manya, H.; Sakai, K.; Kobayashi, K.; Taniguchi, K.; Kawakita, M.; Toda, T.; Endo, T. (2003). Loss-of-function of an *N*-acetylglucosaminyltransferase, POMGnT1, in muscle-eye-brain disease. *Biochem. Biophys. Res. Commun.* 306, 93-97

Manya, H.; Chiba, A.; Yoshida, A.; Wang, X.; Chiba, Y.; Jigami, Y.; Margolis, R.U.; Endo T. (2004). Demonstration of mammalian protein *O*-mannosyltransferase activity: Coexpression of POMT1 and POMT2 required for enzymatic activity. *Proc. Natl. Acad. Sci. USA* 101, 500-505

Martin, P.T. (2005). The dystroglycanopathies: The new disorders of O-linked glycosylation. *Semin Pediatr. Neurol.* 12, 152-158

Masaki T.; Matsumura K. (2010). Biological role of dystroglycan in schwann cell function and its implication in peripheral nervous system diseases. *J Biomed Biotech* doi:10.1155/2010/740403

Mercuri, E.; D'Amico, A.; Tessa, A.; Berardineli, A.; Pane, M.; Messina, S.; van Reeuwijk, J.; Bertini, E.; Muntoni, F.; Santorelli, F.M. (2006). POMT2 mutation in a patient with 'MEB-like' phenotype. *Neuromusc. Disord.* 16, 446-448a

Mercuri, E.; Topaloglu, H.; Brockington, M.; Berardenelli, A.; Pichiecchio, A.; Santorelli, F.; Rutherford, M.; Talim, B.; Ricci, E.; Voit, T.; Muntoni, F. (2006). Spectrum of brain changes in patients with congenital muscular dystrophy and *FKRP* gene mutations. *Arch. Neurol.* 63, 251-257b

Michele, D.E.; Campbell, K.P. (2003). Dystrophin-glycoprotein complex: post-transcriptional processing and dystroglycan function. *J. Biol. Chem.* 278, 15457-15460

Miller, G.; Ladda, R.L.; Towfighi, J. (1991). Cerebro-ocular dysplasia-Muscular dystrophy (Walker Warburg) syndrome. Findings in 20-week-old fetus. *Acta Neuropathol.* 82, 234-238

Moore, S.A.; Saito, F.; Chen, J.; Michele, D.E.; Henry, M.D.; Messing, A.; Cohn, R.D.; Ross-Barta, S.E.; Westra, S.; Williamson, R.A.; Hoshi, T.; Campbell, K.P. (2002). Deletion of brain dystroglycan recapitulates aspects of congenital muscular dystrophy. *Nature* 418, 422-425

Muntoni, F.; Wells, D. (2007). Genetic treatments in muscular dystrophies. *Curr. Opin. Neurol.* 20, 590-594

Murakami, T.; Hayashi, Y.K.; Noguchi, S.; Ogawa, M.; Nonaka, I.; Tanabe, Y.; Ogino, M.; Takada, F.; Eriguchi, M.; Kotooka, N.; Campbell, K.P.; Osawa, M.; Nishino, I. (2006). Fukutin gene mutations cause dilated cardiomyopathy with minimal muscle weakness. *Ann. Neurol.* 60, 597-602

Nakano, I.; Funahashi, M.; Takada, K.; Toda, T. (1996). Are breaches in the glia limitans the primary cause of the micropolygyria in Fukuyama-type congenital muscular dystrophy (FCMD)? Pathological study of the cerebral cortex of an FCMD fetus. *Acta Neuropathol.* 91, 313-321

Oak, S.A.; Zhou, Y.W.; Jarrett, H.W. (2003). Skeletal muscle signaling pathway through the dystrophin glycoprotein complex and Rac1. *J. Biol. Chem.* 278, 39287-39295

Odom, G.L.; Gregorevic, P.; Chamberlain, J.S. (2007). Viral-mediated gene-therapy for the muscular dystrophies: successes, limitations and recent advances. *Biochim. Biophys. Acta* 1772, 243-262

Osawa M.; Sumida S.; Suzuki N.; Arai Y., Ikenaka H., Murasugi H., Shishikura K., Suzuki H., Saito K., Fukuyama Y. (1997). Fukuyama type congenital muscular dystrophy, In: *Congenital Muscular Dystrophies*, Fukuyama Y., Osawa M., Saito K. (Eds.), pp. 31-68, Elsevier, Amsterdam

Pihko, H.; Santavuori, P. (1997). Muscle-eye-brain (MEB) disese – a review. In: *Congenital Muscular Dystrophies*, Fukuyama Y., Osawa M., Saito K. (eds), pp99-104, Elsevier, Amsterdam

Rambukkana, A.; Yamada, H.; Zanazzi, G.; Mathus, T.; Salzer, J.L.; Yurchenco, P.D.; Campbell, K.P.; Fischetti, V.A. (1998). Role of α-dystroglycan as a Schwann cell receptor for *Mycobacterium leprae*. *Science* 282, 2076-2079

Sabatelli, P.; Columbaro, M.; Mura, I.; Capanni, C.; Lattanzi, G.; Maraldi, N.M.; Baltrán-Valero de Bernabé, D.; van Bokoven, H.; Squarzoni, S.; Merlini, L. (2003). Extracellular matrix and nuclear abnormalities in skeletal muscle of a patient with Walker-Warburg syndrome caused by *POMT1* mutation. *Biochim. Biophys. Acta* 1638, 57-62

Saito, F.; Masaki, T.; Saito, Y.; Nakamura, A.; Takeda, S.; Shimizu, T.; Toda, T.; Matsumura, K. (2007). Defective peripheral nerve myelination and neuromuscular junction formation in fukutin-deficient chimeric mice. *J. Neurochem.* 101, 1712-1722

Saito, K.; Osawa, M.; Wang, Z.-P.; Ikeya, K.; Fukuyama, Y.; Kondo-Iida, E.; Toda, T.; Ohashi, H.; Kurosawa, K.; Wakai, S.; Kaneko, K. (2000). Haplotype-phenotype correlation in Fukuyama congenital muscular dystrophy. *Am. J. Med. Genet.* 92, 184-190a

Saito, Y.; Mizuguchi, M.; Oka, A.; Takashima, S. (2000). Fukutin protein is expressed in neurons of the normal developing human brain but is reduced in Fukuyama-type congenital muscular dystrophy brain. *Ann. Neurol.* 47, 756-764b

Saito, Y.; Kobayashi, M.; Itoh, M.; Saito, K.; Mizuguchi, M., Sasaki, H., Arima K., Yamamoto T., Takashima S., Sasaki M., Hayashi K., Osawa M. (2003). Aberrant neuronal migration in the brainstem of Fukuyama-type congenital muscular dystrophy. *J. Neuropathol. Exp. Neurol.* 62, 497-508

Saito, Y.; Yamamoto, T.; Mizuguchi, M.; Kobayashi, M.; Saito, K.; Ohno, K.; Osawa, M. (2006). Altered glycosylation of α-dystroglycan in neurons of Fukuyama congenital muscular dystrophy brains. *Brain Res.* 1075, 223-228

Sasaki, J.; Ishikawa, K.; Kobayashi, K.; Kondo-Iida, E.; Fukayama, M.; Mizusawa, H.; Takashima, S.; Sakakihara, Y.; Nakamura, Y.; Toda, T. (2000). Neuronal expression of the fukutin gene. *Hum. Mol. Genet.* 9, 3083-3090

Satz, J.S.; Ostendorf, A.P.; Hou, S.; Turner, A.; Kusano, H.; Lee, J.C.; Turk, R.; Nguyen, H.; Ross-Barta, S.E.; Westra, S.; Hoshi, T.; Moore, S.A.; Campbell, K.P. (2010). Distinct functions of glial and neuronal dystroglycan in the developing and adult mouse brain. *J Neurosci* 30, 14560-14572

Schessl, J.; Zou, Y.; Bönnemann, C.G. (2006). Congenital muscular dystrophies and the extracellular matrix. *Semin. Pediatr. Neurol.* 13, 80-89

Sgambato, A.; Camerini, A.; Faraglia, B.; Pavoni, E.; Montanari, M.; Spada, D.; Losasso, C.; Brancaccio, A.; Cittadini, A. (2004). Increased expression of dystroglycan inhibits the growth and tumorigenicity of human mammary epithelial cells. *Cancer Biol. Ther.* 3, 967-975

Sgambato, A.; Brancaccio, A. (2005). The dystroglycan complex: From biology to cancer. *J. Cell Physiol.* 205, 163-169

Sotgia, F.; Lee, H.; Bedford, M.T.; Petrucci, T.; Sudol, M.; Lisanti, M.P. (2001). Tyrosine phosphorylation of β-dystroglycan at its WW domain binding motif, PPxY, recruits SH2 domain containing proteins. *Biochemistry* 40, 14585-14592

Takada, K.; Nakamura, H.; Tanaka J. (1984). Cortical dysplasia in congenital muscular dystrophy with central nervous system involvement (Fukuyama type). *J. Neuropathol. Exp. Neurol.* 43, 395-407

Takada, K.; Nakamura, H.; Suzumori, K.; Ishikawa, T.; Sugiyama, N. (1987). Cortical dysplasia in a 23-week fetus with Fukuyama congenial muscular dystrophy (FCMD). *Acta Neuropathol.* 74, 300-306

Takahashi, S.; Sasaki, T.; Manya, H.; Chiba, Y.; Yoshida, A.; Mizuno, M.; Ishida, H.; Ito, F.; Inazu, T.; Kotani, N.; Takasaki, S.; Takeuchi, M.; Endo, T. (2001). A new β1,2-*N*-acetylglucosaminyltransferase that may play a role in the biosynthesis of mammalian *O*-mannosyl glycans. *Glycobiology* 11, 37-45

Taniguchi, K.; Kobayashi, K.; Saito, K.; Yamanouchi, H.; Ohnuma, A.; Hayashi, Y.K.; Manya, H.; Jin D.K.; Lee, M.; Parano, E.; Falsaperla, R.; Pavone, P.; Coster, R.V.; Talim, B.; Steinbrecher, A.; Straub, V.; Nishino, I.; Topaloglu, H.; Voit, T.; Endo, T.; Toda, T. (2003). Worldwide distribution and broder clinical spectrum of muscle-eye-brain disease. *Hum. Mol. Genet.* 12, 527-534

Toda, T.; Ikegawa, S.; Okui, K.; Kondo, E.; Saito, K.; Fukuyama, Y.; Yoshioka, M.; Kumagai, T.; Suzumori, K.; Kanazawa, I.; Nakamura, Y. (1994). Refined mapping of a gene responsible for Fukuyama-type congenital muscular dystrophy: Evidence for strong linkage disequilibrium. *Am. J. Hum. Genet.* 55, 946-950

Ule, J.; Darnell, R.B. (2006). RNA binding proteins and the regulation of neuronal synaptic plasticity. *Curr. Opin. Neurobiol.* 16, 102-110

van Reeuwijk, J.; Janssen, M.; van den Elzen, C.; Beltrán-Valero de Bernabé, D.; Sabatelli, P.; Merlini, L.; Boon, M.; Scheffer, H.; Brockington, M.; Muntoni, F.; Huynen, M.A.; Verrips, A.; Walsh, C.A.; Barth, P.G.; Brunner, H.G.; van Bokhoven, H. (2005). *POMT2* mutations cause α-dystroglycan hypoglycosylation and Walker-Warburg syndrome. *J. Med. Genet.* 42, 907-912

Yamamoto, T.; Toyoda, C.; Kobayashi, M.; Kondo, E.; Saito, K.; Osawa, M. (1997). Pial-glial barrier abnormalities in fetuses with Fukuyama congenital muscular dystrophy. *Brain Dev.* 19, 35-42

Yamamoto, T.; Kato, Y.; Karita, M.; Takeiri, H.; Muramatsu, F.; Kobayashi, M.; Saito, K.; Osawa, M. (2002). Fukutin expression in glial cells and neurons: implication in the brain lesions of Fukuyama congenital muscular dystrophy. *Acta Neuropathol.* 104, 217-224

Yamamoto, T.; Kato, Y.; Shibata, N.; Sawada, T.; Osawa, M.; Kobayashi, M. (2008). A role of fukutin, a gene responsible for Fukuyama type congenital muscular dystrophy, in cancer cells: a possible role to suppress cell proliferation. *Int J Exp Pathol* 89, 332-341

Yamamoto, T.; Shibata, N.; Saito, Y.; Osawa, M.; Kobayashi M. (2010). Functions of fukutin, a gene responsible for Fukuyama type congenital muscular dystrophy, in neuromuscular and other somatic organs. *Cent. Nerv. Syst .Agents Med. Chem.* 10, 169-179

Yang, Y.; Zhang, P.; Xiong, Y.; Li, X.; Qi, Y.; Hu H. (2007). Ectopia of meningeal fibroblasts and reactive gliosis in the cerebral cortex of the mouse model of muscle-eye-brain disease. *J Comp Neurol* 505, 459-477

Yis, U.; Uyanik, G.; Heck, P.B.; Smitka, M.; Nobel, H.; Ebinger, F.; Dirik, E.; Feng, L.; Kurul, S.H.; Brocke, K.; Unalp, A.; Özer, E.; Cakmakci, H.; Sewry, C.; Cirak, S.; Muntoni, F.; Hehr, U.; Morris-Rosendahl, D.J. (2011). *Fukutin* mutations in non-Japanese patients with congenital muscular dystrophy: less severe mutations predominate in patients with a non-Walker-Warburg phenotype. *Neuromusc. Disord.* 21, 20-30

Yoon, J.H.; Chandrasekharan, K.; Xu, R.; Glass, M.; Singhal, N.; Martin, P.T. (2009). The synaptic CT carbohydrate modulates binding and expression of extracellular matrix proteins in skeletal muscle: Partial dependence on utrophin. *Mol. Cell Neurosci.* 41, 448-63

Yoshida, A.; Kobayashi, K.; Manya, H.; Taniguchi, K.; Kano, H;, Mizuno, M.; Inazu, T.; Mitsuhashi, H.; Takahashi, S.; Takeuchi, M.; Herrmann, R.; Straub, V.; Talim, B.; Voit, T.; Topaloglu, H.; Toda, T.; Endo, T. (2001). Muscular dystrophy and neuronal migration disorder caused by mutations in a glycosyltransferase, POMGnT1. *Dev. Cell* 1, 717-724

Yoshida-Moriguchi, T.; Yu, L.; Stalnaker, S.H.; Davis, S.; Kunz, S.; Madson, M.; Oldstone, M.B.A.; Schachter, H.; Wells, L.; Campbell, KP. (2010). *O*-mannosyl phosphorylation of alpha-dystroglycan is required for laminin binding. *Science* 327, 88-92

Yoshioka, M. (2009). Phenotypic spectrum of fukutinopathy: most severe phenotype of fukutinopathy. *Brain Dev.* 31, 419-422

Zhou, Y.; Jiang, D.; Thomason, D.B.; Jarrett, H.W. (2007). Laminin-induced activation of Rac1 and JNKp46 is initiated by src family kinases and mimics the effects of skeletal muscle contraction. *Biochemistry* 46, 14907-14916

Section 2

Pathophysiology and Disease State

5

Duchenne Muscular Dystrophy and Brain Function

J.L. Anderson[1], S.I. Head[2] and J.W. Morley[3]
[1]*Childrens Hospital, Westmead, Sydney,*
[2]*School of Medical Sciences, University of New South Wales, Sydney,*
[3]*School of Medicine, University of Western Sydney, Sydney,*
Australia

1. Introduction

Muscular dystrophies have historically been characterised according to clinical criteria, however in the genomic age the muscular dystrophies are now subdivided into groups according to the primary gene defect. Currently identified are 29 different loci and encoded proteins, giving rise to 34 distinct forms of muscular dystrophy (Dalkilic & Kunkel 2003; Hsu 2004). The majority of these types of muscular dystrophy are caused by perturbations of different components of the dystrophin-glycoprotein complex (DGC) an integral component of the cellular cytoskeleton (see below). Dystrophin is the largest component of the DGC and is absent in Duchenne muscular dystrophy (DMD), and severely truncated with decreased levels in Becker muscular dystrophy (BMD) (Hoffman & Kunkel 1989). DMD and the allelic BMD are the most common forms of muscular dystrophy in humans and together they are termed dystrophinopathies (Kingston et al. 1984; Shaw & Dreifuss 1969). DMD alone accounts for approximately 80% of all the myopathies in the muscular dystrophy group (Culligan et al. 1998).The dystrophin gene is the second largest described to date, totalling 1.5% of the X chromosome, 0.1% of the entire genome. The DMD gene is 99% introns, with a coding sequence of 86 exons (including the promoters) and remains the only known human metagene (Blake et al. 2002; Burmeister et al. 1988; Hamed & Hoffmann 2006; Kenwrick et al. 1987; Koenig et al. 1987; Kunkel et al. 1986; Muntoni et al. 2003; Roberts et al. 1993; Smith et al. 2006; Van Ommen et al. 1987; Wallis et al. 2004). Dystrophin was demonstrated to be localised at the sarcolemma in human skeletal muscle after its' genetic characterisation (Arahata et al. 1988; Sugita et al. 1988; Zubrzycka-Gaarn et al. 1988). This discovery was followed by a report of dystrophin messenger RNA in brain, with the protein being specifically localised at postsynaptic densities (PSD) in the CNS, in particular in the hippocampus, cerebral cortex and in cerebellar Purkinje cells (PC) (Chamberlain et al. 1988; Chelly et al. 1988, 1989; Lidov et al. 1990, Nudel et al. 1988).

From the earliest reports authors have noted a preponderance of cognitive impairment in the Duchenne population and it has been well established that the average IQ of the boys with DMD is 85, one standard deviation below the normal of 100 (Cotton et al. 2005). With a greater understanding of the underlying molecular biology i.e. genotype, the recognised phenotype of dystrophinopathies is expanding (Beggs 1997; Emery 2002, 2002a; Ferlini et al. 1999; Muntoni et al. 1993). More recently investigations into the role of these proteins in the

CNS have commenced. In contrast to skeletal muscle, the function of dystrophin in brain is less well understood in part due to its more recent discovery in the CNS as well as the greater complexity of the dystrophin gene products and DGCs in this location (Culligan et al. 2001). It has been suggested that dystrophin may play a role in anchoring the postsynaptic apparatus, receptor channel clustering and membrane organization (Lidov et al. 1993). This anchoring of molecules, critical for neuronal function, may be achieved by dystrophin/DGC acting as adaptors between the actin cytoskeleton and membrane bound receptors (Yoshihara et al. 2003). It may also play a critical role in the formation and maintenance of macromolecular signalling complexes (Tokarz et al. 1998; Yoshihara et al. 2003). Dystrophin has also been suggested to play a role in stabilizing the postsynaptic apparatus to maintain a certain status of the network after brain maturation and/or episodes of synaptic plasticity (Brunig et al. 2002). Calcium levels have been found to be abnormal in neurons from an animal model of DMD (*mdx* mouse), and in a situation analogous to muscle, this could make these cells more susceptible to necrosis (Culligan et al. 2001). In summary, dystrophin deficiency may significantly alter membrane integrity, ion channel physiology, calcium homeostasis, regional cellular signal integration and structural reorganisation at the synapse (Mehler 2000; Vaillend & Billard 2002; Vaillend et al. 2004). The majority of recent studies support a role for dystrophin in organisation of the mature synapse - particularly GABA-ergic synapses under dynamic conditions. Below is a brief summary of the localisation of dystrophin/DGC in the CNS and a synthesis of the current literature investigating the role of dystrophin in human and murine CNS at the behavioural, morphological, biochemical and electrophysiological level.

1.1 The dystrophin-glycoprotein complex in CNS

Individual members of the DGC show a variety of site-specific specializations leading to many different DGCs (differentiated by binding-partner profile, localization and composition) existing in the CNS. Differences exist between the DGC in muscle and neuromuscular junction and also between both of these DGCs and brain DGCs. Additionally, individual members of the DGC play different roles at different sites. In the brain, unlike in muscle, the association of syntrophin with dystrophin is not crucial for DGC formation (Moukhles & Carbonetto 2001; Waite et al. 2009). Furthermore, Culligan & Ohlendieck (2002) have suggested that the brain DGC consists of four main components, the dystroglycan subcomplex, a dystrophin or utrophin gene product, a dystrobrevin isoform and a syntrophin subcomplex (Fig.1). Complexes including short dystrophin gene products together with syntrophin may also be expressed in both neurons and glia.

A role for the DGC in CNS has been suggested by many investigators, yet unequivocal evidence has yet to emerge. One theory suggests a role for the DGC in cellular communication by acting as a transmembrane signalling complex (Muntoni et al. 2003; Petrof 2002; Rando 2001). Supportive evidence for this theory is seen when mutations of the DGC component genes leads to cell death, thought to be due to a disruption of cell survival pathways and cellular defence mechanisms, both of which are regulated by signalling cascades (Muntoni et al. 2003; Rando 2001). The DGC in CNS may also play a dual function: incorporating both membrane stabilization as well as transmembrane signalling, as has been demonstrated at the neuromuscular junction (Albrecht & Froehner 2002). Additionally, the DGC has been suggested to play a role in the structural/functional organisation and/or stabilization of synapses (Albrecht & Froehner 2002). Dystroglycan and dystrophin, as

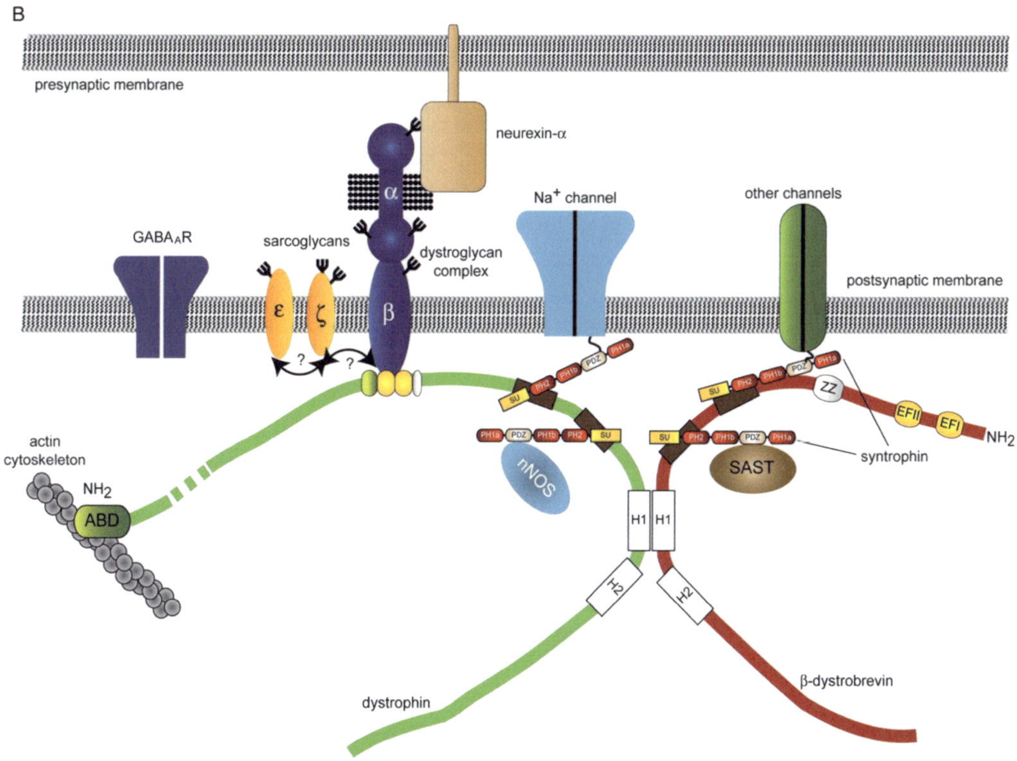

Fig. 1. The molecular organization of the "DGC-like" complexes and associated proteins in neurons (Modified from Waite et al. 2009).

central components of DGCs, have been implicated in the stabilisation of neurotransmitter receptor clusters e.g. GABAergic and cholinergic afferents (Knuesel et al. 1999; Zaccaria et al. 2001). It has been suggested that the DGC may act as a cytoskeletal scaffold on which signalling complexes as well as transmembrane proteins can be assembled and clustered, largely mediated by the syntrophins and dystrobrevins (Albrecht & Froehner 2002; Cavaldesi et al. 1999; Connors et al. 2004; Gee et al. 1998; Hashida-Okumura et al. 1999). Culligan and Ohlendieck (2002) propose that the extracellular component of neuronal DGCs mediates cellular signalling through interactions of specific proteins such as laminin, laminin α2, perlecan, agrin and biglycan. These interactions are believed to play a role in terminal consolidation, integrity and maintenance. Ceccarini et al. (2002) postulate that the DGC may play a role in the neuronal maturation process i.e. in morphological and functional modifications such as neurite outgrowth and synapse formation. Levi et al. (2002) suggest that the DGC may act as a trans-synaptic signal for some aspects of signalling involved in central neuron synaptic differentiation (Levi et al. 2002).

2. Dystrophin and the CNS

2.1 Localization

Dystrophin expression in the CNS is significantly more complicated compared to muscle due to the site specificity, developmental expression and diversity of gene products in this tissue. Levels of dystrophin in the brain are approximately 10% of those found in muscle. However, the CNS has the highest number of different dystrophin gene products of any other organ/tissue in the body (Abdulrazzak et al. 2001; Gorecki et al. 1991, 1992; Gorecki & Barnard 1995; Tokarz et al. 1998). Early studies indicated that in the CNS dystrophin localises primarily to the vascular endothelium, postsynaptic regions, pia and choroid plexus (Kamakura et al. 1994; Lidov et al. 1990; Uchino et al. 1994). Later studies demonstrated that Dp71 a smaller gene product of the dystrophin gene, is present in the wall of blood vessels, but is actually expressed in perivascular astrocyte endfeet (Ueda et al. 2000). Nudel et al. 1998, Chelly et al. (1988 and 1989) and Chamberlain et al. (1988) found dystrophin messenger RNA in brain and suggested that the lack of dystrophin in DMD may be the cause of cognitive impairment known to exist in this population. Lidov et al. (1990) demonstrated that dystrophin was specifically localised at postsynaptic densities (PSD) in the CNS, in particular in the hippocampus, cerebral cortex and in cerebellar Purkinje cells (PC) in rodents. This is in agreement with others who also found Dp427 as well as Dp71 enriched at the PSD (Blake et al. 1999; Jung et al. 1993; Kim et al. 1992; Moukhles & Carbonetto 2001). Uchino et al. (1994) confirmed these findings of PSD localisation in humans in agreement with Kim et al. (1995) and Jancsik & Hajos (1998). This latter group found that dystrophin was in the spines of neurons, with particularly heavy labelling at the PSD (Jancsik & Hajos 1998). There are now known to be three full-length dystrophin gene-products found in the CNS: M-dystrophin has been found in cerebral cortex and hippocampus (CA1, CA2 and CA3), C-dystrophin has also been localised to the cortex (grey matter, parietal layers II-IV, cingulated cortex) and hippocampus (pyramidal layer , layer II of infrahinal cortex, striatum radiatum and striatum oriens). C-dystrophin has also been demonstrated to be present in brainstem (inferior olive and trigeminal complex) and the midbrain (Caudate putamen). The third full-length dystrophin gene product P-dystrophin has been found in foetal cerebral cortex and Purkinje cells from early in the developmental process. Full-length dystrophin gene products are expressed almost exclusively in neurons (Lidov et al. 1990; Waite et al. 2009). The shorter dystrophin-gene products have a nomenclature of 'Dp' followed by their molecular weight: Dp 260 (D'Souza et al. 1995) Dp 140 (Lidov et al. 1995), Dp 116 (Byers et al. 1993; Schofield et al. 1994) and Dp71 (Blake et al. 1992; Iannello et al. 1991; formerly named apo-dystrophin 1 or G-dystrophin). Dp260 is found predominately in the retina (also brain and cardiac tissue) (Cibis et al. 1993; Costa et al. 2007; D'Souza et al. 1995; Pillers et al. 1993). Dp140 is predominately expressed in brain during foetal development and at very low levels in the adult brain, localised to astro-glial processes, vascular endothelium and leptomeningeal surfaces (Bardoni et al. 2000; Lidov et al. 1995). Dp 116 has been localised to adult peripheral nerves, along the Schwann cell membrane and fibroblasts (Byers et al. 1993; Labarque et al. 2008). Dp71 is expressed in a variety of tissues, predominately the CNS (where it is the most abundant dystrophin gene product), it has multiple isoforms each with specific subcellular localisations (Austin et al. 1995, 2000; Bar et al. 1990; Blake & Kroger 2000; Ceccarini et al. 2002; Chamberlain et al. 1988; Greenberg et al. 1996; Holder et al. 1996; Huard et al. 1992; Ilarraza-Lomeli et al. 2007; Lederfein et al. 1992;Miyatake et al. 1991; Rapaport et al. 1992). Dp71 has been localised to hippocampus (CA1 and dentate gyrus), olfactory bulb as well as perivascular astrocyte feet (Daoud et al. 2009). Figure 2 (modified from Blake et al. 2002) is a schematic diagram of the structure of dystrophin gene products. The basic structure consists of four main domains:

i. the N terminal which shares similarities to α-actin and has an actin-binding domain (Byers 1989; Fabbrizio et al. 1995; Koenig et al. 1988).
ii. a central rod domain with 24 spectrin-like triple helical repeats conferring an extended rod shape interrupted by four proline-rich spacer domains thought to act as hinges and conferring flexibility (Arahata et al. 1988; Cross et al. 1990; Koenig & Kunkel 1990, Michalak & Opas et al. 2001; O'Brien & Kunkel 2001; Roberts 2001).
iii. Cysteine-rich domain, separated from the rod domain by a WW domain (a protein-binding module found in several signalling and regulatory molecules). The cysteine-rich domain encompasses the EF1, EF2 and ZZ domains which together are termed the dystroglycan-binding domain. Following the ZZ domain is an α-helical domain important in mediating interactions with syntrophin (Bork & Sudol 1994; Huang et al. 2000; Ishikawa-Sakurai et al. 2004; Jung et al. 1995; Ponting et al. 1996; Rentschler et al. 1999; Suzuki et al. 1994; Winder et al. 1995).
iv. The C-terminal domain which contains binding sites for some dystrophin-associated glycoproteins, as well as putative sites for endogenous protein kinases to act upon (Lederfein et al. 1993; Michalak & Opas et al. 2001; Milner et al. 1993; Zubrzycka-Gaarn et al. 1988).

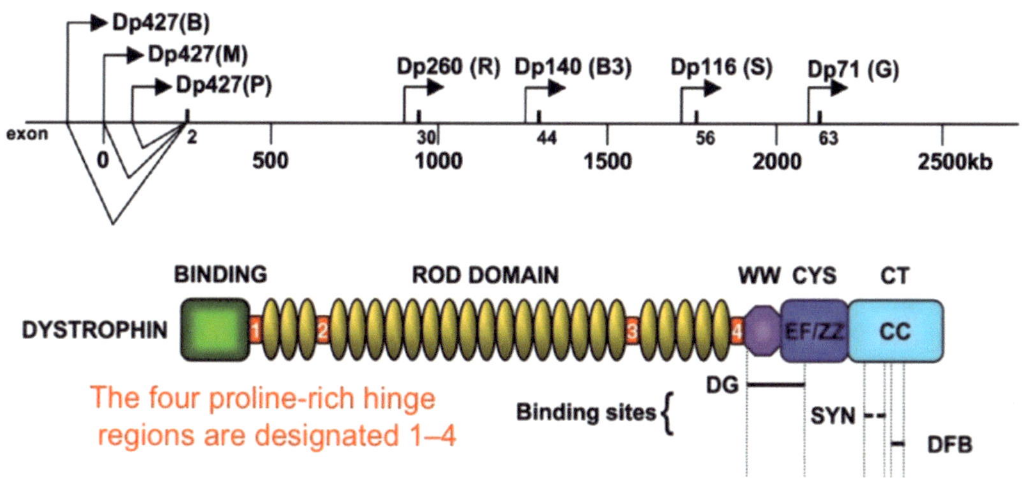

Fig. 2. Schematic showing the organization of the human Duchenne muscular dystrophy (DMD) gene and the dystrophin-related protein family (Modified from Blake et al. 2002).

3. Functional evidence of CNS aberrations in dystrophinopathy

Since the original description of the disease by Duchenne (1868) in which he reported five patients with some degree of cognitive impairment there has been debate as to whether there is a cognitive deficit associated with DMD. A meta-analysis of 32 studies comprising of 1224 patients with DMD with full-scale IQ data available for 1146 DMD patients reported an average IQ of 80.6 (SD 19.3), which was statistically different from the normal population average (Cotton et al. 2001). In this sample 35% of boys had an IQ lower than 70. Of these 79% were characterized as mild, 19% moderate, 1% severe and 0.3% profound (Cotton et al. 2001).

The importance of cognitive impairment in DMD has been demonstrated by a number of reports detailing developmental delay as the first presentation of disease (Essex & Roper 2001;

Kaplan et al. 1986; Mohamed et al. 2000; Smith et al. 1989). Specific subsets in cognitive ability which have been found to be affected in DMD/BMD include: memory/attention/recall (for patterns, numbers and verbal labels, serial position), verbal learning, language/verbal skills/confrontational naming, phonological and graphophonological production, reading, visuospatial organization skills, writing/spelling, comprehension/receptive language, mathematics, locomotor areas, verbal expression/fluency and conceptual ability (Anderson et al. 1988; Billard et al. 1992, 1998; Bresolin et al. 1994; Cotton et al. 1998; D'Angelo & Bresolin 2003; Dorman et al. 1988; Hendriksen & Vles 2006; Hinton et al. 2000, 2001; Karagan et al. 1980; Ogasawara 1989; Palumbo et al. 1996; Savage & Adams 1979; Smith et al. 1989, 1990; Sollee et al. 1985; Whelan 1987). Recent evidence suggests that children with DMD may have a distinct language-based learning deficit, similar to that seen in developmental dysphonetic-dyseidetic dyslexia i.e. problems with phonic analysis and synthesis of words as well as perception of the visual shape of words (Billard et al. 1992, 1998; Cotton et al. 2001). A number of investigators have hypothesized that the cerebellum plays an important role in the manifestation of cognitive deficits in dystrophinopathies (Cyrulnik & Hinton 2008; D'Angelo & Bresolin 2003; Hendriksen & Vles 2006).

Individual studies finding a difference between verbal and performance IQ include Karagan & Zellweger (1976), Karagan & Zellweger (1978), Karagan (1979), Glaub & Mechler (1987), Bresolin et al. (1994), Roccella et al. (2003), and Ogasawara (1989a). In a more recent meta-analysis VIQ and PIQ data was available for >800 children with VIQ = 80.4 +/- 18.8 (SD, n=881) and PIQ 85.4 +/- 16.9 (SD, n=878), both significantly different from the normal population. The discrepancy in VIQ and PIQ was –5.1 +/- 14.4 (SD, n=877). The mean was significantly different from zero but the distribution did not differ significantly from normal and was less than 10, the figure thought to establish clinical significance (Cotton et al. 2001, Wechsler 1997). Although there is a statistical difference between these IQ scores the functional significance is negligible.

Gauld et al. (2005) investigated the influence of IQ on the ability of children with DMD to perform spirometry, as well as assessing the impact of specific interventions for improvement. They found that the mean IQ was 84.7, PIQ 90.6 and VIQ 85.6 in 47 boys tested (mean age 12.6 years). The mean parent reported oppositional behaviour score was 56.3 (range 39 - 87) and mean teacher reported oppositional behaviour score was 56.9 (range 45 - 90) (higher scores on the scale correlate to children more likely to break rules, have problems with authority and who are easily annoyed) (Conners 2000). The oppositional behavioural scores remained stable over a 2.3 year period with a test-retest reliability of $r = 0.54$ (parent-rated) and $r = 0.6$ (teacher-rated), $P < 0.001$ for both (Gauld et al. 2005). They found that the results of spirometry testing were related to the individuals' performance IQ and can be explained by difficulties in understanding or learning to perform the technique required. The use of computer visualised incentives led to an improvement in function of spirometry testing in those shown to have a moderate intellectual or behavioural disturbance (Gauld et al. 2005). Additionally, Uchikawa et al. (2004) found in a group of 7 - 14 year old boys with DMD living in the community, that motor scores were higher in those with good cognitive functioning compared to those with impaired cognitive functioning, even though muscle strength was not significantly different. The authors note that poor cognitive functioning has an adverse effect on activities of daily living in DMD and that this impacts training and performance of these activities. These studies demonstrate the importance of paying attention to the cognitive functioning of individual patients with

DMD, as specific interventions can lead to improved symptom management and quality of life.

The search for a clear genotype-phenotype correlation with the degree of cognitive impairment has been confusing with conflicting reports. A recent study has brought some clarity to this issue. Taylor et al. (2010) have demonstrated that there is a quasi dose-response i.e. the cognitive impairment increases with cumulative loss of dystrophin gene products. A number of studies have suggested a higher incidence of a variety of neuropsychiatric deficits in boys with DMD compared to normal including dysthmic and major depressive disorders, anxiety, attention deficit hyperactivity disorder, obsessive-compulsive disorder and autism spectrum disorder (Fitzpatrick et al. 1986; Hendriksen & Vles 2008; Komoto et al. 1984; Melo et al. 1995; Poysky 2007; Reid & Renwick 2001; Roccella et al. 2003; Sekiguchi 2005; Wu et al. 2005; Young et al. 2008; Zwaigenbaum &Tarnopolsky 2003). As yet Reid & Renwick (2001) have been the only investigators to demonstrate an effect of decreased IQ on mental health in the dystrophinopthies, with no reports to investigate if the converse is true.

3.1 Morphological evidence of a CNS deformity in dystrophinopathy

Morphological studies of the CNS in dystrophinopathy have been inconsistent with some investigators reporting no or minimal changes (Bresolin et al. 1994; Dubowitz and Crome 1969; Rae et al. 1998), cerebral atrophy in later stages of disease (Al-Qudah et al. 1990; Yoshioka et al. 1980), abnormalities in dendritic development and arborisation in visual cortical neurons with extensive Purkinje cell loss (Jagadha & Becker 1988) and pachygyria (Bandoh et al. 1987; Rosman & Kakulas 1966; Wibawa et al. 2000). Some investigators have found a link between morphological abnormalities and impaired cognitive function (Bandoh et al. 1987; Bresolin et al. 1994; Rosman & Kakulas 1966; Septien et al. 1991; Wibawa et al. 2000; Yoshioka et al. 1980), whilst others have not (Al-Qudah et al. 1990).

Sogos et al. (1997) disrupted the expression of dystrophin in human neuronal cultures using *in vitro* techniques. They found a disruption of the morphology of synaptic boutons with alteration of the neuronal cytoskeleton in these cells. This also assessed whether a lack of dystrophin would lead to any perturbations of neuronal NOS (*n*NOS) using similar techniques (Sogos et al. 2003). They found that *n*NOS messenger RNA was significantly decreased (~ 35%) in neurones treated with B-dystrophin antisense. These authors postulated that decreased *n*NOS in neurons deficient for dystrophin may be responsible for alterations in synaptic plasticity (due to known association between *n*NOS and the NMDA receptor). Alternatively, the involvement of *n*NOS in CNS development may mean any perturbation could lead to altered neuronal maturation and abnormal synaptogenesis in developing neurons (Sogos et al. 2003).

3.2 Biochemical evidence of a CNS abnormality in dystrophinopathy

The search for the biochemical mechanisms underlying the cognitive deficit associated with lack of dystrophin in humans has been necessarily limited, however, new technologies allowing *in vivo* analysis has enabled some investigations. Not surprisingly oxygen and carbon dioxide levels have been found to be abnormal (especially during sleep), thought to be due to weakened respiratory function secondary to underlying muscle weakness and rib cage deformation (Khan & Heckmatt 1994; Manni et al. 1991; Misuri et al. 2000; Smith et al. 1988). Glucose hypometabolism has been studied by a number of groups as it is a common feature of disorders with associated cognitive deficits, and is generally indicative of lowered synaptic activity (Jueptner & Weiller 1995). Bresolin et al. (1994) found decreased glucose uptake in the cerebellum in DMD boys using PET imaging. Lee et al. (2002) using PET and MRI found four clusters of decreased glucose metabolism in DMD: medial temporal structures and cerebellum bilaterally, the sensorimotor and lateral temporal cortex on the right side (compared to an adult control group). The authors suggest that these findings may reflect local cytoarchitectural changes and abnormalities associated with altered neural development. Tracey et al. (1995), Kato et al. (1997) and Rae et al. (1998) using magnetic resonance spectroscopy and autopsy studies (Kato et al. 1997) focussed on choline-containing compounds which are seen to be elevated in a number of brain disorders and interpreted as symptomatic of increased membrane turnover or decreased membrane stability (Rae et al. 1998). MRI demonstrated significantly increased choline-containing compounds in the cerebellum, but not the cortex of boys < 13 years (Rae et al. 1998). The ratio of choline-containing compounds to N-acetylaspartyl-containing compounds (Cho/NA) was shown to correlate significantly with scores on the Matrix Analogies Test (MAT). The cerebellar and hippocampal focus of the biochemical lesions in DMD are of interest, due to the normally high expression of dystrophin in neurons found in these regions (Bresolin et al. 1994; Lee et al. 2002; Rae et al. 1998). Both Dorman et al. (1988) and Billard et al. (1998) noted that the reading deficits seen in DMD patients are similar to those seen in phonological dyslexia (Castles & Coltheart, 1993). Persons with phonological dyslexia, either developmental (Nicolson et al. 1999; Rae et al. 1998) or acquired (Levisohn et al. 2000), have been shown to have abnormalities in the right cerebellum. Similarly, deficits in verbal working memory, a large component of the DMD cognitive deficit (Hinton et al. 2001) are known to have a cerebellar focus (Desmond et al. 1997).

3.3 Electrophysiological evidence of a CNS abnormality in dystrophinopathy

EEG abnormalities have been reported in DMD although the only large study with appropriate controls (Barwick et al. 1965) found no association between abnormal EEG and dystrophinopathy. To date no studies have examined genotypically confirmed DMD and EEG abnormalities although an increased incidence of epilepsy has been noted in boys with dystrophinopathies compared to the general population (Etemadifar & Molaei 2004; Goodwin et al. 1997). Motor cortex excitability has also been demonstrated to be affected in DMD with reduced excitability thought to be due to aberrant synaptic functioning (Bresolin et al. 1994; Di Lazzaro et al. 1998; Jueptner & Weiller 1995).

4. Evidence from animal models of dystrophinopathy: the *mdx* mouse

The *mdx* mouse (*m*uscular *d*ystrophy *X*-linked) is the most widely studied animal model of dystrophinopathy (Collins & Morgan 2003; Durbeej & Campbell 2002; Partridge 1991). Although its discovery predated the genotyping of this disorder it has since been proven to be an appropriate model with identification of a premature stop codon terminating translation of murine dystrophin resulting in an absence of all full-length dystrophin-gene products (Bulfield et al. 1984; Chamberlain et al. 1987; Hoffman et al. 1987; Sicinski et al. 1989). This mouse model has aided in investigations of the function of dystrophin, particularly in the CNS as invasive functional investigations can be carried out on these animals. The majority of current knowledge of the role of dystrophin in the CNS comes from this animal model.

4.1 Cognitive functioning

Impairments in passive avoidance learning, long-term recognition memory and procedural learning have all been shown to be adversely affected in *mdx* mice compared to controls. Task acquisition, procedural memory spatial discrimination tasks, novelty-seeking behaviour and exploration in an elevated plus maze have all been shown to be unaffected in the *mdx* mouse (Mehler et al. 1992; Muntoni et al. 1991; Perronnet & Vaillend 2010; Sesay et al. 1996; Vaillend et al. 1995, 1998, 1999, 2004). Most recently Sekiguchi et al. (2009) have demonstrated an enhanced defensive freezing response to a brief restraint as well as enhanced unconditioned and conditioned defensive responses to electrical footshock in *mdx* mice compared to wildtype. This abnormal behaviour was ameliorated with intracerebroventricular administration of antisense morpholino oligonucleotide (which induces skipping of the premature stop codon located at exon 23 in the *mdx* mouse and produces a truncated dystrophin with a 71 amino acid deletion in the mid-rod domain) (Alter et al. 2006; Sekiguchi et al. 2009).

4.2 Morphology

No gross abnormalities in brain or spinal cord in the *mdx* mouse have been found (Bulfield et al. 1984; Dunn & Zaim-Wadghiri 1999; Torres & Duchen 1987; Yoshihara et al. 2003). This was most recently confirmed using MRI by Miranda et al. (2009) who found no major alteration of brain anatomy in *mdx* mice, reporting no significant changes in the cortex, hippocampus or cerebellum (normally dystrophin-positive). At the cellular/axonal level dystrophin has been found to localise to the cell membrane, predominately the soma and postsynaptic densities particularly in hippocampus, neocortex, cerebellum and amygdale (Anderson et al. 2002; Lidov 1996; Perronnet & Vaillend 2010). Anatomical alterations have been found in the *mdx* mouse in various brain regions including decreased cell number, altered cell packing density and changes in cell morphology (Carretta et al. 2001; Sbriccoli et al. 1995). It should be noted that these changes were not demonstrated when investigated in the hippocampus. CA1 pyramidal cell packing density, mean nuclear area and circularity has been found to be unaltered in *mdx* mice (Miranda et al. 2009). PSD length of axospinous perforated excitatory synapses has been found to be larger in *mdx* proximal radiatum of the hippocampus (Miranda et al. 2009). These authors note that perforated synapses are the hallmarks of activity dependent synaptic plasticity (Miranda et al. 2009). A more recent report by this group has demonstrated that the presynaptic ultrastructure of excitatory hippocampal synapses is altered in both *mdx* and Dp71-null mice (Miranda et al. 2011). Again examining the proximal radiatum glutaminergic synapses (normally dystrophin-positive) they report an increased number of docked vesicles, with the number and size of vesicles similar in *mdx* mice compared to controls. They also found a decrease in the number of vesicles in the 'reserve pool' i.e. > 300nm away from the synapse) in *mdx* mice compared to controls. In the Dp71-null mice they found that the number and spatial distribution of vesicles was no different from control (Miranda et al. 2011). In contrast to Dp427-null (*mdx*) mice the number of vesicles in the active zone was decreased and the number of vesicles in the reserve pool was increased compared to controls, whilst the number of docked vesicles remained the same. Alterations in parvalbumin-positive and calbindin-positive interneurons (both calcium binding proteins) have been demonstrated to be significantly increased in particular brain regions of *mdx* compared to wildtype (Carretta et al. 2003, 2004). At the receptor level the glucose transporters GLUT1 and GLUT4, α1 and α2 $GABA_A$ receptor subunit and nicotinic ACh receptor gene expression is decreased in specific brain regions of *mdx* mouse (Wallis et al. 2004). Of particular interest is the strong association of dystrophin with the $GABA_A$ receptor. Knuesel et al. (1999) found co-localization of the $GABA_A$ channel with dystrophin in the mouse cerebellum and hippocampus. In these areas of the *mdx* mouse there was a marked reduction of $GABA_A$ clusters. This decrease in clustering was particularly striking around the soma of cerebellar Purkinje cells. In both the cerebellum and hippocampus the number (but not size) of $GABA_A$ clusters was reduced by ~ 50%. Brunig et al. (2002) found that the DGC and $GABA_A$-gephyrin complexes undergo different clustering mechanisms and that the DGC is unchanged by the absence of gephyrin/$GABA_A$. They suggested that selective signalling from presynaptic GABAergic terminals contributes to DGC clustering (Brunig et al. 2002). The authors postulated that the DGC may stabilise $GABA_A$ clusters, in a developmentally regulated manner. They also suggested functions for the DGC at the synapse: i) by stabilizing the postsynaptic apparatus, the DGC may "freeze" GABAergic synapses in order to maintain a certain status of the network once learning processes have been primarily completed or ii) DGC may provide a scaffold enabling changes in clusters of $GABA_A$ receptor without incurring the loss of the postsynaptic apparatus, as may be required in circuits with a high degree of synaptic plasticity.

Grady et al. (2006) generated α-dystrobrevin, β-dystrobrevin (both members of the DGC) and double mutant α - and β-dystrobrevin knockout mice. They examined the localisation of α and β-dystrobrevin, finding both proteins in the hippocampus and cerebral cortex. They found that all larger β-dystrobrevin-positive puncta on the dendrites (but not somata) of PC were colocalised with gephyrin staining (gephyrin is associated with inhibitory synapses in the CNS). When staining for the $GABA_A$ α1 subunit in β-dystrobrevin knockout mice, they found a decrease in the number of $GABA_A$ α1-positive clusters of 33% and reduction in size by approx 50% in cerebellar PC. This finding is comparable with Knuesel et al. (1999) (no such association in the cerebellum of α-dystrobrevin knockout mice was found). They further demonstrated that, in *mdx* mice, a loss of dystrophin led to a loss of dystrobrevin at these sites and in dystrobrevin knockout mice, a loss of dystrobrevin led to a loss of dystrophin at these sites. This interrelationship between dystrobrevin and dystrophin was not demonstrated in the hippocampus. Another member of the DGC – dystroglycan has also been demonstrated to be clustered at GABAergic synapses. Dystroglycan deficient mice have GABAergic clusters lacking dystrophin, however dystrophin-deficient mice (i.e. *mdx*) as well as gephyrin-deficient mice do not lose colocalisation of dystroglycan and GABAergic synapses (Brunig et al. 2002; Levi et al. 2002; Waite et al. 2009). As will be described below Kueh et al. (2011) demonstrated that there is a reduction in the number of functional receptors localised at the GABAergic synapses in the cerebellar PCs of *mdx* mice and an increase in extrasynaptic $GABA_A$ receptors. Vaillend et al. (2010) have demonstrated a re-expression of a truncated dystrophin in the hippocampus after intra-hippocampal injection of adenovirus-associated vector expressing antisense sequences linked to a modified U7 small nuclear RNA that re-directed the splicing of dystrophin pre-mRNA allowing omission of exon 23 of the dystrophin gene in the *mdx* mouse. This allows restoration of the reading frame and a functional dystrophin protein to be expressed. The levels of expression of the truncated dystrophin reached 15-25% of wildtype. They further investigated whether this 'rescue' of dystrophin expression had an impact on $GABA_A$ receptor clustering. They found that the number of clusters and the area of the α2 subunit of the $GABA_A$ receptor was significantly larger in the treated *mdx* mice compared to untreated *mdx* mice, and was actually no longer significantly different from wildtype (Vaillend et al. 2010) suggesting complete recovery of $GABA_A$ receptor clustering after partial dystrophin-rescue. They conclude that although dystrophin is not involved in synpatogenesis it may be important in maintenance and stabilisation of postsynaptic $GABA_A$ receptors. They note that dystrophin is co-localised with α2-containing $GABA_A$ receptors at a relatively low rate and postulate that the remaining dystrophin may be involved in trafficking/targeting processes, expressed in empty synapses transiently devoid of $GABA_A$ receptors (Vaillend et al. 2010).

The overall protein expression levels of $GABA_A$ receptors containing α1 subunits in a whole membrane preparation of murine cerebellum was investigated by our group and found to be no different from littermate controls (Kueh et al. 2008). This finding supports the theory that it is the organisation of the $GABA_A$ receptor (i.e. altered clustering) rather than the expression (i.e. quantity) that is adversely affected by a lack of dystrophin.

4.3 Biochemistry

A number of reports have examined metabolites in *mdx* CNS. Griffin et al. (2001) identified discernable changes in metabolic pathways: glycolysis, β-oxidation, the TCA cycle, phosphocreatine/ATP cycle and lipid metabolism were all altered in *mdx* cerebral cortex and cerebellum. Young *mdx* mice have been found to have normal levels of N-acetylaspartate and total creatinine content, increased whole-brain levels of choline-containing compounds (glycero- and phosphocholine) and *myo*-inositol, and a decrease in the ATP synthase γ subunit in cerebellum and hippocampi (Tracey et al. 1996; Wallis et al. 2004). In older *mdx* mice a decrease in the total creatinine content, increase in inorganic phosphate to phosphocreatine ratio, increased intracellular brain pH, decreased expression of mitochondrial creatine kinase in *mdx* hippocampi, and increased choline containing compounds in cerebellum and hippocampus of *mdx* brain, but not the cortex, have all been reported (Rae et al. 2002; Tracey et al. 1996; Wallis et al. 2004). Together these results indicate that there are significant differences in *mdx* mice CNS metabolism possibly indicating increased membrane turnover or decreased membrane stability. Furthermore, there is a clear exacerbation of these biochemical abnormalities with age, although there is yet no clear explanation of how a lack of dystrophin leads to these changes and why some of these perturbations are increased and others decreased with age.

Other reports have looked at glucose utilisation in CNS of *mdx* mice. Rae et al. (2002) found significantly decreased free glucose in *mdx*, significantly increased fractional enrichment and increased flux of ^{13}C into metabolites such as glutamate and GABA. These authors noted that this may indicate a faster metabolic rate in dystrophin-deficient brain due to abnormal functioning of $GABA_A$ receptors and, therefore, decreased inhibition (as, in general, excitatory stimulation leads to increased glucose metabolism and inhibitory activation leads to decreased glucose metabolism) (Ito et al. 1994; Rae et al. 2000, 2002). In old *mdx* mice there was abnormal metabolism of [1-^{13}C] glucose (Rae et al. 2002). In a follow-on study this group found no significant difference in glucose metabolism in the young *mdx* mice compared to controls, suggesting that changes in glucose metabolism seen in the old *mdx* mice are due to other factors (i.e. not changes in expression of glucose transporters) (Wallis et al. 2004).

AQP4 and osmotic/cellular volume alterations in *mdx* mice has been reported. Increased extracellular and decreased intracellular volume in *mdx* brain as well as altered osmoregulation was reported by Tracey et al. (1996a) and Griffin et al. (2001). Frigeri et al. (2001) found that although AQP4 mRNA staining pattern was unaltered, the level of this protein was decreased in *mdx* CNS. This decrease grew with age (70% decrease at 12 months). Dp71 has been found to be the major dystrophin gene product responsible for anchoring AQP4 and the DGC at the glial endfeet (Amiry-Moghaddam et al. 2004; Neely et al. 2001; Nicchia et al. 2008; Yokota et al. 2000). Nicchia et al. (2004) reported the unpublished observation of Frigeri et al. (2001) that *mdx* mice also demonstrate a resistance to brain oedema. They postulated that the absence and/or mislocalisation of AQP4 at the perivascular endfeet is protective in induced brain oedema. Nico et al. (2003) found a profoundly altered blood-brain-barrier (BBB). Although initial reports suggested no alteration in response to osmotic stress (hypo-osmotic shock) in *mdx* CNS (Rae et al. 2002). Vajda et al. (2002, 2004) found, in osmotic stress experiments, that the *mdx-βgeo* mice had a delayed decompensation and increased survival time (66.5 min compared to 56 min) indicating that Dp71 is necessary for the polarized distribution of AQP4 in brain.

Interestingly, many of these reports propose a link between the biochemical abnormalities and underlying channel dysfunction secondary to a lack of dystrophin. Rae et al.'s (2002) report suggests that the increased glucose use demonstrated in *mdx* brain may be due to decreased inhibitory input from the subset of abnormally clustered $GABA_A$-receptors. Further Griffin et al. (1999) have proposed this elevation is associated with cellular membranes implying a progressive, degenerative or compensatory process (Rae et al. 2002).

Decreased bioenergetic buffering capacity would be expected to influence susceptibility to hypoxia. Mehler and coworkers (Mehler et al. 1992) reported an increase in sensitivity of hippocampal slices from *mdx* mice to loss of synaptic transmission of CA1 hippocampal pyramidal cells during hypoxia. This was partially ameliorated by blocking both sodium-dependent action potentials as well as low-threshold calcium conductances. Yoshihara et al. (2003) suggested that the increased sensitivity to hypoxia found by Mehler et al. (1992) may be due to impaired function of inhibitory synapses at this site. Another group (Godfraind et al. 1998, 2000) has shown increased susceptibility of *mdx* hippocampal tissue slices to irreversible hypoxic failure when kept in 10 mM glucose, but less susceptibility of *mdx* slices when kept in 4 mM glucose, in agreement with Wallis et al. (2004). The latter group suggest that the decrease in GLUT1 and GLUT3 expression they found is most likely related to decreased synaptic integrity, resulting in decreased activity and decreased glucose utilization. These authors noted that dystrophin may be required to maintain synaptic integrity (Knuesel et al. 2001) rather than being directly involved in anchoring/clustering of the $GABA_A$ receptor itself. Additionally, it is known that the expression of components of the $GABA_A$ receptor relate to synaptic activity (Ives et al. 2002). Thus, Wallis et al. (2004) proposed that the lack of dystrophin in the PSD may impede synaptic activity leading to decreased $GABA_A$ receptor components due to decreased GABAergic demand. Wallis et al. (2004) suggested that dystrophin may be involved in the clustering of this complex of proteins (mitochondrial creatine kinase, adenine nucleotide translocase and the gamma subunit of ATP synthase). Furthermore, Rae et al. (2002) suggested that the regulation of oxidative metabolism during hypoxia was impaired, and that this may be another manifestation of calcium overload in the neuronal mitochondria of *mdx* CNS.

4.4 Electrophysiology

The highest levels of dystrophin gene products are in areas in which neurons maintain a high degree of synaptic plasticity: olfactory bulb, hippocampus, neocortex and cerebellum (Gorecki et al. 1997, 1998; Lidov et al. 1990). Synaptic plasticity has been examined in both the hippocampus and cerebellum and found to be altered in the *mdx* mouse in both of these brain regions (Anderson et al. 2004, 2010; Vaillend et al. 1998, 1999, 2004). Vaillend's group examined the CA1 dendritic layer of the hippocampus and found that NMDA-receptor dependent short-term and long-term potentiation, and long-term depression were abnormally enhanced in *mdx* mice (Perronnet & Vaillend 2010; Vaillend et al. 1998, 1999, 2004). Both our and Vaillend's group have investigated the function of the GABA receptor in the *mdx* cerebellum and hippocampus respectively as it is known to colocalise with dystrophin (Knuesel et al. 1999). In *mdx* mice hippocampus and cerebellum there is a marked reduction of $GABA_A$ clusters, with the number (but not size) of $GABA_A$ clusters being reduced by ~ 50% (Knuesel et al. 1999). In both the cerebellum and hippocampus the $GABA_A$ antagonist had a decreased effect (Anderson et al. 2003; Vaillend et al. 2002). When miniature inhibitory postsynaptic potentials were examined in the cerebellum a decrease in frequency and amplitude was found in contrast to the hippocampus where an increase in frequency was demonstrated (Anderson et al. 2003; Kueh et al. 2008; Graciotti et al. 2008). We have noted however that the reduction in amplitude may lead to a falsely lowered frequency due to lowered amplitude IPSCs being below counting threshold. These results have led to the 'dysfunctional inhibition' hypothesis being postulated as the cause of the cognitive impairment seen in DMD (Perronnet & Vaillend 2010). Dallerac et al. (2011) demonstrated that *mdx* mice treated with U7 small nuclear RNAs modified to encode antisense sequences and expressed from recombinant adeno-associated viral vectors to induce skipping of the premature stop codon at exon 23 of the dystrophin gene normalises hippocampal synaptic plasticity. The vector was injected into the hippocampus and months after two months CA1 hippocampal LTP, which is normally enhanced compared to wildtype, was no longer different from wildtype. In studies of seizure induction in mice, dystrophin deficiency has been found to alter the neuronal excitability of AMPA/kainic-type glutamate receptors suggesting a dysfunctional excitatory-inhibitory balance (De Sarro et al. 2004; Perronnet & Vaillend 2010; Yoshihara et al. 2003). Basolateral nucleus of the amygdale pyramidal neurons have also been studied in the *mdx* mouse and have been demonstrated to have decreased inductions of GABA-ergic IPSCs by noradrenalin. These authors note that in the *mdx* there were cells sensitive to noradrenalin (~40%) and a larger subset of cells insensitive to noradrenalin (~60%). Whilst the regular-spiking non-pyramidal basolateral nucleus of the amygdale neurons had similar proportions of noradrenalin-induced depolarisation and AP firing (~50%) in wildtype and *mdx* demonstrating that the mechanism by which noradrenalin depolarises interneurons beyond AP threshold is not impaired in *mdx* mice. Rather it is more likely that a decrease in the number of normal functioning GABAergic synapses between the noradrenalin-responsive interneurons and pyramidal neurons underlies their findings (Sekiguchi et al. 2009).

Work from our laboratory has similarly demonstrated altered GABA-ergic function in the cerebellum of *mdx* mice. We found that evoked excitatory post-synaptic potentials in cerebellar Purkinje cells show a decreased response (approx 50%) to bicuculline (a GABA antagonist) compared to wildtype (Anderson et al. 2003). We also demonstrated that miniature inhibitory postsynaptic currents had a significantly decreased amplitude in *mdx* cerebellar Purkinje cells compared to wildtype. This difference in amplitude was principally due to the absence of large amplitude miniature inhibitory postsynaptic currents in *mdx* mice. We postulate that this decrease is the result of a decrease in the number of postsynaptic GABA-ergic receptors (Nusser et al. 1997). This finding was reproduced in later studies (Fig. 3; Kueh et al. 2008, 2011). We further went on to investigate the number of $GABA_A$ channels located at the GABAergic synapse of cerebellar Purkinje cells. We found a significant reduction in the number of receptors at the PSD in *mdx* compared with littermate controls determined by non-stationary noise analysis of spontaneous miniature inhibitory postsynaptic currents. Single unitary conductance, rise and decay times of the currents were no different from littermate controls demonstrating that although there is a reduction in the number of channels at the postsynaptic membrane in *mdx* cerebellar Purkinje cells, the $GABA_A$ channels that are present are functioning normally. Further, Gaboxadol, an extrasynaptic GABA agonist, was applied inducing an increase in the holding current of the Purkinje cell. In *mdx* mice this increase was significantly greater (~200%) compared to littermate controls (Kueh et al. 2011), indicating that in *mdx* mice the number of extrasynpatic $GABA_A$ receptors is increased.

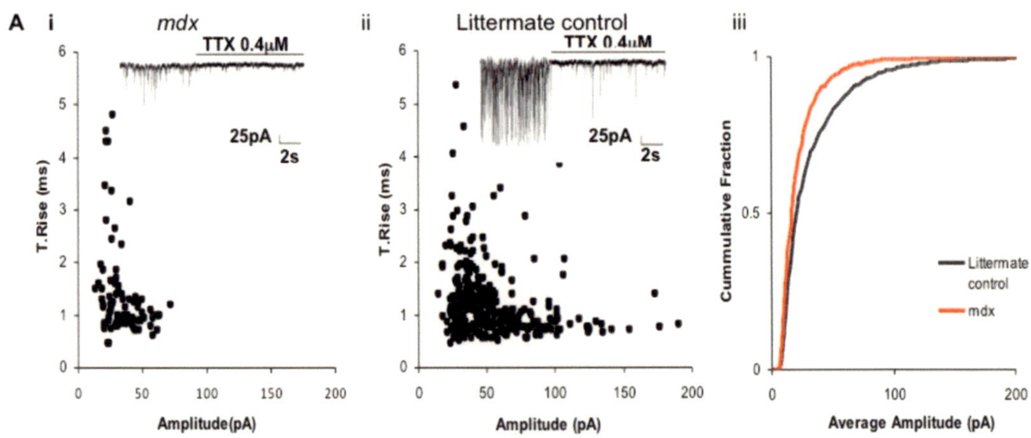

Fig. 3. A scatter plot of rise time versus peak amplitude, showing the distribution of mIPSCs in a (i) *mdx* and a (ii) littermate control mouse. The inserts show a section of the recording in aCSF and when TTX was added to the bath. iii) Cumulative probability of mIPSC amplitudes (average) in *mdx* and littermate control cells. There was a significant difference between mIPSC amplitudes between *mdx* and litermate control cells (Mann Whitney test, p=0.0001) (Modified from Kueh et al. 2011).

Our group has also investigated synaptic plasticity in the *mdx* cerebellum which is uniquely suited to these investigations as the Purkinje cell - the major output neuron of the cerebellum normally expresses a specific full-length dystrophin - P-dystrophin, which is absent in *mdx* mice. The major inputs to the Purkinje cells - parallel fibres and inhibitory interneurons are normally dystrophin negative. Firstly we examined a presynaptic form of synaptic plasticity in the cerebellum - short-term synaptic plasticity mediated at the parallel-fibre to Purkinje cell synapse. We found no difference between wildtype and *mdx* mice in this form of plasticity as expected due to the post-synaptic localisation of

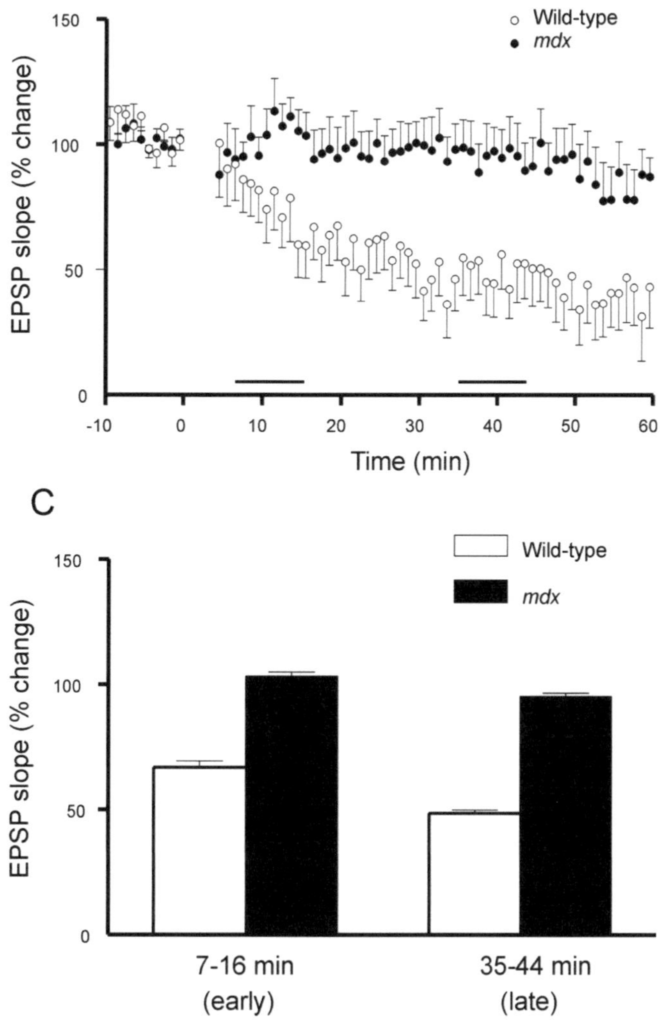

Fig. 4. Long-term depression (LTD) in cerebellar Purkinje cells of wild-type and *mdx* mice. Upper graph shows the average slope of evoked EPSPs in wild-type and *mdx* Purkinje cells before and after LTD induction. Open circles are wildtype Purkinje cells (n=11) and closed circles are *mdx* Purkinje cells (n=12). Slopes are normalised to the average slope for wild-type and *mdx* cells respectively recorded in the 10 minutes preceding LTD induction. Thin horizontal bars above the abscissa represent the two 10 minute time periods during which the EPSP slopes were averaged and represent the magnitude of early and late phases of LTD. Vertical bars are SEM and for clarity are shown on one side of the data points only. Lower bar graph displays the average slope for all wild-type and all *mdx* cells in the early and late phases following LTD induction (Modified from Anderson et al. 2004)

dystrophin. We then went on to examine a post-synaptic mediated form of synaptic plasticity - long-term depression. As postulated the extent of depression was decreased in *mdx* cerebellar Purkinje cells compared to wildtype (Fig, 4; Anderson et al. 2004). We next examined homosynaptic longterm depression at this synapse and found that there was no difference between wildtype and *mdx* cerebellar Purkinje cells in the initial observation period, however the depression was significantly greater in the latter part of the observation period in *mdx* compared to wildtype (Anderson et al. 2010). The three most compelling explanations for the differences demonstrated above are i) an alteration in calcium homeostasis, ii) an indirect effect of altered $GABA_A$ receptor localisation and/or trafficking and iii) an alteration in putative AMPA-receptor localisation/trafficking. The most recent investigations of the multiplicity of effects of the known $GABA_A$ receptor dysfunction on the neurophysiology of the *mdx* mouse is compelling.

Further unpublished data from our laboratory has demonstrated that that short term synaptic plasticity (inhibitory interneuron to Purkinje cell synapse) is no different between *mdx* and wildtype. However rebound potentiation - a form of longterm synaptic plasticity expressed at this synapse is significantly different. Wildtype cerebellar Purkinje cells demonstrated potentiation of the inhibitory postsynaptic potential as previously reported, however the *mdx* cerebellar Purkinje cells depressed. In a pilot study 5/12 wildtype cerebellar Purkinje cells demonstrated rebound potentiation (0 depressed) compared to 0/5 *mdx* cells demonstrating potentiation and 4/5 cells demonstrating depression. Although preliminary, these findings are the first to demonstrate a deficit in GABA-mediated synaptic plasticity. These findings also locate the problem at the post-synaptic (dystrophin-deficient Purkinje cell) locus as the presynaptically-mediated short-term synaptic plasticity of this synapse is preserved. (Anderson 2009).

5. Conclusion

The role of dystrophin in the CNS is complex and incompletely understood. It is clear that the absence of this protein leads to profound functional deficits at the macro-level (behavioural alterations and cognitive impairment) as well as the micro-level (alterations in synaptic plasticity, GABA-ergic functioning). Morphologically there are alterations in cellular architecture and organisation as well as channel localisation. The increase in investigations of the role of dystrophin in the CNS has led to a rapid appreciation of the consequence of its absence in this tissue, however a clear mechanism by which these alterations occur has yet to emerge. The majority of current evidence points convincingly to a link between a lack of dystrophin and alterations in the localisation of $GABA_A$ receptors. Furthermore there is evidence that a lack of dystrophin is associated with abnormal functioning of $GABA_A$ receptor-mediated cellular activity as measured by changes in amplitude of IPSCs. The well-established cognitive-impairment seen in the boys with dystrophinopathies may be due to an underlying abnormality in synaptic plasticity as demonstrated in the *mdx* animal models. However evidence linking the alteration in GABA-ergic localisation and function with alterations in synaptic plasticity is speculative. The postulated dysfunctional excitatory-inhibitory balance - perhaps mediated by chronic alteration of calcium-handling by these neurons, is the most compelling hypothesis to date linking these two major findings (alterations in GABA clustering and function with alterations in synaptic plasticity). Further how a lack of dystrophin leads to the structural alterations seen in found in *mdx* CNS, as well as the plethora of biochemical alterations in seen in both humans and animal models of DMD has yet to emerge. The role of the smaller dystrophin gene products in the brain are now beginning to be appreciated with a recent report demonstrating that a loss of the smallest of these - Dp71, can lead to changes at the behavioural, cell membrane and synaptic levels (Daoud et al. 2009). The role of dystrophin and the dystrophin-glycoprotein complex in the CNS is slowly being elucidated. With a greater understanding of the function of this protein useful therapies may be able to ameliorate the CNS manifestations of Duchenne muscular dystrophy as well as aid in the effort to arrest the devastating muscular degeneration.

6. References

ABDULRAZZAK, H., NORO, N., SIMONS, J. P., GOLDSPINK, G., BARNARD, E. A. & GORECKI, D. C. (2001). Structural diversity despite strong evolutionary conservation in the 5'-untranslated region of the P-type dystrophin transcript. *Molecular & Cellular Neursciences,* 17, 500-13.

ALBRECHT, D. E. & FROEHNER, S. C. (2002). Syntrophins and dystrobrevins: defining the dystrophin scaffold at synapses. *Neurosignals,* 11, 123-9.

AL-QUDAH, A. A., KOBAYASHI, J., CHUANG, S., DENNIS, M. & RAY, P. (1990). Etiology of intellectual impairment in Duchenne muscular dystrophy. *Pediatr Neurol,* 6, 57-9.

ALTER, J., LOU, F., RABINOWITZ, A., YIN, H., ROSENFELD, J., WILTON, S.D., PARTRIDGE, T.A. & LU Q.L. (2006). Systemic delivery of morpholino oligonucleotide restores dystrophin expression bodywide and improves dystrophic pathology. *Nature Medicine* 12, 175-77.

AMIRY-MOGHADDAM, M., XUE, R., FINN-MOGENS, H., NEELY, J.D., BHARDWAJ, A., AGRE, P., ADAMS, M.E., FROEHNER, S.C., MORI, S. & OTTERSEN, O.P. (2004). Alpha-syntrophin deletion removes the perivascular but not the endothelial pool of aquaporin-4 at the blood-brain barrier and delays the development of brain edema in an experimental model of acute hyponatraemia. *The FASEB Journal* 18 542-44.

ANDERSON, J.L. (2009) Cerebellar synaptic plasticity in two animal models of muscular dystrophy. PhD dissertation. University of New South Wales, Sydney Australia.

ANDERSON, J.L., HEAD, S.I., RAE, C. & MORLEY, J.W. (2002). Brain function in Duchenne muscular dystrophy. *Brain* 125: 4-13.

ANDERSON, J.L., HEAD, S.I. & MORLEY, J.W. (2003). Altered inhibitory input to Purkinje cells of dystrophin-deficient mice. *Brain Res* 982: 280-283.

ANDERSON, J.L., HEAD, S.I. & MORLEY, J.W. (2004). Long-term depression is reduced in cerebellar Purkinje cells of dystrophin-deficient mdx mice. *Brain Res* 1019: 289-92.

ANDERSON, J.L., MORLEY, J.W. & HEAD, S.I. (2010). Enhanced homosynaptic LTD in cerebellar Purkinje cells of the dystrophic mdx mouse. *Muscle & Nerve* 41 (3) 329-34.

ANDERSON, S. W., ROUTH, D. K. & IONASESCU, V. V. (1988). Serial position memory of boys with Duchenne muscular dystrophy. *Dev Med Child Neurol,* 30, 328-33.

ARAHATA, K., ISHIURA, S., ISHIGURO, T., TSUKAHARA, T., SUHARA, Y., EGUCHI, C., ISHIHARA, T., NONAKA, I., OZAWA, E. & SUGITA, H. (1988). Immunostaining of skeletal and cardiac muscle surface membrane with antibody against Duchenne muscular dystrophy peptide. *Nature,* 333, 861-3.

AUSTIN, R. C., HOWARD, P. L., D'SOUZA, V. N., KLAMUT, H. J. & RAY, P. N. (1995). Cloning and characterization of alternatively spliced isoforms of Dp71. *Hum Mol Genet,* 4, 1475-83.

AUSTIN, R. C., MORRIS, G. E., HOWARD, P. L., KLAMUT, H. J. & RAY, P. N. (2000). Expression and synthesis of alternatively spliced variants of Dp71 in adult human brain. *Neuromuscul Disord,* 10, 187-93.

BANDOH, T., KAWAI, H., ADACHI, K. & II, K. (1987). [Clinical and pathological studies on intellectual impairment in Duchenne muscular dystrophy, with special reference to patients with severe intellectual impairment]. *Rinsho Shinkeigaku,* 27, 692-701.

BAR, S., BARNEA, E., LEVY, Z., NEUMAN, S., YAFFE, D. & NUDEL, U. (1990). A novel product of the Duchenne muscular dystrophy gene which greatly differs from the known isoforms in its structure and tissue distribution. *Biochem J,* 272, 557-60.

BARDONI, A., FELISARI, G., SIRONI, M., COMI, G., LAI, M., ROBOTTI, M. & BRESOLIN, N. (2000). Loss of Dp140 regulatory sequences is associated with cognitive impairment in the dystrophinopathies. *Neuromuscul Disord* 10(3) 194-199.

BARWICK, D. D., OSSELTON, J. W. & WALTON, J. N. (1965). Electroencephalographic Studies in Hereditary Myopathy. *J Neurol Neurosurg Psychiatry,* 28, 109-14.

BEGGS, A. H. (1997). Dystrophinopathy, the expanding phenotype. Dystrophin abnormalities in X-linked dilated cardiomyopathy. *Circulation,* 95, 2344-7.

BILLARD, C., GILLET, P., SIGNORET, J. L., UICAUT, E., BERTRAND, P., FARDEAU, M., BARTHEZ-CARPENTIER, M. A. & SANTINI, J. J. (1992). Cognitive functions in Duchenne muscular dystrophy: a reappraisal and comparison with spinal muscular atrophy. *Neuromuscul Disord,* 2, 371-8.

BILLARD, C., GILLET, P., BARTHEZ, M., HOMMET, C. & BERTRAND, P. (1998). Reading ability and processing in Duchenne muscular dystrophy and spinal muscular atrophy. *Dev Med Child Neurol,* 40, 12-20.

BLAKE, D. J., LOVE, D. R., TINSLEY, J., MORRIS, G. E., TURLEY, H., GATTER, K., DICKSON, G., EDWARDS, Y. H. & DAVIES, K. E. (1992). Characterization of a 4.8kb transcript from the Duchenne muscular dystrophy locus expressed in Schwannoma cells. *Hum Mol Genet,* 1, 103-9

BLAKE, D. J., HAWKES, R., BENSON, M. A. & BEESLEY, P. W. (1999). Different dystrophin-like complexes are expressed in neurons and glia. *J Cell Biol,* 147, 645-58.

BLAKE, D. J. & KROGER, S. (2000). The neurobiology of duchenne muscular dystrophy: learning lessons from muscle? *Trends Neurosci,* 23, 92-9.

BLAKE, D.J., WEIR, A., NEWEY, S.E. & DAVIES, K.E. (2002). Function and genetics of dystrophin and dystrophin-related proteins in muscle. *Physiol Rev* 82 (2) 291-329.

BORK, P. & SUDOL, M. (1994). The WW domain: a signalling site in dystrophin? *Trends Biochem Sci,* 19, 531-3.

BRESOLIN, N., CASTELLI, E., COMI, G. P., FELISARI, G., BARDONI, A., PERANI, D., GRASSI, F., TURCONI, A., MAZZUCCHELLI, F., GALLOTTI, D. & ET AL. (1994). Cognitive impairment in Duchenne muscular dystrophy. *Neuromuscul Disord,* 4, 359-69.

BRUNIG, I., SUTER, A., KNUESEL, I., LUSCHER, B. & FRITSCHY, J. M. (2002). GABAergic terminals are required for postsynaptic clustering of dystrophin but not of GABA(A) receptors and gephyrin. *J Neurosci,* 22, 4805-13.

BULFIELD, G., SILLER, W. G., WIGHT, P. A. & MOORE, K. J. (1984). X chromosome-linked muscular dystrophy (mdx) in the mouse. *Proc Natl Acad Sci U S A,* 81, 1189-92.

BURMEISTER, M., MONACO, A. P., GILLARD, E. F., VAN OMMEN, G. J., AFFARA, N. A., FERGUSON-SMITH, M. A., KUNKEL, L. M. & LEHRACH, H. (1988). A 10-megabase physical map of human Xp21, including the Duchenne muscular dystrophy gene. *Genomics,* 2, 189-202.

BYERS, T. J., HUSAIN-CHISHTI, A., DUBREUIL, R. R., BRANTON, D. & GOLDSTEIN, L. S. (1989). Sequence similarity of the amino-terminal domain of Drosophila beta spectrin to alpha actinin and dystrophin. *J Cell Biol,* 109, 1633-41.

BYERS, T.J., LIDOV, H.G. & KUNKEL, L.M. (1993). An alternative dystrophin transcript specific to peripheral nerve. *Nat Genet* 4 (1) 77-81.

CARRETTA, D., SANTARELLI, M., VANNI, D., CARRAI, R., SBRICCOLI, A., PINTO, F. & MINCIACCHI, D. (2001). The organisation of spinal projecting brainstem neurons in an animal model of muscular dystrophy. A retrograde tracing study on mdx mutant mice. *Brain Res,* 895, 213-22.

CARRETTA, D., SANTARELLI, M., VANNI, D., CIABATTI, S., SBRICCOLI, A., PINTO, F. & MINCIACCHI, D. (2003). Cortical and brainstem neurons containing calcium-binding proteins in a murine model of Duchenne's muscular dystrophy: selective changes in the sensorimotor cortex. *J Comp Neurol,* 456, 48-59.

CARRETTA, D., SANTARELLI, M., SBRICCOLI, A., PINTO, F., CATINI, C. & MINCIACCHI, D. (2004). Spatial analysis reveals alterations of parvalbumin- and calbindin-positive local circuit neurons in the cerebral cortex of mutant mdx mice. *Brain Res,* 1016, 1-11.

CASTLES, A. & COLTHEART, M. (1993). Varieties of developmental dyslexia. *Cognition,* 47, 149-80.

CAVALDESI, M., MACCHIA, G., BARCA, S., DEFILIPPI, P., TARONE, G. & PETRUCCI, T. C. (1999). Association of the dystroglycan complex isolated from bovine brain synaptosomes with proteins involved in signal transduction. *J Neurochem,* 72, 1648-55.

CECCARINI, M., MACIOCE, P., PANETTA, B. & PETRUCCI, T. C. (2002). Expression of dystrophin-associated proteins during neuronal differentiation of P19 embryonal carcinoma cells. *Neuromuscul Disord,* 12, 36-48.

CHAMBERLAIN, J. S., GRANT, S. G., REEVES, A. A., MULLINS, L. J., STEPHENSON, D. A., HOFFMAN, E. P., MONACO, A. P., KUNKEL, L. M., CASKEY, C. T. & CHAPMAN, V. M. (1987). Regional localization of the murine Duchenne muscular dystrophy gene on the mouse X chromosome. *Somat Cell Mol Genet,* 13, 671-8.

CHAMBERLAIN, J. S., PEARLMAN, J. A., MUZNY, D. M., GIBBS, R. A., RANIER, J. E., CASKEY, C. T. & REEVES, A. A. (1988). Expression of the murine Duchenne muscular dystrophy gene in muscle and brain. *Science,* 239, 1416-8.

CHELLY, J., KAPLAN, J-C., MAIRE, P., GAUTRON, S. & KAHN, A. (1988). Transcription of the dystrophin gene in human muscle and non-muscle tissues. *Nature* 333, 858-60.

CHELLY, J., CONCORDET, J. P., KAPLAN, J. C. & KAHN, A. (1989). Illegitimate transcription: transcription of any gene in any cell type. *Proc Natl Acad Sci U S A,* 86, 2617-21.

CIBIS, G.W., FITZGERALD, K.W., HARRIS, D.J., ROTHBERG, P.G. & RUPANI, M. (1993). The effect of dystrophin gene mutations on the ERG in mice and humans. *Invest Ophthalmol Vis Sci* 34 (13) 3646-52.

COLLINS, C. A. & MORGAN, J. E. (2003). Duchenne's muscular dystrophy: animal models used to investigate pathogenesis and develop therapeutic strategies. *Int J Exp Pathol,* 84, 165-72.

CONNERS, K. (2000). *Technical manual for the Conners rating scales - revised,* North Tonawanda, Multi-Health Systems Inc.

CONNORS, N. C., ADAMS, M. E., FROEHNER, S. C. & KOFUJI, P. (2004). The potassium channel Kir4.1 associates with the dystrophin-glycoprotein complex via alpha-syntrophin in glia. *J Biol Chem,* 279, 28387-92.

COSTA, M.F., OLIVEIRA, A.G., FEITOSA-SANTANA, C., ZATZ, M. & VENTURA, D.F. (2007). Red-green colour vision impairment in Duchenne muscular dystrophy. *Am J Hum Genet* 80 (6) 1064-75.

COTTON, S., CROWE, S. & VOUDOURIS, N. (1998). Neuropsychological Profile of Duchenne Muscular Dystrophy. *Child Neuropsychology,* 4, 110-17.

COTTON, S., VOUDOURIS, N. J. & GREENWOOD, K. M. (2001). Intelligence and Duchenne muscular dystrophy: full-scale, verbal, and performance intelligence quotients. *Dev Med Child Neurol,* 43, 497-501.

COTTON, S. M., VOUDOURIS, N. J. & GREENWOOD, K. M. (2005). Association between intellectual functioning and age in children and young adults with Duchenne muscular dystrophy: further results from a meta-analysis. *Dev Med Child Neurol,* 47, 257-65.

CROSS, R. A., STEWART, M. & KENDRICK-JONES, J. (1990). Structural predictions for the central domain of dystrophin. *FEBS Lett,* 262, 87-92.

CULLIGAN, K. G., MACKEY, A. J., FINN, D. M., MAGUIRE, P. B. & OHLENDIECK, K. (1998). Role of dystrophin isoforms and associated proteins in muscular dystrophy (review). *Int J Mol Med,* 2, 639-48.

CULLIGAN, K., GLOVER, L., DOWLING, P. & OHLENDIECK, K. (2001). Brain dystrophin-glycoprotein complex: persistent expression of beta-dystroglycan, impaired oligomerization of Dp71 and up-regulation of utrophins in animal models of muscular dystrophy. *BMC Cell Biol,* 2, 2.

CULLIGAN, K. & OHLENDIECK, K. (2002). Diversity of the Brain Dystrophin-Glycoprotein Complex. *J Biomed Biotechnol,* 2, 31-36.

CYRULNIK, S. E. & HINTON, V. J. (2008). Duchenne muscular dystrophy: A cerebellar disorder? *Neurosci Biobehav Rev,* 32, 486-96.

D'ANGELO, M. G. & BRESOLIN, N. (2003). Report of the 95th European Neuromuscular Centre (ENMC) sponsored international workshop cognitive impairment in neuromuscular disorders, Naarden, The Netherlands, 13-15 July 2001. *Neuromuscul Disord,* 13, 72-9.

D'SOUZA, V. N., NGUYEN, T. M., MORRIS, G. E., KARGES, W., PILLERS, D. A. & RAY, P. N. (1995). A novel dystrophin isoform is required for normal retinal electrophysiology. *Hum Mol Genet,* 4, 837-42.

DALKILIC, I. & KUNKEL, L. M. (2003). Muscular dystrophies: genes to pathogenesis. *Curr Opin Genet Dev,* 13, 231-8.

DALLERAC, G., PERRONNET, C., CHAGNEAU, C., LEBLANC-VEYRAC, P., SAMSON-DESVIGNES, N., PELTEKIAN, E., DANOS, O., GARCIA LAROCHE, S., BILLARD, J.M. & VAILLEND, C. (2011). Rescue of a dystrophin-like protein by exon skipping normalizes synaptic plasticity in the hippocampus of the mdx mouse. *Neurobiol Dis* 43(3) 635-41.

DAOUD, F., ANGEARD, N., DEMERRE, B., MARTIE, I., BENYAOU, R., LETURCQ, F., COSSÉE, M., DEBURGRAVE, N., SAILLOUR, Y., TUFFERY, S., URTIZBEREA, A., TOUTAIN, A., ECHENNE, B., FRISCHMAN, M., MAYER, M., DESGUERRE, I., ESTOURNET, B., RÉVEILLÈRE, C., PENISSON-BESNIER, CUISSET, J.M., KAPLAN, J.C., HÉRON, D., RIVIER, F. & CHELLY, J. (2009). Analysis of Dp71 contribution in the severity of mental retardation through comparison of Duchenne and Becker patients differing by mutation consequences on Dp71 expression. *Hum Mol Genet* 18 (20) 3779-94.

DE SARRO, G., IBBADU, G. F., MARRA, R., ROTIROTI, D., LOIACONO, A., DONATO DI PAOLA, E. & RUSSO, E. (2004). Seizure susceptibility to various convulsant stimuli in dystrophin-deficient mdx mice. *Neurosci Res,* 50, 37-44.

DESMOND, J. E., GABRIELI, J. D., WAGNER, A. D., GINIER, B. L. & GLOVER, G. H. (1997) Lobular patterns of cerebellar activation in verbal working-memory and finger-tapping tasks as revealed by functional *MRI. J Neurosci, 17, 9675-85.*

DI LAZZARO, V., RESTUCCIA, D., SERVIDEI, S., NARDONE, R., OLIVIERO, A., PROFICE, P., MANGIOLA, F., TONALI, P. & ROTHWELL, J. C. (1998). Functional involvement of cerebral cortex in Duchenne muscular dystrophy. *Muscle Nerve,* 21, 662-4.

DORMAN, C., HURLEY, A. D. & D'AVIGNON, J. (1988). Language and learning disorders of older boys with Duchenne muscular dystrophy. *Dev Med Child Neurol,* 30, 316-27.

DUBOWITZ, V. & CROME, L. (1969). The central nervous system in Duchenne muscular dystrophy. *Brain,* 92, 805-808.

DUCHENNE, G. (1868). Recherche sur la paralysie musculaire pseudo-hypertrophique ou paralysie myosclerosique. *Archives of General Medicine,* 2, 5.

DUNN, J. F. & ZAIM-WADGHIRI, Y. (1999). Quantitative magnetic resonance imaging of the mdx mouse model of Duchenne muscular dystrophy. *Muscle Nerve,* 22, 1367-71.

DURBEEJ, M. & CAMPBELL, K. P. (2002). Muscular dystrophies involving the dystrophin-glycoprotein complex: an overview of current mouse models. *Curr Opin Genet Dev,* 12, 349-61.

EMERY, A. E. (2002). Muscular dystrophy into the new millennium. *Neuromuscul Disord,* 12, 343-9.

EMERY, A. E. (2002a). The muscular dystrophies. *Lancet,* 359, 687-95.

ESSEX, C. & ROPER, H. (2001). Lesson of the week: late diagnosis of Duchenne's muscular dystrophy presenting as global developmental delay. *BMJ,* 323, 37-38.

ETEMADIFAR, M. & MOLAEI, S. (2004). Epilepsy in Boys with Duchenne Muscular Dystrophy. *Journal of Research in Medical Sciences,* 3, 14-17.

FABBRIZIO, E., BONET-KERRACHE, A., LIMAS, F., HUGON, G. & MORNET, D. (1995). Dystrophin, the protein that promotes membrane resistance. *Biochem Biophys Res Commun,* 213, 295-301.

FERLINI, A., SEWRY, C., MELIS, M. A., MATEDDU, A. & MUNTONI, F. (1999). X-linked dilated cardiomyopathy and the dystrophin gene. *Neuromuscul Disord,* 9, 339-46.

FITZPATRICK, C., BARRY, C. & GARVEY, C. (1986). Psychiatric disorder among boys with Duchenne muscular dystrophy. *Dev Med Child Neurol* 28(5):589-95.

FRIGERI, A., NICCHIA, G. P., NICO, B., QUONDAMATTEO, F., HERKEN, R., RONCALI, L. & SVELTO, M. (2001). Aquaporin-4 deficiency in skeletal muscle and brain of dystrophic mdx mice. *Faseb J*, 15, 90-98.

GAULD, L. M., BOYNTON, A., BETTS, G. A. & JOHNSTON, H. (2005). Spirometry is affected by intelligence and behavior in Duchenne muscular dystrophy. *Pediatr Pulmonol*, 40, 408-13.

GEE, S. H., MADHAVAN, R., LEVINSON, S. R., CALDWELL, J. H., SEALOCK, R. & FROEHNER, S. C. (1998). Interaction of muscle and brain sodium channels with multiple members of the syntrophin family of dystrophin-associated proteins. *J Neurosci*, 18, 128-37.

GLAUB, T. & MECHLER, F. (1987). Intellectual function in muscular dystrophies. *Eur Arch Psychiatry Neurol Sci*, 236, 379-82.

GODFRAIND, J.-M., TEKKOK, S. B. & KRNJEVIC, K. (1998). Hypoxia on hippocampal slices from mice deficient in dystrophin (mdx) and dystrophin isoforms (mdx3cv). *Soc Neurosci Abst*

GODFRAIND, J.-M., TEKKOK, S. B. & KRNJEVIC, K. (2000). Hypoxia on Hippocampal Slices From Mice Deficient in Dystrophin (mdx) and Isoforms (mdx3cv). *J Cereb Blood Flow Metab*, 20, 145-152.

GOODWIN, F., MUNTONI, F. & DUBOWITZ, V. (1997). Epilepsy in Duchenne and Becker muscular dystrophies. *Eur J Paediatr Neurol*, 1, 115-9.

GORECKI, D., GENG, Y., THOMAS, K., HUNT, S. P., BARNARD, E. A. & BARNARD, P. J. (1991). Expression of the dystrophin gene in mouse and rat brain. *Neuroreport*, 2, 773-6.

GORECKI, D. C., MONACO, A. P., DERRY, J. M., WALKER, A. P., BARNARD, E. A. & BARNARD, P. J. (1992). Expression of four alternative dystrophin transcripts in brain regions regulated by different promoters. *Hum Mol Genet*, 1, 505-10.

GORECKI, D. C. & BARNARD, E. A. (1995). Specific expression of G-dystrophin (Dp71) in the brain. *Neuroreport*, 6, 893-6.

GORECKI, D. C., ABDULRAZZAK, H., LUKASIUK, K. & BARNARD, E. A. (1997). Differential expression of syntrophins and analysis of alternatively spliced dystrophin transcripts in the mouse brain. *Eur J Neurosci*, 9, 965-76.

GORECKI, D. C., LUKASIUK, K., SZKLARCZYK, A. & KACZMAREK, L. (1998). Kainate-evoked changes in dystrophin messenger RNA levels in the rat hippocampus. *Neuroscience*, 84, 467-77.

GRACIOTTI, L., MINELLI, A., MINCIACCHI, D., PROCOPIO, A. & FULGENZI, G. (2008). GABAergic miniature spontaneous activity is increased in the CA1 hippocampal region of dystrophic mdx mice. *Neuromuscul Disord* 18(3) 220-26.

GRADY, R.M., WOZNIAK, D.F., OHLEMILLER, K.K. & SANES, J.R. (2006). Cerebellar synaptic defects and abnormal motor behavior in mice lacking alpha- and beta-dystrobrevin. *J Neurosci* 26(11) 2841-51.

GREENBERG, D. S., SCHATZ, Y., LEVY, Z., PIZZO, P., YAFFE, D. & NUDEL, U. (1996). Reduced levels of dystrophin associated proteins in the brains of mice deficient for Dp71. *Hum Mol Genet*, 5, 1299-303.

GRIFFIN, J., NICHOLLS, A., MORTSHIRE-SMITH, R., RAE, C. & NICHOLSON, J. (1999). High resolution magic angle spinning ^{1}H NMR of cerebral tissue as applied to a mouse model of Duchenne muscular dystrophy [abstract]. *International Society Magnetic Resonance Medicine.* British Chapter.

GRIFFIN, J. L., WILLIAMS, H. J., SANG, E., CLARKE, K., RAE, C. & NICHOLSON, J. K. (2001). Metabolic profiling of genetic disorders: a multitissue (1)H nuclear magnetic resonance spectroscopic and pattern recognition study into dystrophic tissue. *Anal Biochem,* 293, 16-21.

HAMED, S. A. & HOFFMAN, E. P. (2006). Automated sequence screening of the entire dystrophin cDNA in Duchenne dystrophy: point mutation detection. *Am J Med Genet B Neuropsychiatr Genet,* 141, 44-50.

HASHIDA-OKUMURA, A., OKUMURA, N., IWAMATSU, A., BUIJS, R. M., ROMIJN, H. J. & NAGAI, K. (1999). Interaction of neuronal nitric-oxide synthase with alpha1-syntrophin in rat brain. *J Biol Chem,* 274, 11736-41.

HENDRIKSEN, J. G. & VLES, J. S. (2006). Are males with Duchenne muscular dystrophy at risk for reading disabilities? *Pediatr Neurol,* 34, 296-300.

HENDRIKSEN, J.G. & VLES, J.S. (2008). Neuropsychiatric disorders in males with duchenne muscular dystrophy: frequency rate of attention-deficit hyperactivity disorder (ADHD), autism spectrum disorder, and obsessive--compulsive disorder. *J Child Neurol* 23(5) 477-81.

HINTON, V. J., DE VIVO, D. C., NEREO, N. E., GOLDSTEIN, E. & STERN, Y. (2000). Poor verbal working memory across intellectual level in boys with Duchenne dystrophy. *Neurology,* 54, 2127-32.

HINTON, V. J., DE VIVO, D. C., NEREO, N. E., GOLDSTEIN, E. & STERN, Y. (2001). Selective deficits in verbal working memory associated with a known genetic etiology: the neuropsychological profile of duchenne muscular dystrophy. *J Int Neuropsychol Soc,* 7, 45-54.

HOFFMAN, E. P., BROWN, R. H., JR. & KUNKEL, L. M. (1987). Dystrophin: the protein product of the Duchenne muscular dystrophy locus. *Cell,* 51, 919-28.

HOFFMAN, E. P. & KUNKEL, L. M. (1989). Dystrophin abnormalities in Duchenne/Becker muscular dystrophy. *Neuron,* 2, 1019-29.

HOLDER, E., MAEDA, M. & BIES, R. D. (1996). Expression and regulation of the dystrophin Purkinje promoter in human skeletal muscle, heart, and brain. *Hum Genet,* 97, 232-9.

HOPF, F. W. & STEINHARDT, R. A. (1992). Regulation of intracellular free calcium in normal and dystrophic mouse cerebellar neurons. *Brain Res,* 578, 49-54.

HSU, Y. D. (2004). Muscular dystrophy: from pathogenesis to strategy. *Acta Neurol Taiwan,* 13, 50-8.

HUANG, X., POY, F., ZHANG, R., JOACHIMIAK, A., SUDOL, M. & ECK, M. J. (2000). Structure of a WW domain containing fragment of dystrophin in complex with beta-dystroglycan. *Nat Struct Biol,* 7, 634-8.

HUARD, J. & TREMBLAY, J. P. (1992) Localization of dystrophin in the Purkinje cells of normal mice. *Neurosci Lett,* 137, 105-8.

IANNELLO, R. C., MAR, J. H. & ORDAHL, C. P. (1991). Characterization of a promoter element required for transcription in myocardial cells. *J Biol Chem,* 266, 3309-16.

ILARRAZA-LOMELI, R., CISNEROS-VEGA, B., CERVANTES-GOMEZ, M.D.E. L., MORNET, D. & MONTAÑEZ, C. (2007). Dp71, utrophin and beta-dystroglycan expression and distribution in PC12/L6 cell cocultures. *NEUROREPORT* 18(16):1657-61.

ISHIKAWA-SAKURAI, M., YOSHIDA, M., IMAMURA, M., DAVIES, K. E. & OZAWA, E. (2004). ZZ domain is essentially required for the physiological binding of dystrophin and utrophin to beta-dystroglycan. *Hum Mol Genet,* 13, 693-702.

ITO, K., SAWADA, Y., SUGIYAMA, Y., SUZUKI, H., HANANO, M. & IGA, T. (1994). Linear relationship between GABAA receptor occupancy of muscimol and glucose metabolic response in the conscious mouse brain. Clinical implication based on comparison with benzodiazepine receptor agonist. *Drug Metab Dispos,* 22, 50-4.

IVES, J. H., DREWERY, D. L. & THOMPSON, C. L. (2002). Neuronal activity and its influence on developmentally regulated GABA(A) receptor expression in cultured mouse cerebellar granule cells. *Neuropharmacology,* 43, 715-25.

JAGADHA, V. & BECKER, L. E. (1988). Brain morphology in Duchenne muscular dystrophy: a Golgi study. *Pediatr Neurol,* 4, 87-92.

JANCSIK, V. & HAJOS, F. (1998). Differential distribution of dystrophin in postsynaptic densities of spine synapses. *Neuroreport,* 9, 2249-51.

JUEPTNER, M. & WEILLER, C. (1995). Review: does measurement of regional cerebral blood flow reflect synaptic activity? Implications for PET and fMRI. *Neuroimage,* 2, 148-56.

JUNG, D., FILLIOL, D., METZ-BOUTIGUE, M. H. & RENDON, A. (1993). Characterization and subcellular localization of the dystrophin-protein 71 (Dp71) from brain. *Neuromuscul Disord,* 3, 515-8.

JUNG, D., YANG, B., MEYER, J., CHAMBERLAIN, J. S. & CAMPBELL, K. P. (1995). Identification and characterization of the dystrophin anchoring site on beta-dystroglycan. *J Biol Chem,* 270, 27305-10.

KAMAKURA, K., TADANO, Y., KAWAI, M., ISHIURA, S., NAKAMURA, R., MIYAMOTO, K., NAGATA, N. & SUGITA, H. (1994). Dystrophin-related protein is found in the central nervous system of mice at various developmental stages, especially at the postsynaptic membrane. *J Neurosci Res,* 37, 728-34.

KAPLAN, L. C., OSBORNE, P. & ELIAS, E. (1986). The diagnosis of muscular dystrophy in patients referred for language delay. *J Child Psychol Psychiatry,* 27, 545-9.

KARAGAN, N. J. & ZELLWEGER, H. U. (1976). IQ studies in Duchenne muscular dystrophy II: test-retest performance. *Developmental Medicine and Child Neurology,* 18, 251.

KARAGAN, N. J. & ZELLWEGER, H. U. (1978). Early verbal disability in children with Duchenne muscular dystrophy. *Dev Med Child Neurol,* 20, 435-41.

KARAGAN, N. J. (1979). Intellectual functioning in Duchenne muscular dystrophy: a review. *Psychol Bull,* 86, 250-9.

KARAGAN, N. J., RICHMAN, L. C. & SORENSEN, J. P. (1980). Analysis of verbal disability in Duchenne muscular dystrophy. *J Nerv Ment Dis,* 168, 419-23.

KATO, T., NISHINA, M., MATSUSHITA, K., HORI, E., AKABOSHI, S. & TAKASHIMA, S. (1997). Increased cerebral choline-compounds in Duchenne muscular dystrophy. *Neuroreport,* 8, 1435-7.

KENWRICK, S., PATTERSON, M., SPEER, A., FISCHBECK, K. & DAVIES, K. (1987). Molecular analysis of the Duchenne muscular dystrophy region using pulsed field gel electrophoresis. *Cell,* 48, 351-7.

KHAN, Y. & HECKMATT, J. Z. (1994). Obstructive apnoeas in Duchenne muscular dystrophy. *Thorax,* 49, 157-61.

KIM, T. W., WU, K., XU, J. L. & BLACK, I. B. (1992). Detection of dystrophin in the postsynaptic density of rat brain and deficiency in a mouse model of Duchenne muscular dystrophy. *Proc Natl Acad Sci U S A,* 89, 11642-4.

KIM, T. W., WU, K. & BLACK, I. B. (1995). Deficiency of brain synaptic dystrophin in human Duchenne muscular dystrophy. *Ann Neurol,* 38, 446-9.

KINGSTON, H. M., SARFARAZI, M., THOMAS, N. S. & HARPER, P. S. (1984). Localisation of the Becker muscular dystrophy gene on the short arm of the X chromosome by linkage to cloned DNA sequences. *Hum Genet,* 67, 6-17.

KNUESEL, I., MASTROCOLA, M., ZUELLIG, R. A., BORNHAUSER, B., SCHAUB, M. C. & FRITSCHY, J. M. (1999). Short communication: altered synaptic clustering of GABAA receptors in mice lacking dystrophin (mdx mice). *Eur J Neurosci,* 11, 4457-62.

KNUESEL, I., ZUELLIG, R. A., SCHAUB, M. C. & FRITSCHY, J. M. (2001). Alterations in dystrophin and utrophin expression parallel the reorganization of GABAergic synapses in a mouse model of temporal lobe epilepsy. *Eur J Neurosci,* 13, 1113-24.

KOENIG, M., HOFFMAN, E. P., BERTELSON, C. J., MONACO, A. P., FEENER, C. & KUNKEL, L. M. (1987). Complete cloning of the Duchenne muscular dystrophy (DMD) cDNA and preliminary genomic organization of the DMD gene in normal and affected individuals. *Cell,* 50, 509-17.

KOENIG, M., MONACO, A. P. & KUNKEL, L. M. (1988). The complete sequence of dystrophin predicts a rod-shaped cytoskeletal protein. *Cell,* 53, 219-26

KOENIG, M. & KUNKEL, L. M. (1990). Detailed analysis of the repeat domain of dystrophin reveals four potential hinge segments that may confer flexibility. *J Biol Chem,* 265, 4560-6.

KOMOTO, J., USUI, S., OTSUKI, S. & TERAO, A. (1984). Infantile autism and Duchenne muscular dystrophy. *J Autism Dev Disord,* 14, 191-5.

KUEH, S.L., HEAD, S.I. & MORLEY, J.W. (2008). GABA(A) receptor expression and inhibitory post-synaptic currents in cerebellar Purkinje cells in dystrophin-deficient mdx mice. *Clin Exp Pharmacol Physiol* 35(2):207-10.

KUEH, S.L., DEMPSTER, J., HEAD, S.I. & MORLEY, J.W. (2011). Reduced postsynaptic GABAA receptor number and enhanced gaboxadol induced change in holding currents in Purkinje cells of the dystrophin-deficient mdx mouse. *Neurobiol Dis* 43(3):558-64.

KUNKEL, L. M., MONACO, A. P., BERTELSON, C. J. & COLLETTI, C. A. (1986). Molecular genetics of Duchenne muscular dystrophy. *Cold Spring Harb Symp Quant Biol,* 51 Pt 1, 349-51.

LABARQUE, V., FRESON, K., THYS, C., WITTEVRONGEL, C., HOYLAERTS, M.F., DE VOS, R., GOEMANS, N. & VAN GEET, C. (2008). Increased Gs signalling in platelets and impaired collagen activation, due to a defect in the dystrophin gene, result in increased blood loss during spinal surgery. *Hum Mol Genet* 17(3):357-66.

LEDERFEIN, D., LEVY, Z., AUGIER, N., MORNET, D., MORRIS, G., FUCHS, O., YAFFE, D. & NUDEL, U. (1992). A 71-kilodalton protein is a major product of the Duchenne muscular dystrophy gene in brain and other nonmuscle tissues. *Proc Natl Acad Sci U S A,* 89, 5346-50.

LEDERFEIN, D., YAFFE, D. & NUDEL, U. (1993). A housekeeping type promoter, located in the 3' region of the Duchenne muscular dystrophy gene, controls the expression of Dp71, a major product of the gene. *Hum Mol Genet,* 2, 1883-8.

LEE, J. S., PFUND, Z., JUHASZ, C., BEHEN, M. E., MUZIK, O., CHUGANI, D. C., NIGRO, M. A. & CHUGANI, H. T. (2002). Altered regional brain glucose metabolism in Duchenne muscular dystrophy: a pet study. *Muscle Nerve,* 26, 506-12.

LEVI, S., GRADY, R. M., HENRY, M. D., CAMPBELL, K. P., SANES, J. R. & CRAIG, A. M. (2002). Dystroglycan is selectively associated with inhibitory GABAergic synapses but is dispensable for their differentiation. *J Neurosci,* 22, 4274-85.

LEVISOHN, L., CRONIN-GOLOMB, A. & SCHMAHMANN, J. D. (2000). Neuropsychological consequences of cerebellar tumour resection in children: cerebellar cognitive affective syndrome in a paediatric population. *Brain,* 123 (Pt 5), 1041-50.

LIDOV, H. G., BYERS, T. J., WATKINS, S. C. & KUNKEL, L. M. (1990). Localization of dystrophin to postsynaptic regions of central nervous system cortical neurons. *Nature,* 348, 725-8.

LIDOV, H. G., BYERS, T. J. & KUNKEL, L. M. (1993). The distribution of dystrophin in the murine central nervous system: an immunocytochemical study. *Neuroscience,* 54, 167-87.

LIDOV, H. G., SELIG, S. & KUNKEL, L. M. (1995). Dp140: a novel 140 kDa CNS transcript from the dystrophin locus. *Hum Mol Genet,* 4, 329-35.

LIDOV, H. G. (1996). Dystrophin in the nervous system. *Brain Pathol,* 6, 63-77.

MANNI, R., ZUCCA, C., GALIMBERTI, C. A., OTTOLINI, A., CERVERI, I., BRUSCHI, C., ZOIA, M. C., LANZI, G. & TARTARA, A. (1991). Nocturnal sleep and oxygen balance in Duchenne muscular dystrophy. A clinical and polygraphic 2-year follow-up study. *Eur Arch Psychiatry Clin Neurosci,* 240, 255-7.

MEHLER, M. F., HAAS, K. Z., KESSLER, J. A. & STANTON, P. K. (1992). Enhanced sensitivity of hippocampal pyramidal neurons from mdx mice to hypoxia-induced loss of synaptic transmission. *Proc Natl Acad Sci U S A,* 89, 2461-5.

MEHLER, M. F. (2000). Brain dystrophin, neurogenetics and mental retardation. *Brain Res Brain Res Rev,* 32, 277-307.

MELO, M., LAURIANO, V., GENTIL, V., EGGERS, S., DEL BIANCO, S. S., GIMENEZ, P. R., AKIYAMA, J., OKABAIASHI, H., FROTA-PESSOA, O., PASSOS-BUENO, M. R. & ET AL. (1995). Becker and limb-girdle muscular dystrophies: a psychiatric and intellectual level comparative study. *Am J Med Genet,* 60, 33-8.

MICHALAK, M. & OPAS, M. (2001). *Duchenne muscular dystrophy,* Chichester, John Wiley & Sons LTD.

MILNER, R. E., BUSAAN, J. L., HOLMES, C. F., WANG, J. H. & MICHALAK, M. (1993). Phosphorylation of dystrophin. The carboxyl-terminal region of dystrophin is a substrate for in vitro phosphorylation by p34cdc2 protein kinase. *J Biol Chem,* 268, 21901-5.

MIRANDA, R., SÉBRIÉ, C., DEGROUARD, J., GILLET, B., JAILLARD, D., LAROCHE, S., VAILLEND, C. (2009). Reorganization of inhibitory synapses and increased PSD length of perforated excitatory synapses in hippocampal area CA1 of dystrophin-deficient mdx mice. *Cereb Cortex* 19(4):876-88.

MIRANDA, R., NUDEL, U., LAROCHE, S. & VAILLEND, C. (2011). Altered presynaptic ultrastructure in excitatory hippocampal synapses of mice lacking dystrophins Dp427 or Dp71. *Neurobiol Dis* 43(1):134-41,

MISURI, G., LANINI, B., GIGLIOTTI, F., IANDELLI, I., PIZZI, A., BERTOLINI, M. G. & SCANO, G. (2000). Mechanism of CO(2) retention in patients with neuromuscular disease. *Chest,* 117, 447-53.

MIYATAKE, M., MIIKE, T., ZHAO, J. E., YOSHIOKA, K., UCHINO, M. & USUKU, G. (1991). Dystrophin: localization and presumed function. *Muscle Nerve,* 14, 113-9.

MOHAMED, K., APPLETON, R. & NICOLAIDES, P. (2000). Delayed diagnosis of Duchenne muscular dystrophy. *Eur J Paediatr Neurol,* 4, 219-23.

MOUKHLES, H. & CARBONETTO, S. (2001). Dystroglycan contributes to the formation of multiple dystrophin-like complexes in brain. *J Neurochem,* 78, 824-34.

MUNTONI, F., MATEDDU, A. & SERRA, G. (1991). Passive avoidance behaviour deficit in the mdx mouse. *Neuromuscul Disord,* 1, 121-3.

MUNTONI, F., CAU, M., GANAU, A., CONGIU, R., ARVEDI, G., MATEDDU, A., MARROSU, M. G., CIANCHETTI, C., REALDI, G., CAO, A. & ET AL. (1993). Brief report: deletion of the dystrophin muscle-promoter region associated with X-linked dilated cardiomyopathy. *N Engl J Med,* 329, 921-5.

MUNTONI, F., TORELLI, S. & FERLINI, A. (2003). Dystrophin and mutations: one gene, several proteins, multiple phenotypes. *Lancet Neurol,* 2, 731-40.

NEELY, J. D., AMIRY-MOGHADDAM, M., OTTERSEN, O. P., FROEHNER, S. C., AGRE, P. & ADAMS, M. E. (2001). Syntrophin-dependent expression and localization of Aquaporin-4 water channel protein. *Proc Natl Acad Sci U S A,* 98, 14108-13.

NICCHIA, G.P., NICO, B., CAMASSA, L.M., MOLA, M.G., LOH, N., DERMIETZEL, R., SPRAY, D.C., SVELTO, M. & FRIGERI, A. (2004). The role of aquaporin-4 in the blood-brain barrier development and integrity: studies in animal and cell culture models. *Neuroscience* 129(4):935-45.

NICCHIA, G.P., ROSSI, A., NUDEL, U., SVELTO, M. & FRIGERI, A. (2008). Dystrophin-dependent and -independent AQP4 pools are expressed in the mouse brain. *Glia* 56(8):869-76.

NICO, B., FRIGERI, A., NICCHIA, G. P., CORSI, P., RIBATTI, D., QUONDAMATTEO, F., HERKEN, R., GIROLAMO, F., MARZULLO, A., SVELTO, M. & RONCALI, L. (2003). Severe alterations of endothelial and glial cells in the blood-brain barrier of dystrophic mdx mice. *Glia,* 42, 235-51.

NICOLSON, R. I., FAWCETT, A. J., BERRY, E. L., JENKINS, I. H., DEAN, P. & BROOKS, D. J. (1999). Association of abnormal cerebellar activation with motor learning difficulties in dyslexic adults. *Lancet,* 353, 1662-7.

NUDEL, U., ROBZYK, K. & YAFFE, D. (1988). Expression of the putative Duchenne muscular dystrophy gene in differentiated myogenic cell cultures and in the brain. *Nature,* 331, 635-8.

NUSSER, Z., CULL-CANDY, S. & FARRANT, M. (1997) Differences in synaptic GABA(A) receptor number underlie variation in GABA mini amplitude. *Neuron,* 19, 697-709.

O'BRIEN, K. F. & KUNKEL, L. M. (2001). Dystrophin and muscular dystrophy: past, present, and future. *Mol Genet Metab,* 74, 75-88.

OGASAWARA, A. (1989). Similarity of IQs of siblings with Duchenne progressive muscular dystrophy. *Am J Ment Retard,* 93, 548-50.

OGASAWARA, A. (1989a). Downward shift in IQ in persons with Duchenne muscular dystrophy compared to those with spinal muscular atrophy. *Am J Ment Retard,* 93, 544-7.

PALUMBO, D., PANDYA, S., MOXLEY, R. & SILVERSTEIN, S. (1996). Cognitive Dysfunction in Boys with Duchenne Muscular Dystrophy. *Archives of Clinical Neuropsychology,* 11, 431.

PARTRIDGE, T. (1991). Animal models of muscular dystrophy--what can they teach us? *Neuropathol Appl Neurobiol,* 17, 353-63.

PERRONNET, C. & VAILLEND, C. (2010). Dystrophins, utrophins, and associated scaffolding complexes: role in mammalian brain and implications for therapeutic strategies. J *Biomed Biotechnol* 2010:849426.

PETROF, B. J. (2002). Molecular pathophysiology of myofiber injury in deficiencies of the dystrophin-glycoprotein complex. *Am J Phys Med Rehabil,* 81, S162-74.

PILLERS, D.A., BULMAN, D.E., WELEBER, R.G., SIGESMUND, D.A., MUSARELLA, M.A., POWELL, B.R., MURPHEY, W.H., WESTALL, C., PANTON, C., BECKER, L.E., WORTON, R.G. & RAY, P.N. (1993). Dystrophin expression in the human retina is required for normal function as defined by electroretinography. *Nat Genet* 4(1):82-6.

PONTING, C. P., BLAKE, D. J., DAVIES, K. E., KENDRICK-JONES, J. & WINDER, S. J. (1996). ZZ and TAZ: new putative zinc fingers in dystrophin and other proteins. *Trends Biochem Sci,* 21, 11-13.

POYSKY J. (2007). Behavior patterns in Duchenne muscular dystrophy: report on the Parent Project Muscular Dystrophy behavior workshop 8-9 of December 2006, Philadelphia, USA. *Neuromuscul Disord.* 17(11-12):986-94.

RAE, C., LEE, M. A., DIXON, R. M., BLAMIRE, A. M., THOMPSON, C. H., STYLES, P., TALCOTT, J., RICHARDSON, A. J. & STEIN, J. F. (1998). Metabolic abnormalities in developmental dyslexia detected by 1H magnetic resonance spectroscopy. *Lancet,* 351, 1849-52.

RAE, C., SCOTT, R. B., THOMPSON, C. H., DIXON, R. M., DUMUGHN, I., KEMP, G. J., MALE, A., PIKE, M., STYLES, P. & RADDA, G. K. (1998). Brain biochemistry in Duchenne muscular dystrophy: a 1H magnetic resonance and neuropsychological study. *J Neurol Sci,* 160, 148-57.

RAE, C., LAWRANCE, M. L., DIAS, L. S., PROVIS, T., BUBB, W. A. & BALCAR, V. J. (2000). Strategies for studies of neurotoxic mechanisms involving deficient transport of L-glutamate: antisense knockout in rat brain in vivo and changes in the neurotransmitter metabolism following inhibition of glutamate transport in guinea pig brain slices. *Brain Res Bull,* 53, 373-81.

RAE, C., GRIFFIN, J. L., BLAIR, D. H., BOTHWELL, J. H., BUBB, W. A., MAITLAND, A. & HEAD, S. (2002). Abnormalities in brain biochemistry associated with lack of dystrophin: studies of the mdx mouse. *Neuromuscul Disord,* 12, 121-9.

RANDO, T. A. (2001). The dystrophin-glycoprotein complex, cellular signaling, and the regulation of cell survival in the muscular dystrophies. *Muscle Nerve,* 24, 1575-94.

RAPAPORT, D., LEDERFEIN, D., DEN DUNNEN, J. T., GROOTSCHOLTEN, P. M., VAN OMMEN, G. J., FUCHS, O., NUDEL, U. & YAFFE, D. (1992). Characterization and cell type distribution of a novel, major transcript of the Duchenne muscular dystrophy gene. *Differentiation,* 49, 187-93.

REID, D. T. & RENWICK, R. M. (2001). Relating familial stress to the psychosocial adjustment of adolescents with Duchenne muscular dystrophy. *Int J Rehabil Res,* 24, 83-93.

RENTSCHLER, S., LINN, H., DEININGER, K., BEDFORD, M. T., ESPANEL, X. & SUDOL, M. (1999). The WW domain of dystrophin requires EF-hands region to interact with beta-dystroglycan. *Biol Chem,* 380, 431-42.

ROBERTS, R. G., COFFEY, A. J., BOBROW, M. & BENTLEY, D. R. (1993). Exon structure of the human dystrophin gene. *Genomics,* 16, 536-8.

ROBERTS, R. G. (2001). Dystrophins and dystrobrevins. *Genome Biol,* 2, REVIEWS3006.

ROCCELLA, M., PACE, R. & DE GREGORIO, M. T. (2003). Psychopathological assessment in children affected by Duchenne de Boulogne muscular dystrophy. *Minerva Pediatr,* 55, 267-73, 273-6.

ROSMAN, N. P. & KAKULAS, B. A. (1966). Mental deficiency associated with muscular dystrophy. A neuropathological study. *Brain,* 89, 769-88.

SAVAGE, R. & ADAMS, M. (1979). Cognitive Functioning and Neurological Deficit: Duchenne Muscular Dystrophy and Cerebral Palsy. *Australian Psychologist* 14, 59-75.

SBRICCOLI, A., SANTARELLI, M., CARRETTA, D., PINTO, F., GRANATO, A. & MINCIACCHI, D. (1995). Architectural changes of the cortico-spinal system in the dystrophin defective mdx mouse. *Neurosci Lett,* 200, 53-6.

SCHOFIELD, J. N., BLAKE, D. J., SIMMONS, C., MORRIS, G. E., TINSLEY, J. M., DAVIES, K. E. & EDWARDS, Y. H. (1994). Apo-dystrophin-1 and apo-dystrophin-2, products of the Duchenne muscular dystrophy locus: expression during mouse embryogenesis and in cultured cell lines. *Hum Mol Genet,* 3, 1309-16.

SEKIGUCHI, M. (2005). The role of dystrophin in the central nervous system: a mini review. *Acta Myol,* 24, 93-7.

SEKIGUCHI, M., ZUSHIDA, K., YOSHIDA, M., MAEKAWA, M., KAMICHI, S., YOSHIDA, M., SAHARA, Y., YUASA, S., TAKEDA, S. & WADA, K. (2009). A deficit of brain dystrophin impairs specific amygdala GABAergic transmission and enhances defensive behaviour in mice. *Brain* 132(Pt 1):124-35.

SEPTIEN, L., GRAS, P., BORSOTTI, J. P., GIROUD, M., NIVELON, J. L. & DUMAS, R. (1991). [Mental development in Duchenne muscular dystrophy. Correlation of data of the brain scanner]. *Pediatrie,* 46, 817-9.

SESAY, A. K., ERRINGTON, M. L., LEVITA, L. & BLISS, T. V. (1996). Spatial learning and hippocampal long-term potentiation are not impaired in mdx mice. *Neurosci Lett,* 211, 207-10.

SHAW, R. F. & DREIFUSS, F. E. (1969). Mild and severe forms of X-linked muscular dystrophy. *Arch Neurol,* 20, 451-60.

SICINSKI, P., GENG, Y., RYDER-COOK, A. S., BARNARD, E. A., DARLISON, M. G. & BARNARD, P. J. (1989). The molecular basis of muscular dystrophy in the mdx mouse: a point mutation. *Science,* 244, 1578-80.

SMITH, D. I., ZHU, Y., MCAVOY, S. & KUHN, R. (2006). Common fragile sites, extremely large genes, neural development and cancer. *Cancer Lett,* 232, 48-57.

SMITH, P. E., CALVERLEY, P. M. & EDWARDS, R. H. (1988). Hypoxemia during sleep in Duchenne muscular dystrophy. *Am Rev Respir Dis,* 137, 884-8.

SMITH, R. A., SIBERT, J. R., WALLACE, S. J. & HARPER, P. S. (1989). Early diagnosis and secondary prevention of Duchenne muscular dystrophy. *Arch Dis Child,* 64, 787-90.

SMITH, R. A., SIBERT, J. R. & HARPER, P. S. (1990). Early development of boys with Duchenne muscular dystrophy. *Dev Med Child Neurol,* 32, 519-27.

SOGOS, V., ENNAS, M. G., MUSSINI, I. & GREMO, F. (1997). Effect of dystrophin antisense oligonucleotides on cultured human neurons. *Neurochem Int,* 31, 447-57.

SOGOS, V., REALI, C., FANNI, V., CURTO, M. & GREMO, F. (2003). Dystrophin antisense oligonucleotides decrease expression of nNOS in human neurons. *Brain Res Mol Brain Res,* 118, 52-9.

SOLLEE, N. D., LATHAM, E. E., KINDLON, D. J. & BRESNAN, M. J. (1985). Neuropsychological impairment in Duchenne muscular dystrophy. *J Clin Exp Neuropsychol,* 7, 486-96.

SUGITA, H., ARAHATA, K. & ISHIGURO, T. (1988). Negative immunostaining of Duchenne muscular dystrophy (DMD) and mdx muscle surface membrane with antibody against synthetic peptide fragment predicted from DMD cDNA. *Proc Jap Acad,* 64, 37-39.

SUZUKI, A., YOSHIDA, M., HAYASHI, K., MIZUNO, Y., HAGIWARA, Y. & OZAWA, E. (1994). Molecular organization at the glycoprotein-complex-binding site of dystrophin. Three dystrophin-associated proteins bind directly to the carboxy-terminal portion of dystrophin. *Eur J Biochem,* 220, 283-92.

TAYLOR, P.J., BETTS, G.A., MAROULIS, S., GILISSEN, C., PEDERSEN, R.L., MOWAT, D.R., JOHNSTON, H.M. & BUCKLEY, M.F. (2010). Dystrophin gene mutation location and the risk of cognitive impairment in Duchenne muscular dystrophy. *PLOS ONE* 20;5(1):e8803.

TOKARZ, S. A., DUNCAN, N. M., RASH, S. M., SADEGHI, A., DEWAN, A. K. & PILLERS, D. A. (1998). Redefinition of dystrophin isoform distribution in mouse tissue by RT-PCR implies role in nonmuscle manifestations of duchenne muscular dystrophy. *Mol Genet Metab,* 65, 272-81.

TORRES, L. F. & DUCHEN, L. W. (1987). The mutant mdx: inherited myopathy in the mouse. Morphological studies of nerves, muscles and end-plates. *Brain,* 110 (Pt 2), 269-99.

TRACEY, I., SCOTT, R. B., THOMPSON, C. H., DUNN, J. F., BARNES, P. R., STYLES, P., KEMP, G. J., RAE, C. D., PIKE, M. & RADDA, G. K. (1995). Brain abnormalities in Duchenne muscular dystrophy: phosphorus-31 magnetic resonance spectroscopy and neuropsychological study. *Lancet,* 345, 1260-4.

TRACEY, I., DUNN, J. F. & RADDA, G. K. (1996). Brain metabolism is abnormal in the mdx model of Duchenne muscular dystrophy. *Brain,* 119 (Pt 3), 1039-44.

TRACEY, I., DUNN, J. F., PARKES, H. G. & RADDA, G. K. (1996a). An in vivo and in vitro H-magnetic resonance spectroscopy study of mdx mouse brain: abnormal development or neural necrosis? *J Neurol Sci,* 141, 13-8.

UCHIKAWA, K., LIU, M., HANAYAMA, K., TSUJI, T., FUJIWARA, T. & CHINO, N. (2004). Functional staus and muscle strength in people with Duchenne muscular dystrophy living in the community. *Journal of Rehabilitation Medicine,* 36, 124-129.

UCHINO, M., YOSHIOKA, K., MIIKE, T., TOKUNAGA, M., UYAMA, E., TERAMOTO, H., NAOE, H. & ANDO, M. (1994). Dystrophin and dystrophin-related protein in the brains of normal and mdx mice. *Muscle Nerve,* 17, 533-8.

UEDA, H., BABA, T., KASHIWAGI, K., IIJIMA, H. & OHNO, S. (2000) Dystrobrevin localization in photoreceptor axon terminals and at blood-ocular barrier sites. *Invest Ophthalmol Vis Sci,* 41, 3908-14.

VAILLEND, C., RENDON, A., MISSLIN, R. & UNGERER, A. (1995). Influence of dystrophin-gene mutation on mdx mouse behavior. I. Retention deficits at long delays in spontaneous alternation and bar-pressing tasks. *Behav Genet,* 25, 569-79.

VAILLEND, C., BILLARD, J. M., CLAUDEPIERRE, T., RENDON, A., DUTAR, P. & UNGERER, A. (1998). Spatial discrimination learning and CA1 hippocampal synaptic plasticity in mdx and mdx3cv mice lacking dystrophin gene products. *Neuroscience,* 86, 53-66.

VAILLEND, C., UNGERER, A. & BILLARD, J.M. (1999). Facilitated NMDA receptor-mediated synaptic plasticity in the hippocampal CA1 area of dystrophin-deficient mice. *Synapse* 33(1):59-70.

VAILLEND, C. & BILLARD, J. M. (2002). Facilitated CA1 hippocampal synaptic plasticity in dystrophin-deficient mice: role for GABAA receptors? *Hippocampus,* 12, 713-7.

VAILLEND, C., BILLARD, J. M. & LAROCHE, S. (2004). Impaired long-term spatial and recognition memory and enhanced CA1 hippocampal LTP in the dystrophin-deficient Dmd(mdx) mouse. *Neurobiol Dis,* 17, 10-20.

VAILLEND, C., PERRONNET, C., ROS, C., GRUSZCZYNSKI, C., GOYENVALLE, A., LAROCHE, S., DANOS, O., GARCIA, L. & PELTEKIAN, E. (2010). Rescue of a dystrophin-like protein by exon skipping in vivo restores GABAA-receptor clustering in the hippocampus of the mdx mouse. *Mol Ther* 8(9):1683-8.

VAJDA, Z., PEDERSEN, M., FUCHTBAUER, E. M., WERTZ, K., STODKILDE-JORGENSEN, H., SULYOK, E., DOCZI, T., NEELY, J. D., AGRE, P., FROKIAER, J. & NIELSEN, S. (2002). Delayed onset of brain edema and mislocalization of aquaporin-4 in dystrophin-null transgenic mice. *Proc Natl Acad Sci U S A,* 99, 13131-6.

VAJDA, Z., PEDERSEN, M., DOCZI, T., SULYOK, E. & NIELSEN, S. (2004). Studies of mdx mice. *Neuroscience,* 129, 993-8.

VAN OMMEN, G. J., BERTELSON, C., GINJAAR, H. B., DEN DUNNEN, J. T., BAKKER, E., CHELLY, J., MATTON, M., VAN ESSEN, A. J., BARTLEY, J., KUNKEL, L. M. & ET AL. (1987). Long-range genomic map of the Duchenne muscular dystrophy (DMD) gene: isolation and use of J66 (DXS268), a distal intragenic marker. *Genomics,* 1, 329-36.

WAITE, A., TINSLEY, C.L., LOCKE, M. & BLAKE DJ. (2009). The neurobiology of the dystrophin-associated glycoprotein complex. *Ann Med* 1(5):344-59.

WALLIS, T., BUBB, W. A., MCQUILLAN, J. A., BALCAR, V. J. & RAE, C. (2004). For want of a nail. ramifications of a single gene deletion, dystrophin, in the brain of the mouse. *Front Biosci,* 9, 74-84.

WECHSLER, D. (1997). *WAIS-III/WMS-III Technical Manual,* San Antonio TX, Psychological Corporation.

WHELAN, T. B. (1987) Neuropsychological performance of children with Duchenne muscular dystrophy and spinal muscle atrophy. *Dev Med Child Neurol,* 29, 212-20.

WIBAWA, T., TAKESHIMA, Y., MITSUYOSHI, I., WADA, H., SURONO, A., NAKAMURA, H. & MATSUO, M. (2000). Complete skipping of exon 66 due to novel mutations of the dystrophin gene was identified in two Japanese families of Duchenne muscular dystrophy with severe mental retardation. *Brain Dev,* 22, 107-12.

WINDER, S. J., GIBSON, T. J. & KENDRICK-JONES, J. (1995). Dystrophin and utrophin: the missing links! *FEBS Lett,* 369, 27-33.

WU, J. W., KUBAN, K. C. K., ALLRED, E., SHAPIRO, F. & DARRAS, B. T. (2005). Association of Duchenne Muscular Dystrophy With Autism Spectrum Disorder. *Journal of Child Neurology,* 20, 790-795.

YOKOTA, T., MIYAGOE, Y., HOSAKA, Y., TSUKITA, K., KAMEYA, S., SHIBUYA, S., MATSUDA, R., WAKAYAMA, Y. & TAKEDA, S. (2000). Aquaporin-4 is absent at the sarcolemma and at perivascular astrocyte endfeet in .ALPHA.1-syntrophin knockout mice. *Proceedings of the Japanese Academy Series B,* 76B, 22-27.

YOSHIHARA, Y., ONODERA, H., IINUMA, K. & ITOYAMA, Y. (2003). Abnormal kainic acid receptor density and reduced seizure susceptibility in dystrophin-deficient mdx mice. *Neuroscience,* 117, 391-5.

YOSHIOKA, M., OKUNO, T., HONDA, Y. & NAKANO, Y. (1980). Central nervous system involvement in progressive muscular dystrophy. *Arch Dis Child,* 55, 589-94.

YOUNG, H.K., BARTON, B.A., WAISBREN, S., PORTALES DALE, L., RYAN, M.M., WEBSTER, R.I. & NORTH, K.N. (2008). Cognitive and psychological profile in males with Becker muscular dystrophy. *J Child Neurol* 23(2):155-62.

ZACCARIA, M. L., PERRONE-CAPANO, C., MELUCCI-VIGO, G., GAETA, L., PETRUCCI, T. C. & PAGGI, P. (2001). Differential regulation of transcripts for dystrophin Isoforms, dystroglycan, and alpha3AChR subunit in mouse sympathetic ganglia following postganglionic nerve crush. *Neurobiol Dis,* 8, 513-24.

ZUBRZYCKA-GAARN, E. E., BULMAN, D. E., KARPATI, G., BURGHES, A. H., BELFALL, B., KLAMUT, H. J., TALBOT, J., HODGES, R. S., RAY, P. N. & WORTON, R. G. (1988). The Duchenne muscular dystrophy gene product is localized in sarcolemma of human skeletal muscle. *Nature,* 333, 466-9.

ZWAIGENBAUM, L. & TARNOPOLSKY, M. (2003). Two children with muscular dystrophies ascertained due to referral for diagnosis of autism. *J Autism Dev Disord,* 33, 193-9.

6

Proteomic Analysis of Signalling Pathway Deregulation in Dystrophic Dog Muscle

Marie Féron[1], Karl Rouger[2] and Laetitia Guével[1,2]
[1]*University of Nantes CNRS UMR6204,*
[2]*ONIRIS/INRA UMR 703,*
France

1. Introduction

During recent years, considerable effort has been made to develop proteomics technologies, with the aim of providing a complementary approach to the genomics tools already used in biomedical settings. This development has been extremely fast, and a number of emerging methodological proteomics tools now allow scientists to study the variable aspects of proteins in particular cell types, tissues or disease states. These tools include antibody arrays, two-dimensional-gel electrophoresis (2D-GE) and mass spectrometry (MS), the latter knowing an increasing use. In particular, candidate or non-candidate-based analyses of cell signalling represent powerful approaches for the investigation of the answers developed by cells in response to genetic modifications. Signalling molecules are key players in the regulation of the numerous and various biological processes occurring in a cell, and the alteration of signalling pathways has been associated with multiple diseases. Alterations in individual signalling pathways have been described in neuromuscular disorders, however, little information is available regarding their putative implication in Duchenne Muscular Dystrophy (DMD).

DMD is an X-linked neuromuscular disorder that affects 1 newborn in 3500. This recessive disease represents the most common and severe form of muscular dystrophy. Although the genetic basis of the disease is well resolved, the cellular mechanisms associated with the physiopathology remain largely unknown. Increasing evidence suggests that mechanisms secondary to the dystrophin deficiency at the basis of the disease, such as alterations in key signalling pathways, may play an important role. Proteomic profiling of dystrophic *vs* healthy skeletal muscle can help to generate a DMD-specific proteomic signature. Understanding which particular signal transduction pathways are involved in muscular dystrophy might provide a basis for new target and therapeutic agents discovery. This chapter examines signalling pathways status in skeletal muscles from the Golden Retriever Muscular Dystrophy (GRMD) dog, the only clinically relevant animal model for DMD (Valentine et al., 1988; Cooper et al., 1988). More specifically, we will describe how proteomic studies were successfully used to identify reliable biomarkers of the disease in animal models.

2. Signalling pathways and DMD

In dystrophic muscles, the absence of dystrophin, and the consequent destabilization of the dystrophin-glycoprotein associated complex DGC (a multiprotein transmembrane complex), lead to the loss of sarcolemma integrity, calcium overload, calpains activation and finally, necrosis of the myofibers (Muntoni et al., 2003). Besides providing mechanical stability, the DGC interacts with several proteins, including growth factor receptor-bound protein 2 (Grb2) (Yang et al., 1995), neuronal nitric oxide synthase (nNOS) (Brenman et al., 1995), calmodulin (Madhavan et al., 1992), focal adhesion kinase (FAK) (Cavaldesi et al., 1999) and caveolin-3 (Crosbie et al., 1998), that play a role in cell signalling. Grb2 has been identified as a component of the Ras/ mitogen-activated protein kinases (MAPK) signalling pathway and both FAK and Grb2 function as mediators of survival signalling in various cell types, often working through the phosphatidyl inositol 3-kinase (PI3K)/Akt pathway (Langenbach&Rando, 2002). Even if this mechanism can, in part, account for the degenerative phenotype observed in DMD, it seems increasingly obvious that the deregulation of intracellular signalling pathways also plays a role. These pathways, which are implicated in the regulation of crucial processes such as the balance between apoptosis and cell survival or the equilibrium between atrophy and hypertrophy, involve cascades of phosphorylation/dephosphorylation events. Protein kinases represent key enzymes responsible for the phosphorylation of specific targets. Moreover, altered cell signalling is thought to increase the susceptibility of muscle fibers to secondary triggers, such as functional ischemia and oxidative stress, and free-radical scavengers can have a direct impact on the activity/phosphorylation of some components of the MAPK cascades (Hnia et al., 2007). In progressive muscular dystrophy, muscles are characterized by hypertrophy in the early phase, while atrophic changes are observed with aging (Noguchi, 2005).

Studies of the X chromosome-linked muscular dystrophy (*mdx*) mouse model of DMD (Bulfield et al., 1984) revealed modulations in MAPK signalling cascades, as dystrophic animals exhibited increased phosphorylation of extracellular signal-regulated kinases 1 and 2 (ERK1/2) (Kumar et al., 2004; Lang et al., 2004) and c-jun N-terminal kinases 1 and 2 (JNK1/2) (Kolodziejczyk et al., 2001; Nakamura et al., 2005; St-Pierre et al., 2004), and decreased phosphorylation of p38 (Lang et al., 2004). The PI3K/Akt signalling pathway has also been shown to be affected in the *mdx* mouse, with an increased synthesis and phosphorylation of Akt observed (Dogra et al., 2006; Peter&Crosbie, 2006). Studies finally demonstrated that directly modulating signalling pathways activity could improve *mdx* muscle function (Kim et al., 2010; Tang et al., 2010). More specifically, increasing Akt activity by transgenic overexpression of the activated kinase itself has been shown to be able to reverse the dystrophic phenotype (Blaauw et al., 2009; Peter et al., 2009).

Moreover, the phosphorylation status of Akt was shown to be altered in human and canine dystrophic biopsies (Peter&Crosbie, 2006; Feron et al., 2009). Enhanced expression and activity of the phosphatidylinositol-3,4,5-trisphosphate 3-phosphatase (PTEN) has been observed in dystrophin-deficient dog muscle, and proposed to be at the origin of Akt inactivation (Feron et al., 2009). Indeed, PTEN opposes PI3K action by dephosphorylating phosphatidylinositol (3,4,5)-triphosphate (PtdIns(3,4,5)P_3) (Maehama&Dixon, 1998) and the increased activity detected in GRMD muscle would presumably lead to a decreased level of the phosphoinositide, which should limit the recruitment and activation of Akt (see Figure 1 for a schematic representation of the signalling pathway deregulation in dystrophic dog muscle).

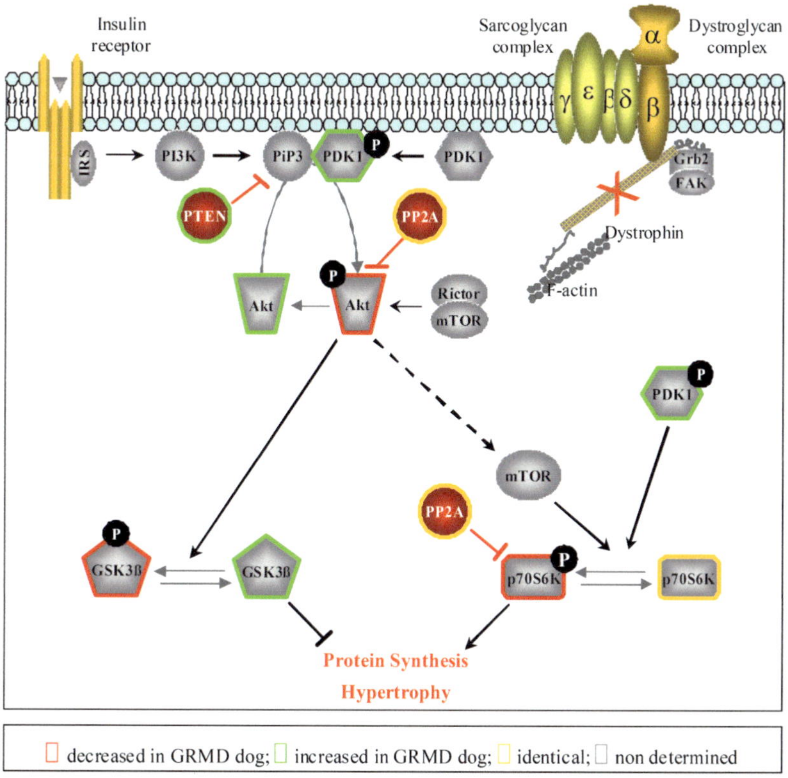

Fig. 1. Schematic diagram of signalling in the PI3K/Akt pathway and deregulations detected in GRMD skeletal muscle. Proteins shown in red, green and yellow indicate decreased, increased and unchanged level of expression or activity of these enzymes in GRMD *vs.* healthy muscle, respectively. As protein phosphatase 2A (PP2A) activity was not statistically modulated in GRMD muscle, the protein is shown in yellow. The deregulations detected in GRMD skeletal muscle could lead to decreased protein synthesis and block compensatory hypertrophy.

Akt directly phosphorylates glycogen synthase kinase-3 (GSK3β) at Ser9, thereby repressing its activity (Cross et al., 1995), and catalyses, *via* the mammalian target of rapamycin (mTOR), 70-kDa ribosomal protein S6 kinase (p70S6K) phosphorylation and activation (Chung et al., 1992; Glass, 2005; Inoki et al., 2002; Inoki et al., 2005; Price et al., 1992) (Figure 1). The PI3K/Akt/GSK3β and PI3K/Akt/mTOR/p70S6K pathways have been implicated in the regulation of skeletal muscle mass. Akt/mTOR signals were found to be upregulated during hypertrophy and downregulated during atrophy and the activation of Akt or p70S6K (or inactivation of GSK3β) appeared to be sufficient to induce hypertrophy. Moreover, in addition to acting as an inductive cue for hypertrophy, activation of the Akt/mTOR pathway could also prevent muscle atrophy *in vivo* (Bodine et al., 2001; Rommel et al., 2001). Furthermore, it has been shown *in vitro* that the overexpression of Src homology 2 (SH2) domain-containing inositol-5′-phosphatase 2 (SHIP-2), which, like PTEN, decreases PIP3 level, led to atrophy whereas the overexpression of a dominant negative mutant, which increases PIP3 level, induced hypertrophy (Rommel et al., 2001). The overexpression of

SHIP-2 in healthy mice muscle had no effect on fiber size but the overexpression of the phosphatase in a model of compensatory hypertrophy completely blocked the hypertrophy response (Bodine et al., 2001). It is thereby likely that the overexpression and increased activity of PTEN detected in GRMD muscle (by decreasing Akt activity and p70S6K phosphorylation, and by activating GSK3β) could prevent compensatory muscle hypertrophy. More recently, the peroxisome proliferator-activated receptor-gamma co-activator 1 alpha (PGC-1α) and PTEN inhibitor DJ-1/Parkinson disease (autosomal recessive early-onset) 7 (PARK7) appeared substantially reduced in GRMD *vs* healthy muscle (Feron et al., 2009; Guevel et al., 2011). Given the role of DJ-1 in the regulation of PTEN, this suggests that PTEN activation in GRMD dog muscle may originate from the under-expression of DJ-1. Noteworthy, in addition to its role in PTEN's regulation, DJ-1 also promotes the activity of PGC-1α (Zhong&Xu, 2008). As such, DJ-1 sensitive signalling pathways may provide high priority targets for the development of novel drug therapies for DMD.

Thus, compelling evidence suggest that alterations in signal transduction pathways may represent significant contributing factors to the progression of DMD. Proteomic profiling performed on the *mdx* mouse (Doran et al., 2006; Lewis et al., 2009; Ohlendieck, 2011) and GRMD dog models (Feron et al., 2009; Guevel et al., 2011) identified signalling proteins and reliable biomarkers of the secondary changes taking place in dystrophic muscles.

3. Proteomic analysis of dystrophic dog muscle

Proteomic approaches have been developed in order to try to identify putative biomarkers of DMD. The proteome-wide investigation of proteins requires technological efforts in three essential steps: the separation, the identification and the quantification of multiple proteins. Reversible protein phosphorylation is arguably the most common and significant mechanism for the dynamic control of biological processes. Phosphorylation can dramatically alter a protein's biological location and/or activity and recent studies clearly highlighted the involvement of phosphoproteins and kinases in DMD (Kolodziejczyk et al., 2001; Kumar et al., 2004; Lang et al., 2004; Peter&Crosbie, 2006; Feron et al., 2009). Although up to one-third of the total proteome might be phosphorylated, the absolute levels of any single protein specie might be very low. In contrast to the traditional biochemical study of single proteins or isolated pathways in the context of muscular dystrophy, technical advances in the high-throughput screening by MS and array-based technology have established new ways of identifying entire cellular proteins populations in one shift analytical approach.

Global identification of signalling proteins can be done by a dedicated approach using antibody arrays. Antibody arrays also serve as an attractive option to carry out phosphoproteomic profiling in disease (Feron et al., 2009; Gembitsky et al., 2004; Kingsmore, 2006). Phospho-specific antibody arrays commercially available facilitate the investigation of specific activated pathways in muscular disorders. On the other hand, a considerable number of proteomic studies have employed unbiased technology such as 2D-GE and stable isotope-labelling techniques combined with MS. To construct an accurate model of the proteome variations occurring in dystrophic dog muscle, complementary proteomic screenings have been done (Figure 2).

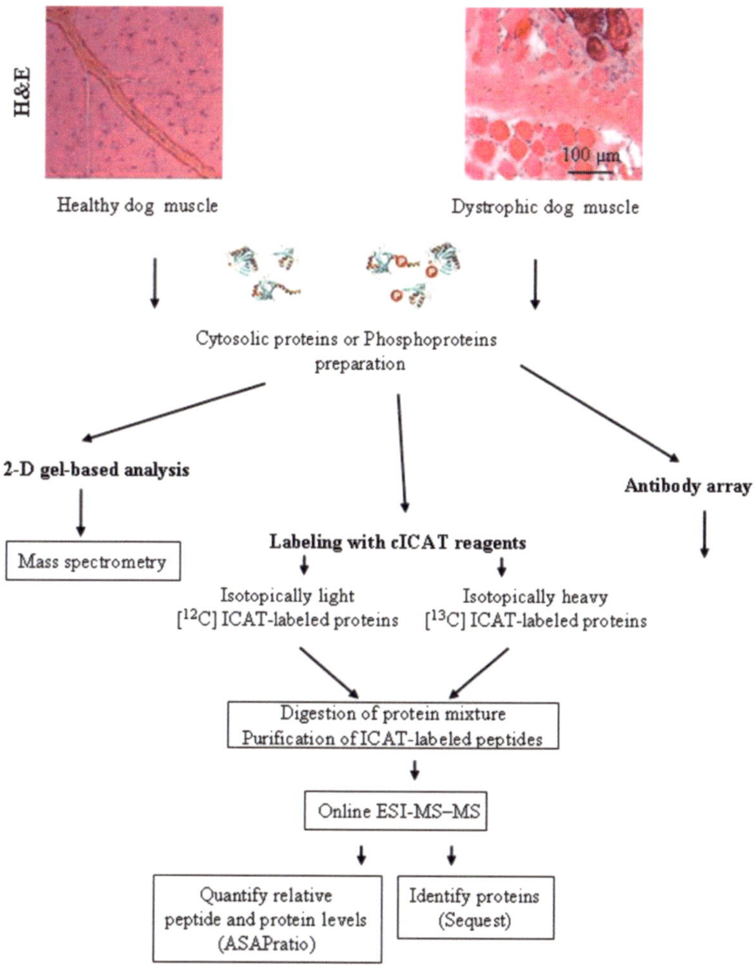

Fig. 2. Schematic diagram of the proteomic analysis of dystrophic dog muscle. H&E (hematoxylin and eosin) staining showing classical pathological changes of DMD, including fiber size variation, fiber splitting, and central nucleation in skeletal muscle. 2D-GE, isotope-coded affinity tag (ICAT) quantitative proteomic analysis and antibody array of proteins purified from 4-month-old healthy and GRMD dog muscle.

3.1 Protein array profiling

Biomedical research of the 21st century will largely be based on the results of studies focusing on the evaluation of gene expression and performed in order to develop molecular tools for the diagnosis and treatment of human diseases. Currently, DNA arrays represent the most commonly used means to follow gene expression in health and disease, and in muscular dystrophies in particular (Chen et al., 2000; Rouger et al., 2002). However, gene expression studies are limited by several aspects: i) gene expression levels do not necessarily reflect the level of proteins (that can also be regulated by degradation), ii) the activity of some proteins is regulated by posttranslational modifications (PTM) such as phosphorylation, glycosylation, carbonylation, acetylation and ubiquitylation, or by allosteric modifications and iii) localization changes can also play roles in this regulation. On the other hand, a lot of studies have been focusing on single proteins, protein complexes or isolated pathways, limiting the understanding of the pathogenesis of DMD at the organism level. In order to obtain this information and to be able to measure in parallel the expression and the state of activation of several hundreds of proteins, it was important to develop new approaches. Protein array-based approaches can provide not only data complementary to DNA microarrays but also provide unique information about the functional state of proteins under normal and pathological conditions (Hanash, 2003; MacBeath, 2002). Miniaturized protein array technology has opened a new chapter in biotechnology due to its ability to compare, characterize and quantify simultaneously a large number of proteins in the form of spots, thus replacing numerous individual protein by protein tests.It also allows parallel evaluation of several parameters in complex biological solutions. Moreover, a minute spot with immobilized protein sample on an array slide provides greater sensitivity for the detection of molecular interactions compared to other binding assays (Ekins&Chu, 1999). For the first time, antibody arrays were used by Anderson group to look for protein expression changes in spinal muscular atrophy (Anderson&Davison, 1999). A relatively small number of differences were found within a group of proteins that function as both RNA binding proteins and transcription factors. A second group used microarrays to profile the level of proteins associated with calcium regulation in sarcoplasmic reticulum isolated from muscle (Schulz et al., 2006). They used a reverse-phase protein array printed with proteins from genotyped animals and probed with seven target proteins important in calcium regulation. Reverse-phase arrays have been used for profiling phosphorylated proteins in various cancers (Grubb et al., 2003; Sheehan et al., 2005), and it was hoped that these arrays would become a powerful clinical tool for diagnosis and therapy guidance in different diseases.

More recently, the antibody array technology was used to assess the phosphorylation status of key proteins of the MAPK and PI3K/Akt signalling pathways in the *Vastus lateralis* muscle from 4-month old GRMD *vs* healthy dogs. The antibody array technology represents a powerful tool for the semi-quantitative comparison of the expression and/or phosphorylation level of a high number of proteins in a limited number of samples (Sakanyan, 2005; Yeretssian et al., 2005). The main advantage resides in the gain of time that it provides, as a high number of proteins can be studied in just one experiment. Moreover (and in contrary to the ICAT technology for example), antibody arrays give access to information about PTM, such as phosphorylation, which is of course crucial in the context of cell signalling. Though it represents a biased technique (data is obtained only for the antibodies initially spotted on the membrane) but, as hundreds of different antibodies can be spotted onto the same membrane, it can easily be used for screening purposes such asfor disease diagnosis using disease biomarkers. This study indicated that Akt1, GSK3β and p70S6K, as well as ERK1/2 and the p38δ and γ kinases all displayed a decreased phosphorylation level in canine dytrophic muscle (Figure 3). Antibody arrays allow the detection of the presence of specific proteins, and the level of expression of phospho-proteins in disease tissue (Cahill, 2001), thus having a potential for biomedical and diagnostic applications. However, it had not been possible to address the systematic analysis of proteins using this dedicated approach.

A lot of evidence now indicates that various signalling and metabolic pathways are altered in DMD, and a global, unbiased, proteomics study was necessary to identify these perturbations. In order to characterize the complete dystrophic proteome, the use the recent 2D-GE technology coupled to MS became favorable.

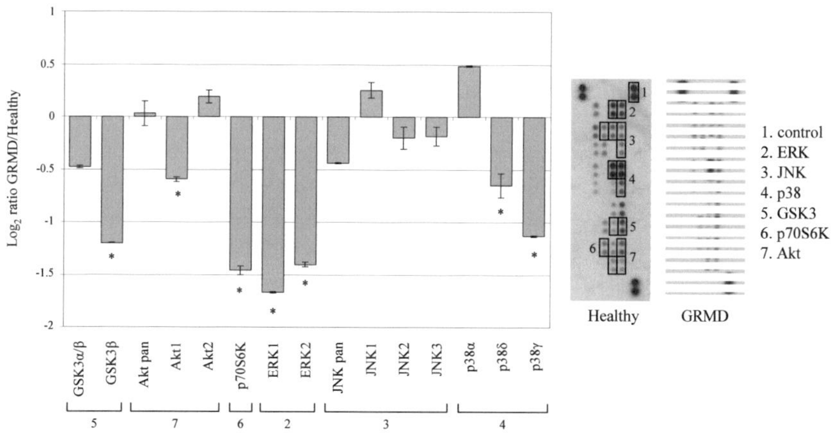

Fig. 3. Antibody array analysis revealed PI3K/Akt and MAPK signalling pathway modulation in GRMD skeletal muscle. Healthy and GRMD muscle extracts from 4-month-old dogs were incubated with two antibody arrays. A ratio of signal intensity (GRMD/healthy) was calculated, and log transformed (base2). A cutoff value was determined by ANOVA analysis at 95% confidence level ($p<0.05$). * - significantly different from healthy muscle.

3.2 Mass spectrometry-based proteomic analyses

MS-based proteomics represents an unbiased approach allowing the comprehensive cataloging of the whole protein alterations associated with a specific disease. This chapter outlines the findings from recent applications of MS-based proteomics for studying alterations in dystrophic dog muscle, and examines novel strategies to establish DMD-specific biomarkers.

3.2.1 Separation of muscle proteins by two-dimensional gel electrophoresis

2D-GE represents a highly reproducible and discriminatory technique that allows the analysis of the accessible (meaning soluble and abundant) muscle proteins. The proteins that appear differentially expressed between the different samples analyzed are then identified by high-throughput MS (matrix-assisted laser desorption/ionization time-of-flight - MALDI-ToF or electrospary ionization - ESI). Proteomics dataset are finally interlinked with international web-based gel electrophoretic and protein sequence databanks for comparative analysis. Modern mass spectrometers produce and separate ions according to their mass-to-charge ratio (m/z) with an extraordinary resolving power. MS-based analysis of the skeletal muscle proteome has already been successfully used in the context of muscle development, fiber type specification, fast-to-slow transformation, muscle growth and aging, and in the context of denervation-induced fiber damage, atrophy, obesity, diabetes and muscular dystrophies (Ohlendieck, 2010). Detailed 2D maps of the major soluble muscle proteome, including proteins involved in actomyosin apparatus, regulation of contraction, ion homeostasis, signalling, cytosolic and mitochondrial metabolism and stress response, have been established for various mammals (Doran et al., 2009a). The results obtained by this high-throughput technology should then be confirmed by more classical techniques such as western immunoblotting and immunohistochemistry. For example, the *mdx* mouse model was employed in recent proteomics profiling studies which revealed new disease markers in dystrophin-deficient fibres (Doran et al., 2004; Doran et al., 2006a, 2006b; Gardan-Salmon et al., 2011). A differential in-gel analysis (DIGE) analysis of *mdx vs* normal diaphragm muscle revealed a drastic differential expression pattern of 35 proteins, with 21 proteins being decreased (including the F-box only protein 11 - Fbxo11, adenylate kinase 1 – AK1, and the calcium-binding protein regucalcin) and 14 proteins being increased, including the small cardiovascular heat shock protein cvHSP and muscle proteins such as vimentin, desmin and myosin heavy chain (MHC) (Doran et al., 2006a).

More recently, the GRMD dog model was used to profile changes in protein abundance associated with DMD using 2D-GE. To eliminate the structural and contractile proteins that are over-abundant in crude protein extracts prepared from skeletal muscle, and to enrich the samples in signalling proteins, the study restricted the analysis to the cytosolic and phospho-enriched proteins of the *Vastus lateralis* muscle removed from 4-month-old healthy and dystrophic dogs. Among the differentially expressed proteins , 8 were chosen, according to their high level of dysregulation, for further identification by MS. This led to the identification of skeletal muscle markers involved in the contractile function and mitochondrial proteins involved in energy metabolism (Guevel et al., 2011). Although 2D-GE analysis represents an efficient technique to identify relative changes in protein expression, it is not well suited for studying low-abundant proteins, which are often important regulators of cell signalling. The high abundance of cytoskeletal, contractile and chaperone proteins identified in the phospho-enriched sample combined with dynamic range issues associated with the 2D-GE approach hampered studies on skeletal muscle analysis. Recently, Hojlund and colleague used 1D-GE and high-performance liquid chromatography (HPLC)-ESI-MS/MS to characterize the proteome of human skeletal muscle (Hojlund et al., 2008). The proteins identified in this study provide a representation of the major biological function of healthy human skeletal muscle. To elucidate changes in the proteome associated with DMD, and to overcome disadvantages of 2D-GE, peptide-centric approach can be used, which allows quantitative comparison of two samples. Numerous stable isotope-labelling techniques have been employed in quantitative shotgun proteomics, including isobaric tag for relative and absolute quantification (iTRAQ); isotope-coded affinity tag (ICAT); and stable isotope labelling by amino-acids in cell culture (SILAC) (Ohlendieck, 2011). In dystrophic skeletal muscle, the ICAT labelling approach has been used for the quantitative proteomic profiling of healthy and GRMD dog muscles.

3.2.2 Quantitative proteomic analysis

ICAT labelling followed by LC-MS/MS was used to analyze the quantitative variations of the proteome in both a cytoplasmic and a phospho-enriched fraction prepared from the *Vastus lateralis* muscle of 4-month old healthy and GRMD dogs (Guevel et al., 2011). A total of 84 proteins appeared significantly altered (61 proteins from the cytosolic fraction and 36 proteins from the phospho-enriched fraction, with an overlap of 13 proteins). These proteins were classified into 7 major categories including: i) muscle development and contraction, ii) glycolytic metabolism, iii) oxidative metabolism, iv) calcium ion homeostasis, v) intracellular signalling, vi) regulation of apoptosis, and vii) other functions. Gene Ontology

(GO) annotation of the altered proteome led to several key findings which might reflect the ongoing muscle regeneration taking place in dystrophic muscle. Among the proteins altered in the intracellular signalling category in the dystrophic muscle, protein phosphatase 1 (PP1) and DJ-1 appear particularly interesting. PP1, which is present in skeletal muscle, is known to regulate both glycogen and fatty metabolism, while promoting the dephosphorylation of myosin. The protein DJ-1 (also called PARK7) was recently described as a negative regulator of PTEN (Kim et al., 2005; Villa-Moruzzi et al., 1996). Interestingly, the under-expressed proteins primarily composed of metabolic proteins, many of which have been shown to be regulated by PGC-1α. Interestingly, among the several PGC-1α targets identified to be under-expressed in dystrophic dog muscle, 5 (namely 6-phosphofructokinase, phosphoglucomutase-1, aconitase 2, cytochrome c1 and fatty acid binding protein 3) have already been identified in a different transcriptomic study as under-expressing in DMD compared to healthy human biopsies (Pescatori et al., 2007). PGC-1α has been described as a potent regulator of mitochondrial biogenesis and oxidative metabolism in skeletal muscle (Wu et al., 1999; Lin et al., 2002). In addition, activation of the peroxysome proliferator-activated receptor (PPAR)/PGC-1α pathway has been shown, by preventing the bioenergetic deficit observed, to efficiently improve a mitochondrial myopathy phenotype (Wenz et al., 2008), suggesting that PGC-1α mediated improvement of dystrophic muscle may rely (in part) on the restoration of PGC-1α mitochondrial targets (Handschin et al., 2007). Interestingly, a recent study has shown that pharmacologic activation of PPARβ/δ also leads to an upregulation in the expression of utrophin A, which was concurrent with a partial correction of the dystrophic phenotype (Miura et al., 2009). Taken together, these results provide compelling new evidence that defects in PTEN and PGC-1α contribute to profound signalling pathway deregulation in the canine model of DMD as well as to the disease progression. In addition, they demonstrate that proteomics tools are of particular interest for the study of muscular disorders. Recently, the combination of proteomics, metabolomics and fluoximics has confirmed the existence in the *mdx* mouse of perturbations that reflect mitochondrial energetic alterations (Griffin&Des Rosiers, 2009). The broad aim of these studies has been two-fold, first the identification of co-founding factors that promote or limit the disease progression and second, the identification of new biomarkers that could be used to more accurately define the disease status.

4. Reliable biomarkers of DMD, with a special focus on signalling proteins

As previously mentioned, the absence of a single protein (dystrophin) in muscle has devastating consequences. Despites the tremendous efforts that have been made for more than 20 years in order to try to understand how this initial genetic defect could lead to the progressive and irreversible muscle wasting observed, the pathogenesis of DMD has not been fully characterized. Furthermore, no curative treatment is yet available and DMD patients are still dying during early adulthood. The identification, at the proteome level, of the alterations associated with DMD is important for at least five reasons. By providing a better understanding of the pathogenesis of DMD, they should i) improve diagnosis, ii) enable a better monitoring of disease progression, iii) lead to the proposal of new therapeutic targets (in the perspective of a pharmacological treatment - alone or in combination with a gene or cell therapy approach), iv) enable the fast and efficient evaluation of the benefits provided by the treatments currently under study (are they able to reverse the secondary changes associated with the absence of dystrophin?) and v) in some cases, they could even enable the improvement of a given therapy. Ideally, serum biomarkers should be identified (Cacchiarelli et al., 2011) allowing an easy and non invasive analysis, but a muscle muscular biopsy could always be used if necessary.

Skeletal muscle proteomics represents a new and powerful analytical tool for the swift separation and identification of new biomarkers and, in the recent years, several reviews written mainly by Doran, Ohlendieck and their colleagues focused on the proteomics analysis, by 2D-GE and high-throughput MS, of skeletal muscle during aging or disease (Lewis et al., 2009; Griffin&Des Rosiers, 2009; Doran et al., 2009a; Doran et al., 2007a, 2007b). Although being extremely powerful for the identification of new biomarkers, the proteomics analysis of skeletal muscle encounters some limitations. In the particular case of DMD, some complications are also due to the increase in endomysial fat and connective tissue, changes in the interstitial volume, infiltration by immune cells, residual blood components or drastic transformations in contractile fiber types. However, MS is so sensitive that it can differentiate these effects in heterogeneous cell mixtures. On the other hand, it is not always easy to distinguish between a DMD-specific biomarker and a biomarker that is more linked to muscle degeneration in general. The detailed analysis of the overlapping results obtained in the studies of DMD *vs* dysferlinopathies *vs* age-induced muscle wasting may help to distinguish between common and more specific biomarkers. In parallel to 2D-GE, we successfully used the antibody array technology to compare cell signalling in dystrophic *vs* healthy dog skeletal muscle (Feron et al., 2009). Finally, metabolomics and fluxomics (metabolic flux anlysis) studies have been successfully performed on skeletal muscle (Griffin&Des Rosiers, 2009).

In 2003, Ge and colleagues published the results of a proteomic analysis, using 2D-GE/MS, of *mdx* hindlimb skeletal muscle (Ge et al., 2003). Among the 60 proteins identified as differentially expressed in dystrophic *vs* healthy muscle (40 in the cytosolic fraction and 20 in the microsomal one), AK1 (cytosolic fraction) appeared to be of particular interest, because of its dramatic decrease (> four-fold) and because of its role, along with creatine kinase (CK), in the regulation of nucleotide ratios and energy metabolism. The expression and activity of AK1 was reduced in *mdx* muscle at different stages (one, three and six months), suggesting a direct link with the deficiency in dystrophin. Decreased AK1 activity in *mdx* muscle could contribute to the energetic defect, the decreased force and the increased fatigability exhibited. At the same time, the redistribution of energy flow through the alternative and compensatory CK phosphotransfer system could limit cellular energy failure. In DMD patients, lower ATP levels and impaired energy metabolism had been reported very early, and several studies suggest that defects in energy metabolism could contribute to DMD pathogenesis.

Ge and colleagues, in 2004, also published a study in which they compared by 2D-GE the proteome of *mdx vs* control hindlimb muscles at different stages of the disease (Ge et al., 2004). Among the 46 differentially expressed cytosolic proteins detected at three months (10 down- and 36 up-regulated proteins), 24 could be identified by MS. These proteins belong to five different functional categories, and illustrate the increase in protein turnover caused by the cycles of degeneration/regeneration characteristic of *mdx* muscles. Concerning metabolism and energy production (i), the reduction in AK1 was confirmed and an increase in the expression level of the CK, ATP synthase, ATP succinyl-CoA synthetase and pyrophosphatase enzymes was detected, highlighting the general mitochondrial dysfunction and metabolism crisis taking place in dystrophic muscles. Concerning the serine protease inhibitor family (ii), an up-regulation was detected for protease inhibitor member 1a and serine protease inhibitors 3, 6 and 1-5, suggesting a partial inhibition of proteolysis in *mdx* muscles. Concerning growth and differentiation (iii), an increase was detected in the expression level of PP1, cofilin 2 (CFL2) and ε 14-3-3, indicating active proliferation and differentiation. Of interest, an increase in CFL2 had also been observed in human DMD biopsies. As far as calcium homeostasis is concerned (iv), the up-regulation of PP1 can also be cited, as the phosphatase binds to the ryanodine-sensitive calcium release channel protein to regulate calcium flux. The calcium-binding protein annexin V was also increased. Finally, and concerning cytoskeleton reorganization and biogenesis (v), RhoGDI-1, γ-actin and tropomyosin 1 were found to be up-regulated in *mdx* muscles, indicating cytoskeleton remodeling. At one and six months, 62 and 48 differentially expressed proteins were detected, respectively. At one month, most of the proteins detected were down-regulated whereas at six months (as it was the case at three months), most of them were up-regulated. These results confirmed the specificity of the one month stage ("DMD-like" crisis) in the evolution of the disease in the *mdx* mouse. Six proteins were detected as differentially expressed in *mdx vs* healthy muscles at the three stages tested: AK1 (down-regulated), CK (up-regulated), myosin light chain 2 (MLC2, up-regulated), annexin V, tropomyosin and ε 14-3-3 (all down-regulated at one month and up-regulated at three and six months). Some of these changes thus appear directly linked to the absence of dystrophin whereas some others appear more dependent of the phenotype on the muscle. The elevation detected in MLC2 levels could reflect the proliferation/differentiation processes occurring in *mdx* muscles, as the protein is involved in muscle differentiation, and its consistent elevation during the progression of the disease suggests that *mdx* muscles may assume a chronic or abnormal differentiation state.

In another study, Doran and colleagues performed a 2D-GE/MS-based subproteomics analysis of calcium-binding proteins by using the cationic carbocyanine dye 'Stains-All' (Doran et al., 2004). Among the 8 dye-positive proteins identified as greatly reduced in *mdx vs* healthy skeletal muscle, calsequestrin was present. Calsequestrin represents the main luminal sarcoplasmic reticulum calcium reservoir protein. It is a terminal cisternae constituent with high-capacity and medium-affinity, and acts as a mediator of the excitation-contraction-relaxation cycle, both as a luminal ion trap and an endogenous regulator of the ryanodine receptor. The authors could also confirm the reduction in sarcalumenin, a calcium-shuttle element of the longitudinal tubules. These results of course confirm the calcium hypothesis of DMD. The reduction in calsequestrin could explain the impaired calcium buffering capacity of dystrophic sarcoplasmic reticulum, which is known to cause an increase in free cytosolic calcium level and thus in proteolysis. Previous microsomal study had not detected any change in the expression level of calsequestrin, highlighting the power of the technique used here.

More recently, Doran and colleagues could also show, using 2D-GE/MS again, that another protein involved in calcium homeostasis, regucalcin, was reduced in young and aged *mdx vs* healthy diaphragm, limb and heart muscles (Doran et al., 2006a). Regucalcin represented the most interesting hit in respect to the calcium hypothesis of DMD as its reduced level could render *mdx* fibers more susceptible to necrosis. Regucalcin is a cytosolic calcium-handling protein involved in signalling. By enhancing the calcium-pumping activity in the plasma membrane, endoplasmic reticulum and mitochondria, regucalcin appears as an important regulator that maintains low cytosolic calcium levels. Its reduced expression level could be confirmed by immunoblotting in the diaphragm muscle from 3-week-, 9-week-, 11-month- and 20-month-old *mdx* mice. At 9 weeks, a reduced level of the protein could also be observed in hindlimb and heart muscles. Doran and colleagues finally used the powerful DIGE technique and identified 2398 proteins among which 35 exhibited a differential expression level in *mdx vs* healthy diaphragm muscle (Doran et al., 2006b). These proteins are involved in muscle contraction, cytoskeleton formation, mitochondrial function, metabolism, ion homeostasis and chaperone function. The most interesting finding concerned the dramatic increase in the expression level of the small heat shock protein cvHSP (highest fold change). This drastic increase could be observed in 9-week- and 11-month-old *mdx* diaphragm muscles (it increases with the age – in correlation with the severity of the phenotype). Whereas the protein was concentrated in subsarcolemmal regions in healthy muscle, it was shown to be present throughout the cytoplasm of *mdx* fibers, with a typical striated appearance suggesting an association with contractile elements and/or cytoskeletal components and a role in the stress response developed by *mdx* damaged fibers. This increase in cvHSP was associated with the differential expression of others key heat shock proteins (HSP20, GRP75, HSP90 and HSP110), emphasizing stress response as an important mechanism in DMD pathogenesis, and suggesting that it could be targeted by new pharmacological treatments. Heat shock chaperon proteins can be activated, besides by heat shock *per se*, by other stress factors such as inflammation, ischemia, oxidative stress, exposure to heavy metals or certain amino acids analogs. They prevent the aggregation of misfolded proteins as well as they influence the transport of mature proteins. The up-regulation of cvHSP observed in *mdx* diaphragm indicates an attempt of damaged muscle fibers to repair their cytoskeletal network. The change observed in the localization of the protein also suggests a protective role in muscle fiber degeneration. The up-regulation of chaperones probably represents an autoprotective mechanism, whereby the stress response can be considered as a reaction to the pathological increase in abnormally folded muscle proteins.

More recently, a magnetic bead fractionation and MS-based serum protein profiling was performed in the *mdx* mouse and described coagulation Factor XIIIa, previously identified in human serum, as a potential biomarker of muscular dystrophy (Alagaratnam et al., 2008). Factor XIIIa plays roles in coagulation and cardiovascular biology, possibly through macrophage activation, and macrophages are known to infiltrate dystrophic muscles. Because blood serum analysis is fast, economical and non invasive, this type of study is of high interest, and a study with serum from DMD patients should be performed. However, this factor alone may not be sufficient to distinguish between DMD and other inflammatory context.

Finally, our lab identified two signalling molecules (PTEN and PGC1-α) as biomarkers in GRMD dog model, strongly reinforcing the hypothesis that signalling pathways alteration could play a role in DMD pathogenesis. In a first study (Feron et al., 2009), we were able to show that an increase in the activity of PTEN, a phosphatase that counteracts Akt activation by dephosphorylating the PIP3 generated by PI3K (Maehama&Dixon, 1998), in dystrophin-deficient dog muscle leads to a profound and long-term deregulation of the PI3K/Akt signalling pathway. All the GSK3β$^+$ fibers observed in dystrophic muscle appeared to exhibite a strong accumulation of PTEN, whereas the fibers with weak PTEN labelling were systematically GSK3β$^-$. In order to see if the alterations initially detected at 4-months were specific of this age, the double labelling experiment was repeated at 3 months (when the morphological features of muscular dystrophy are yet very few) and 36 months (which corresponds to a very advanced stage). PTEN$^+$/GSK3β$^+$ fibers could be observed at all stages, and we demonstrated that the alteration of the pathway could not be attributed only to a feature or regeneration or to a consequence of inflammatory changes. In conclusion, increased PTEN activity revealed to be a signature of muscular dystrophy pathogenesis in dog, leading to long-term and deep PI3K/Akt signalling pathway alteration. This dysregulation probably limits compensatory hypertrophy, thus exacerbating muscle degeneration, and these results could open the door to new potential therapeutic targets for the treatment of DMD.

In a second analysis, a quantitative proteomic analysis of dystrophic *vs* healthy dog muscle was performed using the ICAT technology coupled to LC/MS/MS (Guevel et al., 2011). This study, performed on both a cytoplasmic and a phospho-enriched fractions, identified 84 proteins as being differentially represented in GRMD *vs* healthy dog muscle. Interestingly, many of the under-expressed proteins detected have been previously shown to be regulated by PGC-1α, and we were able to show that PGC1-α expression was indeed dramatically reduced in GRMD *vs* healthy muscle. These results confirmed that defective energy metabolism is a central hallmark of the disease in the canine model, and reinforced once more the hypothesis that secondary changes may play an active role in DMD pathogenesis.

In conclusion, proteomics studies performed in the recent years on dystrophic *vs* healthy muscles led to the identification of new biomarkers of DMD, such as AK1 (nucleotide metabolism), calsequestrin, regucalcin (calcium homeostais) and cvHSP (cellular stress response) in the *mdx* mouse and PTEN and PGC-1α (cell signalling: atrophy/hypertrophy and energy metabolism) in the GRMD dog. Other putative biomarkers were also identified in the following processes: nucleotide metabolism (CK, Atp5b), calcium homeostasis (sarcalumenin), cellular stress response (αBC, chaperonins), muscle contraction (MHC and MLC, troponin, actin), intermediate filament formation (vimentin, desmin), glycolysis (glyceraldehyde-3-phosphate dehydrogenase, aldolase), polyol pathway of glucose metabolism (sorbitol dehydrogenase), citric acid cycle (isocitrate dehydrogenase), fatty acid oxidation (electron transferring flavoprotein), aldehyde metabolism (aldehyde reductase, aldehyde dehydrogenase), formation of acetyl-coenzyme A (dihydrolipoamide dehydrogenase), remethylation pathway of homocysteine homeostasis (betaine-homocysteine methyltransferase), acid-base balance (carbonic anhydrase), oxygen transport (β-haemoglobin, α-globin), protein ubiquitination (Fbxo11) and transcriptional control (Jmjd1a). Taken together, these results indicate a drastic reduction in key metabolic regulators and a compensatory up-regulation of structural elements.

5. Proteomic profiling of experimental therapy

As previously mentioned, no curative treatment is yet available for DMD patients that can benefit only from palliative care and generally die during early adulthood. Two therapeutic strategies can be envisaged to treat, or at least to alleviate the symptoms of DMD: try to restore dystrophin expression in dystrophic muscle fibers (through gene or cell therapy approaches), or target the molecular pathways lying downstream of dystrophin (through pharmacological treatments). Several strategies have been recently set up in order to rescue dystrophin synthesis in animal models of DMD and some of them have now entered clinical trials (Kinali et al., 2009; van Deutekom et al., 2007). One of the major problems in comparing the benefit of different therapeutic treatments is to find common outcome measurements. This paragraph does not aim at describing in details the therapies currently under study [for a review, please see (Sugita&Takeda, 2010; Guglieri&Bushby, 2010; Zhang et al., 2007)], but rather to show how proteomic profiling could be used to evaluate the efficiency of therapeutic treatments. Recently, Doran and colleagues (Doran et al., 2009b) used DIGE analysis to evaluate the efficiency of an exon skipping-based strategy in the *mdx* mouse.

The idea behind the study is that, as secondary mechanisms such as abnormal signalling, energy metabolism defects, alterations in ion homeostasis or in excitation-contraction coupling, probably play a crucial role in DMD pathogenesis, any novel therapeutic strategy should be evaluated on several aspects: re-expression of dystrophin (except for therapeutic treatments targeting downstream events), muscle function tests, but also correction of the secondary changes previously detected in the above mentioned processes.

Proteomic profiling of exon skipping-treated *mdx* muscles showed that the re-expression of dystrophin led to the correction of the previously detected alterations in calcium handling, nucleotide metabolism, bioenergetic pathways, acid-base balance and cellular stress response. More precisely, the re-expression of dystrophin was associated with the restoration of β-dystroglycan and nNOS (two proteins associated with the DGC at the sarcolemma), and with a normal expression level of some biomarkers previously identified (namely calsequestrin, adenylate kinase, aldolase, mitochondrial creatine kinase and cvHsp).

Both the primary and secondary abnormalities provoked by the absence of dystrophin were reversed, reinforcing the interest of the exon skipping strategy for the treatment of DMD. This study reinforced the role ofsecondary mechanisms in DMD pathogenesis, and it demonstrated for the first time the utility of evaluation of the effect of any novel therapeutic approach on both the re-expression of dystrophin and the indirect alterations associated with its absence. AK1, that had previously been reported as down-regulated in *mdx* diaphragm muscle (Ge et al., 2003), was restored after the antisense-induced exon skipping. Also, the down-regulation of the mitochondrial isozyme of CK was partially reversed. Accordingly, the known down-regulation of two others metabolic enzymes, namely aldolase and isocitrate dehydrogenase (Doran et al., 2006b) was also partially reversed. Conversely, the major increase previously reported in the level of cvHSP in *mdx* diaphragm was significantly reduced after treatment. As far as the acid-base balance is concerned, the expression level of carbonic anhydrase was also restored after treatment. For calsequestrin, an immunoblotting experiment (as DIGE is not well suited for the analysis of membrane proteins) was performed that revealed that exon skipping treatment was again able to restore its expression (Doran et al., 2004), suggesting a partial abolishment of the secondary changes in calcium homeostasis associated with DMD. The exon skipping strategy presented here effectively reverses both the metabolic crisis and the compensatory up-regulation of different chaperones and enzymes associated with muscular dystrophy in the mouse.

Lastly, miRNAs specifically expressed in muscle cells and known to be released in the blood of DMD patients in a way proportional to the extent of muscle degeneration, could be used as biomarkers in the evaluation of therapeutic strategies (Cacchiarelli et al., 2011).

To sum up, even though many different DMD therapeutic approaches are now entering clinical trials, a unifying method for assessing the benefit of different treatments is still lacking.

6. Conclusion

In conclusion, proteomics analysis plays a significant role in our ability to understand molecular mechanisms associated with DMD. Various technological platforms are now available for proteomic studies enabling us to address different aspects of dystrophic muscle governed by signalling pathways. We foresee proteomics emerging as a vital technique in clinical research to assist us in understanding which particular signal transduction pathways are involved in muscular dystrophy and to evaluate the benefit of clinical trials.

7. Acknowledgment

Research in the author's laboratory on proteomics handling in Duchenne muscular dystrophy was supported by projects grants from the AFM (Association Française contre les Myopathies).

8. References

Alagaratnam, S.;Mertens, B. J.;Dalebout, J. C.;Deelder, A. M.;Van Ommen, G. J.;Den Dunnen, J. T. & T Hoen, P. A. (2008) Serum protein profiling in mice: identification of Factor XIIIa as a potential biomarker for muscular dystrophy. *Proteomics,* 8, 8, pp. 1552-63, ISSN 1615-9861

Anderson, L. V. & Davison, K. (1999) Multiplex Western blotting system for the analysis of muscular dystrophy proteins. *Am J Pathol,* 154, 4, pp. 1017-22

Blaauw, B.;Canato, M.;Agatea, L.;Toniolo, L.;Mammucari, C.;Masiero, E.;Abraham, R.;Sandri, M.;Schiaffino, S. & Reggiani, C. (2009) Inducible activation of Akt increases skeletal muscle mass and force without satellite cell activation. *FASEB J,* ISSN 1530-6860

Bodine, S. C.;Stitt, T. N.;Gonzalez, M.;Kline, W. O.;Stover, G. L.;Bauerlein, R.;Zlotchenko, E.;Scrimgeour, A.;Lawrence, J. C.;Glass, D. J. & Yancopoulos, G. D. (2001) Akt/mTOR pathway is a crucial regulator of skeletal muscle hypertrophy and can prevent muscle atrophy in vivo. *Nat Cell Biol,* 3, 11, pp. 1014-9

Brenman, J. E.;Chao, D. S.;Xia, H.;Aldape, K. & Bredt, D. S. (1995) Nitric oxide synthase complexed with dystrophin and absent from skeletal muscle sarcolemma in Duchenne muscular dystrophy. *Cell,* 82, 5, pp. 743-52

Bulfield, G;Siller, W.G;Wight , P.A.G. & Moore, K.J (1984) X chromosome-linked muscular dystrophy (mdx) in the mouse. *Proc Natl Acad Sci U S A,* 81, pp. 1189-1192

Cacchiarelli, D.;Legnini, I.;Martone, J.;Cazzella, V.;D'amico, A.;Bertini, E. & Bozzoni, I. (2011) miRNAs as serum biomarkers for Duchenne muscular dystrophy. *EMBO Mol Med,* 3, 5, pp. 258-65, ISSN 1757-4684

Cahill, D. J. (2001) Protein and antibody arrays and their medical applications. *J Immunol Methods,* 250, 1-2, pp. 81-91, ISSN 0022-1759

Cavaldesi, M.;Macchia, G.;Barca, S.;Defilippi, P.;Tarone, G. & Petrucci, T. C. (1999) Association of the dystroglycan complex isolated from bovine brain synaptosomes with proteins involved in signal transduction. *J Neurochem,* 72, 4, pp. 1648-55

Chen, Y. W.;Zhao, P.;Borup, R. & Hoffman, E. P. (2000) Expression profiling in the muscular dystrophies: identification of novel aspects of molecular pathophysiology. *J Cell Biol,* 151, 6, pp. 1321-36

Chung, J.;Kuo, C. J.;Crabtree, G. R. & Blenis, J. (1992) Rapamycin-FKBP specifically blocks growth-dependent activation of and signaling by the 70 kd S6 protein kinases. *Cell,* 69, 7, pp. 1227-36, ISSN 0092-8674

Cooper, B. J.;Winand, N. J.;Stedman, H.;Valentine, B. A.;Hoffman, E. P.;Kunkel, L. M.;Scott, M. O.;Fischbeck, K. H.;Kornegay, J. N.;Avery, R. J. & Et Al. (1988) The homologue of the Duchenne locus is defective in X-linked muscular dystrophy of dogs. *Nature,* 334, 6178, pp. 154-6

Crosbie, R. H.;Yamada, H.;Venzke, D. P.;Lisanti, M. P. & Campbell, K. P. (1998) Caveolin-3 is not an integral component of the dystrophin glycoprotein complex. *FEBS Lett,* 427, 2, pp. 279-82, ISSN 0014-5793

Cross, D. A.;Alessi, D. R.;Cohen, P.;Andjelkovich, M. & Hemmings, B. A. (1995) Inhibition of glycogen synthase kinase-3 by insulin mediated by protein kinase B. *Nature,* 378, 6559, pp. 785-9

Dogra, C.;Changotra, H.;Wergedal, J. E. & Kumar, A. (2006) Regulation of phosphatidylinositol 3-kinase (PI3K)/Akt and nuclear factor-kappa B signaling pathways in dystrophin-deficient skeletal muscle in response to mechanical stretch. *J Cell Physiol,* 208, 3, pp. 575-85

Doran, P.;Donoghue, P.;O'connell, K.;Gannon, J. & Ohlendieck, K. (2007a) Proteomic profiling of pathological and aged skeletal muscle fibres by peptide mass fingerprinting (Review). *Int J Mol Med,* 19, 4, pp. 547-64, ISSN 1107-3756

Doran, P.;Donoghue, P.;O'connell, K.;Gannon, J. & Ohlendieck, K. (2009a) Proteomics of skeletal muscle aging. *Proteomics,* 9, 4, pp. 989-1003, ISSN 1615-9861

Doran, P.;Dowling, P.;Donoghue, P.;Buffini, M. & Ohlendieck, K. (2006a) Reduced expression of regucalcin in young and aged mdx diaphragm indicates abnormal cytosolic calcium handling in dystrophin-deficient muscle. *Biochim Biophys Acta,* 1764, 4, pp. 773-85

Doran, P.;Dowling, P.;Lohan, J.;Mcdonnell, K.;Poetsch, S. & Ohlendieck, K. (2004) Subproteomics analysis of Ca+-binding proteins demonstrates decreased calsequestrin expression in dystrophic mouse skeletal muscle. *Eur J Biochem,* 271, 19, pp. 3943-52, ISSN 0014-2956

Doran, P.;Gannon, J.;O'connell, K. & Ohlendieck, K. (2007b) Proteomic profiling of animal models mimicking skeletal muscle disorders. *Proteomics Clin Appl,* 1, 9, pp. 1169-84, ISSN 1862-8346

Doran, P.;Martin, G.;Dowling, P.;Jockusch, H. & Ohlendieck, K. (2006b) Proteome analysis of the dystrophin-deficient MDX diaphragm reveals a drastic increase in the heat shock protein cvHSP. *Proteomics,* 6, 16, pp. 4610-21

Doran, P.;Wilton, S. D.;Fletcher, S. & Ohlendieck, K. (2009b) Proteomic profiling of antisense-induced exon skipping reveals reversal of pathobiochemical abnormalities in dystrophic mdx diaphragm. *Proteomics,* 9, 3, pp. 671-85, ISSN 1615-9861

Ekins, R. & Chu, F. W. (1999) Microarrays: their origins and applications. *Trends Biotechnol,* 17, 6, pp. 217-8

Feron, M.;Guevel, L.;Rouger, K.;Dubreil, L.;Arnaud, M. C.;Ledevin, M.;Megeney, L. A.;Cherel, Y. & Sakanyan, V. (2009) PTEN contributes to profound PI3K/Akt signaling pathway deregulation in dystrophin-deficient dog muscle. *Am J Pathol,* 174, 4, pp. 1459-70, ISSN 1525-2191

Gardan-Salmon, D.;Dixon, J. M.;Lonergan, S. M. & Selsby, J. T. (2011) Proteomic assessment of the acute phase of dystrophin deficiency in mdx mice. *Eur J Appl Physiol,* ISSN 1439-6327

Ge, Y.;Molloy, M. P.;Chamberlain, J. S. & Andrews, P. C. (2003) Proteomic analysis of mdx skeletal muscle: Great reduction of adenylate kinase 1 expression and enzymatic activity. *Proteomics,* 3, 10, pp. 1895-903, ISSN 1615-9853

Ge, Y.;Molloy, M. P.;Chamberlain, J. S. & Andrews, P. C. (2004) Differential expression of the skeletal muscle proteome in mdx mice at different ages. *Electrophoresis,* 25, 15, pp. 2576-85, ISSN 0173-0835

Gembitsky, D. S.;Lawlor, K.;Jacovina, A.;Yaneva, M. & Tempst, P. (2004) A prototype antibody microarray platform to monitor changes in protein tyrosine phosphorylation. *Mol Cell Proteomics,* 3, 11, pp. 1102-18

Glass, D. J. (2005) Skeletal muscle hypertrophy and atrophy signaling pathways. *Int J Biochem Cell Biol,* 37, 10, pp. 1974-84, ISSN 1357-2725

Griffin, J. L. & Des Rosiers, C. (2009) Applications of metabolomics and proteomics to the mdx mouse model of Duchenne muscular dystrophy: lessons from downstream of the transcriptome. *Genome Med,* 1, 3, pp. 32, ISSN 1756-994X

Grubb, R. L.;Calvert, V. S.;Wulkuhle, J. D.;Paweletz, C. P.;Linehan, W. M.;Phillips, J. L.;Chuaqui, R.;Valasco, A.;Gillespie, J.;Emmert-Buck, M.;Liotta, L. A. & Petricoin, E. F. (2003) Signal pathway profiling of prostate cancer using reverse phase protein arrays. *Proteomics,* 3, 11, pp. 2142-6

Guevel, L. ;Lavoie, Jr.;Perez-Iratxeta, C. ;Rouger, K. ;Dubreil, L. ;Feron, M. ;Talon, S. ;Brand, M. & Megeney, L. (2011) Quantitative proteomic analysis of dystrophic dog muscle. *J Proteome Res.,* 10, 5, pp. 2465-78, ISSN 1535-3907

Guglieri, M. & Bushby, K. (2010) Molecular treatments in Duchenne muscular dystrophy. *Curr Opin Pharmacol,* 10, 3, pp. 331-7, ISSN 1471-4973

Hanash, S. (2003) Disease proteomics. *Nature,* 422, 6928, pp. 226-32

Handschin, C.;Kobayashi, Y. M.;Chin, S.;Seale, P.;Campbell, K. P. & Spiegelman, B. M. (2007) PGC-1alpha regulates the neuromuscular junction program and ameliorates Duchenne muscular dystrophy. *Genes Dev,* 21, 7, pp. 770-83, ISSN 0890-9369

Hnia, K.;Hugon, G.;Rivier, F.;Masmoudi, A.;Mercier, J. & Mornet, D. (2007) Modulation of p38 Mitogen-Activated Protein Kinase Cascade and Metalloproteinase Activity in Diaphragm Muscle in Response to Free Radical Scavenger Administration in Dystrophin-Deficient Mdx Mice. *Am J Pathol,* 170, 2, pp. 633-43

Hojlund, K.;Yi, Z.;Hwang, H.;Bowen, B.;Lefort, N.;Flynn, C. R.;Langlais, P.;Weintraub, S. T. & Mandarino, L. J. (2008) Characterization of the human skeletal muscle proteome by one-dimensional gel electrophoresis and HPLC-ESI-MS/MS. *Mol Cell Proteomics,* 7, 2, pp. 257-67, ISSN 1535-9484

Inoki, K.;Li, Y.;Zhu, T.;Wu, J. & Guan, K. L. (2002) TSC2 is phosphorylated and inhibited by Akt and suppresses mTOR signalling. *Nat Cell Biol,* 4, 9, pp. 648-57, 1465-7392

Inoki, K.;Ouyang, H.;Li, Y. & Guan, K. L. (2005) Signaling by target of rapamycin proteins in cell growth control. *Microbiol Mol Biol Rev,* 69, 1, pp. 79-100, ISSN 1092-2172

Kim, M. H.;Kino-Oka, M.;Saito, A.;Sawa, Y. & Taya, M. (2010) Myogenic induction of human mesenchymal stem cells by culture on dendrimer-immobilized surface with d-glucose display. *J Biosci Bioeng,* 109, 1, pp. 55-61, ISSN 1347-4421

Kim, R. H.;Peters, M.;Jang, Y.;Shi, W.;Pintilie, M.;Fletcher, G. C.;Deluca, C.;Liepa, J.;Zhou, L.;Snow, B.;Binari, R. C.;Manoukian, A. S.;Bray, M. R.;Liu, F. F.;Tsao, M. S. & Mak, T. W. (2005) DJ-1, a novel regulator of the tumor suppressor PTEN. *Cancer Cell,* 7, 3, pp. 263-73

Kinali, M.;Arechavala-Gomeza, V.;Feng, L.;Cirak, S.;Hunt, D.;Adkin, C.;Guglieri, M.;Ashton, E.;Abbs, S.;Nihoyannopoulos, P.;Garralda, M. E.;Rutherford, M.;Mcculley, C.;Popplewell, L.;Graham, I. R.;Dickson, G.;Wood, M. J.;Wells, D. J.;Wilton, S. D.;Kole, R.;Straub, V.;Bushby, K.;Sewry, C.;Morgan, J. E. & Muntoni, F. (2009) Local restoration of dystrophin expression with the morpholino oligomer AVI-4658 in Duchenne muscular dystrophy: a single-blind, placebo-controlled, dose-escalation, proof-of-concept study. *Lancet Neurol,* 8, 10, pp. 918-28, ISSN 1474-4465

Kingsmore, S. F. (2006) Multiplexed protein measurement: technologies and applications of protein and antibody arrays. *Nat Rev Drug Discov,* 5, 4, pp. 310-20, ISSN 1474-1776

Kolodziejczyk, S. M.;Walsh, G. S.;Balazsi, K.;Seale, P.;Sandoz, J.;Hierlihy, A. M.;Rudnicki, M. A.;Chamberlain, J. S.;Miller, F. D. & Megeney, L. A. (2001) Activation of JNK1 contributes to dystrophic muscle pathogenesis. *Curr Biol,* 11, 16, pp. 1278-82

Kumar, A.;Khandelwal, N.;Malya, R.;Reid, M. B. & Boriek, A. M. (2004) Loss of dystrophin causes aberrant mechanotransduction in skeletal muscle fibers. *FASEB J,* 18, 1, pp. 102-13

Lang, J. M.;Esser, K. A. & Dupont-Versteegden, E. E. (2004) Altered activity of signaling pathways in diaphragm and tibialis anterior muscle of dystrophic mice. *Exp Biol Med (Maywood),* 229, 6, pp. 503-11

Langenbach, K. J. & Rando, T. A. (2002) Inhibition of dystroglycan binding to laminin disrupts the PI3K/AKT pathway and survival signaling in muscle cells. *Muscle Nerve,* 26, 5, pp. 644-53

Lewis, C.;Carberry, S. & Ohlendieck, K. (2009) Proteomic profiling of x-linked muscular dystrophy. *J Muscle Res Cell Motil,* 30, 7-8, pp. 267-9, ISSN 1573-2657

Lin, J.;Wu, H.;Tarr, P. T.;Zhang, C. Y.;Wu, Z.;Boss, O.;Michael, L. F.;Puigserver, P.;Isotani, E.;Olson, E. N.;Lowell, B. B.;Bassel-Duby, R. & Spiegelman, B. M. (2002) Transcriptional co-activator PGC-1 alpha drives the formation of slow-twitch muscle fibres. *Nature,* 418, 6899, pp. 797-801, ISSN 0028-0836

Macbeath, G. (2002) Protein microarrays and proteomics. *Nat Genet,* 32 Suppl, pp. 526-32

Madhavan, R.;Massom, L. R. & Jarrett, H. W. (1992) Calmodulin specifically binds three proteins of the dystrophin-glycoprotein complex. *Biochem Biophys Res Commun,* 185, 2, pp. 753-9

Maehama, T. & Dixon, J. E. (1998) The tumor suppressor, PTEN/MMAC1, dephosphorylates the lipid second messenger, phosphatidylinositol 3,4,5-trisphosphate. *J Biol Chem,* 273, 22, pp. 13375-8, ISSN 0021-9258

Miura, P.;Chakkalakal, J. V.;Boudreault, L.;Belanger, G.;Hebert, R. L.;Renaud, J. M. & Jasmin, B. J. (2009) Pharmacological activation of PPAR{beta}/{delta} stimulates utrophin A expression in skeletal muscle fibers and restores sarcolemmal integrity in mature mdx mice. *Hum Mol Genet*, ISSN 1460-2083

Muntoni, F.;Torelli, S. & Ferlini, A. (2003) Dystrophin and mutations: one gene, several proteins, multiple phenotypes. *Lancet Neurol*, 2, 12, pp. 731-40

Nakamura, A.;Yoshida, K.;Ueda, H.;Takeda, S. & Ikeda, S. (2005) Up-regulation of mitogen activated protein kinases in mdx skeletal muscle following chronic treadmill exercise. *Biochim Biophys Acta*, 1740, 3, pp. 326-31, ISSN 0006-3002

Noguchi, S. (2005) The biological function of insulin-like growth factor-I in myogenesis and its therapeutic effect on muscular dystrophy. *Acta Myol*, 24, 2, pp. 115-8,

Ohlendieck, K. (2010) Proteomics of skeletal muscle differentiation, neuromuscular disorders and fiber aging. *Expert Rev Proteomics*, 7, 2, pp. 283-96

Ohlendieck, K. (2011) Skeletal muscle proteomics: current approaches, technical challenges and emerging techniques. *Skeletal muscle*, 1, 6, pp. 1-15

Pescatori, M.;Broccolini, A.;Minetti, C.;Bertini, E.;Bruno, C.;D'amico, A.;Bernardini, C.;Mirabella, M.;Silvestri, G.;Giglio, V.;Modoni, A.;Pedemonte, M.;Tasca, G.;Galluzzi, G.;Mercuri, E.;Tonali, P. A. & Ricci, E. (2007) Gene expression profiling in the early phases of DMD: a constant molecular signature characterizes DMD muscle from early postnatal life throughout disease progression. *FASEB J*, 21, 4, pp. 1210-26, ISSN 1530-6860

Peter, A. K. & Crosbie, R. H. (2006) Hypertrophic response of Duchenne and limb-girdle muscular dystrophies is associated with activation of Akt pathway. *Exp Cell Res*, 312, 13, pp. 2580-91

Peter, A. K.;Ko, C. Y.;Kim, M. H.;Hsu, N.;Ouchi, N.;Rhie, S.;Izumiya, Y.;Zeng, L.;Walsh, K. & Crosbie, R. H. (2009) Myogenic Akt signaling upregulates the utrophin-glycoprotein complex and promotes sarcolemma stability in muscular dystrophy. *Hum Mol Genet*, 18, 2, pp. 318-27, ISSN 1460-2083

Price, D. J.;Grove, J. R.;Calvo, V.;Avruch, J. & Bierer, B. E. (1992) Rapamycin-induced inhibition of the 70-kilodalton S6 protein kinase. *Science*, 257, 5072, pp. 973-7, ISSN 0036-8075

Rommel, C.;Bodine, S. C.;Clarke, B. A.;Rossman, R.;Nunez, L.;Stitt, T. N.;Yancopoulos, G. D. & Glass, D. J. (2001) Mediation of IGF-1-induced skeletal myotube hypertrophy by PI(3)K/Akt/mTOR and PI(3)K/Akt/GSK3 pathways. *Nat Cell Biol*, 3, 11, pp. 1009-13

Rouger, K.;Le Cunff, M.;Steenman, M.;Potier, M. C.;Gibelin, N.;Dechesne, C. A. & Leger, J. J. (2002) Global/temporal gene expression in diaphragm and hindlimb muscles of dystrophin-deficient (mdx) mice. *Am J Physiol Cell Physiol*, 283, 3, pp. C773-84

Sakanyan, V. (2005) High-throughput and multiplexed protein array technology: protein-DNA and protein-protein interactions. *J Chromatogr B Analyt Technol Biomed Life Sci*, 815, 1-2, pp. 77-95, ISSN 1570-0232

Schulz, J. S.;Palmer, N.;Steckelberg, J.;Jones, S. J. & Zeece, M. G. (2006) Microarray profiling of skeletal muscle sarcoplasmic reticulum proteins. *Biochim Biophys Acta*, 1764, 9, pp. 1429-35

Sheehan, K. M.;Calvert, V. S.;Kay, E. W.;Lu, Y.;Fishman, D.;Espina, V.;Aquino, J.;Speer, R.;Araujo, R.;Mills, G. B.;Liotta, L. A.;Petricoin, E. F., 3rd & Wulfkuhle, J. D. (2005)

Use of reverse phase protein microarrays and reference standard development for molecular network analysis of metastatic ovarian carcinoma. *Mol Cell Proteomics,* 4, 4, pp. 346-55

St-Pierre, S. J.;Chakkalakal, J. V.;Kolodziejczyk, S. M.;Knudson, J. C.;Jasmin, B. J. & Megeney, L. A. (2004) Glucocorticoid treatment alleviates dystrophic myofiber pathology by activation of the calcineurin/NF-AT pathway. *Faseb J,* 18, 15, pp. 1937-9

Sugita, H. & Takeda, S. (2010) Progress in muscular dystrophy research with special emphasis on gene therapy. *Proc Jpn Acad Ser B Phys Biol Sci,* 86, 7, pp. 748-56, ISSN 1349-2896

Tang, Y.;Reay, D. P.;Salay, M. N.;Mi, M. Y.;Clemens, P. R.;Guttridge, D. C.;Robbins, P. D.;Huard, J. & Wang, B. (2010) Inhibition of the IKK/NF-kappaB pathway by AAV gene transfer improves muscle regeneration in older mdx mice. *Gene Ther,* 17, 12, pp. 1476-83, ISSN 1476-5462

Valentine, B. A.;Cooper, B. J.;De Lahunta, A.;O'quinn, R. & Blue, J. T. (1988) Canine X-linked muscular dystrophy. An animal model of Duchenne muscular dystrophy: clinical studies. *J Neurol Sci,* 88, 1-3, pp. 69-81, ISSN 0022-510X

Van Deutekom, J. C.;Janson, A. A.;Ginjaar, I. B.;Frankhuizen, W. S.;Aartsma-Rus, A.;Bremmer-Bout, M.;Den Dunnen, J. T.;Koop, K.;Van Der Kooi, A. J.;Goemans, N. M.;De Kimpe, S. J.;Ekhart, P. F.;Venneker, E. H.;Platenburg, G. J.;Verschuuren, J. J. & Van Ommen, G. J. (2007) Local dystrophin restoration with antisense oligonucleotide PRO051. *N Engl J Med,* 357, 26, pp. 2677-86, ISSN 1533-4406

Villa-Moruzzi, E.;Puntoni, F. & Marin, O. (1996) Activation of protein phosphatase-1 isoforms and glycogen synthase kinase-3 beta in muscle from mdx mice. *Int J Biochem Cell Biol,* 28, 1, pp. 13-22, ISSN 1357-2725

Wenz, T.;Diaz, F.;Spiegelman, B. M. & Moraes, C. T. (2008) Activation of the PPAR/PGC-1alpha pathway prevents a bioenergetic deficit and effectively improves a mitochondrial myopathy phenotype. *Cell Metab,* 8, 3, pp. 249-56, ISSN 1932-7420

Wu, Z.;Puigserver, P.;Andersson, U.;Zhang, C.;Adelmant, G.;Mootha, V.;Troy, A.;Cinti, S.;Lowell, B.;Scarpulla, R. C. & Spiegelman, B. M. (1999) Mechanisms controlling mitochondrial biogenesis and respiration through the thermogenic coactivator PGC-1. *Cell,* 98, 1, pp. 115-24, ISSN 0092-8674

Yang, B.;Jung, D.;Motto, D.;Meyer, J.;Koretzky, G. & Campbell, K. P. (1995) SH3 domain-mediated interaction of dystroglycan and Grb2. *J Biol Chem,* 270, 20, pp. 11711-4

Yeretssian, G.;Lecocq, M.;Lebon, G.;Hurst, H. C. & Sakanyan, V. (2005) Competition on nitrocellulose-immobilized antibody arrays: from bacterial protein binding assay to protein profiling in breast cancer cells. *Mol Cell Proteomics,* 4, 5, pp. 605-17, ISSN 1535-9476

Zhang, S.;Xie, H.;Zhou, G. & Yang, Z. (2007) Development of therapy for Duchenne muscular dystrophy. *Zhongguo Xiu Fu Chong Jian Wai Ke Za Zhi,* 21, 2, pp. 194-203, ISSN 1002-1892

Zhong, N. & Xu, J. (2008) Synergistic activation of the human MnSOD promoter by DJ-1 and PGC-1alpha: regulation by SUMOylation and oxidation. *Hum Mol Genet,* 17, 21, pp. 3357-67, ISSN 1460-2083

7

Abnormal Ion Homeostasis and Cell Damage in Muscular Dystrophy

Yuko Iwata and Shigeo Wakabayashi
National Cerebral and Cardiovascular Center Research Institute
Japan

1. Introduction

Disruption of cytoskeletal organization caused by genetic defects in the components of the dystrophin-glycoprotein complex (DGC) results in muscular dystrophy and/or cardiomyopathy in human patients and animal models. Accumulating evidence obtained from studies by using skeletal muscle fibers, cultured myotubes, and cardiac muscle preparations from dystrophic animals suggest that defects in DGC components cause altered membrane properties in the sarcolemma of myocytes. For example, disruption of the DGC can cause increased susceptibility to mechanical stress or increased permeability to ions such as Ca^{2+} and Na^+, leading to a chronic increase in the concentrations of intracellular Ca^{2+} ($[Ca^{2+}]_i$) and Na^+ ($[Na^+]_i$). Abnormal ion homeostasis, especially under conditions of mechanical stress, is thought to be a key molecular event in the pathology of muscular dysgenesis. In this chapter, we will review the stretch-induced cell damage pathways that result in abnormal Ca^{2+} and Na^+ concentrations. In particular, we will focus on stretch-activated channels, transient receptor potential cation channels, and Na^+-dependent ion transporters, which have been reported to be of critical pathological significance. We will also discuss the therapeutic potential of these ion handling membrane proteins for the treatment of muscular dystrophy.

2. Sarcolemmal weakness and abnormal ion homeostasis in muscular dystrophy

Table 1 shows the genes and their products, which are involved in muscular dystrophy. Disruption of some genes (highlighted in pink) lead to heart failure, most often caused by dilated cardiomyopathy, as well as muscular dystrophy. In Duchenne muscular dystrophy (DMD), in which the protein dystrophin is defective, expression of dystrophin-associated proteins is also greatly reduced (Ervasti and Campbell, 1991). In addition, other types of muscular dystrophy are caused by mutations in genes encoding the components of the DGC (Campbell, 1995; Duclos et al., 1998; Nigro et al., 1997). The DGC is a multi-subunit complex (Campbell, 1995; Campbell & Kahl, 1989; Tinsley et al., 1994) that spans the sarcolemma to structurally link extracellular matrix proteins such as laminin to the actin cytoskeleton (Ervasti & Campbell, 1993), providing mechanical strength to the muscle cell membranes. Therefore, disruption of the DGC could significantly destroy membrane integrity or stability during contraction/relaxation, and cause cell damage. Importantly, defects in different genes cause similar end-stage symptoms, i.e., muscle dysgenesis. Understanding the pathway that leads to cell damage is important for the development of common therapeutic strategies, not only for muscular dystrophy, but also for inherited and non-inherited cases of dilated cardiomyopathy. Two animal models are commonly used for the study of muscular dystrophy: the dystrophin-deficient mouse (*mdx*), which is representative of human DMD, and the delta-sarcoglycan-deficient hamster (BIO14.6), which is a model for human delta-sarcoglycanopathy.

inheritance	disease	gene	gene product	locus	OMIM number
X-linked	Duchenne Muscular Dystrophy	*DMD*	dystrophin	Xp21.2	300377
	Becker Muscular Dystrophy	*BMD*	dystrophin	Xp21.2	300376
	Emery-Dreifus Muscular Dystrophy	*EMD,FHL1*	emerin, FHL1	Xq28, Xq27.2	310300
Autosomal Recessive	Fukuyana-type	*FCMD*	fukutin	9q31-q33	607440
	Merosin-deficient	*LAMA2*	laminin α-2 chain	6q22-q23	156225
	Integrin-deficient	*ITGA7*	integrin α-7	12q13	600536
	Ullrich	*COL6A1,2,3*	collagenVI	2q37, 21q22.3	254090
	Muscle-eye-brain (MEB)	*POMGNT1*	POMGNT1	1p34-p33	606822
	Walker-Warburg syndrome(WWS)	*POMT1,2*	POMT1,2	9q34.1, 14q24.3	236670
	Limb-girdle				
	Calpainopathy	*CAPN3*	calpain-3	15q15.1-q21.1	114240
	Dysferlinopathy, Miyoshi distal	*DYSF*	dysferlin	2p13	603009
	Gamma-sarcoglycanopathy	*SGCG*	γ-sarcoglycan	13q12	253700
	Alpha-sarcoglycanopathy	*SGCA*	α-sarcoglycan	17q21	600119
	Beta-sarcoglycanopathy	*SGCB*	β-sarcoglycan	4q12	600900
	Delta-sarcoglycanopathy	*SGCD*	δ-sarcoglycan	5q33	601411
	Telethoninopathy	*TCAP*	telethonin	17q12	604488
	LGMD2H	*TRIM32*	E3 ubiquitin-protein ligase	9q31-q34.1	254110
	LGMD2I	*FKRP*	fukutin-related protein	19q13.32	606596
	LGMD2J	*TTN*	titin	2q31	608807
	LGMD2K	*POMT1*	POMT1	9q34.1	609308
	LGMD2L	*ANO5*	$Ca2^{+}$ activated Cl^{-} channel	11p12-p13	611307
	LGMD2M	*FKTN*	fukutin	9q31	607440
	LGMD2N	*POMT2*	POMT2	14q24.3	607439
	LGMD2O	*POMGNT1*	POMGNT1	1p34-p33	606822
Autosomal Dominant	Limb-girdle				
	Myotilinopathy(LGMD1A)	*MYOT*	myotilin	5q31	604103
	LGMD1B	*LMNA*	lamin A/C	1q21.2	150330
	Caveolinopathy(LGMD1C)	*CAV3*	caveolin-3	3p25	601253
	LGMD1D	*unknown*	unknown	6q23	603511
	Facioscapulohumeral (FSHD)	*DUX4*	DUX4	4q35	158900
	Myotonic dystrophy	*DMPK*	myotonica protein kinase	19q13.2-q13.3	605377
	Myoclonus dystonia	*SGCE*	ε-sarcoglycan	7q21.3	604149

OMIM number: National Center for Biotechnology Information (http://www.ncbi.nlm.nih.gov/)

[pink shading] Common gene and gene product of cardiomyopathy

POMGNT;protein O-mannose beta 1,2-N-acetylglucosaminyltransferase

POMT ; protein O-mannosyltransferase

Table 1. Genes and their products responsible for muscular dystrophy

In an initial investigation, we found that sarcolemma from BIO14.6 hamster cardiomyopathic hearts has a fragile nature and is highly susceptible to mechanical stress, as evidenced by the ease of extraction of sarcolemma and T-tubules by relatively weak mechanical homogenization in low strength homogenization buffer (Tawada-Iwata et al., 1993). As a result, the amount of dystrophin extracted from BIO14.6 hamsters was 5 times more than that extracted from control hamsters, despite similar or lower dystrophin expression levels in BIO14.6 hamsters (Iwata et al., 1993a). The physical association between dystrophin and dystroglycan in BIO14.6 hearts was very weak (Iwata et al., 1993b). Mechanical membrane weakness was also observed in the skeletal muscle myotubes from BIO14.6 hamsters. Under hypo-osmotic stress (70% osmolarity), extensive cell bleb formation was seen in cultured BIO14.6 myotubes; however, this was not observed in control myotubes (Fig.1 A). Similarly, bleb formation was also seen in *mdx* mouse fibers, but not in control fibers (Fig.1 B). Upon cyclic stretching of up to 20% elongation for 1 h, creatine phosphokinase (CK) efflux (a marker of cell damage) was elevated with increasing strength of stretch in BIO14.6 myotubes, but not in controls (Fig.1 C). Such cell damage in *mdx* myotubes has also been reported by other groups (Menke & Jockusch, 1991; Petrof et al., 1993). These data suggest that skeletal and cardiac muscle is highly sensitive to mechanical stretch in animal models of DGC deficiency.

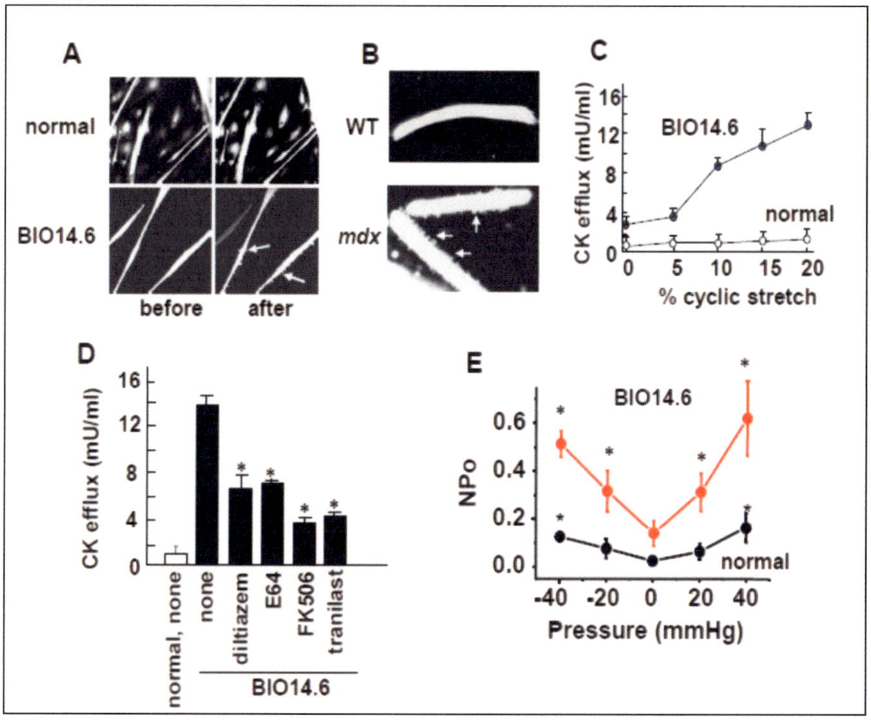

(A) Hypo-osmotic stress-induced cell damage in cultured dystrophic myotubes. Normal and BIO14.6 myotubes were preloaded with 5 mM calcein-AM and exposed to hypo-osmotic medium (70% osmolarity) for 17 min. Extensive bleb formation was observed in BIO14.6 myotubes (arrow). (B) Hypo-osmotic stress-induced cell damage in the single skeletal muscle fibers from WT and *mdx* muscle. Note the extensive bleb formation in *mdx* fibers. (C) Cyclic stretch of up to 20% for 1 h induced CK efflux from BIO14.6 myotubes, indicating the high susceptibility of dystrophic myotubes to mechanical stress. (D) Effect of various agents on stretch-induced CK efflux. The TRPV2 inhibitor tranilast effectively blocked CK efflux. The Ca^{2+} channel blocker diltiazem, the Ca^{2+}-dependent protease calpain inhibitor E64, and the Ca^{2+}-dependent phosphatase calcineurin inhibitor FK506 also blocked CK efflux, suggesting that these Ca^{2+} handling and Ca^{2+} effector proteins are involved in stretch-induced membrane damage. (E) A stretch-induced Ca^{2+}-permeable channel is activated in BIO14.6 myotubes. Positive or negative pressures were applied to the pipette using cell-attached patches that were held at -60 mV. $BaCl_2$ (110 mM) was used as the charge carrier. Note the higher open probability (NP_o) in BIO14.6 myotubes.

Fig. 1. Mechanical membrane weakness in the DGC-defective myotubes

It has been reported that myocyte degeneration may be caused by increased membrane permeability to Ca^{2+}, which is probably linked with membrane weakness. Many studies have reported chronic elevations in $[Ca^{2+}]_i$ underneath the sarcolemma, or within other intracellular compartments, in the skeletal muscle fibers or myotubes from DMD patients and *mdx* mice

(Brown, 1997; Mallouk et al., 2000; Robert et al., 2001). Elevated $[Ca^{2+}]_i$ has been causally linked to a greater rate of protein degradation, catalyzed by the Ca^{2+}-dependent protease calpain (Alderton & Steinhardt, 2000a; MacLennan et al., 1991; Spencer et al., 1995; Turner et al., 1988). Concurrently, myocyte contractile activity would cause physical damage to the sarcolemma, leading to leakage of cytosolic enzymes such as CK. The $[Ca^{2+}]_i$ in the muscle tissue is regulated by numerous ion channels, Ca^{2+} pumps, and transporters in the sarcolemma and sarcoplasmic reticulum (SR). Of these, the sarcolemmal Ca^{2+}-permeable channels (Ca^{2+}-specific leak channels) or the mechanosensitive non-selective cation channels, which contribute to abnormal Ca^{2+} handling in dystrophic myocytes, have been the focus of attention.

In 1990, the Steinhardt group (Fong et al., 1990) reported the existence of Ca^{2+} leak channels with a higher open probability in myotubes from *mdx* mice or DMD patients. These channels were activated by the L-type Ca^{2+} channel blocker nifedipine, but inhibited by the other dihydropyridine compounds AN406 and AN1043 (Alderton et al., 2000a). Treatment with the calpain inhibitor leupeptin decreased opening probabilities of the leak channels and prevented elevation in resting $[Ca^{2+}]_i$ in *mdx* myotubes (Turner et al., 1993). The leak channels were activated by store depletion in control myotubes (Hopf et al., 1996). From these data, Steinhardt et al. proposed a mechanism of myocyte degeneration caused by leak channel activation; contraction-induced sarcolemmal tears in dystrophin-deficient myotubes lead to localized Ca^{2+} entry, which initiates the repair of the defect. Activation of proteolysis is thought to be essential for the activation of leak channels, which accelerate Ca^{2+} entry and further increase Ca^{2+}–dependent proteolysis, the final common pathway of cell damage (Alderton & Steinhardt, 2000b). However, molecular identification and characterization of Ca^{2+} leak channels has not been carried out.

Mechanosensitive stretch-activated channels (SACs) have been described to contribute to increased Ca^{2+} permeability in dystrophic myotubes. The open probability of these channels increases when negative pressure is applied to a patch pipette. This is observed in both control and *mdx* muscle, but to a greater extent in *mdx* myotubes and fibers (Franco-Obregon & Lansman, 1994). SACs are non-selective cation channels permeable to Na^+, K^+, Ca^{2+}, and Ba^{2+}, and have a conductance of 13 pS when a patch pipette is filled with 110 mM Ca^{2+} (Franco & Lansman, 1990). In addition, a stretch-inactivated channel has been reported to exist only in *mdx* muscle cells (Franco et al., 1990), which was later reported to have identical conductance properties to SACs (Franco-Obregon & Lansman, 2002). These channels are blocked by Gd^{3+}, streptomycin (Hamill & McBride, 1996), and the spider venom toxin GsMtx4 (Suchyna et al., 2000). Abnormalities in SACs have been detected in the recordings from the muscle biopsy samples of DMD patients (Vandebrouck et al., 2001; Vandebrouck et al., 2002a). These results suggest that SACs are important for pathological Ca^{2+} entry into the dystrophin-deficient muscle, at early stages of the pathogenesis.

Research has shown that store-operated Ca^{2+} channels (SOCs) may also be involved in the pathogenesis of muscular dystrophy. SOCs have voltage-independent properties and a unitary conductance between 7 and 8 pS (with 110 mM Ca^{2+} in a patch pipette). Their open probability increases when luminal Ca^{2+} in the SR is depleted by the Ca^{2+} pump inhibitor thapsigargin. SOC activity was reported to be about twice as high in *mdx* compared to wild-type mice, and contributes to increased $[Ca^{2+}]_i$ in DMD (Vandebrouck et al., 2002b). Recently, Ca^{2+}-independent phospholipase A2 was found to be localized in the sarcolemma of *mdx* muscle, and its enzymatic product, lysophosphatidylcholine, was found to trigger Ca^{2+} entry through SOCs (Boittin et al., 2006). SACs and SOCs share several biophysical and pharmacological properties in adult muscle fibers; they have the same unitary conductance, and a similar sensitivity to Gd^{3+}, SKF-96365, 2-aminoethoxydiphenyl borate (2-APB), GsMTx4 toxin, and IGF-1 stimulation (Ducret et al., 2006). These observations suggest that SACs and SOCs may share common constituents, although molecular identification of these components is still required.

3. Therapeutic targets for muscular dystrophy

3.1 TRPV channels

Since a large body of evidence indicates the pathological significance of increased $[Ca^{2+}]_i$ in muscular dystrophy, much effort has been made to identify the genes responsible for abnormal Ca^{2+} handling in this disease. Our group has shown that stretch-sensitive cation-selective channels, similar to those recorded in *mdx* skeletal muscle, are active in cultured myotubes prepared from BIO14.6 hamsters (Nakamura et al., 2001). Positive or negative pressure increases the open probability of this channel in BIO14.6 myotubes (Fig.1 E). To identify the Ca^{2+} entry pathway responsible for myocyte degeneration, we searched for mammalian homologs of the *Drosophila* stretch sensor *NompA,* which were expressed in the striated muscle. We were successful in identifying a candidate that belongs to the transient receptor potential (TRP) channel family, which is similar to *NompA*. Many members of this family are Ca^{2+}-permeable cation channels sensitive to physical stimuli such as osmotic stress or heat (Montell et al., 2002). The candidate channel was previously reported as growth factor responsive channel (GRC) (Kanzaki et al., 1999), and later renamed TRP vanilloid type 2 (TRPV2) channel. We showed that TRPV2 is activated by mechanical stimuli and plays a critical role in the pathogenesis of muscular dystrophy and cardiomyopathy (Iwata et al., 2003; Muraki et al., 2003). TRPV2 is normally localized in the intracellular membrane compartment, but translocates to the plasma membrane in response to stretch or growth factor stimulation. Importantly, TRPV2 was observed to accumulate in the sarcolemma of the skeletal muscle from human patients with muscular dystrophy, BIO14.6 hamsters, and *mdx* mice (Fig.2) (Iwata et al., 2003), thus contributing to a sustained increase in $[Ca^{2+}]_i$ in diseased myocytes.

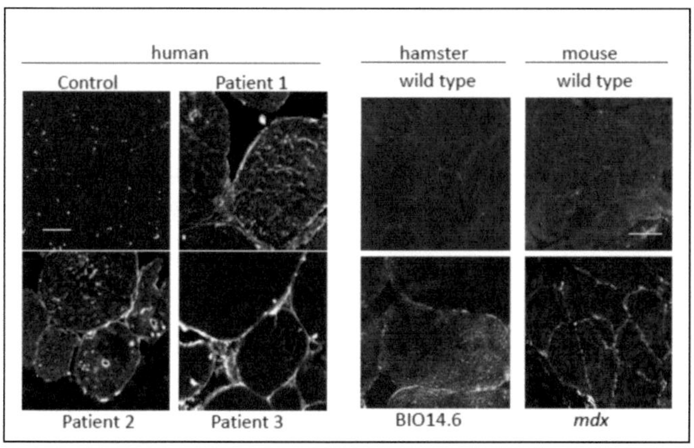

TRPV2 was immunolocalized in the frozen sections of the skeletal muscle from dystrophic patients and a non-dystrophic control, or from wild-type and dystrophic animals (Iwata et al., 2003). Note extensive sarcolemmal localization of TRPV2 in dystrophic patients and animal models. Bars, 50 μm.

Fig. 2. Immunohistochemical localization of TRPV2

In order to determine whether TRPV2 contributes to Ca^{2+}-induced muscle damage, we used a dominant-negative mutant strategy. We produced loss-of-function TRPV2 mutants in the pore region of the protein, which have a dominant-negative effect on the channel function by forming a non-functional oligomer, thereby abrogating the activity of endogenous TRPV2 (Fig.3 A). This dominant-negative TRPV2 mutant was incorporated into *mdx* mice by using a transgenic strategy or into BIO14.6 hamsters by adenoviral transfer. We found that these approaches significantly reduced resting $[Ca^{2+}]_i$ as well as the increase in $[Ca^{2+}]_i$ induced by high Ca^{2+} and the TRPV2 agonist 2-APB observed in dystrophic muscles (Fig.3 B).

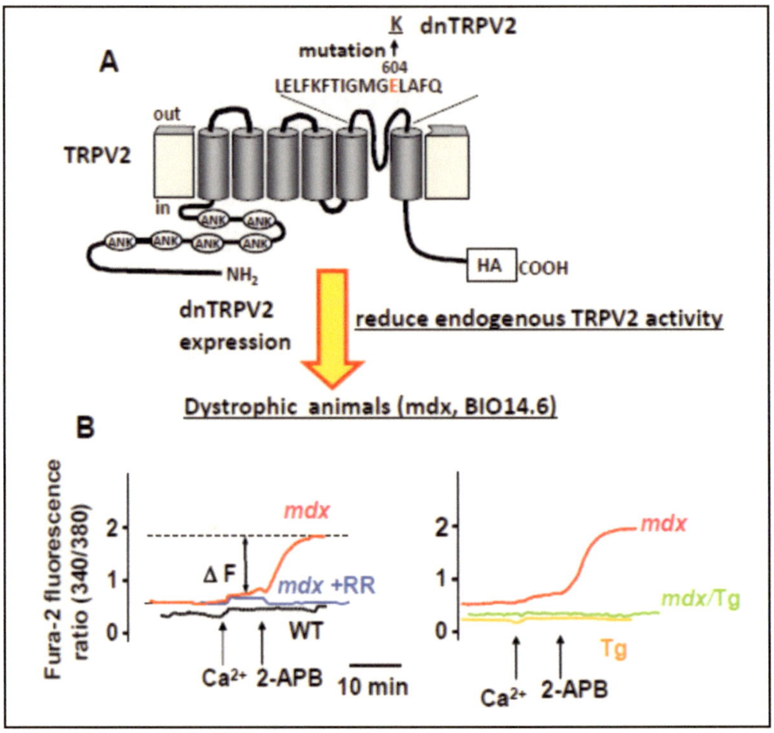

(A) Transgenic (Tg) mice overexpressing the TRPV2 mutant with a mutation in the putative pore region (Glu604) were produced, and crossed with *mdx* mice to introduce dnTRPV2 and inhibit endogenous TRPV2 activity. ANK, ankyrin repeat domain. HA, epitope tag. (B) Agonist (2-APB)-induced $[Ca^{2+}]_i$ increase in the isolated flexor digitorum brevis fibers of *mdx* mice, which is inhibited by ruthenium red (RR) (left). Note that no large $[Ca^{2+}]_i$ increase was detected in the fibers from wild-type mice. Such $[Ca^{2+}]_i$ increases in the *mdx* fibers were markedly reduced by expression of dnTRPV2 (*mdx*/Tg) (right) (Iwata et al., 2009).

Fig. 3. Production of a dominant-negative (dn) TRPV2 mutant

Transgenic or adenoviral expression of dnTRPV2 resulted in a 40%–70% reduction of impaired muscle function, as determined by an increased number of central nuclei and improvements in fiber size variability, fibrosis, apoptosis, elevated serum creatine kinase levels, and reduced muscle performance in dystrophic animals (Fig.4 A) (Iwata et al., 2009). Furthermore, *mdx* muscles were largely protected from eccentric work-induced force drop by the same transgenic strategy (Zanou et al., 2009). These results suggest that the entry of Ca^{2+} through TRPV2 channels precedes and is involved in membrane damage. Interestingly, expression of dnTRPV2 also promoted the removal of endogenous TRPV2 from the sarcolemma (Fig.4 B), suggesting that Ca^{2+} entering the cell via TRPV2 is required for the sarcolemmal retention of TRPV2 expression in dystrophic muscles. The pathological importance of TRPV2 was also verified using a pharmacological approach. A non-selective cation channel blocker tranilast was shown to be an effective inhibitor of TRPV2 (Iwata et al., 2005). Oral administration of tranilast reduced various symptoms of muscular dystrophy, such as elevated serum CK levels, progressive muscle degeneration, and increased infiltration of immune cells (Fig.5 A) (Iwata et al., 2005). Therefore, specific inhibitors of TRPV2 could be potentially useful and effective treatments for various muscle degenerative diseases, including hereditary diseases.

Although the relationship between muscular dystrophy and other types of TRPV channel has not yet been investigated, TRPV4 was recently identified as a responsive gene in inherited neurodegenerative disease, which indirectly causes muscle atrophy (Deng et al., 2010; Landoure et al., 2010).

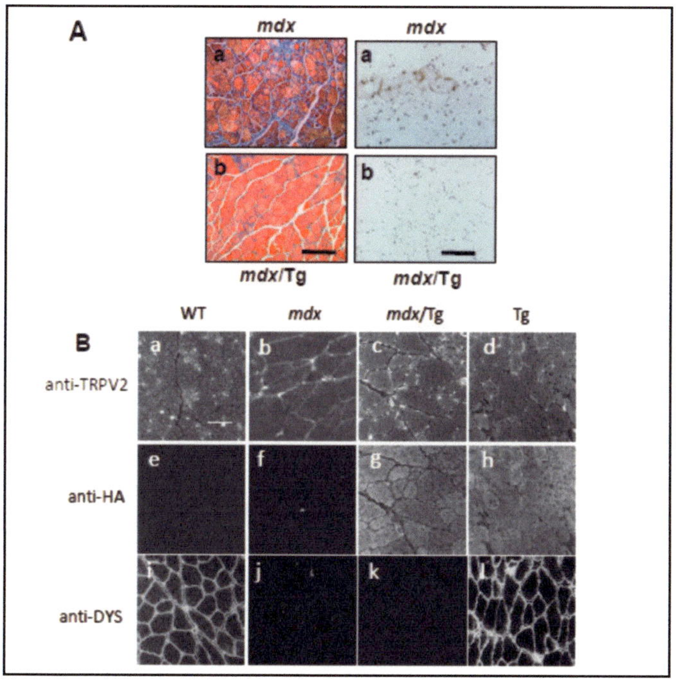

(A) Masson's trichrome staining (left) or TUNEL labeling (right) of the gastrocnemius muscle sections from *mdx* (a) or *mdx*/Tg (b) mice. Note the beneficial effect of dnTRPV2 (*mdx*/Tg). Scale bar, 100 μm. (B) Immunohistochemical analysis of TRPV2 (a-d) and dystrophin (i-l) in frozen cross sections of skeletal muscle. Dominant negative TRPV2 was immunolocalized with rat anti-HA (e-h). Note the removal of TRPV2 from the sarcolemma promoted by dnTRPV2 (*mdx*/Tg). Scale bar, 50 μm.

Fig. 4. Dominant-negative TRPV2 prevents muscle degeneration in *mdx* mice

3.2 TRPC channels

TRPC channels represent another important candidate for a therapeutic target in the treatment of muscular dystrophy. TRPC1, 4, and 6 are expressed in the sarcolemma of the skeletal muscle (Vandebrouck et al., 2002b). Knockdown of TRPC1 and TRPC4, but not TRPC6, was reported to reduce abnormal Ca^{2+} influx in dystrophic fibers (Vandebrouck et al., 2002b). TRPC1 has been shown to form the stretch-activated channel (Maroto et al., 2005), although contrary data also exists (Gottlieb et al., 2008). TRPC1, together with its binding partner caveolin-3, accumulates at higher levels in the sarcolemma of the dystrophin-deficient muscle and contributes to abnormal Ca^{2+} influx, which is activated by reactive oxygen species and Src kinase (Allen & Whitehead, 2011; Gervasio et al., 2008). Furthermore, mice lacking the scaffolding protein Homer-1, which interacts with TRPC1, exhibit myopathy associated with increased spontaneous cation influx (Stiber et al., 2008b). A recent study (Millay et al., 2009) also showed that overexpression of TRPC3 resulted in a phenotype of muscular dystrophy nearly identical to that observed in dystrophic animal models with abnormal DGC. Transgene-mediated inhibition of TRPC channels dramatically reduced the dystrophic phenotype in this animal model. These results suggest that Ca^{2+} entry through TRPC channels is sufficient to induce muscular dystrophy *in vivo*, and that TRPC channels are also promising therapeutic targets for muscular dysgenesis.

3.3 STIM1 and Orai1

Recently, the molecules involved in store-operated Ca^{2+} entry (SOCE) were identified. Stromal interaction molecules (STIM) were identified as the endoplasmic reticulum (ER) Ca^{2+} sensor, and found to interact with sarcolemmal Orai1 channels after Ca^{2+} store depletion to trigger SOCE. STIM1 and Orai1 are highly expressed in skeletal muscle: STIM1 is pre-localized at junctions of the SR with the T-tubule system, which contains pre-localized Orai1 (Stiber et al., 2008a). STIM1/Orai1 couples with TRPC channels (Dirksen, 2009) and the resulting STIM1/Orai1/TRPC1 ternary complexes have been shown to assemble during store depletion, thereby contributing to SOCE (Yuan et al., 2007; Zeng et al., 2008). Recently, the amount of STIM1/Orai1 proteins was reported to be upregulated in *mdx* muscle fibers, and the thresholds for the activation and deactivation of SOCE shifted to higher SR Ca^{2+} concentrations. This contributes to increased Ca^{2+} influx during long stimulation periods in *mdx* muscles (Edwards et al., 2010). In contrast, knockdown or inhibition of STIM1/Orai1 function was reported to cause myopathy resulting from impaired muscle development, which is different to muscular dystrophy caused by DGC defects. For example, mice lacking either STIM1 or Orai1 display skeletal muscle myopathy (Stiber et al., 2008a), and severe combined immunodeficiency patients characterized by loss-of-function mutations in STIM1/Orai1 signaling display similar skeletal muscle myopathy (Feske et al., 2006). Knockdown of STIM1 or expression of the Orai1 dominant negative E106Q caused a marked decrease in SOCE in skeletal muscle myotubes (Lyfenko & Dirksen, 2008). These findings suggest that STIM1/Orai1 proteins are involved in the fine-tuning of Ca^{2+} regulation, and physiological levels are required for normal skeletal muscle function.

3.4 Na^{+}-dependent ion transporters

In addition to $[Ca^{2+}]_i$, $[Na^{+}]_i$ is also reported to be elevated in skeletal muscle of *mdx* mice (Dunn et al., 1993). The increase in $[Na^{+}]_i$ is accompanied by a compensatory increase in membrane-bound Na^{+}/K^{+} ATPase contents (Dunn et al., 1995). A possible cause of increased $[Na^{+}]_i$ in the *mdx* skeletal muscle may be enhanced activity of stretch-activated channels, since it was inhibited by Gd^{3+} and streptomycin, which are known to be broad inhibitors of this channel type (Yeung et al., 2003a; Yeung et al., 2003b). It has also been shown that increases in $[Na^+]_i$ under the sarcolemma in *mdx* mice may be due to alterations in localization and gating properties of Nav1.4; the skeletal muscle isoform of the voltage-gated sodium channel may be correlated with increased cell death because $[Na^+]_i$ overload is reversed by tetrodotoxin, a specific Nav1.4 blocker (Hirn et al., 2008).

Recently, we have shown that the sarcolemmal Na^+/H^+ exchanger (NHE), which is known to be stimulated in response to various stimuli, including growth factors and osmotic stress, is significantly activated in dystrophic myocytes (from BIO14.6 hamsters). This is evidenced by an alkaline shift in the intracellular pH (pH_i) dependent on NHE activity, enhanced $^{22}Na^+$ influx, and elevated $[Na^+]_i$ (Iwata et al., 2007). In dystrophic myotubes, NHE was found to be a major Na^+ influx pathway, since the specific NHE inhibitor cariporide markedly (65%) inhibited it. Interestingly, NHE inhibition also significantly reduced the increase in intracellular Ca^{2+} and stretch-induced CK release in dystrophic myotubes, and ameliorated myopathic damage *in vivo* (Fig.5 B) (Iwata et al., 2007), indicating that the inhibition of NHE protects muscle cells against injury. Elevation in $[Na^+]_i$ may contribute to abnormal Ca^{2+} homeostasis by influencing the activity of the Na^+/Ca^{2+} exchanger.

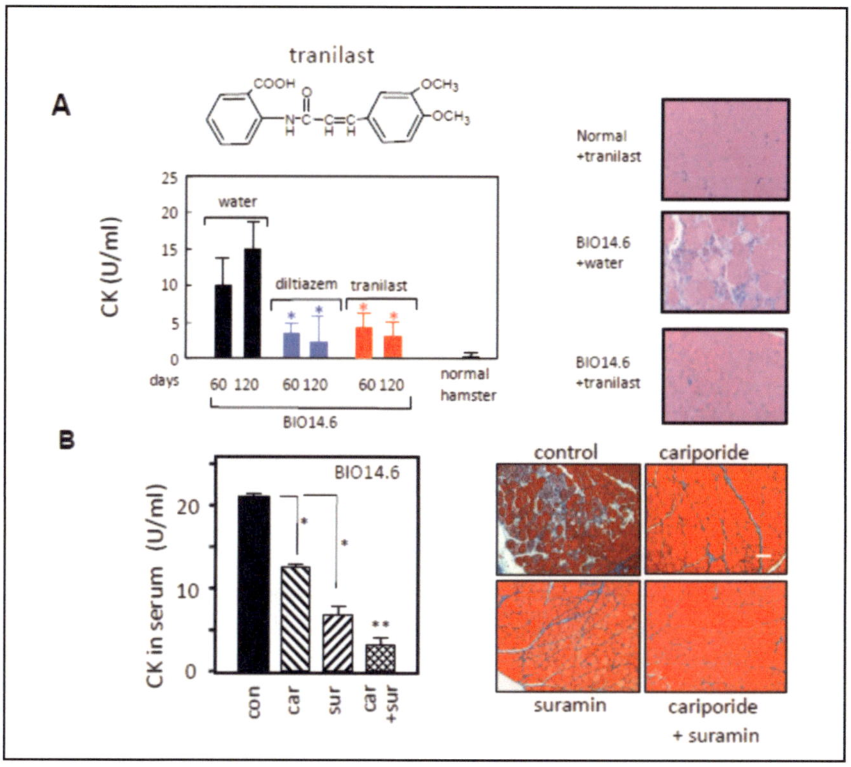

(A) Beneficial effect of the Ca^{2+}-handling drugs diltiazem and tranilast. Chemicals were administered orally to 30-day-old BIO14.6 hamsters for 60 or 120 days. The TRPV2 inhibitor tranilast effectively reduces CK release (left) and prevents muscle degeneration (H&E staining, right) (Iwata et al., 2005). (B) Beneficial effect of the P2 receptor antagonist suramin (sur) and the NHE inhibitor cariporide (car). In particular, note an excellent amelioration of muscle degeneration by combined administration of the two chemicals (Masson's trichrome staining of the quadriceps muscle sections, right) (Iwata et al., 2007). Scale bar, 100 μm.

Fig. 5. Effects of pharmacological agents on muscle degeneration in BIO14.6 hamsters

Furthermore, ATP was released more easily from the dystrophic myotubes in response to mechanical stretch. Thus, it is likely that P2 receptor stimulation with ATP activates the NHE, thereby leading to $[Ca^{2+}]_i$ overload (Iwata et al., 2007). These molecules also represent good targets for muscular dystrophy therapy. In fact, combined treatment with the P2 receptor antagonist suramin and the NHE1-specific inhibitor cariporide resulted in efficient amelioration of muscular dystrophy in BIO14.6 hamsters (Fig.5 B).

3.5 SR proteins

Recently, the occurrence of increased Ca^{2+} sparks, an indication of abnormalities in the SR Ca^{2+} release channel ryanodine receptor (RyR1), was reported in dystrophic fibers (Bellinger et al., 2009; Wang et al., 2005). RyR1 from *mdx* mice were shown to be excessively cystein-nitrosylated, which was coupled with depletion of calstabin-1 (calcium channel-stabilizing binding protein-1, also known as FKBP12) from RyR1. As a consequence, this led to increased spontaneous RyR1 openings (Ca^{2+} sparks), and reduced specific muscle force. Prevention of calstabin-1 depletion from RyR1 inhibited SR Ca^{2+} leak, reduced muscle damage, improved muscle function, and increased exercise performance in *mdx* mice (Bellinger et al., 2009).

One strategy to reduce the effects associated with chronic Ca^{2+} leak from activated channels and membrane rupture is to increase the rate of Ca^{2+} reuptake into the SR, by overexpression of the SR Ca^{2+} pump SERCA1. Indeed, transgenic overexpression of SERCA1 dramatically rescued the dystrophic phenotype of delta-sarcoglycan-null mice (Goonasekera et al., 2011). Furthermore, Ca^{2+} removal by adenovirus-mediated overexpression of SERCA1a reduced susceptibility to contraction-induced damage in *mdx* mice (Morine et al., 2010). These results suggest that Ca^{2+} is a common risk factor in the transmission of most genetic defects to downstream necrosis pathways in muscular dystrophy. Thus, control of $[Ca^{2+}]_i$ would provide a universal therapeutic strategy that reduces the dystrophic phenotype.

3.6 Other candidates

Dystrophic muscles are always exposed to oxidative and immune stress, as well as mechanical stress. Although not discussed in detail in this chapter, there are many important stress-dependent factors leading to muscle injury in muscular dystrophy (Lawler, 2011; Tidball & Wehling-Henricks, 2007). For example, NADPH oxidase in the muscles was recently reported to be an important source of oxidative stress, which stimulates stretch-activated Ca^{2+} entry in dystrophic muscles (Whitehead et al., 2010). Futhermore, nitric oxide (NO) synthase in macrophages may be another risk factor that promotes membrane injury in dystrophic muscles (Villalta et al., 2009). Therapeutic interventions that regulate stress pathways may be useful in protecting against dystrophic phenotypes.

4. Conclusion

As described above, disruption of the DGC results in increased mechanical stress and abnormal ion homeostasis. Sustained increases in $[Ca^{2+}]_i$ are the key pathological event leading to muscle degeneration (Fig.6). Many key players contribute to abnormal Ca^{2+} handling. Among these molecules, we consider TRPV2 to have high therapeutic potential for the treatment of muscular dystrophy, because most TRPV2 localizes to the intracellular

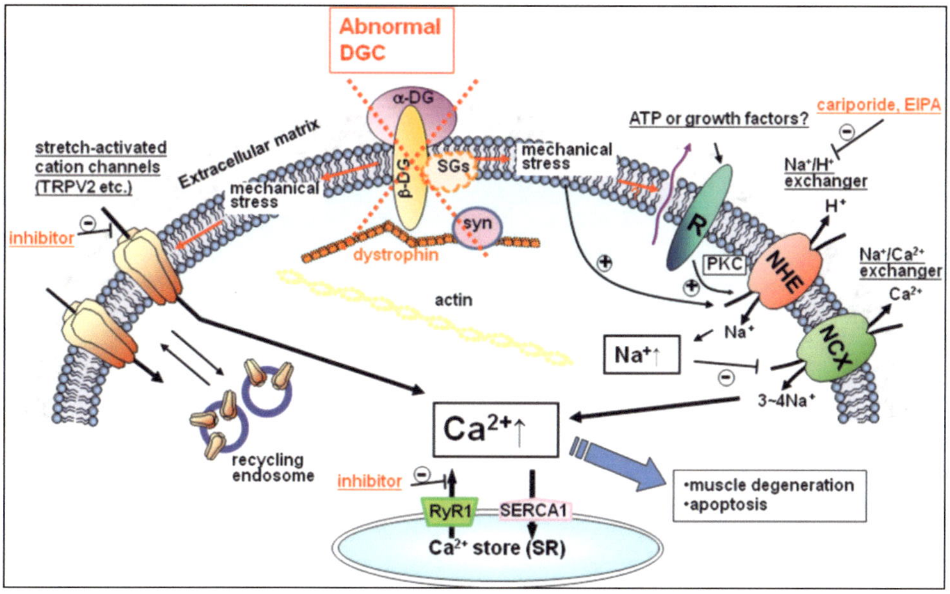

Fig. 6. Schematic drawing showing a possible pathway leading to abnormal Ca^{2+} handling and subsequent muscle degeneration in DGC-defective dystrophic muscles, according to our recent studies (Iwata et al., 2003; 2009; 2007; 2005) Increased mechanical stress caused by DGC defects induces sarcolemmal translocation and TRPV2 activation, leading to sustained $[Ca^{2+}]_i$ increase. On the other hand, mechanical stress also induces release of bioactive substances such as ATP and growth factors, which, in turn, activates NHE, increases $[Na^+]_i$, and results in further increase in $[Ca^{2+}]_i$ via inhibition of the NCX forward mode. Ca^{2+} handling proteins in the SR may also contribute to cytosolic Ca^{2+} overload. Therapeutic intervention at the level of Ca^{2+}-handling proteins would be useful for reducing the dystrophic phenotype.

membranes in the healthy skeletal muscles, while it translocates to the surface membrane upon muscle degeneration. Hence, specific inhibitors against TRPV2 are expected to act only on degenerative muscles. Given the lack of a definitive strategy to cure muscular dystrophy, identifying new therapeutic targets appears to be extremely important. We hope that this chapter might help to provide an opportunity to promote such studies.

5. Acknowledgments

We thank all the members of our laboratory who participated in the studies described in this chapter for their contribution and advice. We also thank the staff in the National Cerebral and Cardiovascular Center and the National Center of Neurology and Psychiatry for financial support and helpful suggestions.

6. References

Alderton, J. M. & Steinhardt, R. A. 2000a. Calcium influx through calcium leak channels is responsible for the elevated levels of calcium-dependent proteolysis in dystrophic myotubes. *Journal of Biological Chemistry*, 275(13): 9452-9460.

Alderton, J. M. & Steinhardt, R. A. 2000b. How calcium influx through calcium leak channels is responsible for the elevated levels of calcium-dependent proteolysis in dystrophic myotubes. *Trends in Cardiovascular Medicine*, 10(6): 268-272.

Allen, D. G. & Whitehead, N. P. 2011. Duchenne muscular dystrophy--what causes the increased membrane permeability in skeletal muscle? *International Journal of Biochemistry and Cell Biology*, 43(3): 290-294.

Bellinger, A. M.; Reiken, S.; Carlson, C.; Mongillo, M.; Liu, X.; Rothman, L.; Matecki, S.; Lacampagne, A. & Marks, A. R. 2009. Hypernitrosylated ryanodine receptor calcium release channels are leaky in dystrophic muscle. *Nature Medicine*, 15(3): 325-330.

Boittin, F. X.; Petermann, O.; Hirn, C.; Mittaud, P.; Dorchies, O. M.; Roulet, E. & Ruegg, U. T. 2006. Ca^{2+}-independent phospholipase A2 enhances store-operated Ca^{2+} entry in dystrophic skeletal muscle fibers. *Journal of Cell Science*, 119(Pt 18): 3733-3742.

Brown, R. H., Jr. 1997. Dystrophin-associated proteins and the muscular dystrophies. *Annual Review of Medicine*, 48: 457-466.

Campbell, K. P. 1995. Three muscular dystrophies: loss of cytoskeleton-extracellular matrix linkage. *Cell*, 80(5): 675-679.

Campbell, K. P. & Kahl, S. D. 1989. Association of dystrophin and an integral membrane glycoprotein. *Nature*, 338(6212): 259-262.

Deng, H. X.; Klein, C. J.; Yan, J.; Shi, Y.; Wu, Y.; Fecto, F.; Yau, H. J.; Yang, Y.; Zhai, H.; Siddique, N.; Hedley-Whyte, E. T.; Delong, R.; Martina, M.; Dyck, P. J. & Siddique, T. 2010. Scapuloperoneal spinal muscular atrophy and CMT2C are allelic disorders caused by alterations in TRPV4. *Nature Genetics*, 42(2): 165-169.

Dirksen, R. T. 2009. Checking your SOCCs and feet: the molecular mechanisms of Ca^{2+} entry in skeletal muscle. *J Physiol*, 587(Pt 13): 3139-3147.

Duclos, F.; Straub, V.; Moore, S. A.; Venzke, D. P.; Hrstka, R. F.; Crosbie, R. H.; Durbeej, M.; Lebakken, C. S.; Ettinger, A. J.; van der Meulen, J.; Holt, K. H.; Lim, L. E.; Sanes, J. R.; Davidson, B. L.; Faulkner, J. A.; Williamson, R. & Campbell, K. P. 1998. Progressive muscular dystrophy in alpha-sarcoglycan-deficient mice. *Journal of Cell Biology*, 142(6): 1461-1471.

Ducret, T.; Vandebrouck, C.; Cao, M. L.; Lebacq, J. & Gailly, P. 2006. Functional role of store-operated and stretch-activated channels in murine adult skeletal muscle fibres. *J Physiol*, 575(Pt 3): 913-924.

Dunn, J. F.; Bannister, N.; Kemp, G. J. & Publicover, S. J. 1993. Sodium is elevated in mdx muscles: ionic interactions in dystrophic cells. *Journal of the Neurological Sciences*, 114(1): 76-80.

Dunn, J. F.; Burton, K. A. & Dauncey, M. J. 1995. Ouabain sensitive Na^+/K^+-ATPase content is elevated in mdx mice: implications for the regulation of ions in dystrophic muscle. *Journal of the Neurological Sciences*, 133(1-2): 11-15.

Edwards, J. N.; Friedrich, O.; Cully, T. R.; von Wegner, F.; Murphy, R. M. & Launikonis, B. S. 2010. Upregulation of store-operated Ca^{2+} entry in dystrophic mdx mouse muscle. *Am J Physiol Cell Physiol*, 299(1): C42-50.

Ervasti, J. M. & Campbell, K. P. 1993. A role for the dystrophin-glycoprotein complex as a transmembrane linker between laminin and actin. *Journal of Cell Biology*, 122(4): 809-823.

Feske, S.; Gwack, Y.; Prakriya, M.; Srikanth, S.; Puppel, S. H.; Tanasa, B.; Hogan, P. G.; Lewis, R. S.; Daly, M. & Rao, A. 2006. A mutation in Orai1 causes immune deficiency by abrogating CRAC channel function. *Nature*, 441(7090): 179-185.

Fong, P. Y.; Turner, P. R.; Denetclaw, W. F. & Steinhardt, R. A. 1990. Increased activity of calcium leak channels in myotubes of Duchenne human and mdx mouse origin. *Science*, 250(4981): 673-676.

Franco-Obregon, A., Jr. & Lansman, J. B. 1994. Mechanosensitive ion channels in skeletal muscle from normal and dystrophic mice. *J Physiol*, 481 (Pt 2): 299-309.

Franco-Obregon, A. & Lansman, J. B. 2002. Changes in mechanosensitive channel gating following mechanical stimulation in skeletal muscle myotubes from the mdx mouse. *J Physiol*, 539(Pt 2): 391-407.

Franco, A., Jr. & Lansman, J. B. 1990. Calcium entry through stretch-inactivated ion channels in mdx myotubes. *Nature*, 344(6267): 670-673.

Gervasio, O. L.; Whitehead, N. P.; Yeung, E. W.; Phillips, W. D. & Allen, D. G. 2008. TRPC1 binds to caveolin-3 and is regulated by Src kinase - role in Duchenne muscular dystrophy. *Journal of Cell Science*, 121(Pt 13): 2246-2255.

Goonasekera, S. A.; Lam, C. K.; Millay, D. P.; Sargent, M. A.; Hajjar, R. J.; Kranias, E. G. & Molkentin, J. D. 2011. Mitigation of muscular dystrophy in mice by SERCA overexpression in skeletal muscle. *Journal of Clinical Investigation*, 121(3): 1044-1052.

Gottlieb, P.; Folgering, J.; Maroto, R.; Raso, A.; Wood, T. G.; Kurosky, A.; Bowman, C.; Bichet, D.; Patel, A.; Sachs, F.; Martinac, B.; Hamill, O. P. & Honore, E. 2008. Revisiting TRPC1 and TRPC6 mechanosensitivity. *Pflugers Archiv. European Journal of Physiology*, 455(6): 1097-1103.

Hamill, O. P. & McBride, D. W., Jr. 1996. The pharmacology of mechanogated membrane ion channels. *Pharmacological Reviews*, 48(2): 231-252.

Hirn, C.; Shapovalov, G.; Petermann, O.; Roulet, E. & Ruegg, U. T. 2008. Nav1.4 deregulation in dystrophic skeletal muscle leads to Na^+ overload and enhanced cell death. *Journal of General Physiology*, 132(2): 199-208.

Hopf, F. W.; Turner, P. R.; Denetclaw, W. F., Jr.; Reddy, P. & Steinhardt, R. A. 1996. A critical evaluation of resting intracellular free calcium regulation in dystrophic mdx muscle. *American Journal of Physiology*, 271(4 Pt 1): C1325-1339.

Iwata, Y.; Katanosaka, Y.; Arai, Y.; Komamura, K.; Miyatake, K. & Shigekawa, M. 2003. A novel mechanism of myocyte degeneration involving the Ca^{2+}-permeable growth factor-regulated channel. *Journal of Cell Biology*, 161(5): 957-967.

Iwata, Y.; Katanosaka, Y.; Arai, Y.; Shigekawa, M. & Wakabayashi, S. 2009. Dominant-negative inhibition of Ca^{2+} influx via TRPV2 ameliorates muscular dystrophy in animal models. *Human Molecular Genetics*, 18(5): 824-834.

Iwata, Y.; Katanosaka, Y.; Hisamitsu, T. & Wakabayashi, S. 2007. Enhanced Na^+/H^+ Exchange Activity Contributes to the Pathogenesis of Muscular Dystrophy via Involvement of P2 Receptors. *American Journal of Pathology*, 171(5):1576-1587.

Iwata, Y.; Katanosaka, Y.; Shijun, Z.; Kobayashi, Y.; Hanada, H.; Shigekawa, M. & Wakabayashi, S. 2005. Protective effects of Ca^{2+} handling drugs against abnormal Ca^{2+} homeostasis and cell damage in myopathic skeletal muscle cells. *Biochemical Pharmacology*, 70(5): 740-751.

Iwata, Y.; Nakamura, H.; Fujiwara, K. & Shigekawa, M. 1993a. Altered membrane-dystrophin association in the cardiomyopathic hamster heart muscle. *Biochemical and Biophysical Research Communications*, 190(2): 589-595.

Iwata, Y.; Nakamura, H.; Mizuno, Y.; Yoshida, M.; Ozawa, E. & Shigekawa, M. 1993b. Defective association of dystrophin with sarcolemmal glycoproteins in the cardiomyopathic hamster heart. *FEBS Letters*, 329(1-2): 227-231.

Kanzaki, M.; Zhang, Y. Q.; Mashima, H.; Li, L.; Shibata, H. & Kojima, I. 1999. Translocation of a calcium-permeable cation channel induced by insulin-like growth factor-I. *Nat Cell Biol*, 1(3): 165-170.

Landoure, G.; Zdebik, A. A.; Martinez, T. L.; Burnett, B. G.; Stanescu, H. C.; Inada, H.; Shi, Y.; Taye, A. A.; Kong, L.; Munns, C. H.; Choo, S. S.; Phelps, C. B.; Paudel, R.; Houlden, H.; Ludlow, C. L.; Caterina, M. J.; Gaudet, R.; Kleta, R.; Fischbeck, K. H. & Sumner, C. J. 2010. Mutations in TRPV4 cause Charcot-Marie-Tooth disease type 2C. *Nature Genetics*, 42(2): 170-174.

Lawler, J. M. 2011. Exacerbation of pathology by oxidative stress in respiratory and locomotor muscles with Duchenne muscular dystrophy. *J Physiol*, 589(Pt 9): 2161-2170.

Lyfenko, A. D. & Dirksen, R. T. 2008. Differential dependence of store-operated and excitation-coupled Ca^{2+} entry in skeletal muscle on STIM1 and Orai1. *J Physiol*, 586(Pt 20): 4815-4824.

MacLennan, P. A.; McArdle, A. & Edwards, R. H. 1991. Effects of calcium on protein turnover of incubated muscles from mdx mice. *American Journal of Physiology*, 260(4 Pt 1): E594-598.

Mallouk, N.; Jacquemond, V. & Allard, B. 2000. Elevated subsarcolemmal Ca^{2+} in mdx mouse skeletal muscle fibers detected with Ca^{2+}-activated K^+ channels. *Proceedings of the National Academy of Sciences of the United States of America*, 97(9): 4950-4955.

Maroto, R.; Raso, A.; Wood, T. G.; Kurosky, A.; Martinac, B. & Hamill, O. P. 2005. TRPC1 forms the stretch-activated cation channel in vertebrate cells. *Nat Cell Biol*, 7(2): 179-185.

Menke, A. & Jockusch, H. 1991. Decreased osmotic stability of dystrophin-less muscle cells from the *mdx* mouse. *Nature*, 349(6304): 69-71.

Millay, D. P.; Goonasekera, S. A.; Sargent, M. A.; Maillet, M.; Aronow, B. J. & Molkentin, J. D. 2009. Calcium influx is sufficient to induce muscular dystrophy through a TRPC-dependent mechanism. *Proceedings of the National Academy of Sciences of the United States of America*, 106(45): 19023-19028.

Montell, C.; Birnbaumer, L. & Flockerzi, V. 2002. The TRP channels, a remarkably functional family. *Cell*, 108(5): 595-598.

Morine, K. J.; Sleeper, M. M.; Barton, E. R. & Sweeney, H. L. 2010. Overexpression of SERCA1a in the *mdx* diaphragm reduces susceptibility to contraction-induced damage. *Human Gene Therapy*, 21(12): 1735-1739.

Muraki, K.; Iwata, Y.; Katanosaka, Y.; Ito, T.; Ohya, S.; Shigekawa, M. & Imaizumi, Y. 2003. TRPV2 is a component of osmotically sensitive cation channels in murine aortic myocytes. *Circulation Research*, 93(9): 829-838.

Nakamura, T. Y.; Iwata, Y.; Sampaolesi, M.; Hanada, H.; Saito, N.; Artman, M.; Coetzee, W. A. & Shigekawa, M. 2001. Stretch-activated cation channels in skeletal muscle myotubes from sarcoglycan-deficient hamsters. *Am J Physiol Cell Physiol*, 281(2): C690-699.

Nigro, V.; Okazaki, Y.; Belsito, A.; Piluso, G.; Matsuda, Y.; Politano, L.; Nigro, G.; Ventura, C.; Abbondanza, C.; Molinari, A. M.; Acampora, D.; Nishimura, M.; Hayashizaki, Y. & Puca, G. A. 1997. Identification of the Syrian hamster cardiomyopathy gene. *Human Molecular Genetics*, 6(4): 601-607.

Petrof, B. J.; Shrager, J. B.; Stedman, H. H.; Kelly, A. M. & Sweeney, H. L. 1993. Dystrophin protects the sarcolemma from stresses developed during muscle contraction. *Proceedings of the National Academy of Sciences of the United States of America*, 90(8): 3710-3714.

Robert, V.; Massimino, M. L.; Tosello, V.; Marsault, R.; Cantini, M.; Sorrentino, V. & Pozzan, T. 2001. Alteration in calcium handling at the subcellular level in *mdx* myotubes. *Journal of Biological Chemistry*, 276(7): 4647-4651.

Spencer, M. J.; Croall, D. E. & Tidball, J. G. 1995. Calpains are activated in necrotic fibers from *mdx* dystrophic mice. *Journal of Biological Chemistry*, 270(18): 10909-10914.

Stiber, J.; Hawkins, A.; Zhang, Z. S.; Wang, S.; Burch, J.; Graham, V.; Ward, C. C.; Seth, M.; Finch, E.; Malouf, N.; Williams, R. S.; Eu, J. P. & Rosenberg, P. 2008a. STIM1 signalling controls store-operated calcium entry required for development and contractile function in skeletal muscle. *Nat Cell Biol*, 10(6): 688-697.

Stiber, J. A.; Zhang, Z. S.; Burch, J.; Eu, J. P.; Zhang, S.; Truskey, G. A.; Seth, M.; Yamaguchi, N.; Meissner, G.; Shah, R.; Worley, P. F.; Williams, R. S. & Rosenberg, P. B. 2008b. Mice lacking Homer 1 exhibit a skeletal myopathy characterized by abnormal transient receptor potential channel activity. *Molecular and Cellular Biology*, 28(8): 2637-2647.

Suchyna, T. M.; Johnson, J. H.; Hamer, K.; Leykam, J. F.; Gage, D. A.; Clemo, H. F.; Baumgarten, C. M. & Sachs, F. 2000. Identification of a peptide toxin from Grammostola spatulata spider venom that blocks cation-selective stretch-activated channels. *Journal of General Physiology*, 115(5): 583-598.

Tawada-Iwata, Y.; Imagawa, T.; Yoshida, A.; Takahashi, M.; Nakamura, H. & Shigekawa, M. 1993. Increased mechanical extraction of T-tubule/junctional SR from cardiomyopathic hamster heart. *American Journal of Physiology*, 264(5 Pt 2): H1447-1453.

Tidball, J. G. & Wehling-Henricks, M. 2007. The role of free radicals in the pathophysiology of muscular dystrophy. *Journal of Applied Physiology*, 102(4): 1677-1686.

Tinsley, J. M.; Blake, D. J.; Zuellig, R. A. & Davies, K. E. 1994. Increasing complexity of the dystrophin-associated protein complex. *Proceedings of the National Academy of Sciences of the United States of America*, 91(18): 8307-8313.

Turner, P. R.; Schultz, R.; Ganguly, B. & Steinhardt, R. A. 1993. Proteolysis results in altered leak channel kinetics and elevated free calcium in *mdx* muscle. *Journal of Membrane Biology*, 133(3): 243-251.

Turner, P. R.; Westwood, T.; Regen, C. M. & Steinhardt, R. A. 1988. Increased protein degradation results from elevated free calcium levels found in muscle from *mdx* mice. *Nature*, 335(6192): 735-738.

Vandebrouck, C.; Duport, G.; Cognard, C. & Raymond, G. 2001. Cationic channels in normal and dystrophic human myotubes. *Neuromuscular Disorders*, 11(1): 72-79.

Vandebrouck, C.; Duport, G.; Raymond, G. & Cognard, C. 2002a. Hypotonic medium increases calcium permeant channels activity in human normal and dystrophic myotubes. *Neuroscience Letters*, 323(3): 239-243.

Vandebrouck, C.; Martin, D.; Colson-Van Schoor, M.; Debaix, H. & Gailly, P. 2002b. Involvement of TRPC in the abnormal calcium influx observed in dystrophic (*mdx*) mouse skeletal muscle fibers. *Journal of Cell Biology*, 158(6): 1089-1096.

Villalta, S. A.; Nguyen, H. X.; Deng, B.; Gotoh, T. & Tidball, J. G. 2009. Shifts in macrophage phenotypes and macrophage competition for arginine metabolism affect the severity of muscle pathology in muscular dystrophy. *Human Molecular Genetics*, 18(3): 482-496.

Wang, X.; Weisleder, N.; Collet, C.; Zhou, J.; Chu, Y.; Hirata, Y.; Zhao, X.; Pan, Z.; Brotto, M.; Cheng, H. & Ma, J. 2005. Uncontrolled calcium sparks act as a dystrophic signal for mammalian skeletal muscle. *Nat Cell Biol*, 7(5): 525-530.

Whitehead, N. P.; Yeung, E. W.; Froehner, S. C. & Allen, D. G. 2010. Skeletal muscle NADPH oxidase is increased and triggers stretch-induced damage in the *mdx* mouse. *PLoS One*, 5(12): e15354.

Yeung, E. W.; Ballard, H. J.; Bourreau, J. P. & Allen, D. G. 2003a. Intracellular sodium in mammalian muscle fibers after eccentric contractions. *Journal of Applied Physiology*, 94(6): 2475-2482.

Yeung, E. W.; Head, S. I. & Allen, D. G. 2003b. Gadolinium reduces short-term stretch-induced muscle damage in isolated *mdx* mouse muscle fibres. *J Physiol*, 552(Pt 2): 449-458.

Yuan, J. P.; Zeng, W.; Huang, G. N.; Worley, P. F. & Muallem, S. 2007. STIM1 heteromultimerizes TRPC channels to determine their function as store-operated channels. *Nat Cell Biol*, 9(6): 636-645.

Zanou, N.; Iwata, Y.; Schakman, O.; Lebacq, J.; Wakabayashi, S. & Gailly, P. 2009. Essential role of TRPV2 ion channel in the sensitivity of dystrophic muscle to eccentric contractions. *FEBS Letters*, 583(22): 3600-3604.

Zeng, W.; Yuan, J. P.; Kim, M. S.; Choi, Y. J.; Huang, G. N.; Worley, P. F. & Muallem, S. 2008. STIM1 gates TRPC channels, but not Orai1, by electrostatic interaction. *Molecular Cell*, 32(3): 439-448.

8

Mitogen-Activated Protein Kinases and Mitogen-Activated Protein Kinase Phosphatases in Regenerative Myogenesis and Muscular Dystrophy

Hao Shi[1] and Anton M. Bennett[1,2]
[1]*Department of Pharmacology*
[2]*Program in Integrative Cell Signaling and Neurobiology of Metabolism, Yale University School of Medicine, United States*

1. Introduction

The mitogen-activated protein kinase (MAPK) signal transduction pathway is required to promote skeletal myogenesis and maintain skeletal muscle function. Although it has been long appreciated that the MAPK pathway plays a critical role in skeletal myogenesis it is still unclear as to whether the MAPKs are involved in the development of skeletal muscle diseases such as muscular dystrophies. Much evidence has demonstrated that MAPK activation is important for skeletal myogenesis. The cessation of MAPK activity is also an important part of the process of skeletal myogenesis. The MAPK phosphatases (MKPs) are responsible for inactivating the MAPKs. The role of the MKPs in physiological and pathophysiological functions of skeletal muscle remains to be fully understood. In this review, we will summarize the current state of understanding of the functional roles of the MAPKs, and the emerging role of the MKPs in the regulation of physiological skeletal muscle function, and their potential involvement in skeletal muscle diseases.

2. Mitogen-activated Protein Kinase signaling and myogenesis

The mitogen-activated protein kinase (MAPK) cascade plays an essential role in conveying extracellular signals from growth factors, stress, and cytokines into biological responses that include differentiation, proliferation, apoptosis and cell motility (Cuevas et al., 2007; Pearson et al., 2001). Up until now, at least 4 MAPK signaling pathways have been identified: 1) extracellular signal-regulated kinase 1 and 2 (ERK1/2), 2) p38α/β/γ/δ MAPK, 3) c-Jun NH_2-terminal kinases 1, 2, and 3 (JNK1/2/3) and 4) ERK5 (Bogoyevitch, 2006; Bogoyevitch and Court, 2004; Whitmarsh, 2006; Zarubin and Han, 2005). MAPKs when phosphorylated on their regulatory threonine and tyrosine residues by their upstream MAPK kinases become activated. Once activated, these MAPKs phosphorylate substrates that include transcription factors, phospholipases, protein kinases and cytoskeletal proteins (Johnson and Lapadat, 2002; Turjanski et al., 2007).

A large body of data suggests that the p38 MAPK pathway is pro-myogenic. p38 MAPK promotes myogenesis through 1) interaction with transcription factors. At the early stage of differentiation, p38 MAPK phosphorylates E-protein E47, which dimerizes with the transcription factor MyoD to activate muscle-specific gene expression (Lluis et al., 2005). Whereas, at later stages of differentiation, p38 MAPK phosphorylates the transcription factor MRF4 thereby repressing its transcriptional activity (Suelves et al., 2004). 2) phosphorylation of the SWI/SNF chromatin-remodeling complex, recruiting this complex to myogenic loci (Simone et al., 2004); 3) phosphorylation of the transcription factor myocyte enhancer factor-2 (MEF2) thereby enhancing its transcriptional activity (Black and Olson, 1998; Zetser et al., 1999); 4) stabilization of myogenic mRNA by directly phosphorylating KSRP, an important factor for decaying AU-rich element mRNA, and compromising its function to promote mRNA decay (Briata et al., 2005). These observations provide strong mechanistic insight into how p38 MAPK couples to the myogenic machinery.

Evidence derived from mouse models also supports the functional role of p38 MAPK in muscle differentiation (Perdiguero et al., 2007). In an effort to dissect the role of different p38 MAPK isoforms in myogenesis, Perdiguero *et al* used p38α, p38β, p38γ, and p38δ-deficient mice and analyzed the function of each. p38α rather than p38β and p38γ-deficient myoblasts failed to form multinucleated myotubes, whereas p38δ-deficient myoblasts exhibited attenuated differentiation (Perdiguero et al., 2007). Although a wide body of evidence supports the pro-myogenic role of p38 MAPK, several reports also imply the involvement of p38 MAPK in muscle cell proliferation. The concomitant activation of p38 MAPKα/β and satellite cells imply that p38 MAPK may also be involved in satellite cell activation, since blockade of p38 MAPK by pharmacological inhibitors of p38 MAPK prevents both satellite cell proliferation and differentiation (Jones et al., 2005; Shi et al., 2010). A recent study using p38γ-deficient mice revealed that muscles lacking this isoform of p38 MAPK contain 50% less satellite cells, and these cells exhibit reduced proliferation (Gillespie et al., 2009) implying that this p38 MAPK isoform may also be an important regulator of satellite cell deposition and proliferation.

Although a critical role for ERK1/2 in satellite cell proliferation is established, surprisingly the role of ERK1/2 in myogenesis has not been well defined. Conflicting data from various groups suggest that this pathway may be tailored to respond to distinct cellular and extracellular conditions. Using 10T1/2 fibroblasts, Gredinger el showed that MEK1 and/or Raf1 positively regulates myogenesis by enhancing MyoD transcriptional activity, addition of the MEK inhibitor PD098059 represses MyoD-responsive genes (Gredinger et al., 1998). PD098059 also partially inhibits the formation of multinucleated myotubes in C2 myoblasts (Gredinger et al., 1998). In contrast, others have reported a negative effect of ERK1/2 in the regulation of myogenesis (Dorman and Johnson, 1999; Weyman and Wolfman, 1998). In 23A2 and C2C12 myoblasts, IGF-1 and FGF-2 inhibit myoblast differentiation through ERK1/2 signaling as PD098059 blocked this effect (Kontaridis et al., 2002; Weyman and Wolfman, 1998). Persistent activation of Raf/MEK/ERK1/2 by overexpression of a constitutively active Raf inhibits the fusion of embryonic chick myoblasts into multinucleated myotubes. This inhibition can be rescued by addition of PD098059 (Dorman and Johnson, 1999). Yet there is another layer of regulation of Ras/Raf/ERK1/2 on myogenesis. A novel regulator of the Ras-Raf interaction, named DA-Raf, lacks the Raf kinase domain and interferes with the binding of Ras to other targets. It was found that DA-

Raf serves as a positive regulator of myogenic differentiation (Yokoyama et al., 2007). A recent study revealed that Grb2-associated binder 1 (Gab1) interacts with the protein tyrosine phosphatase SHP-2 to activate downstream ERK signaling, thereby inhibiting IGF-1-mediated myogenic differentiation (Koyama et al., 2008). These results are consistent with other data in which conditional deletion of SHP-2 in skeletal muscle impairs skeletal muscle growth (Fornaro et al., 2006). Taken together, these findings tend to support the notion that ERK1/2 signaling promotes myoblast proliferation and inhibits myogenic differentiation. However, further genetic data using ERK-deficient mice needs to be provided to fully conclude the relevance of ERK1/2 in myoblast proliferation and differentiation.

ERK5 is a novel member of the MAPK family and its physiological function in myogenesis remains to be fully defined. ERK5 is enriched in skeletal muscle, it is activated upon myogenic differentiation, and anti-sense RNA to ERK5 blocks entry into myogenesis (Dinev et al., 2001). A recent study revealed an essential role of ERK5 in muscle cell fusion through the transcription factors Sp1 and Klf2/4 (Sunadome et al., 2011). ERK5 has also been shown to be responsible for muscle cell fusion without interference with other differentiation processes (Sunadome et al., 2011).

Although the JNK pathway has been implicated in myoblast proliferation (Perdiguero et al., 2007) its role in myogenic differentiation remains controversial. JNK has been demonstrated to be either dispensable or negative for myogenesis (Gallo et al., 1999; Khurana and Dey, 2004; Meriane et al., 2002). It would be extremely informative if myoblasts derived from mice lacking either of the JNK isoforms were analyzed for their effects on cell proliferation and differentiation to resolve these issues.

3. Duchenne muscular dystrophy

The most common form of muscular dystrophy is Duchenne muscular dystrophy (DMD) which affects up to 1:3,500 males in the United States (Porter, 2000). The regenerative capacity of skeletal muscle in DMD-stricken patients is impaired due to the loss of dystrophin (Davies and Nowak, 2006). DMD patients lose muscle strength and mobility and the disease often results in death. There is neither a cure, nor an effective treatment for DMD, or similar skeletal muscle degenerative diseases (Bhatnagar and Kumar, 2010; Tedesco et al., 2010). DMD is caused by the loss or partial deficiency in the dystrophin protein, which serves as a critical component of the dystrophin glycoprotein complex (DGC) linking the cytoskeleton of the muscle fibers to that of the extracellular matrix. The loss of dystrophin cripples the functionality of the DGC rendering the muscle fiber more susceptible to stress-induced injury. Although the primary defect of DMD is the loss of dystrophin, there are multiple secondary events that contribute to the progression of the disease. These include profound inflammatory responses, extracellular matrix degradation and fibrosis. Strategies therefore that curtail some of these secondary responses have been considered as potential therapeutic avenues to treating the progression of the disease in DMD patients.

Although the DGC and its components such as dystrophin appear to primarily serve structural roles to couple the muscle fiber to the extracellular matrix, there is clearly an important intracellular role played by providing a platform from which signaling pathways are launched. These links to downstream pathways suggest that the DGC engages active signaling in order to regulate muscle fiber function. Hence, DGC dysregulation may lead to alterations in intracellular signaling cascades, which may contribute to the pathogenesis of the muscular dystrophies. In this regard, understanding the signaling pathways such as the MAPKs in skeletal muscle function and muscular dystrophy may provide important insight into new avenues of therapies for these diseases.

4. MAPKs and Muscular dystrophy

A link between the MAPKs and muscular dystrophy has been indirectly suggested by the fact that the DGC not only functions as a mechanical infrastructure to stabilize skeletal muscle cell membranes, but it also serves as a bridge between stimuli from the extracellular matrix and intracellular signaling through physically interacting with distinct proteins (Rando, 2001). For example, Grb2, an adapter protein involved in MAPK signal transduction and cytoskeletal organization, interacts with β-dystroglycan at the C-terminal proline-rich domains (Yang et al., 1995). Furthermore, β-dystroglycan can physically interact with MAPK kinase 2 (MEK2) and its downstream kinase ERK1/2 in a yeast two-hybrid screen (Spence et al., 2004). These findings imply that MAPK signaling may play an important role in the mechano- and signal transduction of extracellular stimuli to intracellular biological responses that control muscle fiber viability. However, the reports regarding the activity of the MAPKs in the pathogenesis of muscular dystrophy remain inconclusive and vary in different experimental settings. For example, it has been reported that JNK1 is highly activated in a mouse model of DMD (*mdx* mouse) and compound intercrosses between an *mdx* mouse and a MyoD-deficient mouse (*mdx/MyoD*$^{-/-}$) contributes to the progressive dystrophinopathy without appreciable changes in either ERK1/2 or p38 MAPK activities (Kolodziejczyk et al., 2001). In contrast, stable over-expression of the JNK1-specific upstream kinase MKK7 disrupts the formation of myotubes in C2C12 skeletal myoblasts and H9C2 cardiac myoblasts (Kolodziejczyk et al., 2001). Adenoviral infection of the JNK1 specific inhibitor JIP1 (JNK interacting protein) increased the diameter of myofibers (Kolodziejczyk et al., 2001), suggesting that the MAPKs can affect the structural integrity of the myofiber. In an attempt to test whether loss of dystrophin causes aberrant mechanotransduction, Kumar et al measured the activity of the MAPKs following stretching of *mdx* and wild type diaphragm muscles. ERK1/2, but not JNK or p38 MAPKs were significantly activated in the muscles derived from *mdx* mice (Kumar et al., 2004). In addition, the downstream effector of ERK1/2, AP-1 was highly up-regulated (Kumar et al., 2004). In another exercise model, *mdx* mice were subjected to treadmill exercise, p38 MAPK and ERK1/2, but not JNK1 were highly elevated in *mdx* cardiac muscles in comparison with wild type muscles (Nakamura et al., 2002). Elevated p38 MAPK was also observed in utrophin-dystrophin double knock-out cardiac muscles (Nakamura et al., 2001). Together, these findings suggest that MAPK signaling is likely involved in the pathogenesis of muscular dystrophy, but to what extent and how exactly MAPK contributes at the molecular level to the pathogenesis of DMD remains to be established.

5. MAPK phosphatases in skeletal muscle function and muscular dystrophy

Equally important as the activation of the MAPKs is their inactivation, which is catalyzed by the MKPs. The MKPs belong to a sub-class of protein tyrosine phosphatases known as the dual-specificity protein phosphatases (DUSP) (Boutros et al., 2008; Soulsby and Bennett,

2009; Tonks, 2006). The DUSPs are characterized by a consensus signature motif represented by $HC(X)_5R$ which defines the active site of these enzymes (Soulsby and Bennett, 2009; Tonks, 2006). MKPs inactivate the MAPKs by directly dephosphorylating the MAPKs on its regulatory threonine and tyrosine residues. The MKPs share largely the same structure comprising of a cdc25 homology domain and a MAPK binding domain in the NH_2 terminus and a COOH-terminus PTP catalytic domain. The NH_2 terminus of the MKPs controls MAPK binding and sub-cellular targeting (Wu et al., 2005), both of these attributes contribute to MAPK signaling specificity. In this regard, although the MKPs dephosphorylate the MAPKs they do so with varying degrees of potency that depends upon both their MAPK binding affinity and sub-cellular localization. There are 10 catalytically active members in this group and they exhibit distinct sub-cellular localization, responses to extracellular stimuli, tissue distribution and affinity to their substrates (Boutros et al., 2008; Groom et al., 1996; Ishibashi et al., 1994; Misra-Press et al., 1995; Muda et al., 1997; Noguchi et al., 1993; Rohan et al., 1993).

Binding of MKPs to their MAPK substrates increases phosphatase activity (Camps et al., 1998a; Hutter et al., 2000; Slack et al., 2001) and this is due to stabilization of the active enzyme-substrate complex (Field et al., 2000). MKP-3 exhibits high fidelity to its substrate ERK1/2 and upon binding its catalytic activity is enhanced (Camps et al., 1998b). Despite the fact that the MKPs dephosphorylate a common pool of MAPKs these enzymes exhibit remarkably unique physiological effects (Chi et al., 2006; Christie et al., 2005; Wu et al., 2006). Studies from MKP knock-out mice provide convincing genetic evidence to support the notion that these MKPs function in distinct ways (Nunes-Xavier et al., 2011). The complexity of the signaling pathways and biological responses that the MKPs are involved with strongly suggest that these enzymes serve as central players in the regulation of the MAPKs. Therefore, the MKPs, which have the capacity to regulate multiple MAPKs simultaneously, represent a critical signaling node of MAPK convergence. Molecules that act as signalling (before nodes) in signal transduction can be defined as those which represent a point of convergence of multiple pathways, and one that is represented by several isoforms that are both positively and negatively involved in divergent signaling. We propose that the MKPs satisfy these criteria and constitute a critical signaling node in the MAPK pathway. Given the established role of the MAPKs in skeletal myogenesis, the actions of the MKPs as critical signaling nodes of the MAPKs is likely to make them important players in this system.

MKPs in skeletal myogenesis and skeletal muscle function. Studies of the MKPs in myogenesis and skeletal muscle function remain mainly an uncharted area. Much of the work on the MKPs in skeletal muscle function has focused on the role of MKP-1. The first MKP to be implicated in skeletal muscle function was MKP-1 (Bennett and Tonks, 1997). MKP-1 is a ubiquitously expressed, nuclear localized dual-specificity phosphatase, whose substrates include predominantly p38 MAPK, JNK and to a lesser extent, ERK1/2 (Boutros et al., 2008; Owens and Keyse, 2007). MKP-1 is an immediate-early gene and is induced by numerous stresses (Owens and Keyse, 2007). Initial reports demonstrated that MKP-1-deficient mice exhibit an unremarkable phenotype, suggesting that the MKPs largely serve redundant physiological roles (Dorfman et al., 1996). However, we have shown that mice lacking MKP-1 exhibit enhanced ERK1/2, JNK and p38 MAPK activities in skeletal muscle, as well as in other tissues, demonstrating that MKP-1 plays an essential physiological role as a negative regulator of the MAPKs (Wu et al., 2006). The earliest suggestion that MKP-1, and hence the MAPKs, participate in myogenic regulation emerged from studies in which conditional overexpression of MKP-1 was shown to stimulate precocious myogenesis in the context of the inhibitory actions of growth factors (Bennett and Tonks, 1997). MKP-1 expression levels in proliferating myoblasts are initially high, at levels presumably sufficient to allow cell proliferation but not differentiation, and declines upon the onset of myogenesis, suggesting that extinguishing the expression of MKP-1 might be a prerequisite for myogenic entry and/or progression (Bennett and Tonks, 1997; Kondoh et al., 2007; Perdiguero et al., 2007). Consistent with this, overexpression of MKP-1 when myoblasts have become irrevocably committed to myogenesis inhibits multinucleated myotube formation (Bennett and Tonks, 1997; Kondoh et al., 2007). Hence, MKP-1 plays both positive and negative roles in myogenesis in a temporal manner by selectively regulating one or more MAPKs (**Figure 1**). MKP-1 appears to be directly coupled to the myogenic transcriptional machinery as studies have shown that MKP-1 is a target for upregulation by MyoD (Shi et al., 2010). Within the proximal promoter of MKP-1 there resides an E-box binding site that serves to mediate MKP-1 activation by MyoD (Shi et al., 2010). Hence, upon the initiation of myogenesis the activation of MyoD leads to an initial upregulation of MKP-1, which may be required to inactivate ERK1/2 and thus facilitate cell cycle exit in the transition towards myogenic entry. Later on during myogenesis MyoD was shown to uncouple from the MKP-1 promoter and hence downregulate MKP-1 expression (**Figure 1**). Downregulation of MKP-1 during the later stages of myogenesis may facilitate the increased p38 MAPK activation, which is important for multinucleated myotube formation. As such, the complexity of the outcome through which MKP-1 integrates multiple MAPK activities cannot be simply inferred by the implied actions of a single MAPK family member. These results using cultured myoblast cell lines are supported by *in vivo* data where it has been shown that regenerative myogenesis in response to cardiotoxin-induced injury is impaired in MKP-1-deficient mice (Shi et al., 2010). These results support the notion that MKP-1 is an important regulator of myogenesis.

MKP-1 is also implicated in adult skeletal muscle fiber specialization (Shi et al., 2008). Overexpression of MKP-1 in adult type IIb (glycolytic) myofibers converts these fibers to slower-twitch type IIa or type I (oxidative) fibers, suggesting that MKP-1-mediated dephosphorylation of MAPK signaling is required to maintain the glycolytic fiber phenotype through the repression of slow myofibers (Shi et al., 2008). Consistent with these data, it has been shown that MKP-1-deficient mice are protected from the loss of oxidative myofibers during high fat diet-induced obesity (Roth et al., 2009). Hence, decreased MKP-1 expression results in enhanced MAPK signaling, which protects from the loss of glycolytic myofibers by driving oxidative myofiber conversion. The mechanistic basis for these data is based upon the observation that MKP-1 mediates p38 MAPK phosphorylation of the peroxisome proliferator-activated receptor γ co-activator 1α (PGC-1α) (Roth et al., 2009), which is required to promote oxidative myofiber conversion. Collectively, these results suggest that MKP-1 plays an essential role in the maintenance of glycolytic/oxidative myofiber composition. MKP-1 is also suggested to be involved in the maintenance of muscle mass (Shi et al., 2009). Overexpression of MKP-1 in slow-twitch soleus muscles and in fast-twitch gastrocnemius muscles reduces muscle fiber size, though this reduction in fiber size may go through distinct molecular mechanisms (Shi et al., 2009).

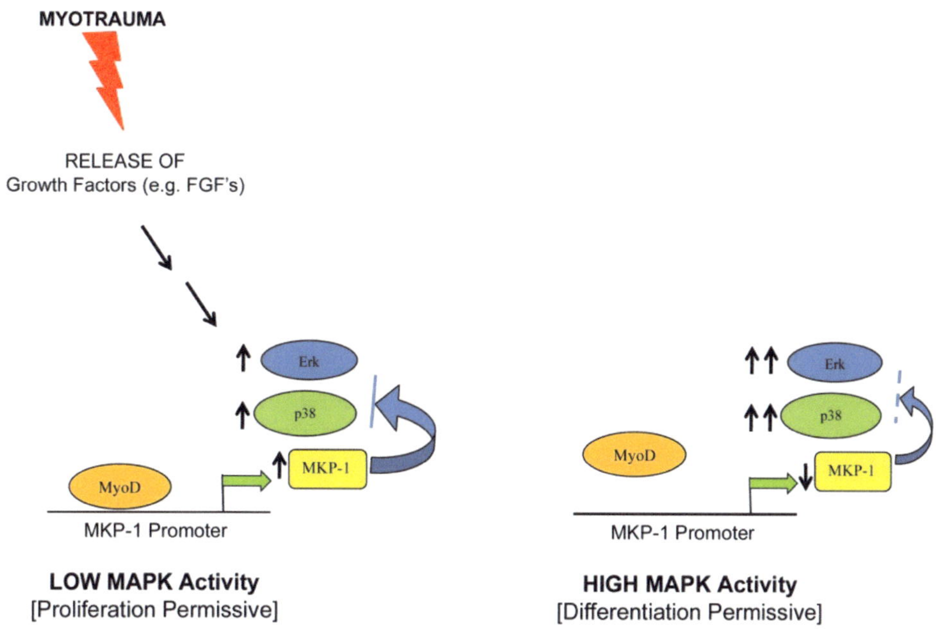

Fig. 1. MAPK/MKP signaling coordinates myogenesis. Following myotrauma the MAPKs become activated to drive cell proliferation. MKP-1 is upregulated by these MAPKs and MyoD. MKP-1 sets the threshold of MAPK activity that permits myoblast proliferation [Proliferation Permissive] but not differentiation. Upon the initiation of differentiation, MyoD uncouples from the MKP-1 promoter causing its expression levels to fall, thereby removing the inhibitory actions of MKP-1 on the MAPKs. This allows for higher levels of MAPK activity to be achieved, in particular p38 MAPK, which promotes differentiation [Differentiation Permissive].

MKP-1 also plays a regulatory role in estrogen-related receptor α (ERRα) and PGC-1α mediated myogenic differentiation. Direct up-regulation of MKP-1 by ERRα and PGC-1α at the early stage of myogenesis inactivate ERK1/2 signaling and facilitate the progression of myogensis as MEK inhibition rescues the myogenic defect in ERRα$^{-/-}$ myoblasts (Murray and Huss, 2011). Recent work from this laboratory suggests that other MKPs, in addition to MKP-1, also contribute to the regulation of skeletal muscle function. Mice lacking MKP-5, which interestingly also dephosphorylates predominately p38 MAPK and JNK, exhibit enhanced skeletal muscle regeneration distinct from that observed with MKP-1-deficient mice (H.S. and A.M.B., *unpublished observations*). These results suggest that the MKPs might play distinct roles in not only coordinating myogenic activation and progression but they may do so through specific and non-overlapping mechanisms.

A role for MKP-1 in muscular dystrophy. The generation, maintenance, and repair of adult skeletal muscle is critically dependent upon the activation and self-renewal of satellite cells (Wagers and Conboy, 2005). In response to skeletal muscle injury, myofiber-released growth factors and cytokines stimulate satellite cell proliferation, migration and differentiation by activating signaling cascades including the MAPK pathway. It is thought that the depletion of satellite cells during the progression of DMD is a major factor that precipitates the ultimate failure of muscle function. Therefore, by modulating satellite cell activation, differentiation and/or self-renewal DMD can theoretically be improved.

Several reports have addressed the role of the MAPKs in *mdx* mice, however there is no underlying consensus as to whether the MAPKs are definitively involved in the pathogenesis of the dystrophic phenotype. Some reports show upregulation of ERK1/2, JNK2 and p38 MAPK (Nakamura et al., 2005), whereas others have shown a downregulation of p38 MAPK and an upregulation of ERK1/2 (Lang et al., 2004), yet others find no consistent differences in p38 MAPK (Nakamura et al., 2001). To study the pathophysiological role of MKP-1 in Duchenne muscular dystrophy, we inter-crossed MKP-1 knockout mice into the *mdx* background in order to determine whether loss of MKP-1 ameliorates or exacerbates the dystrophic phenotype. The advantage of generating an MKP-1-deficient animal model is that instead of studying an individual MAPK, we examined the integration of several MAPKs that become hyperactivated due to the lack of MKP-1. We found that *mdx/mkp-1*$^{-/-}$ mice have reduced body weight and muscle mass in comparison with *mdx/mkp-1*$^{+/+}$ mice (Shi et al., 2010). The reduction of body weight may be attributed to the chronic elevated levels of inflammation or it is also likely that this is due to an underlying metabolic defect that we have observed in mice lacking MKP-1 that is related to increased energy expenditure (Roth et al., 2009; Wu et al., 2006). Histological analysis of muscle sections from *mdx/mkp-1*$^{-/-}$ mice revealed that MKP-1 deficiency exacerbates the pathogenesis of muscular dystrophy (Shi et al., 2010). This exacerbation may be accounted for by a combination of two factors that are cell autonomous and/or directly related to defects in satellite cell function as well as a contribution from a hyperactivated immune response. Satellite cells from MKP-1-deficient muscles exhibit reduced proliferative capacity whereas precocious differentiation was evident even under high serum conditions (Shi et al., 2010). Additionally, increased levels of macrophage and neutrophil infiltrates into damaged myofibers in *mdx/mkp-1*$^{-/-}$ mice compared to MKP-1 wild type *mdx* mice, this was observed along with serum and skeletal muscle cytokine levels that are significantly increased in *mdx/mkp-1*$^{-/-}$ mice (Shi et al., 2010). Collectively, these findings suggest that MKP-1 is critical for the regulation of muscle regeneration in DMD by modulating both immune responses and satellite cell proliferation and differentiation (**Figure 2**). Further studies employing conditional deletion of MKP-1 in the satellite cell and hematopoietic compartments will be required in order to determine the contribution of MKP-1 in these tissues to the overall skeletal muscle regenerative defect.

6. Therapeutic targeting of MAPK/MKPs in muscular dystrophy

Research on MKP-1 and its involvement in regenerative myogenesis and muscular dystrophy suggests that MKP-1 may play an important role in the progression of muscular dystrophy and possibly other degenerative skeletal muscle diseases. Therefore, targeting the MAPK/MKP signaling pathway in order to ameliorate skeletal muscle disease and specifically, muscular dystrophy, merits further investigation. However, definitive validation that the MAPK/MKP module is a valid therapeutic target for muscular dystrophy is still lacking. There has been some suggestion that interference with the MAPK/MKP signaling module may have therapeutic value. It has been shown that adenoviral delivery of the JNK1 inhibitory protein, JIP1, can attenuate the pathogenesis of dystrophic fibers (Kolodziejczyk et al., 2001), implying that inhibition of JNK1 may serve as

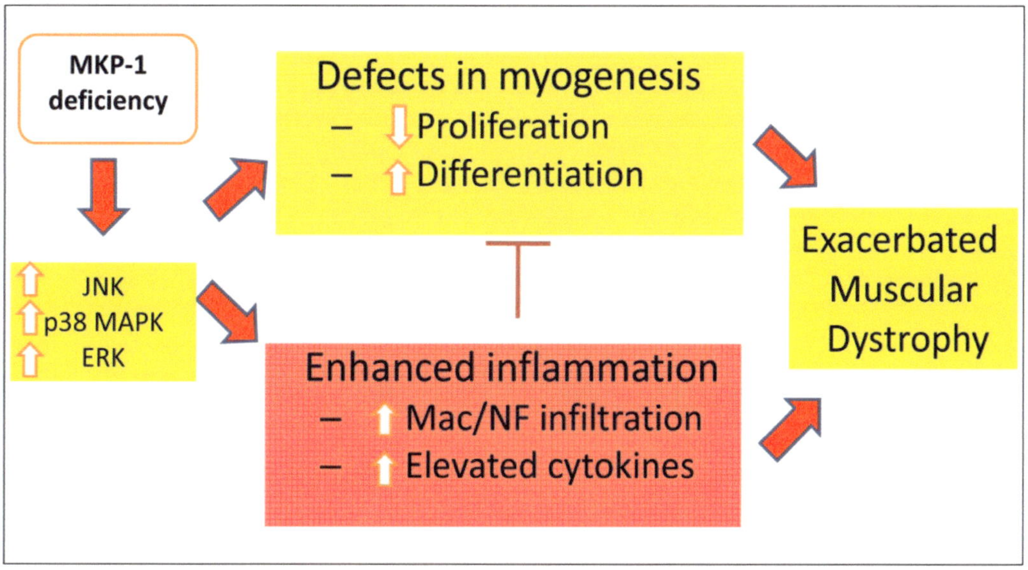

Fig. 2. MKP-1 and Duchenne Muscular Dystrophy. MKP-1 regulates both myoblast proliferation and differentiation (see Figure 1). Loss of MKP-1 in a mouse model of Duchennes' muscular dystrophy exacerbates the dystrophic phenotype due to enhanced MAPK activity, which inhibits myoblast proliferation, and ectopically enhances differentiation. In conjunction, MKP-1 has a profound effect in macrophages (Mac) and neutrophils (NF), which as a result of enhanced MAPK activity, in the absence of MKP-1 become hyper-responsive leading to increased inflammatory responses. Together, both the increased inflammatory response and dysfunctional myoblast proliferation and differentiation exacerbates the dystrophic phenotype.

a potential therapeutic target for the treatment of certain dystrophies. However, given the uncertain role played by JNK in skeletal muscle regeneration this target should be approached cautiously. A recent study shows that treating dystrophic mice with the free radical scavenger α-lipoic acid and L-carnitine improved muscular dystrophy with a concomitant repression of ERK1/2, JNK and p38 MAPK activation (Hnia et al., 2007). This is quite a provocative result since reactive oxygen species have been shown to inhibit the actions of certain protein tyrosine phosphatases through modification of the catalytic cysteine residue (Tonks, 2005). Therefore, treatment of dystrophic muscle with free radical scavengers would be predicted to ameliorate the loss of PTP activity, including MKP activity, resulting in increased inactivation of MAPKs. However, it is not yet clear whether the improved myopathy is caused by the decreased activation of a particular MAPK and/or a combination thereof. In an Emery-Dreyfuss muscular dystrophy mouse model, which lacks the inner nuclear membrane protein A-type lamins (LMNA), JNK and ERK1/2 are highly activated in heart tissue and cardiomycytes (Muchir et al., 2007). Inhibition of the ERK1/2 upstream kinase MEK by PD098059 improves cardiomyopathy in *Lmna* mutant knock-in mice (Muchir et al., 2009), implying that molecules in the ERK1/2 pathway have therapeutic potential for the treatment of human Emery-Dreyfuss muscular dystrophy and potentially related disorders.

Although the MAPK/MKP pathway represents a potentially attractive therapeutic target to treat muscular dystrophy, it is a challenging one given the fact that the MAPK/MKP module is a universal pathway serving a number of common control points in the regulation of cell proliferation, differentiation, migration, and survival. The challenge will be to identify MAPK/MKP family members that exhibit signaling preferences to skeletal muscle with those functions further selectively controlling the appropriate physiological response in dystrophic skeletal muscle tissue. Given the importance of p38 MAPK in promoting regenerative myogenesis an attractive strategy could involve enhancing p38 MAPK activity so as to promote either satellite cell activation, proliferation and/or differentiation in dystrophic tissue. This could conceivably be achieved either through activation of p38 MAPK itself or through inhibition of the MKP that opposes the physiologically relevant pool of p38 MAPK in these cells. Clearly, significant gaps in our knowledge need to be filled in this area, nevertheless it is an important goal given the devastating nature of these skeletal muscle diseases that still lack a successful treatment.

7. Acknowledgements

A.M.B. is supported by the National Institutes of Health and H.S. by a grant from the Muscular Dystrophy Association.

8. References

Bennett, A.M., and N.K. Tonks. 1997. Regulation of distinct stages of skeletal muscle differentiation by mitogen-activated protein kinases. *Science*. 278:1288-1291.

Bhatnagar, S., and A. Kumar. 2010. Therapeutic targeting of signaling pathways in muscular dystrophy. *J Mol Med (Berl)*. 88:155-166.

Black, B.L., and E.N. Olson. 1998. Transcriptional control of muscle development by myocyte enhancer factor-2 (MEF2) proteins. Annu Rev Cell Dev Biol. 14:167-196.

Bogoyevitch, M.A. 2006. The isoform-specific functions of the c-Jun N-terminal Kinases (JNKs): differences revealed by gene targeting. *Bioessays*. 28:923-934.

Bogoyevitch, M.A., and N.W. Court. 2004. Counting on mitogen-activated protein kinases--ERKs 3, 4, 5, 6, 7 and 8. *Cell Signal*. 16:1345-1354.

Boutros, T., E. Chevet, and P. Metrakos. 2008. Mitogen-activated protein (MAP) kinase/MAP kinase phosphatase regulation: roles in cell growth, death, and cancer. *Pharmacol Rev*. 60:261-310.

Briata, P., S.V. Forcales, M. Ponassi, G. Corte, C.Y. Chen, M. Karin, P.L. Puri, and R. Gherzi. 2005. p38-dependent phosphorylation of the mRNA decay-promoting factor KSRP controls the stability of select myogenic transcripts. *Mol Cell*. 20:891-903.

Camps, M., C. Chabert, M. Muda, U. Boschert, C. Gillieron, and S. Arkinstall. 1998a. Induction of the mitogen-activated protein kinase phosphatase MKP3 by nerve growth factor in differentiating PC12. *FEBS Lett*. 425:271-276.

Camps, M., A. Nichols, C. Gillieron, B. Antonsson, M. Muda, C. Chabert, U. Boschert, and S. Arkinstall. 1998b. Catalytic activation of the phosphatase MKP-3 by ERK2 mitogen-activated protein kinase. *Science*. 280:1262-1265.

Chi, H., S.P. Barry, R.J. Roth, J.J. Wu, E.A. Jones, A.M. Bennett, and R.A. Flavell. 2006. Dynamic regulation of pro- and anti-inflammatory cytokines by MAPK phosphatase 1 (MKP-1) in innate immune responses. *Proc Natl Acad Sci U S A*. 103:2274-2279.

Christie, G.R., D.J. Williams, F. Macisaac, R.J. Dickinson, I. Rosewell, and S.M. Keyse. 2005. The dual-specificity protein phosphatase DUSP9/MKP-4 is essential for placental function but is not required for normal embryonic development. *Mol Cell Biol*. 25:8323-8333.

Cuevas, B.D., A.N. Abell, and G.L. Johnson. 2007. Role of mitogen-activated protein kinase kinase kinases in signal integration. *Oncogene*. 26:3159-3171.

Davies, K.E., and K.J. Nowak. 2006. Molecular mechanisms of muscular dystrophies: old and new players. *Nat Rev Mol Cell Biol*. 7:762-773.

Deconinck, N., and B. Dan. 2007. Pathophysiology of duchenne muscular dystrophy: current hypotheses. *Pediatr Neurol*. 36:1-7.

Dorfman, K., D. Carrasco, M. Gruda, C. Ryan, S.A. Lira, and R. Bravo. 1996. Disruption of the erp/mkp-1 gene does not affect mouse development: normal MAP kinase activity in ERP/MKP-1-deficient fibroblasts. *Oncogene*. 13:925-931.

Dorman, C.M., and S.E. Johnson. 1999. Activated Raf inhibits avian myogenesis through a MAPK-dependent mechanism. *Oncogene*. 18:5167-5176.

Field, C.J., C.A. Thomson, J.E. Van Aerde, A. Parrott, A. Euler, E. Lien, and M.T. Clandinin. 2000. Lower proportion of CD45R0+ cells and deficient interleukin-10 production by formula-fed infants, compared with human-fed, is corrected with supplementation of long-chain polyunsaturated fatty acids. *J Pediatr Gastroenterol Nutr*. 31:291-299.

Fornaro, M., P.M. Burch, W. Yang, L. Zhang, C.E. Hamilton, J.H. Kim, B.G. Neel, and A.M. Bennett. 2006. SHP-2 activates signaling of the nuclear factor of activated T cells to promote skeletal muscle growth. *J Cell Biol*. 175:87-97.

Gallo, R., M. Serafini, L. Castellani, G. Falcone, and S. Alema. 1999. Distinct effects of Rac1 on differentiation of primary avian myoblasts. *Mol Biol Cell*. 10:3137-3150.

Gillespie, M.A., F. Le Grand, A. Scime, S. Kuang, J. von Maltzahn, V. Seale, A. Cuenda, J.A. Ranish, and M.A. Rudnicki. 2009. p38-{gamma}-dependent gene silencing restricts entry into the myogenic differentiation program. *J Cell Biol*. 187:991-1005.

Gredinger, E., A.N. Gerber, Y. Tamir, S.J. Tapscott, and E. Bengal. 1998. Mitogen-activated protein kinase pathway is involved in the differentiation of muscle cells. *J Biol Chem*. 273:10436-10444.

Groom, L.A., A.A. Sneddon, D.R. Alessi, S. Dowd, and S.M. Keyse. 1996. Differential regulation of the MAP, SAP and RK/p38 kinases by Pyst1, a novel cytosolic dual-specificity phosphatase. *Embo J*. 15:3621-3632.

Hammer, M., J. Mages, H. Dietrich, A. Servatius, N. Howells, A.C. Cato, and R. Lang. 2006. Dual specificity phosphatase 1 (DUSP1) regulates a subset of LPS-induced genes and protects mice from lethal endotoxin shock. *J Exp Med*. 203:15-20.

Hnia, K., G. Hugon, F. Rivier, A. Masmoudi, J. Mercier, and D. Mornet. 2007. Modulation of p38 mitogen-activated protein kinase cascade and metalloproteinase activity in diaphragm muscle in response to free radical scavenger administration in dystrophin-deficient Mdx mice. *Am J Pathol*. 170:633-643.

Hutter, D., P. Chen, J. Barnes, and Y. Liu. 2000. Catalytic activation of mitogen-activated protein (MAP) kinase phosphatase-1 by binding to p38 MAP kinase: critical role of the p38 C-terminal domain in its negative regulation. *Biochem J*. 352 Pt 1:155-163.

Ishibashi, T., D.P. Bottaro, P. Michieli, C.A. Kelley, and S.A. Aaronson. 1994. A novel dual specificity phosphatase induced by serum stimulation and heat shock. *J Biol Chem*. 269:29897-29902.

Johnson, G.L., and R. Lapadat. 2002. Mitogen-activated protein kinase pathways mediated by ERK, JNK, and p38 protein kinases. *Science*. 298:1911-1912.

Jones, N.C., K.J. Tyner, L. Nibarger, H.M. Stanley, D.D. Cornelison, Y.V. Fedorov, and B.B. Olwin. 2005. The p38alpha/beta MAPK functions as a molecular switch to activate the quiescent satellite cell. *J Cell Biol*. 169:105-116.

Khurana, A., and C.S. Dey. 2004. Involvement of c-Jun N-terminal kinase activities in skeletal muscle differentiation. *J Muscle Res Cell Motil*. 25:645-655.

Kolodziejczyk, S.M., G.S. Walsh, K. Balazsi, P. Seale, J. Sandoz, A.M. Hierlihy, M.A. Rudnicki, J.S. Chamberlain, F.D. Miller, and L.A. Megeney. 2001. Activation of JNK1 contributes to dystrophic muscle pathogenesis. *Curr Biol*. 11:1278-1282.

Kondoh, K., K. Sunadome, and E. Nishida. 2007. Notch signaling suppresses p38 MAPK activity via induction of MKP-1 in myogenesis. *J Biol Chem*. 282:3058-3065.

Kontaridis, M.I., X. Liu, L. Zhang, and A.M. Bennett. 2002. Role of SHP-2 in fibroblast growth factor receptor-mediated suppression of myogenesis in C2C12 myoblasts. *Mol Cell Biol*. 22:3875-3891.

Koyama, T., Y. Nakaoka, Y. Fujio, H. Hirota, K. Nishida, S. Sugiyama, K. Okamoto, K. Yamauchi-Takihara, M. Yoshimura, S. Mochizuki, M. Hori, T. Hirano, and N. Mochizuki. 2008. Interaction of scaffolding adaptor protein Gab1 with tyrosine phosphatase SHP2 negatively regulates IGF-I-dependent myogenic differentiation via the ERK1/2 signaling pathway. *J Biol Chem*. 283:24234-24244.

Kumar, A., N. Khandelwal, R. Malya, M.B. Reid, and A.M. Boriek. 2004. Loss of dystrophin causes aberrant mechanotransduction in skeletal muscle fibers. *Faseb J*. 18:102-113.

Lang, J.M., K.A. Esser, and E.E. Dupont-Versteegden. 2004. Altered activity of signaling pathways in diaphragm and tibialis anterior muscle of dystrophic mice. *Exp Biol Med (Maywood)*. 229:503-511.

Lluis, F., E. Ballestar, M. Suelves, M. Esteller, and P. Munoz-Canoves. 2005. E47 phosphorylation by p38 MAPK promotes MyoD/E47 association and muscle-specific gene transcription. *Embo J*. 24:974-984.

Meriane, M., S. Charrasse, F. Comunale, and C. Gauthier-Rouviere. 2002. Transforming growth factor beta activates Rac1 and Cdc42Hs GTPases and the JNK pathway in skeletal muscle cells. *Biol Cell*. 94:535-543.

Misra-Press, A., C.S. Rim, H. Yao, M.S. Roberson, and P.J. Stork. 1995. A novel mitogen-activated protein kinase phosphatase. Structure, expression, and regulation. *J Biol Chem*. 270:14587-14596.

Muchir, A., P. Pavlidis, V. Decostre, A.J. Herron, T. Arimura, G. Bonne, and H.J. Worman. 2007. Activation of MAPK pathways links LMNA mutations to cardiomyopathy in Emery-Dreifuss muscular dystrophy. *J Clin Invest*. 117:1282-1293.

Muchir, A., J. Shan, G. Bonne, S.E. Lehnart, and H.J. Worman. 2009. Inhibition of extracellular signal-regulated kinase signaling to prevent cardiomyopathy caused by mutation in the gene encoding A-type lamins. *Hum Mol Genet*. 18:241-247.

Muda, M., U. Boschert, A. Smith, B. Antonsson, C. Gillieron, C. Chabert, M. Camps, I. Martinou, A. Ashworth, and S. Arkinstall. 1997. Molecular cloning and functional characterization of a novel mitogen-activated protein kinase phosphatase, MKP-4. *J Biol Chem*. 272:5141-5151.

Murray, J., and J.M. Huss. 2011. Estrogen-related receptor {alpha} regulates skeletal myocyte differentiation via modulation of the ERK MAP kinase pathway. *Am J Physiol Cell Physiol*. 301:C630-645.

Nakamura, A., G.V. Harrod, and K.E. Davies. 2001. Activation of calcineurin and stress activated protein kinase/p38-mitogen activated protein kinase in hearts of utrophin-dystrophin knockout mice. *Neuromuscul Disord*. 11:251-259.

Nakamura, A., K. Yoshida, S. Takeda, N. Dohi, and S. Ikeda. 2002. Progression of dystrophic features and activation of mitogen-activated protein kinases and calcineurin by physical exercise, in hearts of mdx mice. *FEBS Lett.* 520:18-24.

Nakamura, A., K. Yoshida, H. Ueda, S. Takeda, and S. Ikeda. 2005. Up-regulation of mitogen activated protein kinases in mdx skeletal muscle following chronic treadmill exercise. *Biochim Biophys Acta.* 1740:326-331.

Noguchi, T., R. Metz, L. Chen, M.G. Mattei, D. Carrasco, and R. Bravo. 1993. Structure, mapping, and expression of erp, a growth factor-inducible gene encoding a nontransmembrane protein tyrosine phosphatase, and effect of ERP on cell growth. *Mol Cell Biol.* 13:5195-5205.

Nunes-Xavier, C., C. Roma-Mateo, P. Rios, C. Tarrega, R. Cejudo-Marin, L. Tabernero, and R. Pulido. 2011. Dual-specificity MAP kinase phosphatases as targets of cancer treatment. *In* Anticancer Agents Med Chem. Vol. 11. 109-132.

Owens, D.M., and S.M. Keyse. 2007. Differential regulation of MAP kinase signalling by dual-specificity protein phosphatases. *Oncogene.* 26:3203-3213.

Pearson, G., F. Robinson, T. Beers Gibson, B.E. Xu, M. Karandikar, K. Berman, and M.H. Cobb. 2001. Mitogen-activated protein (MAP) kinase pathways: regulation and physiological functions. *Endocr Rev.* 22:153-183.

Perdiguero, E., V. Ruiz-Bonilla, L. Gresh, L. Hui, E. Ballestar, P. Sousa-Victor, B. Baeza-Raja, M. Jardi, A. Bosch-Comas, M. Esteller, C. Caelles, A.L. Serrano, E.F. Wagner, and P. Munoz-Canoves. 2007. Genetic analysis of p38 MAP kinases in myogenesis: fundamental role of p38alpha in abrogating myoblast proliferation. *Embo J.* 26:1245-1256.

Porter, J.D. 2000. Introduction to muscular dystrophy. *Microsc Res Tech.* 48:127-130.

Rando, T.A. 2001. The dystrophin-glycoprotein complex, cellular signaling, and the regulation of cell survival in the muscular dystrophies. *Muscle Nerve.* 24:1575-1594.

Rohan, P.J., P. Davis, C.A. Moskaluk, M. Kearns, H. Krutzsch, U. Siebenlist, and K. Kelly. 1993. PAC-1: a mitogen-induced nuclear protein tyrosine phosphatase. *Science.* 259:1763-1766.

Roth, R.J., A.M. Le, L. Zhang, M. Kahn, V.T. Samuel, G.I. Shulman, and A.M. Bennett. 2009. MAPK phosphatase-1 facilitates the loss of oxidative myofibers associated with obesity in mice. *J Clin Invest.* 119:3817-3829.

Salojin, K.V., I.B. Owusu, K.A. Millerchip, M. Potter, K.A. Platt, and T. Oravecz. 2006. Essential role of MAPK phosphatase-1 in the negative control of innate immune responses. *J Immunol.* 176:1899-1907.

Shi, H., E. Boadu, F. Mercan, A.M. Le, R.J. Flach, L. Zhang, K.J. Tyner, B.B. Olwin, and A.M. Bennett. 2010. MAP kinase phosphatase-1 deficiency impairs skeletal muscle regeneration and exacerbates muscular dystrophy. *Faseb J.* 24:2985-2997.

Shi, H., J.M. Scheffler, J.M. Pleitner, C. Zeng, S. Park, K.M. Hannon, A.L. Grant, and D.E. Gerrard. 2008. Modulation of skeletal muscle fiber type by mitogen-activated protein kinase signaling. *Faseb J.* 22:2990-3000.

Shi, H., J.M. Scheffler, C. Zeng, J.M. Pleitner, K.M. Hannon, A.L. Grant, and D.E. Gerrard. 2009. Mitogen-activated protein kinase signaling is necessary for the maintenance of skeletal muscle mass. *Am J Physiol Cell Physiol.* 296:C1040-1048.

Simone, C., S.V. Forcales, D.A. Hill, A.N. Imbalzano, L. Latella, and P.L. Puri. 2004. p38 pathway targets SWI-SNF chromatin-remodeling complex to muscle-specific loci. *Nat Genet.* 36:738-743.

Slack, D.N., O.M. Seternes, M. Gabrielsen, and S.M. Keyse. 2001. Distinct binding determinants for ERK2/p38alpha and JNK map kinases mediate catalytic activation and substrate selectivity of map kinase phosphatase-1. *J Biol Chem*. 276:16491-16500.

Soulsby, M., and A.M. Bennett. 2009. Physiological signaling specificity by protein tyrosine phosphatases. *Physiology (Bethesda)*. 24:281-289.

Spence, H.J., A.S. Dhillon, M. James, and S.J. Winder. 2004. Dystroglycan, a scaffold for the ERK-MAP kinase cascade. *EMBO Rep*. 5:484-489.

Suelves, M., F. Lluis, V. Ruiz, A.R. Nebreda, and P. Munoz-Canoves. 2004. Phosphorylation of MRF4 transactivation domain by p38 mediates repression of specific myogenic genes. *Embo J*. 23:365-375.

Sunadome, K., T. Yamamoto, M. Ebisuya, K. Kondoh, A. Sehara-Fujisawa, and E. Nishida. 2011. ERK5 regulates muscle cell fusion through Klf transcription factors. *Dev Cell*. 20:192-205.

Tedesco, F.S., A. Dellavalle, J. Diaz-Manera, G. Messina, and G. Cossu. 2010. Repairing skeletal muscle: regenerative potential of skeletal muscle stem cells. *J Clin Invest*. 120:11-19.

Tonks, N.K. 2005. Redox redux: revisiting PTPs and the control of cell signaling. *Cell*. 121:667-670.

Tonks, N.K. 2006. Protein tyrosine phosphatases: from genes, to function, to disease. *Nat Rev Mol Cell Biol*. 7:833-846.

Turjanski, A.G., J.P. Vaque, and J.S. Gutkind. 2007. MAP kinases and the control of nuclear events. *Oncogene*. 26:3240-3253.

Wagers, A.J., and I.M. Conboy. 2005. Cellular and molecular signatures of muscle regeneration: current concepts and controversies in adult myogenesis. *Cell*. 122:659-667.

Weyman, C.M., and A. Wolfman. 1998. Mitogen-activated protein kinase kinase (MEK) activity is required for inhibition of skeletal muscle differentiation by insulin-like growth factor 1 or fibroblast growth factor 2. *Endocrinology*. 139:1794-1800.

Whitmarsh, A.J. 2006. The JIP family of MAPK scaffold proteins. *Biochem Soc Trans*. 34:828-832.

Wu, J.J., R.J. Roth, E.J. Anderson, E.-G. Hong, M.-K. Lee, C.S. Choi, P.D. Neufer, G.I. Shulman, J.K. Kim, and A.M. Bennett. 2006. Mice lacking MAP kinase phosphatase-1 have enhanced MAP kinase activity and resistance to diet-induced obesity. *Cell Metab*. 4:61-73.

Wu, J.J., L. Zhang, and A.M. Bennett. 2005. The noncatalytic amino terminus of mitogen-activated protein kinase phosphatase 1 directs nuclear targeting and serum response element transcriptional regulation. *Mol Cell Biol*. 25:4792-4803.

Yang, B., D. Jung, D. Motto, J. Meyer, G. Koretzky, and K.P. Campbell. 1995. SH3 domain-mediated interaction of dystroglycan and Grb2. *J Biol Chem*. 270:11711-11714.

Yokoyama, T., K. Takano, A. Yoshida, F. Katada, P. Sun, T. Takenawa, T. Andoh, and T. Endo. 2007. DA-Raf1, a competent intrinsic dominant-negative antagonist of the Ras-ERK pathway, is required for myogenic differentiation. *J Cell Biol*. 177:781-793.

Zarubin, T., and J. Han. 2005. Activation and signaling of the p38 MAP kinase pathway. *Cell Res*. 15:11-18.

Zetser, A., E. Gredinger, and E. Bengal. 1999. p38 mitogen-activated protein kinase pathway promotes skeletal muscle differentiation. Participation of the Mef2c transcription factor. *J Biol Chem*. 274:5193-5200.

Zhao, Q., X. Wang, L.D. Nelin, Y. Yao, R. Matta, M.E. Manson, R.S. Baliga, X. Meng, C.V. Smith, J.A. Bauer, C.H. Chang, and Y. Liu. 2006. MAP kinase phosphatase 1 controls innate immune responses and suppresses endotoxic shock. *J Exp Med*. 203:131-140.

9

Synaptic Changes at the Spinal Cord Level and Peripheral Nerve Regeneration During the Course of Muscular Dystrophy in MDX Mice

Gustavo Ferreira Simões and Alexandre Leite Rodrigues de Oliveira
University of Campinas (UNICAMP), Brasil

1. Introduction

Muscular dystrophies are part of a group of degenerative diseases of the muscular system, which are characterized by muscle degeneration and structural changes at the neuromuscular junction. The most common form is Duchenne Muscular Dystrophy (DMD) (Whitehead et al., 2006), which affects approximately 1 in every 3500 live births (Balaban et al., 2005; Judge et al., 2005; Withehead et al., 2006; Radley et al., 2007). It is a severe X-linked recessive disorder, where the X chromosome is mutated in the region of the gene Xp21, which encodes for the production of dystrophin (Pearce, 2005).

Dystrophin is a protein located adjacent to the sarcolemma of myocytes (Arahata et al., 1988; Chelly et al., 1988; Carretta et al., 2001). The dystrophin-glycoprotein complex has the functions of maintaining links between the cytoskeleton and the extracellular matrix (Figure 1), maintaining the integrity of the sarcoplasmic membrane, distributing the lateral forces between the muscle fibers and communicating via the intra-and extracellular environment (Lowe et al., 2006). Its absence is characterized by progressive degeneration and weakness of the skeletal muscles, and an inability to properly repair the muscular tissue, which is gradually replaced by fat and connective tissue (Whitehead et al., 2006).

DMD is usually diagnosed between 2 and 5 years old (Balaban et al., 2005), being inexorably fatal, and the patients usually die around the second decade of life due to impairment of the cardiac and diaphragm muscle (Judge et al., 2005; Whitehead et al., 2006).Duchenne muscular dystrophy is characterized in MDX mice (an animal model for the study of Duchenne Muscular Dystrophy) by a set of muscle degeneration fibers with intense infiltrate inflammation (Nonaka, 1998). The MDX mice myonecrosis is often preceded by a collapse and detachment of the basal lamina of the sarcolemma, and subsequent muscle fiber degeneration associated with an extensive inflammatory process. Macrophages, CD4 + and CD8 + T cells represent the main constituents of the population of inflammatory cells that surround the myofiber degeneration process (Mcdowall et al., 1990; Spencer et al., 2001). Concerning this aspect, Lagrota-Candido et al. (2002) revealed that during the process of muscle degeneration, there is an accumulation of CD4 + and CD8 cells in the skeletal muscles of 4-week old MDX mice. Moreover, during the period of muscle regeneration, there is a proliferation of B lymphocytes and secretion of IFN-β by lymphocytes.

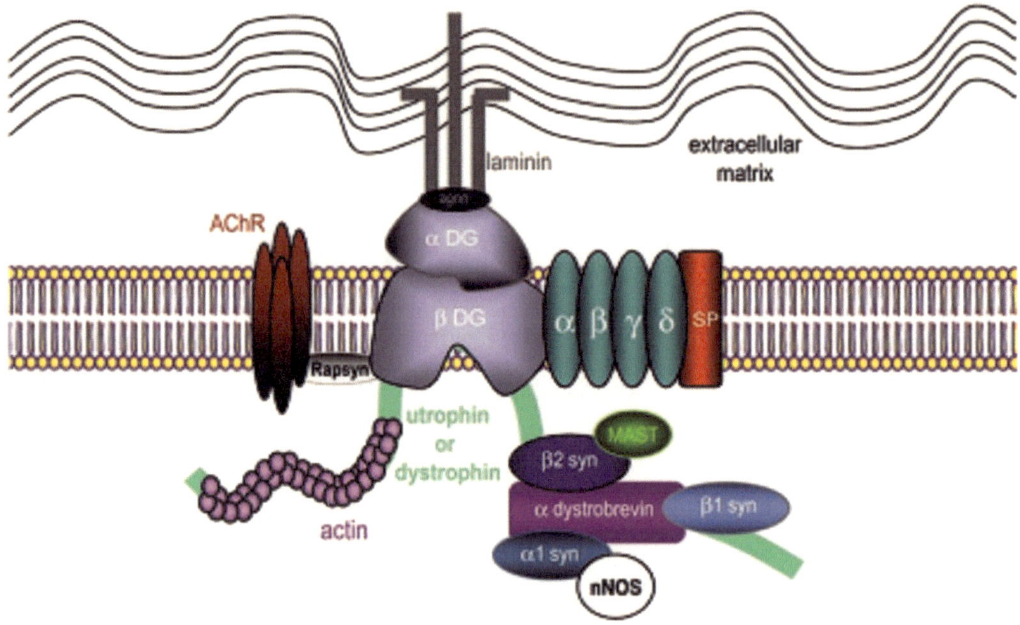

Fig. 1. Composition and schematic organization of the dystrophin glycoprotein complex (DGC) at the neuromuscular junction. Dystrophin or utrophin bind to actin filaments via their **N** terminus. At the C terminus, dystrophin or utrophin are associated with integral and peripheral membrane proteins that can be classified as the dystroglycan complex, the sarcoglycan-sarcospan complex and the cytoplasmic complex. *Role of dystrophin and utrophin for assembly and function of the dystrophin glycoprotein complex in non-muscle tissue* – review from Cellular and Molecular Life Sciences; 63 (2006) 1614–1631.

Currently, much is known about the muscle involvement during the course of DMD, but few studies have focused on the effects on the CNS, specifically in the microenvironment of the spinal motoneurons. It is known that during the course of the disease, axonal terminals enter a cycle of denervation (retraction) and reinnervation (sprouting), and this cycle can pass in a retrograde manner to the cell bodies of the spinal alpha-motoneurons. After an injury resulting in disruption of the contact between the motoneurons and their target muscle fibers, a series of changes occurs in the cell body of the neuron (for example, the presence of edema in the cell body, displacement of the nucleus to the periphery of the cell body and a decrease in electron density along with the dissolution of Nissl corpuscles), which, together, is called chromatolysis (Romanes, 1946; Lieberman, 1971; Aldskogius & Svensson, 1993) - Figure 2.

Pastoret & Sebille (1994) investigated the cycles of muscle degeneration and regeneration as from the second week and up to 104 weeks of life in MDX mice. Their results showed that in the second week of life, some abnormalities could be found in muscle fibers of the tibialis anterior, extensor digitorum longus, muscle longus plantar and soleus muscle. These changes included small scattered foci of degenerated muscle fibers surrounded by cellular infiltrates, "pale" muscle fibers and small groups of regenerated muscle fibers with a central nucleus. By the third week of life these abnormalities were evident and widespread in all the

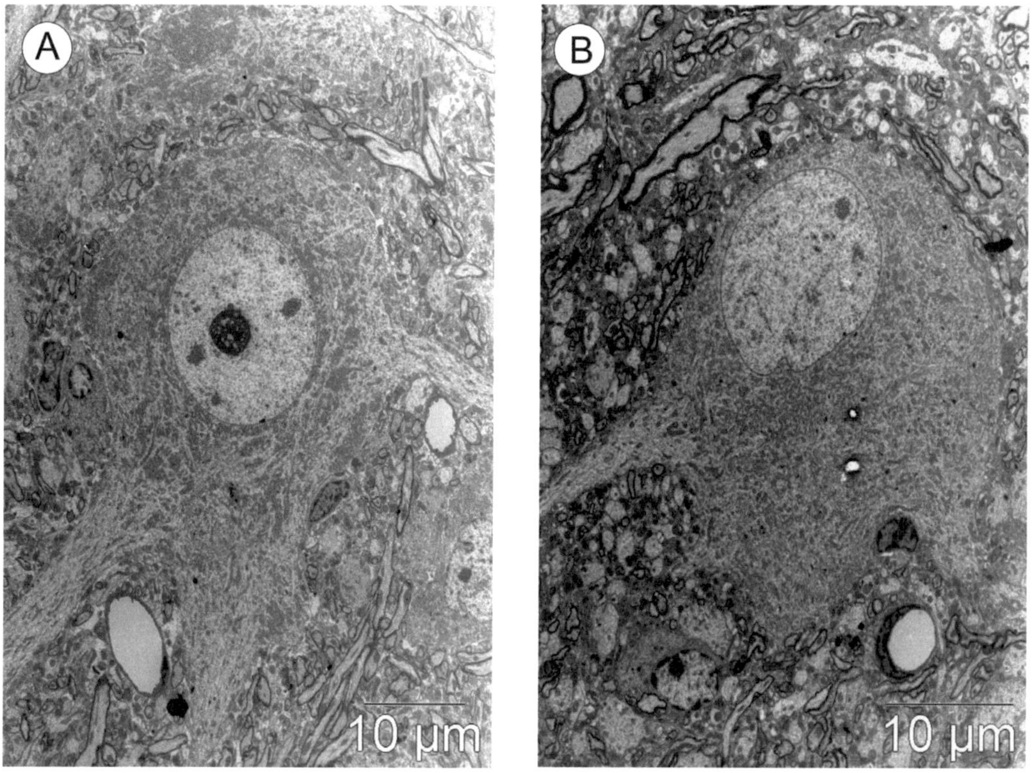

Fig. 2. B and C respectively, a motoneuron subjected to peripheral axotomy and a normal motoneuron, both observed under transmission electron microscopy. Scale = 10µm. *(Expression of class I major histocompatibility complex (MHC I) in the central nervous system: role in synaptic plasticity and regeneration* - review from Coluna/Columna. 2010; 9(2):193-198).

muscles studied by these authors. These same authors showed that in the sixth week of life, about 50% of the muscle fibers of the lower limb muscles presented a central nucleus, and by the eighth week of life, all the muscles showed hypertrophic fibers coexisting with foci of small fibers in various stages of maturation, providing an increase in the variety of fiber diameters. Huard et al. (1992) demonstrated the expression of dystrophin in the cerebellum, cerebral cortex, hippocampus and spinal cord of the central nervous system (CNS) of humans and monkeys. However, Lidove et al. (1993) demonstrated that in mice, dystrophin is expressed almost exclusively in the pyramidal cells and in other neurons of the cerebral cortex and in the Purkinje cells. Sbriccoli et al. (1995) suggested that the dystrophin localized in the CNS has an important role in developing and maintaining the structural and functional properties in the interconnections between neurons. Evidence of abnormal connections in the adult MDX mouse brain has been demonstrated primarily by Carretta et al. (2001). Sbriccoli et al. (1995) showed that in MDX mice, there are decreased numbers of cortico-spinal tract axons. This change in the cortico-spinal tract can be justified by the role of dystrophin in the cerebral cortex, and the complete loss of its expression in MDX mice. Therefore, it plays an important role in the migration and maturation of neurons in the cerebral cortex.

Bearing in mind the possible repercussions of the process of muscle degeneration and regeneration in the spinal microenvironment, unilateral axotomy of the sciatic nerve followed by analysis of the spinal motoneurons was used in MDX mice (Figure 3). This experimental model of peripheral nerve injury was chosen, keeping in mind that the transection of a peripheral nerve, such as the sciatic nerve, is a well-established experimental model to study the correlation between glial reactivity and neuronal response to injury at the anterior column level of the spinal cord (Lundberg et al., 2001). This is due to the fact that in this model, the only elements directly affected by the injury are the axons of spinal neurons. Thus any changes observed in the vicinity of motoneuron bodies, including reactive astrogliosis and the activation of MHC I molecules (histocompatibility complex type I), are reflections of direct communication between the neuron and the glia.

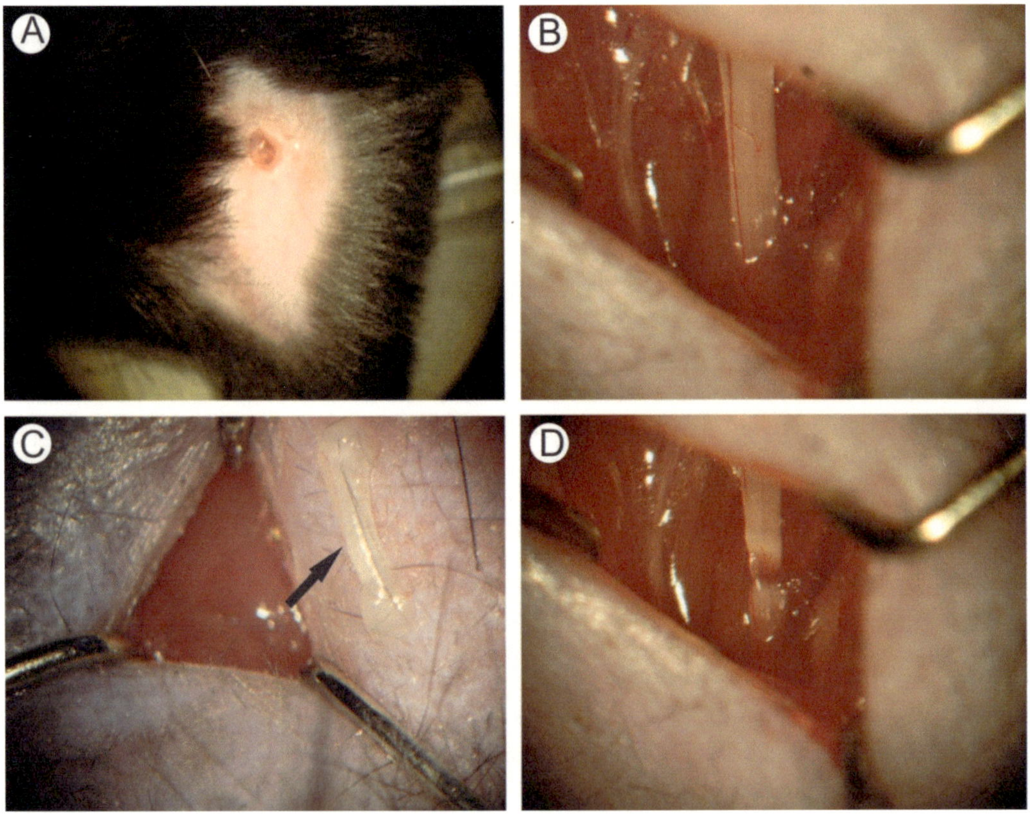

Fig. 3. A - Shaving in the region of the posterior left thigh and an incision in the skin of the mid-thigh, and then parallel to the femur using a scalpel. B - The skin and thigh muscle were carefully retracted, exposing the sciatic nerve to be transected. C - Figure showing the transected sciatic nerve. D – Crushed sciatic nerve.

Distal axotomy also induces, in addition to astroglial activation, the retraction of presynaptic terminals in contact with the cell body (Figure 4) and dendrites of the spinal alpha-motoneurons (Brännström & Kellerth, 1998: Aldskogious et al., 1999). This retraction is more intense in the synaptic terminals of the motoneuron cell body (Brännström & Kellerth, 1998), and occurs in the acute phase of injury, being influenced by the change in physiological state of the neurons, that pass from the transmission state condition to the survival and regeneration condition (Piehl et al., 1998). Reier et al. (1989) have proposed that the astrocytes act as a barrier to axon growth by way of the formation of scar tissue, but may promote its regeneration by releasing neurotrophic factors (Baba, 1998). Therefore the astrocytes directly influence the dynamics of synaptic contacts (Walz, 1989: Araque & Perea, 2004) and may thus influence the processes of synaptic reorganization after injury (Aldskogius et al., 1999).

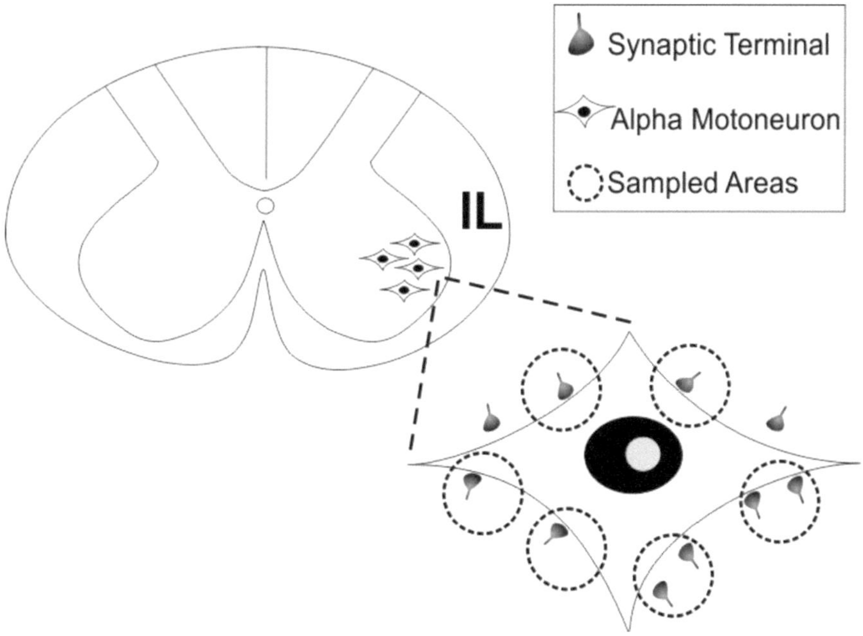

Fig. 4. Schematic representation of the sciatic nerve pool in the ventral horn of the spinal cord. One motoneuron is shown in detail with apposed presynaptic terminals. The dashed circles represent the areas where synaptic retraction is present. 2010 Blackwell Publishing Ltd, *Neuropathology and Applied Neurobiology,* **36** , 55–70.

2. Results and discussion

The immunohistochemistry and transmission electron microscopy results demonstrated that glial reactivity varies between the two strains. In MDX mice with no injury, an increase in GFAP immunoreactivity can be seen as compared to the same group in C57BL/10 mice (Figure 5A and 5B, respectively). The MDX and C57BL/10 ipsilateral groups showed a significant increase in reactive astrogliosis (GFAP) in relation to the contralateral groups in both strains (Figures 5E and 5F, respectively). However, with respect to this, there was evidence of increased astrocyte activity in the MDX contralateral group, as demonstrated by astrogliosis in the region of the spinal alpha-motoneurons (Figure 5D). This increase was approximately 49.5% higher than in the same side of the C57BL/10 strain. The analysis showed a significant increase in ipsilateral activity of the astrocytes in MDX mice, about 65.2% higher as compared to the C57BL/10 mice. Increased astrogliosis at the level of the anterior column of the spinal cord correlates with significant synaptic plasticity in the process of regeneration of injured neurons, as demonstrated by Emirandetti et al. (2006).

However, when the ipsi/contralateral ratio of the GFAP expression was analyzed, it was confirmed that there was no significant difference between the strains studied.

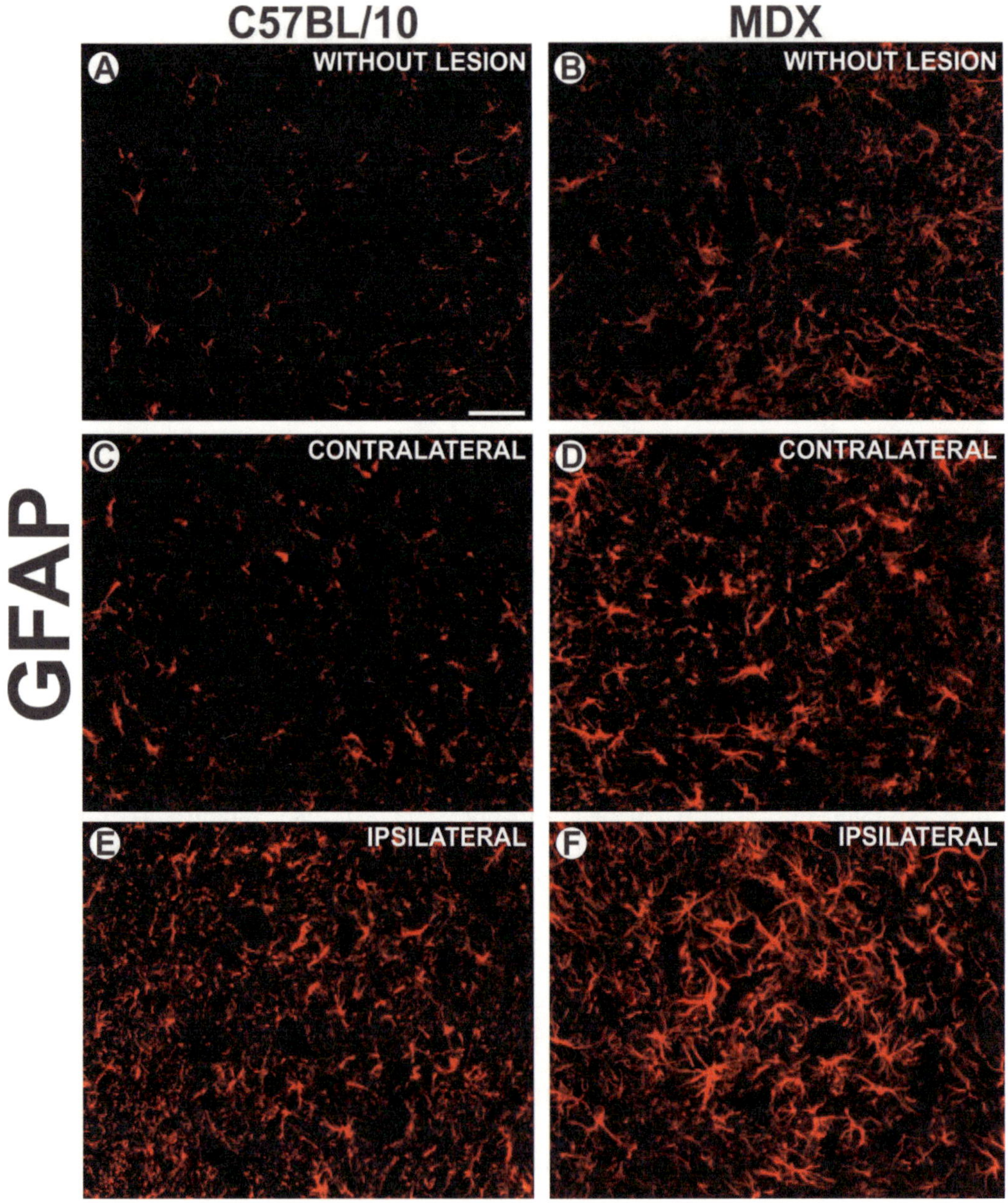

Fig. 5. Anti-GFAP immunostaining. A and B show non-injured animals (C57BL/10 and MDX, respectively). C and D show contralateral groups seven days after axotomy (C57BL/10 and MDX, respectively). E and F show ipsilateral sides, seven days after axotomy (C57BL/10 and MDX, respectively). Note that in general there is a greater expression of GFAP in the MDX strain in relation to the C57BL/10 strain. 2010 Blackwell Publishing Ltd, *Neuropathology and Applied Neurobiology*, **36** , 55–70.

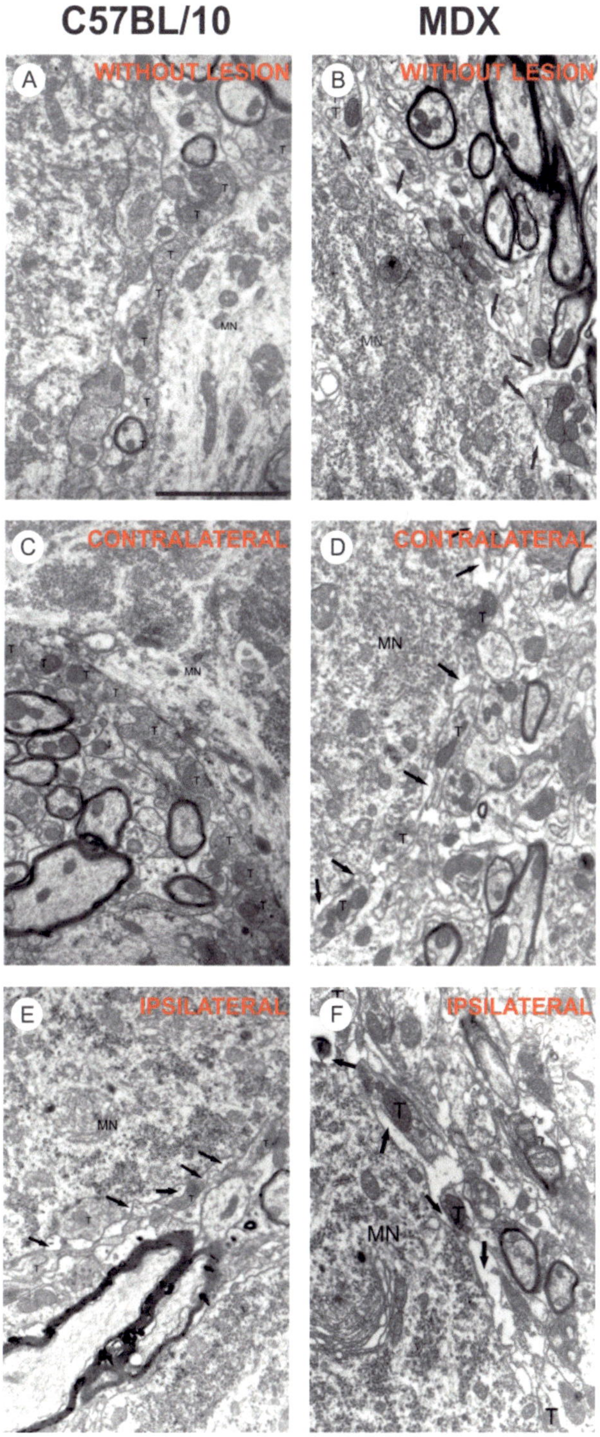

Fig. 6. Ultrastructure of the surface of without lesion spinal cord alpha motoneurons (MN). A – C57BL/10; B – MDX. Observe the normal C57BL/10 terminal apposition on the

postsynaptic membrane. In contrast, the MDX inputs (presynaptic terminals – T) to the motoneurons are partially detached (arrows), with a reduced area of apposition. C – Synaptic covering in the C57BL/10 contralateral side one week after axotomy. E – Synaptic elimination following axotomy in C57BL/10 mice. The arrows represent astroglial processes and T represents the synaptic boutons. D – Synaptic covering in the MDX contralateral side. F - Synaptic elimination following axotomy in MDX mice. The arrows represent astroglial processes and T represents the synaptic boutons. Observe a more intense synaptic loss in MDX mice, also present on without lesion at the contralateral side of the lesion, indicating that the course of the disease had an impact on the spinal cord circuits. Scale = 2 μm. 2010 Blackwell Publishing Ltd, *Neuropathology and Applied Neurobiology,* **36** , 55–70.

Although there was no statistical difference between the ipsi/contralateral ratios of the two strains, it is evident that the MDX mice present a greater astrocyte response in relation to the C57BL/10 mice, taking into account the difference in astrogliosis between the ipsilateral and contralateral sides of each strain. The fact that the MDX mice showed a superior basal level of GFAP in relation to the C57/BL10 mice, suggests that the effects of Ducehnne Muscular Dystrophy are directly reflected in the spinal cord microenvironment, resulting in significant changes in the spinal circuits. It is suggested that such changes in the MDX mice contribute to the progress of the disease by affecting the functionality of the motoneurons.

An ultrastructural analysis of the alpha-motoneurons plasma membrane showed the presence of synaptic elimination processes in both sides (injured and uninjured) on MDX mice. In the ipsilateral side, the two strains exhibited significant synaptic retraction, and the MDX mice showed less synaptic elimination when evaluating the percentage of synaptic covering before and after axotomy (MDX - 14.61% and C57/BL10 - 23.60 % approximately, Figure 6E and 6F). This fact demonstrates that in addition to the synaptic elimination resulting from the disease, the MDX mice probably have a lower potential for response to peripheral nerve injury. This may be related to the fact that these animals show a lower expression of MHC I (Simões & Oliveira, 2009).

These results show a correlation between glial reactivity, subsequent to the axotomy process, and the synaptic retraction that occurs at the spinal cord (Emirandetti et al., 2006), more evident in the MDX strain.

The communication between neurons and glia through MHC I signaling, probably involves receptors that may be able to translate the signal from MHC I to the neurons, and also from the astrocytes and microglia. In an attempt to understand the functional role of MHC I molecules in the CNS, specifically in synaptic plasticity and the regeneration of neurons in adult animals, Oliveira et al. (2004), performed sciatic nerve transection in knock out mice for the β2 microglobulin protein expression, a subunit of the complex of MHC I. In this study, these authors demonstrated that MHC I plays an important role in maintaining selective inhibitory terminals in apposition to axotomized neurons (Figure 8).

The absence or lower expression of MHC I results in a minor retraction of presynaptic boutons thus reducing the regenerative potential of injured neurons (Oliveira et al., 2004). This fact is consistent with that shown in MDX mice, keeping in view the relative synaptic elimination after axotomy. Similarly, Sabha et al. (2008) showed that the lower expression of

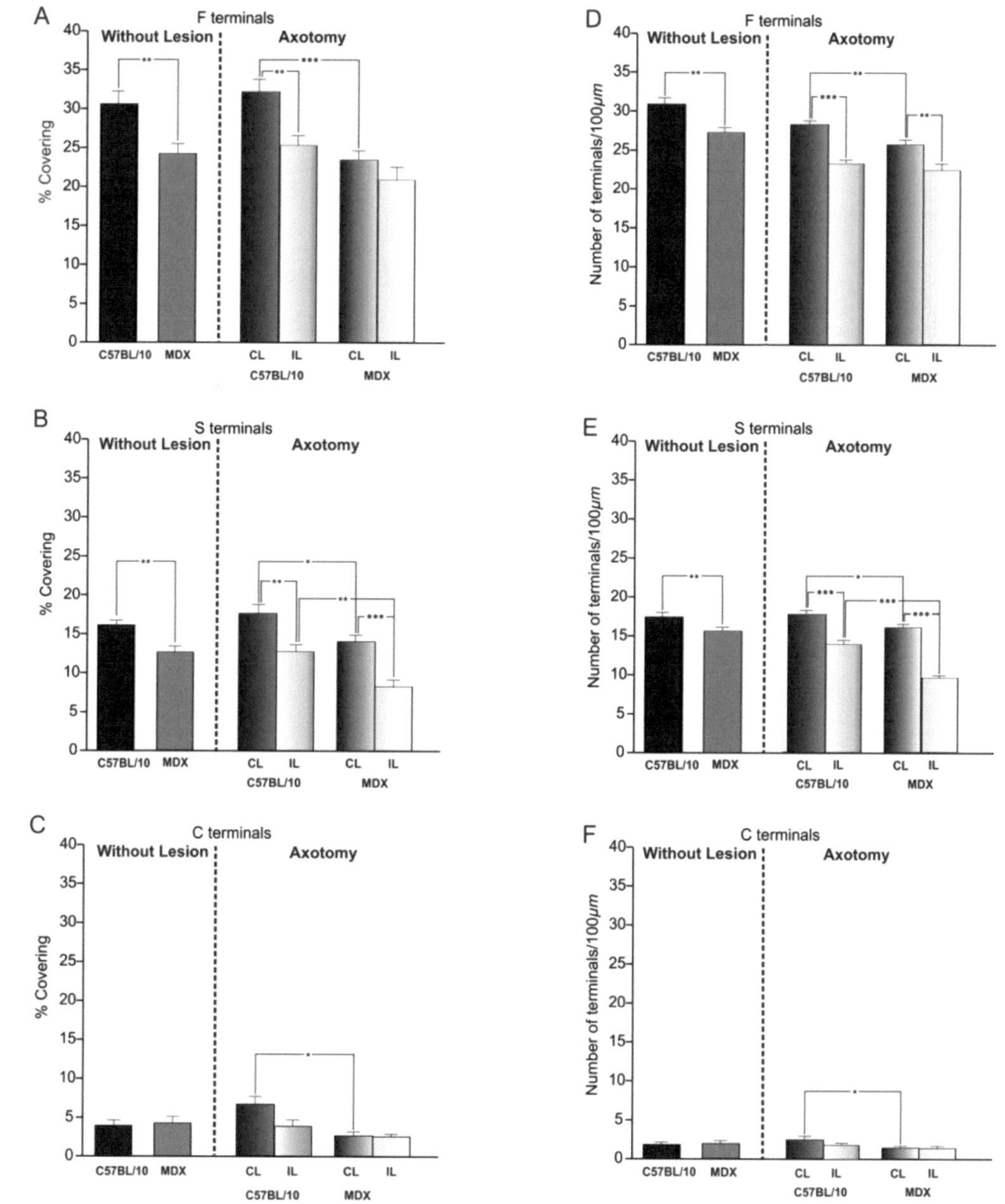

Fig. 7. Representation of the quantitative ultrastructural analysis of the percentage of covering by F, S and C synaptic terminals, and the quantitative ultrastructural analysis of the number of terminals (F, S and C) in apposition/100µm. A, B and C - show the covering of the F, S and C terminals as a percentage, for, respectively, those without injury and the contralateral and axotomized sides of both strains. D, E and F - show the number of presynaptic F, S and C terminals, respectively, in apposition to the neuronal membrane/100µm, for those without injury, and for the control and axotomized groups of both strains. Note that in the MDX mice, the F and S terminals are reduced before and after axotomy in both groups. 2010 Blackwell Publishing Ltd, *Neuropathology and Applied Neurobiology*, **36** , 55–70.

MHC I in C57/BL6J mice results in lower regenerative capacity in relation to A/J mice, which showed a higher expression of MHC I. Thus one can suggest that MDX mice show a lower potential axonal regeneration after peripheral nerve injuries, reflecting the evolution of the disease associated with a lower capacity to express MHC I (Figure 9).

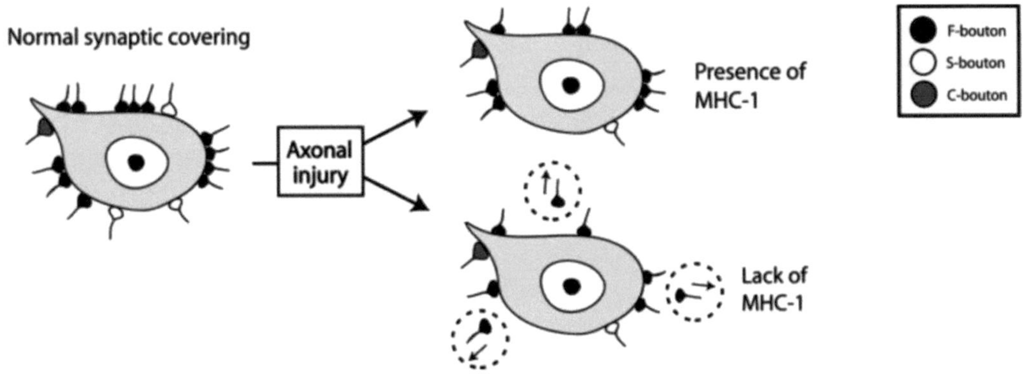

Fig. 8. Scheme showing the synaptic retraction process in motoneurons with the presence and absence of MHC-I. Note the retraction of the boutons in the motoneuron with the absence of MHC-I as compared to the motoneuron with MHC-I. Oliveira et al., *PNAS, 101(51): 17843-17848, 2004.*

This hypothesis was tested by the sciatic nerve crush, another type of peripheral nerve injury, followed by an analysis of motor recovery using the walking track test (Figure 10). After crushing, the animals were monitored for three weeks, every day up to the tenth day after injury, and then on alternate days from the eleventh to the twenty-first day after injury. The results show that MDX mice have a motor deficit compared with C57BL/10 mice, even before injury (MDX, -35.14 ± 3.82, mean + SD; C57BL/10, -7.63 ± 0.94, $p < 0.001$). The motor recovery curve was similar for the two strains, but the MDX mice showed a significant reduction in motor function after three weeks (MDX, -27.76 ± 5.03; C57BL/10, -7.71 ± 2.99, $p < 0.01$).

With regard to synaptic immunoreactivity, a study of the expression of synaptophysin showed there was reduced immunoreactivity in the MDX strain, both ipsilateral and contralateral to the lesion (Figure 13). A significant decrease in the expression of synaptophysin was observed in the MDX mice contralateral to the lesion, approximately 27% lower as compared to the same side in the C57BL/10 strain.

The immunohistochemical evaluation showed an increase in immunoreactivity for the neurofilaments (Figure 11) and the $p75^{NTR}$ - low affinity receptor for neurotrophins - (Figure 12) in both strains after crushing. It can also be seen that the MDX mice showed an increased expression of the neurofilament and $p75^{NTR}$ contralateral to the lesion. Similarly, immunostaining showed a better reorganization of regenerated fibers in the C57BL/10 mice. These results suggest that the reduction in motor function in the MDX mice could be related to the cycles of muscle degeneration that directly affect the neuromuscular junctions.

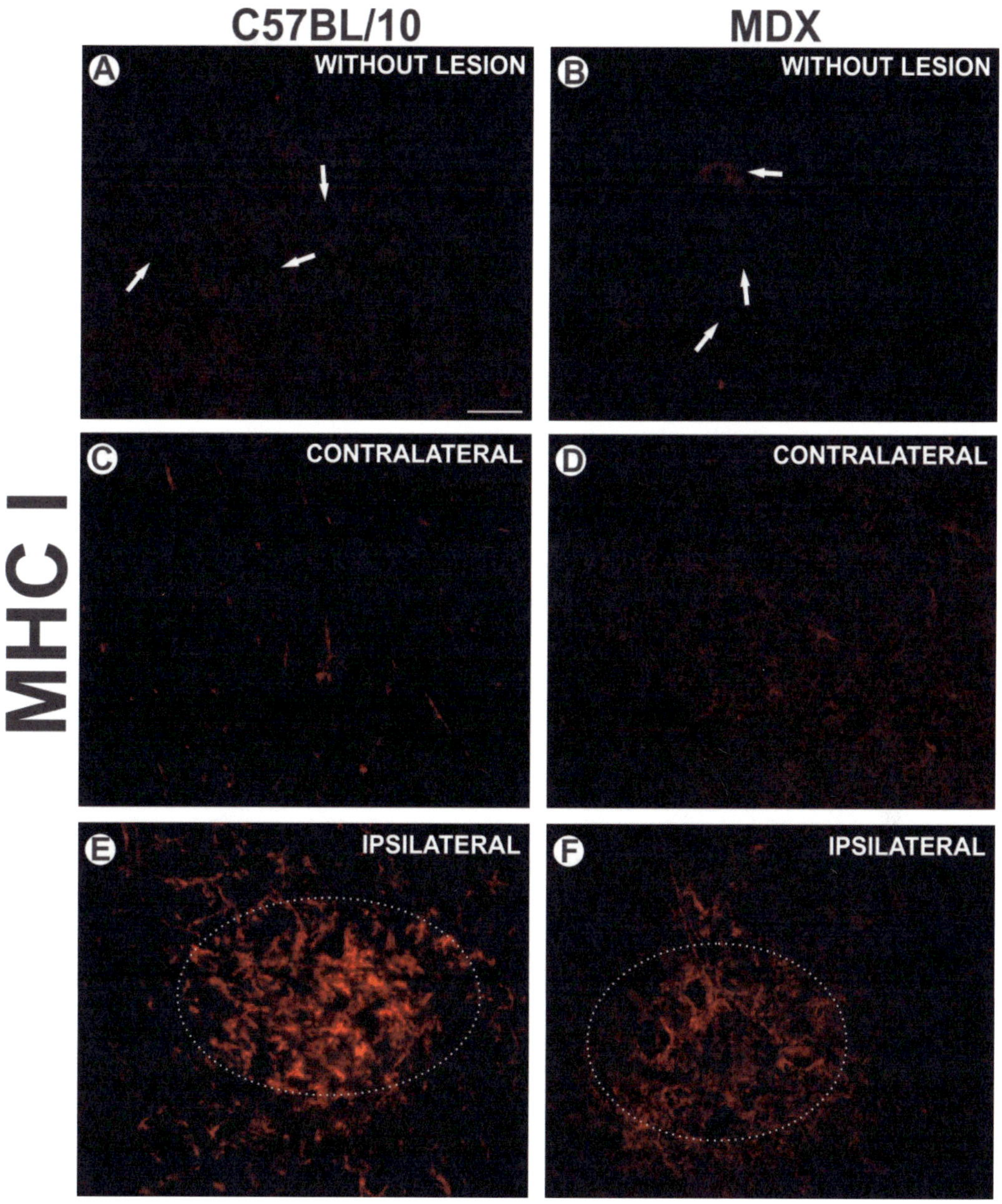

Fig. 9. A and B - Major histocompatibility complex of class I (MHC I) expression in non-injured C57BL/10 and MDX mice, respectively. C and D - Immunolabeling against the MHC I complex on the contralateral (CL) (non-injured) side of the spinal cord. Note the low basal expression of MHC I in both strains. E and F - Immunolabeling against the MHC I protein complex on the ipsilateral (IL) side of the spinal cord 1 week after axotomy, showing an increased expression in both strains, especially in the motoneuron surroundings and adjacent neuropil (dashed areas). The arrows indicate the cell body of the motoneurons. Scale = 50 mm. 2010 Blackwell Publishing Ltd, 9 *Neuropathology and Applied Neurobiology*, 36 , 55–70. 10

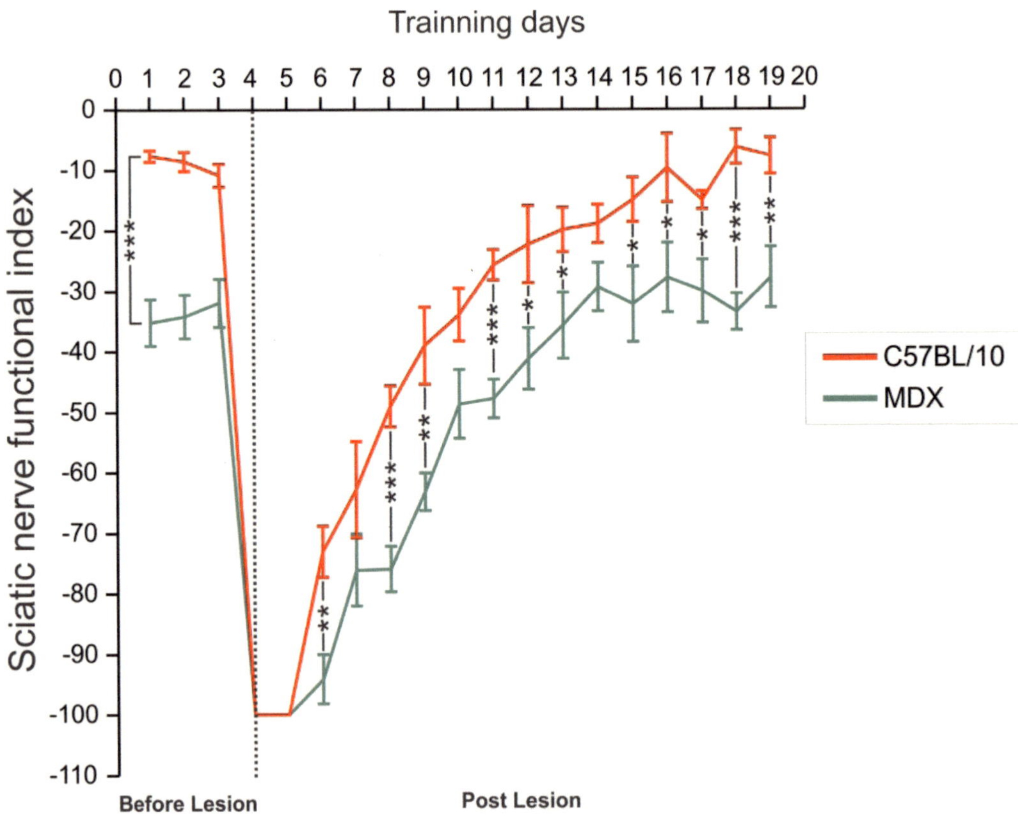

Fig. 10. Graph showing the motor function recovery of the two strains. Note that the MDX mice showed weakened motor function in relation to the C57BL/10 mice, both before and after the sciatic nerve crush.

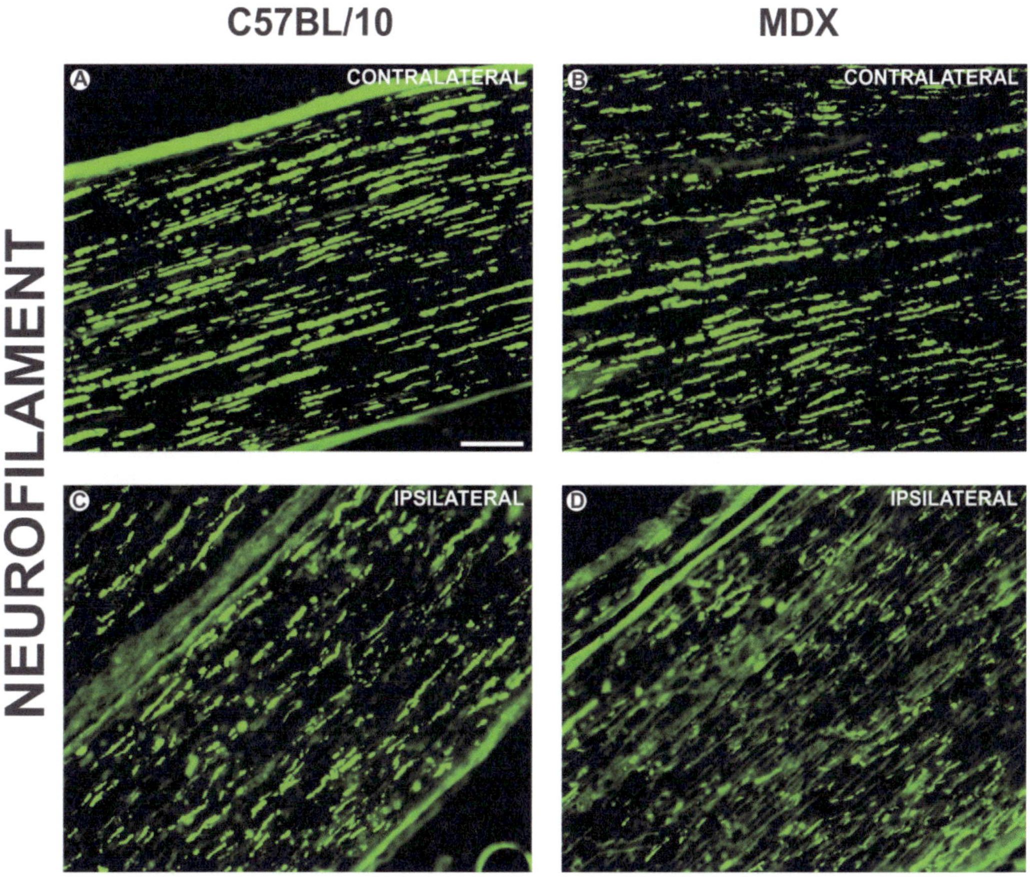

Fig. 11. Anti-neurofilament immunostaining three weeks after the sciatic nerve crush. A and B show the contralateral nerve. C and D show the ipsilateral nerve. Note that there is better organization in the axon fibers after nerve crush in the C57BL/10 mice as compared to the MDX strain.

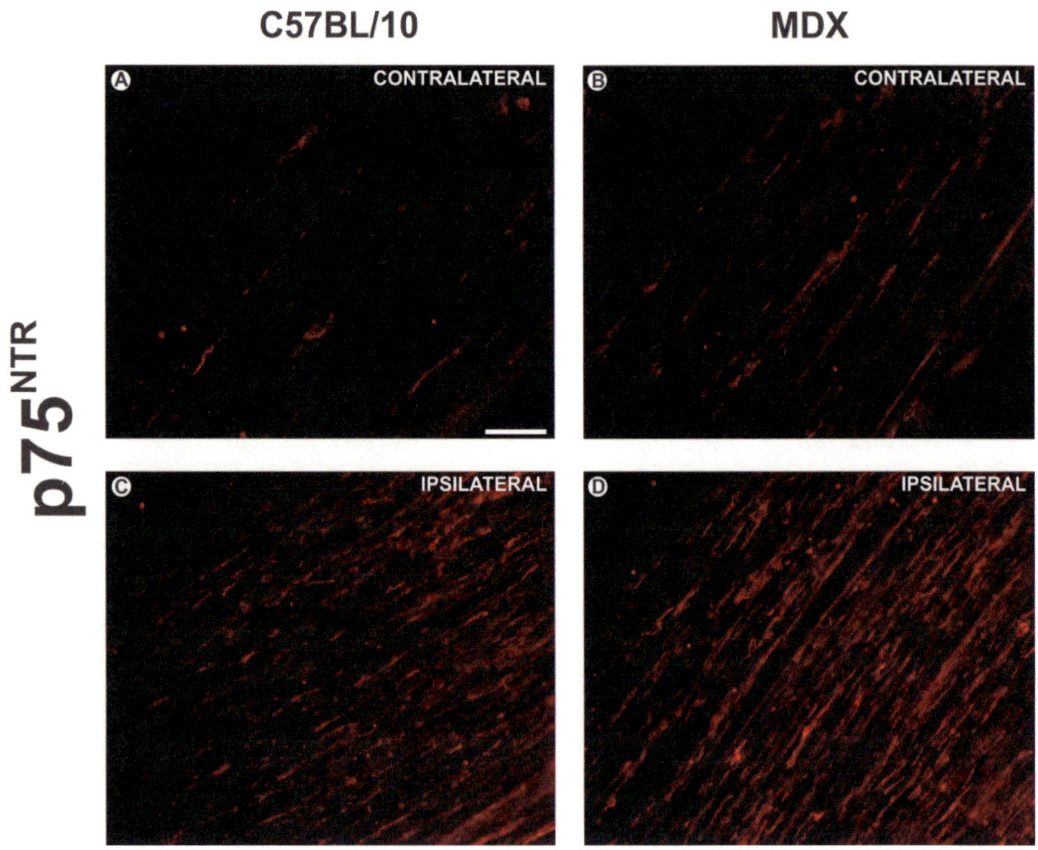

Fig. 12. Immunostaining of the anti- p75^{NTR} (low affinity receptor for neurotrophins) three weeks after sciatic nerve crush. A and B show the contralateral nerves in both strains. C and D show the ipsilateral nerves. Note that there is greater immunoreactivity in the MDX mice as compared to the C57BL/10 mice before and after nerve crushing.

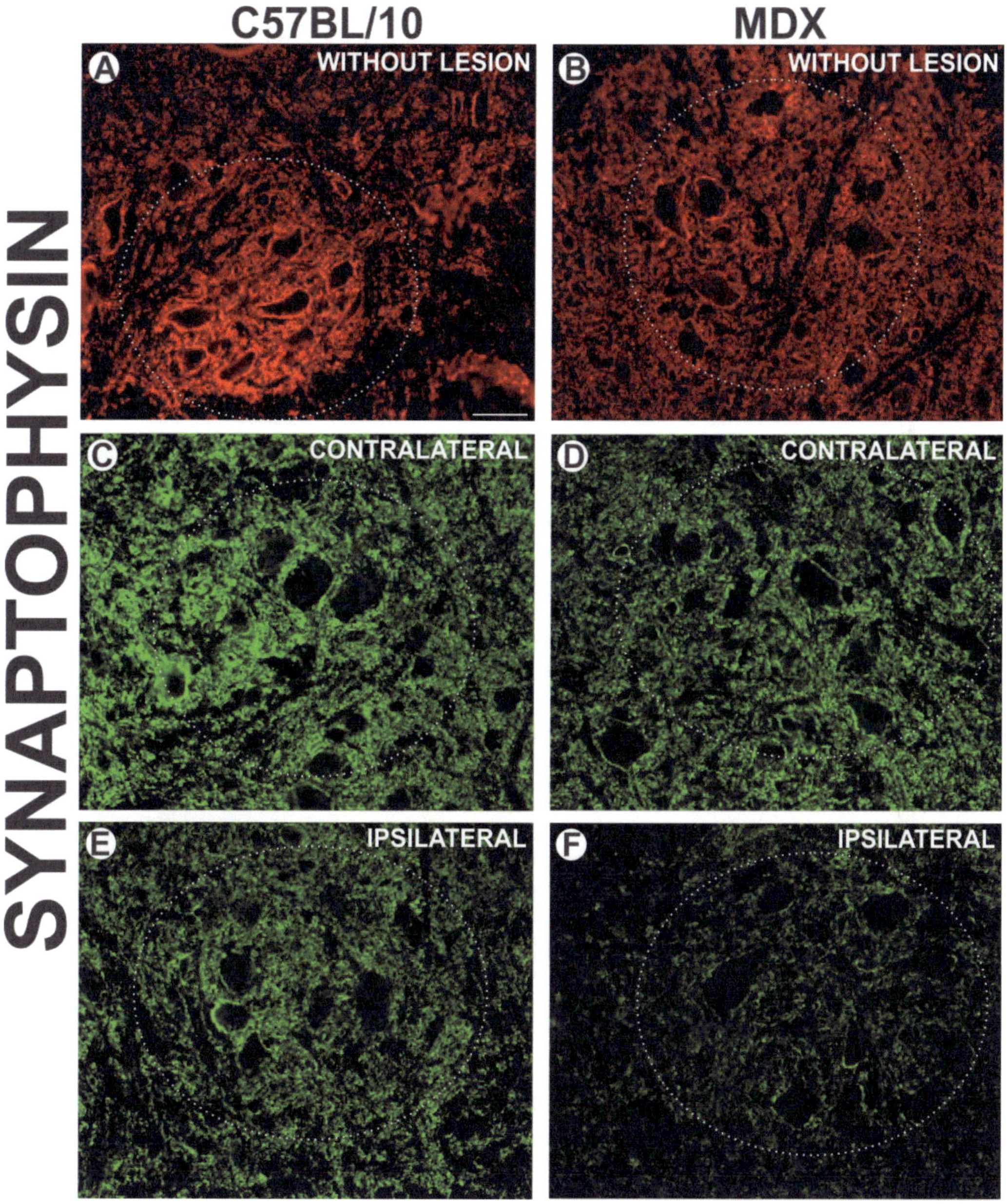

Fig. 13. A and B - Synaptophysin Immunolabeling in non-injured animals. C and D - Synaptophysin immunolabelling of the spinal cord contralateral to the injury 1 week after axotomy. Note the lower synaptic covering in the MDX mice. E and F - the lumbar spinal cord ispsilateral to the injury, 1 week after axotomy, showing an overall decrease in synaptophysin expression around the axotomized motor neuron. The areas containing axotomized motor neurones are highlighted by dashed circles. Scale = 50 mm. 2010 Blackwell Publishing Ltd, *Neuropathology and Applied Neurobiology,* **36** , 55–70.

Altogether, the results described herein indicate that the reduction of inputs in the spinal alpha-motoneurons resulted from a partial disconnection between the motoneuron axon and the muscle targeted during the cycles of muscle degeneration and regeneration that occurred after the second week postnatal. It should be noted that when the animals underwent axotomy at six weeks old, there was a clear central nucleus (indicative of regeneration) in approximately 50% of the muscle fibers (Pastoret & Sebille, 1994). Moreover, in the MDX mice there was a decrease in the number of cells in the cortico-spinal tract (Sbriccoli et al., 1995) and this could also reduce the number of inputs to the spinal alpha-motoneurons and thus cause a decrease in synaptic covering. The present results showing a decrease in protein expression of the synaptophysin and synaptic covering when compared with the findings of Oliveira et al. (2004), are consistent with the idea that the MHC I acts on the stability of the synaptic terminals. Nevertheless, considering its role in signaling between the presynaptic terminals and the motoneurons, as well as taking part in the communication of these with the glia, the greater expression of this protein in the C57BL/10 mice could promote a greater nerve regeneration process as compared to the MDX mice.

As demonstrated by Oliveira et al. (2004), after a nerve injury, MHC I plays a key role in stabilizing the selective inhibitory synapses, which contributes to the presynaptic terminal retraction process occurring in a specific way. Sabha et al. (2008) correlated an increased expression of MHC I with an intensification of the synaptic elimination process seven days after peripheral axotomy in the spinal cord microenvironment. This was evident in both C57BL/10 and MDX strains, but with a lower expression of MHC I in the MDX mice. One hypothesis for this occurrence is that the muscle degeneration and regeneration process already proceeding in these mice at a young age (Pastoret & Sebille, 1994), promotes a "partial disconnection" of the sciatic nerve with its target muscle, possibly stimulating an increased expression of MHC I molecules in these animals. This fact may contribute to the differentiated response of the MDX mice in comparison with that normally seen in the C57BL/10mice, similarly to what was shown in the work of Sabha et al. (2008), where the MHC I expression remained high over a period of up to 3 weeks after axotomy. Thus it is suggested that the lower expression of MHC I in MDX mice may indicate a reduced capacity for adjustment of the inputs by the motoneurons, indicating a lower regenerative potential after nerve injury.

3. References

Aldskogius, H. & Svensson, M. 1993. Neuronal and glial responses to axon injury. In S.K. Malhotra (eds): Advances in structural biology. Greenwich, Connecticut: JAI Press.

Aldskogius, H.; Liu, L.; Svensson, M, 1999. *Glial responses to synaptic damage and plasticity.* Journal Neuroscience Research, 58:33-41.

Arahata, K.: Ishihara, T.; Nonaka, I.; Ozawa, E.; Sugita, H. 1988. *Imunnostaining of skeletal and cardiac muscle surface membrane with antibody against Duchenne muscular dystrophy peptide.* Nature, 333:861-868.

Araque, A. & Perea, G. 2004. *Glial modulation of synaptic transmission in culture.* Glia. 47:241-248.

Baba, A. 1998. *Role of endothelin B receptor signals in reactive astrocytes.* Life Sci., 62 (17/18):1711-1715.

Balaban, B.; Matthews DJ.; Clayton, GH.; Carry T. 2005. *Corticosteroid treatment an functional improvement in Duchenne Muscular Dystrophy: long-term effect.* Am J Phys Med Rehabil., 84:843-850.

Brännström, T. & Kellerth, J.O. 1998. *Changes in synaptology of adult cat spinal alpha-motoneurons after axotomy.* Experimental Brain Research, 118:1-13.

Carreta, D.; Santarelli, M.; Vanni, D.; Carrai, R.; Sbriccoli, A.; Pinto, F.; Minciacchi, D. 2001 *The organization of spinal projecting brainstem neurons in an animal modelo f muscular dystrophy: A retrograde tracinig study on mdx mutante mice.* Brain Research, 895:213-222.

Chelly, J.; Kaplan, J.C.; Maire, P.; Gautron, S.; Kahn, A. 1988. *Transcription of the dystrophy (mdx) in the mouse.* Proc. Natl. Acad. Sci. USA, 81:1189-1192.

Emirandetti, A.; Zanon, R.G.; Sabha, M.J.; Oliveira, A.L.R. 2006. *Astrocyte reactivity influences the number of presynaptic terminals apposed to spinal motoneurons after axotomy.* Brain Research, 1095:35-42.

Haenggi T. & Fritschy J.M. 2006. *Role of dystrophin and utrophin for assembly and function of the dystrophin glycoprotein complex in non-muscle tissue.* Cell Mol Life Sci. 2006 Jul;63(14):1614-31.

Huard, J.; Coté, P.Y.; Parent, A.; Bouchard, J.P.; Tremblay, J.P. 1992. *Dystrophin-like immunoreactivity in monkey and human brain areas involved in learning and motor functions.* Neuroscience Lett., 141:181-186.

Judge, L.M.; Haraguchi, M.; Chamberlain, J.S. 2005. *Dissecting the signaling and mechanical functions of the dystrophin-glycoprotein complex.* Journal of Cell Science., 119:1537-1546.

Lagrota-Candido, J.; Vasconcellos, R.; Cavalcanti, M.; Bozza, M.; Savino, W.; Quirico-Santos, T. 2002. *Resolution of skeletal muscle inflammation in mdx dystrophic mouse is accompanied by increased immunoglobulin and interferon-gama production.* Int. J. Exp. Path., 83:121-132.

Lidov, H.G.; Byers, T.J.; Kunkel, L.M. 1993. *The distribuition of dystrphin in the murine central nervous system: an immunocytochemical study.* Neuroscience, 54:167-187.

Lieberman, A. R. 1971. *The axon reaction: a review of the principal features of perikaryal responses to axon injury.* Int. Rev. Neurobiol., 14:49-124.

Lindå, H.; Piehl, F.; Dagerlind, A.; Verge, V. M.; Arvidsson, U.; Cullheim, S.; Risling, M.; Ulfhake, B.; Hokfelt, T. 1992. *Expression of GAP-43 mRNA in the adult mammalian spinal cord under normal conditions and after different types of lesions, with special reference to motoneurons.* Exp. Brain Res. 91, 284-295.

Lindå, H.; Hammarberg, H.; Cullheim, S.; Levinovitz, A.; Khademi, M.; Olsson, T. 1998. *Expression of MHC class I and β2 – Microglobulin in rat spinal motoneurons: regulatory influences by IFN – gamma and axotomy.* Exp. Neurol., 150, 282-295.

Lowe, Dawn A.; Willians, Brian O.; Thomas, David D. and Grange, Robert. 2006. *Molecular and cellular contractile dysfunction of dystrophic muscle from young mice.* Muscle & Nerve., 34:92-100.

Lundberg, C.; Lidman, O.; Holmdahl, R; Olsson, T; Piehl, F.2001. *Neurodegeneration and glial activation patterns after mechanical nerve injury are differentially regulated by non-MHC genes in congenic inbred rat strains.* J Comp Neurol., 26;431(1):75-87.

Mcdowall, R.M.; Dunn, M.J.; Billiau, A. 1990. *Nature of the mononuclear infiltrate and the mechanism of muscle damage in juvenile dermatomyositis and Duchenne muscular dystrophy.* J. Neurol. Science, 99:199-217.

Nonaka, I. 1998. Animals models of muscular dystrophies. Loboratory Anim. Sci. 48:8-16.

Oliveira, A.L.; Thams, S.; Ldman, O.; Piehl, F.; Hökfelt, T.; Kärre, Lindå, H.; Cullhem, 2004. *A role for MHC class I molecules in synaptic plasticity and regeneration of neurons after axotomy*. PNAS. 101(51):17843-17848.

Pastoret, C. & Sebille, A. 1994. *MDX mice show progressive weakness and muscle deterioration whith age*. Journal of Neurological Sciences, 129:97-105.

Pearce, J.M.S. 2005. *Early Observations on Duchenne-Meryon muscular dystrophy*. Eur Neurol., 54: 46-48.

Piehl, F.; Hammarberg, H.; Hokfelt, T.; Cullheim, S. 1998. *Regulatory effects of trophic factors on expression and distribuition of CGRP and GAP-43 in rat motoneurons*. J. Neurosci., 5:1321-1333.

Radley, H.G.; Davies, M.J.; Grounds, M.D. 2007. *Reduced muscles necrosis and long-term benefits in dystrophic mdx mice after cV1q (blockade of TNF) treatment*. Neuromuscular Disorders, 18:227-238

Reier, P.J.; Eng, L.F.; Jakeman, L. 1989. *Reactive astrocyte and axonal outgrowth in the injured CNS: is gliosis really an impediment to regeneration?* Neur. Reg. Transpl. Front. Clinical Neuroscience, 6;193-209.

Romanes, G. 1946. *Motor localization and the effects of nerve injury on the ventral horn cells of the spinal cord*. J Anat., 80:117-131.

Sabha, M.JR.; Emirandetti, A.; Cullheim, S.; Oliveira, A.L.R. 2008. *MHC I expression and synaptic plasticity ind different mice strains after axotomy*. Synapse, 62:137-148.

Sbriccoli, A.; Santarelli, M.; Carreta, D.; Pinto, F.; Granato, A.; Minciacchi, D. 1995. Architectural changes of the cortiço-spinal system in the dystrophin defective mdx mice. Neuroscience Letters, 200:53-56.

Simões G.F. & Oliveira, A.L. 2010. *Alpha motoneurone input changes in dystrophic MDX mice after sciatic nerve transection*. Neuropathol Appl Neurobiol., 36(1):55-70.

Spencer, M.J.; Montecino-Rodrigues, E.; Dorshkind, K.; Tidball, J.G. 2001. *Helper (CD4+) and cytotoxic (CD8+) T cells promote the pathology of dystrophin-deficient muscle*. Clin. Immunol., 989:235-243.

Wals, W. 1989 Role of glial cells in the regulation of the brain ion microenvironment. Prog. Neurobiol., 33(4):309-333.

Whitehead, N.P.; Yeung, E.W. and Allen, D. 2006. *Muscle damage in MDX (dystrophic) mice: role of calcium and reactive oxygen species*. Clinical and Experimental Pharmacology and Physiology. 33:657-662.

Zanon, R.G.; Emirandetti, A.; Simões, G.F.; Freria, C.M.; Victório, S.C.; Cartarozzi, L.P.; Barbizan, R.; Oliveira, A.L.R. 2010. *Expressão do complexo de histocompatilidade principal de classe I (MHC I) no sistema nervoso central: plasticidade sináptica e regeneração*. COLUNA/COLUMNA.; 9(2):193-198

10

Altered Gene Expression Pathways in Duchenne Muscular Dystrophy

Nevenka Juretić, Francisco Altamirano,
Denisse Valladares and Enrique Jaimovich
*Centro de Estudios Moleculares de la Célula, Facultad de Medicina,
Universidad de Chile, Santiago,
Chile*

1. Introduction

Duchenne muscular dystrophy (DMD) is caused by the absence of functional dystrophin (Blake et al. 2002). Dystrophin is a cytoskeleton protein normally expressed in the inner face of the plasma membrane (Ahn and Kunkel 1993). In normal skeletal muscle, dystrophin is associated with a complex of glycoproteins known as dystrophin-associated proteins (DAPs), providing a linkage between the extracellular matrix (ECM) and cytoskeleton (Batchelor and Winder 2006). Lack of dystrophin in dystrophic muscle results in loss of the complex integrity and allegedly impairs the stability of the plasma membrane causing mechanical stress fragility, and an increase in Ca^{2+} permeability (Alderton and Steinhardt 2000). But the pathophysiology of muscular dystrophy is not only explained by this increased mechanical fragility and a role for dystrophin and DAPs has been suggested as being part of a protein signaling complex involved in cell survival (Rando 2001). In this chapter we discuss evidence of such a role, which may evidence possible interactions between dystrophin and proteins other than those involved in DAP and possible cell location of dystrophin in regions other than the sarcolemma cytoskeleton.

2. Calcium homeostasis

Ca^{2+} is a highly versatile second messenger that can regulate several cellular functions. Skeletal muscles use Ca^{2+} for contraction process and as regulatory signaling molecule. Subsequently, muscle plasticity is closely related with calcium signals (Berchtold et al. 2000).

Under resting conditions, wild type *(wt)* skeletal muscle cells maintain the cytosolic calcium concentration ($[Ca^{2+}]_i$) around 100-120 nM (Lopez et al. 1987; Eltit et al. 2010). Since the chemical gradient between $[Ca^{2+}]_i$ and extracellular medium or sarcoplasmic reticulum (SR) is about 10,000 fold, to constantly keep the $[Ca^{2+}]_i$ in the nM range, skeletal muscle cells uses a complex machinery to finely regulate calcium concentration. Plasma membrane Ca^{2+}-ATPase (PMCA), Na^+/Ca^{2+} exchanger (NCX) in the plasma membrane and the SR Ca^{2+}-ATPase (SERCA) extrudes the Ca^{2+} to extracellular space or to SR, respectively. These functions are opposed, under resting conditions, for the SR Ca^{2+} leak type-1 ryanodine receptor (RyR1) channels and the basal sarcolemma Ca^{2+} influx (Eltit et al. 2010).

2.1 Altered resting calcium in DMD

Several reports demonstrate that the $[Ca^{2+}]_i$ is elevated in *mdx* mice and DMD human fibers (Lopez et al. 1987; Yeung et al. 2005; Allen et al. 2010). Lopez et al. (1987) have shown that the $[Ca^{2+}]_i$ in DMD muscle fibers is 370 nM, while in normal muscle fibers was around 100 nM (Lopez et al. 1987). Similar results were obtained in *mdx* adult fibers compared with the *wt* counterpart (Yeung et al. 2005; Allen et al. 2010). The authors demonstrated that $[Ca^{2+}]_i$ was elevated under resting conditions in *mdx* fibers and when the fibers were exposed to stretch-induced damage, $[Ca^{2+}]_i$ increased to higher levels, around 700 nM (Yeung et al. 2005; Allen et al. 2010).

Increased $[Ca^{2+}]_i$ has been related with necrosis through calpain activation and mitochondrial permeability transition pore (MPTP) (Turner et al. 1988; Spencer et al. 1995; Millay et al. 2008).

The mechanism that has been proposed for dystrophin function involves a role in sarcolemma stabilization, so in muscle fibers that lack this protein, membrane damage would be recurrent (Petrof et al. 1993; Mokri and Engel 1998). These evidences suggested the hypothesis of Ca^{2+} leak into the cell through damaged membrane. There are several evidences in *mdx* muscle fibers that relate the calcium entry with the transient receptor potential channels (TRPC1) and the store-operated calcium entry (SOCE) mechanism. TRPC1-dependent calcium entry is increased in *mdx* muscle fibers (Vandebrouck et al. 2002; Yeung et al. 2005; Gervasio et al. 2008). The blockage of these cationic channels with streptomycin or spider venom toxin (GsMTx4) reduced $[Ca^{2+}]_i$ and prevented the rise of the $[Ca^{2+}]_i$ following stretch (eccentric) contractions. This maneuver, partially reduced the decline in both the tetanic Ca^{2+} increase and force (Yeung et al. 2005; Allen et al. 2010). Gervasio et al. 2008 showed that TRPC1, caveolin-3 and Src-kinase protein levels are increased in *mdx* muscle (Gervasio et al. 2008). The authors propose that the stretch-induced muscle damage and the increase in the $[Ca^{2+}]_i$ is produced by the ROS production, activation of Src-kinase and TRPC-induced Ca^{2+} entry. Furthermore, administration of streptomycin reduced muscle damage and increased myofiber regeneration (Yeung et al. 2005).

More recently, store-operated calcium entry has been implicated in the exacerbated resting Ca^{2+} entry observed in *mdx* fibers (Boittin et al. 2006; Vandebrouck et al. 2006; Edwards et al. 2010). These Ca^{2+} entries are modulated by a Ca^{2+}-independent phospholipase A_2, which is overexpressed in dystrophic fibers (Boittin et al. 2006). Vandebrouck et al. (2005) demonstrate that the high store-operated Ca^{2+} transients observed in dystrophin-deficient myotubes were associated with sustained cytosolic Ca^{2+} transients and high intra-mitochondrial entries, that can be reduced by mini-dystrophin expression or FCCP (uncoupler of oxidative phosphorylation) (Vandebrouck et al. 2006). In addition, the thresholds for SOCE activation and deactivation occur at higher $[Ca^{2+}]_{SR}$ and the proteins levels of STIM1 and Orai1 was 3-fold increased in *extensor digitorum longus* (EDL) muscles from *mdx* mice (Edwards et al. 2010).

2.2 SR Ca^{2+} loading capacity

There is a controversy about the loading capacity of the SR $[Ca^{2+}]_{SR}$ in dystrophic skeletal muscle cells compared with normal skeletal muscle cells. Roberts et al. (2001), using a Ca^{2+}-sensitive photoprotein aequorin chimera with SR destination sequence, show that after SR

Ca^{2+} depletion, the re-addition of Ca^{2+} to the media increases the $[Ca^{2+}]_{SR}$ rapidly up to a steady state that is 50% higher that the *wt* myotubes (Robert et al. 2001). In contrast, Culligan et al. (2002) shows a reduction in Ca^{2+} binding in the SR microsomes from *mdx* mice, associated with a drastic reduction in the calsequestrin-like proteins and normal SERCA1 expression and activity (Culligan et al. 2002). However, a reduction in SERCA activity has been observed in dystrophic muscle (Kargacin and Kargacin 1996; Divet et al. 2005), which could account for the increased $[Ca^{2+}]_i$. SERCA1a overexpression in *mdx* diaphragm muscle by adeno-associated virus gene transfer, resulted in a reduction of centrally located nuclei and reduced susceptibility to eccentric contraction-induced damage (Morine et al. 2010). More recently, δ-sarcoglycan-null and *mdx* mice transgenic animals that overexpress SERCA1, show a reduction in myofiber central nucleation, tissue fibrosis and serum creatine kinase levels. In addition SERCA1 overexpression enhances excitation-contraction (E-C) coupling and restore the $[Ca^{2+}]_i$ and $[Ca^{2+}]_{SR}$ in both dystrophic models (Goonasekera et al. 2011).

2.3 Excitation-Contraction (E-C) coupling

The proteins involved in E-C coupling are normally expressed in dystrophic muscle. The expression of α1-, α2- and β-subunits of the dihydropyridine receptor (DHPR) are similar in microsomes from control and *mdx* mice (Culligan et al. 2002). RyR1 and SERCA1 are also found in comparable amounts in control and dystrophin-deficient muscles (Culligan et al. 2002).

In skeletal muscle cells, membrane depolarization induces a conformational change in Cav1.1 DHPRs that is transmitted to the ryanodine receptor (RyR1), causing it to release Ca^{2+} from the SR, that it is necessary for the contraction process.

Several evidences indicate that the dystrophic skeletal muscle cells have an unpaired E-C coupling. Comparisons of the cytosolic calcium transients evoked by single action potential have shown that the calcium transients are reduced in *mdx* fibers compared with *wt* fibers (Woods et al. 2004; Hollingworth et al. 2008). Recently, similar results have been found in fibers from *utr* $^{-/-}$ *mdx* mice (Capote et al. 2010). Muscle weakness observed in isolated fibers from *mdx* mice and DMD patients has not been fully explained. The reduction in the Ca^{2+} transient evoked by single action potential, reduction in $[Ca^{2+}]_{SR}$ and increased $[Ca^{2+}]_i$ could provide a mechanism for contractile dysfunction and impaired force production in DMD patients.

3. Excitation-Transcription (E-T) coupling

We have previously described that membrane depolarization of skeletal myotubes evokes a fast Ca^{2+} transient during the stimuli, that promotes a contractile response through "E-C coupling", and a slow Ca^{2+} transient peaking 60-100 seconds later, mostly associated to cell nuclei (Jaimovich et al. 2000; Estrada et al. 2001; Powell et al. 2001; Araya et al. 2003; Cardenas et al. 2005). Slow Ca^{2+} transients are involved in the "E-T coupling" mechanism, which relates membrane depolarization with gene expression (Powell et al. 2001; Araya et al. 2003; Carrasco et al. 2003; Juretic et al. 2006; Juretic et al. 2007). The signaling pathway begins at the DHPR, which by a mechanism involving G protein (Eltit et al. 2006), activates

PI3 kinase and PLC to produce inositol 1,4,5-trisphosphate (IP_3) that diffuses in the cytosol and reaches IP_3 receptors (IP_3Rs) located both at the SR membrane and at the nuclear envelope, promoting Ca^{2+} release (Araya et al. 2003). IP_3 mediated Ca^{2+} signals induce both a transient activation of ERK½ and transcription factor CREB, and an increase in early genes (*c-fos, c-jun* and *egr-1)* and in late genes (troponin I, interleukin-6, hmox and hsp70) mRNA levels after depolarization of normal skeletal muscle cells (Carrasco et al. 2003; Juretic et al. 2006; Juretic et al. 2007; Jorquera et al. 2009). Moreover, in electrically stimulated adult muscle fibers, slow Ca^{2+} signals mediate the frequency-dependent activation of slow-phenotype muscle fiber genes (slow troponin I, TnIs) and repression of fast-phenotype ones (TnIf) (Casas et al. 2010). These evidences link slow Ca^{2+} transients with muscular effects of nerve activity and with the process of muscle cell plasticity.

Recently we described a new role for ATP signaling in skeletal muscle in a process called "E-T" coupling (Buvinic et al. 2009, see Fig.1). We were able to show that the main ATP efflux pathway is through pannexin 1 hemichannels. We know that DHPR receptors and pannexin 1 interact with each other but it is not clear whether it is a direct interaction. The ATP released will locally activate the purinergic receptors P2X and P2Y localized in the membrane. This activation induces a transient increase in intracellular Ca^{2+} with specific kinetics. We demonstrated that ATP participates in the fast calcium transient related to contraction because apyrase (catalyses the hydrolysis of ATP) reduced the depolarization-evoked Ca^{2+} transient by about 20%. We can speculate that activation of P2X receptors may contribute to improve the skeletal muscle cells Ca^{2+} availability needed to sustain contractions. Moreover, we could also show that ATP participates in "E-T" coupling due to the total inhibition by apyrase of the second Ca^{2+} transient induced by depolarization. Additionally, the use of apyrase during the electrical stimulation completely abolished the increase in gene expression related with muscle plasticity (unpublished data). We can conclude that gene expression is regulated through activation of P2Y receptors mediated by the ATP released during depolarization.

3.1 Extracellular ATP: a major mediator for signal transduction

ATP for a long time was considering as a molecule that was involved with energy and metabolism of many cells. Nevertheless in the last few years ATP has been considered as an extracellular messenger for autocrine and paracrine signaling (Corriden and Insel 2010). It has been described as a regulator of inflammation, in embryonic and stem cell development, ischemia, among others (Bours et al. 2006; Burnstock and Ulrich 2011). In skeletal muscle ATP has been implicated in the regulation of proliferation, differentiation and regeneration (Ryten et al. 2002; Ryten et al. 2004) and also promoting the stabilization of the neuromuscular junction (Jia et al. 2007).

ATP release is induced in response to several kinds of stress in many cells type, including hypoxia, ischemia, osmotic swelling and mechanical stimulation (Corriden and Insel 2010). ATP can exit cells using several different purinergic signal efflux pathways (Fitz 2007). The main source of extracellular ATP is cell lysis, which occurs when massive cell death takes place during trauma, injury or inflammation. A non-lytic source of ATP is the release of secretory granules during stimulated exocytosis, which occurs in secretory cell types like epithelial cells of the liver, lung, kidney, neurons and astrocytes (Volonte and D'Ambrosi

2009). A non-lytic, and also non-exocytotic release of ATP can occur by channel- or transporter-mediated mechanisms, such as: (a) hemichannels, such as connexins and pannexin (Dubyak 2009); (b) anion channels, such as plasmalemma voltage dependent anion channel, voltage-dependent maxi-anion channel, volume sensitive Cl^- channel and P2X7 receptor (Sabirov and Okada 2005; Suadicani et al. 2006; Liu et al. 2008); (c) ATP-binding cassette transporters, such as cystic fibrosis transmembrane conductance regulator Cl^- channel and P-glycoprotein (Campbell et al. 2003; Sabirov and Okada 2005); and (d) exchange carriers such as ADP/ATP exchange carrier (Sabirov and Okada 2005; Volonte and D'Ambrosi 2009). Several studies have recently demonstrated that ATP can be released by pannexin hemichannels in a variety of cells types that include myotubes (D'Hondt et al. 2011). Pannexin is widely distributed among tissues with cell communication via calcium waves (Shestopalov and Panchin 2008). The channel formed by this protein can be opened by mechanical perturbation at the resting membrane potential. The channel is permeable for ATP and it can be opened at physiological calcium concentration (Barbe et al. 2006). These properties make pannexin 1 (Panx1) a very attractive candidate for an ATP-releasing channel. The widespread distribution of Panx1 has been confirmed in a variety of human tissues, with the highest levels being found in skeletal muscle (Baranova et al. 2004). Results of our laboratory indicate that this hemichannel is expressed in myotubes and adult fibers of rat and mouse.

Once released, ATP acts as an extracellular signal trough the binding to purinergic receptors expressed in most cell types. Purinergic receptors comprise both ionotropic P2X receptor subtypes and G-protein-coupled P2Y receptor subtypes (Burnstock 2004). Between the purinergic receptors and the purine-generating reactions, there exist purino-converting enzymes. These enzymes named ectonucleotidases, consist of several different families with well-characterized molecular and functional features (Yegutkin 2008). They operate to metabolize nucleotides down to the respective nucleoside analogues, thus having the potential to decrease the extracellular concentrations of nucleotides. Consequently these enzymes modulate ligand availability at both nucleotide and nucleoside receptors (Yegutkin 2008). The contribution of the diverse ectonucleotidases to the modulation of purinergic signaling depends on their availability of different ectonucleotidases and their selectivity for substrates, but also on their abundance and cell distribution (Volonte and D'Ambrosi 2009).

ATP signaling has been implicated in many cell functions ranging from proliferation, differentiation, toxic actions, neurotransmission, smooth and cardiac muscle contraction, vasodilation, chemosensory signaling and secretion, to complex phenomena such as immune responses, male reproduction, fertilization, embryonic development, and so on (Burnstock 2004). This vast heterogeneity of their biological responses is influenced by different parameters such as the presence of endogenous ligands at receptor sites and the time and distance from the source of release; the concentration gradient of a ligand that simultaneously can activate more than one receptor subtype; the different composition of purinergic receptors in a given cell, or even more the composition in the diverse sub membrane compartments in which each ligand operates (Volonte and D'Ambrosi 2009).

3.2 Purinergic receptors

Purinergic receptors are subdivided into two major groups: eight G-protein-coupled seven-transmembrane P2Y subunits ($P2Y_{1,\ 2,\ 4,\ 6,\ 11\text{-}14}$), and seven P2X ligand-gated ion channels

($P2X_{1\text{-}7}$). These two types of receptor have larger differences in their aminoacid sequences, molecular/physiological properties and relative sensitivities to ATP, with ranges of nanomolar for P2Y, low micromolar for most P2X, to high micromolar for P2X7. Moreover the complexity of these receptors is augmented because both subtypes can form homomers and heteromers and these different combinations can change the agonist and antagonist selectivity, transmission signaling, channel and desensitization properties (Nakata et al. 2004).

P2X receptors are ATP-gated ion channels that mediate sodium influx, potassium efflux and, to varying extents, calcium influx, leading to depolarization of the cell membrane. Membrane depolarization subsequently activates voltage-gated calcium channels, thus causing accumulation of calcium ions in the cytoplasm. The predicted structure of the P2X subunits is a transmembrane protein with two membrane spanning domains that are involved in gating the ion channel and lining the ion pore (Surprenant and North 2009). Functional P2X receptor ion channels are now thought to consist of three subunits that could be homomers and heteromers (North 2002). The different combinations present different desensitization and permeability properties, as well as agonist and antagonist specificities. P2X receptors are widely distributed, and in neurons, glial cells, bone, muscle, endothelium, epithelium, and hematopoietic cells, they have functional roles. Moreover, several studies have implicated these receptors in the pathophysiology of Parkinson's disease, Alzheimer's disease, and multiple sclerosis (Jarvis and Khakh 2009).

P2Y receptors are G-protein-coupled receptors (GPCRs) that are activated by purine and/or pyrimidine nucleotides. Like other members of the GPCR superfamily, they are composed of seven transmembrane spanning regions that assist in forming the ligand binding pocket and also the purinergic receptor (Abbracchio et al. 2006). Stimulation leads to activation of heterotrimeric G proteins and their dissociation into α and $\beta\gamma$ subunits that can then interact with a variety of effector proteins. Some of P2Y receptors are activated mainly by nucleoside diphosphates ($P2Y_{1,6,12}$), while others are activated mainly by nucleoside triphosphates ($P2Y_{2,4}$). Otherwise, some P2Y receptors are activated by both purine and pyrimidine nucleotides ($P2Y_{2,4,6}$), and others only by purine nucleotides ($P2Y_{1,\ 11,\ 12}$) (Jacobson et al. 2009). Each individual P2Y receptor subtypes can couple to distinct G proteins that are specific for each cell type or tissue. The abilities to activate different G proteins were inferred from their capability to induce increases in inositol tris-phosphate, cytoplasmic Ca^{2+}, or cyclic AMP levels, and determination of sensitivity to the Gi/o protein inhibitors pertussis toxin (PTX) (Abbracchio et al. 2006). P2Y receptors can also be coupled to the activation of monomeric G proteins like Rac and RhoA. Even more, in the last few years many studies have revealed that a cross-talk exist between different GPCRs and their downstream effectors as well as between GPCRs and other signaling proteins, such as ion channels, integrins, and receptor and non-receptor tyrosine kinases (von Kugelgen 2006). These properties explain how the activation of particular P2Y receptors can lead to the induction of more than one signaling pathway in the same cell type. These receptors are able to regulate many different functions in a variety of cell types, and for that reason an intense effort has been developed to design selective agonist and antagonist ligands, both as pharmacological tools and as potential therapeutic agents (Abbracchio et al. 2003; Brunschweiger and Muller 2006). For cystic fibrosis, dry eye disease, and thrombosis the application of P2Y receptor ligands has been tested as drug candidates. The development of new chemical compounds will provide new opportunities for therapeutics of several diseases, including cardiovascular diseases, inflammatory diseases, and neurodegeneration (Jacobson and Boeynaems 2010).

Between the many functions that P2 receptors can regulate is ion channel activity. The studies have been performed mainly in neurons, in which specific P2 subtype can regulate the N-type Ca^{2+} channel and the M-current K^+ channel. Nevertheless, recent studies have demonstrated that P2 receptors can induce fast inhibitory junction potential in rat colon (Grasa et al. 2009), membrane hyperpolarization in vascular endothelial cells (Raqeeb et al. 2011), Ca^{2+} influx mediated contraction in intestinal myofibroblasts (Nakamura et al. 2011), and contraction induced by electrical field stimulation in smooth muscle (Cho et al. 2010). These data suggest that ATP signaling is important in excitable cells for their normal function. In skeletal muscle there are many evidences of the importance of ATP signaling. The activation of P2 receptors has been associated with modulation of Ca^{2+} influx and signaling (Sandona et al. 2005; May et al. 2006), activation of the ERK½ (May et al. 2006), muscle contractility (Sandona et al. 2005; Grishin et al. 2006), and regulation of excitability of muscle fibers (Voss 2009; Broch-Lips et al. 2010). Also extracellular nucleotides play important functions during skeletal muscle development and regeneration (Ryten et al. 2002; Ryten et al. 2004). Importantly, it has been shown that ATP promotes differentiation of rat skeletal muscle satellite cells (Araya et al. 2004; Banachewicz et al. 2005).

4. Alterations in both IP_3Rs and E-T coupling in DMD models

We have described that the amount of IP_3Rs, as well as the total mass of IP_3, are largely increased in both an *mdx* mice derived cell line and in a human DMD derived cell line compared to normal cells (Liberona et al. 1998). In dystrophic skeletal muscle, it has been suggested that an alteration of Ca^{2+} homeostasis occurs and might be responsible for muscle degeneration (Turner et al. 1988; Turner et al. 1991). Several studies indicate that IP_3 pathways could be involved in the DMD pathophysiology (Liberona et al. 1998; Balghi et al. 2006a; Balghi et al. 2006b). We recently found that both expression and localization of IP_3Rs are different in normal and dystrophic human skeletal muscle and cell lines (Cárdenas et al. 2010). On the other hand, experiments performed using two types of myotubes originated from the same Sol8 cell line - dystrophin deficient myotubes, SolC1(-), and myotubes transfected to express the minidystrophin, SolD(+) - show that Ca^{2+} rise evoked by potassium depolarization was higher in SolC1(-) than in SolD(+) myotubes (Balghi et al. 2006a). Analysis of the kinetics of the Ca^{2+} rise, reveals that the slow IP_3-dependent release may be increased in the SolC1(-) as compared to the SolD(+), suggesting an inhibitory effect of mini-dystrophin on IP_3R-dependent K^+-evoked Ca^{2+} release (Balghi et al. 2006a). Moreover, it has been described that IP_3 production after membrane depolarization is significantly elevated in dystrophin-deficient myotubes and that the presence of mini-dystrophin under the membrane leads to reduced IP_3 production (Balghi et al. 2006a). In fact, we have recently demonstrated, using normal (RCMH) and dystrophic (RCDMD) human skeletal muscle cell lines, that IP_3 dependent, slow Ca^{2+} transients evoked by electrical stimulation are faster in dystrophic cells, compared to normal myotubes (Cárdenas et al. 2010). Electrical stimulation induced an important phosphorylation of ERK½ in normal but not in dystrophic cells, and a differential pattern of gene expression between cell lines.

In normal adult mice skeletal muscle, we observed that IP_3R immuno-labeling follows distinctive patters resembling the SR (types 1, 2 and 3 IP_3Rs), sarcolemmal (types 1 and 3 IP_3Rs) or nuclear localizations (types 1 and 3 IP_3Rs) (Casas et al. 2010). The labeling for both type 1 and type 2 IP_3Rs subtypes showed a fiber type-specific distribution with much higher expression in fast (type II) muscle fibers, whereas type 3 IP_3R showed a uniform distribution in both fiber types, as shown by co-labeling with slow myosin heavy chain antibody. Likewise, mice muscle fibers show a characteristic mosaic pattern for type 1 IP_3R (Casas et al. 2010). When human muscle was studied, type II muscle fibers showed a much more intense labeling for the IP_3R subtype 1 compared to type I (slow) fibers. In biopsies from DMD patients, we found that $24 \pm 7\%$ of type II fibers have totally lost type 1 IP_3R labeling, compared to age-matched control biopsies (Cárdenas et al. 2010). On the other hand, RCDMD cells show a five-fold over expression of type 2 IP_3Rs and down regulation of type 3 IP_3Rs compared to normal RCMH cells (Cárdenas et al. 2010). Unlike normal muscle cells, type 2 IP_3R locate in the nucleus in RCDMD cells, while type 1 and type 3 IP_3Rs also display a particular subcellular location for each line (Cárdenas et al. 2010). These results showed that IP_3Rs expression and localization are different in muscle affected by DMD.

5. Signaling by extracellular nucleotides in dystrophic skeletal muscle

A number of skeletal muscle pathologies have been associated with alterations in the metabolism of extracellular ATP, changes in the sensitivity towards ATP and altered expression of purinergic receptors; among these pathologies we have DMD. In recent works, ATP signaling has been implicated in abnormal calcium homeostasis in dystrophic muscle and proposed to have implications in the pathogenesis of muscular dystrophies. Moreover, in myoblasts of a dystrophin negative muscle cell line, exposure to extracellular ATP elicited a strong increase in cytoplasmic Ca^{2+} concentrations. This increased susceptibility to ATP was due to changes in expression and function of P2X receptors and proposed to be a significant contributor to pathogenic Ca^{2+} entry in dystrophic mouse muscle (Yeung et al. 2006). The plasma membrane Na^+/H^+ exchanger (NHE) has been proposed to be involved in the pathogenesis of muscular dystrophy, most probably through the sustained increase in intracellular Ca^{2+}. The mechanism by which NHE is constitutive activated appears to be through stimulation of P2 receptors with ATP being continuously released in response to stretching (Iwata et al. 2007).

Nevertheless, these works failed to explain the mechanism by which ATP is released from skeletal muscle. ATP in skeletal muscle was proposed to be co-released with acetylcholine from motor nerve terminals during nerve activation (Smith 1991; Silinsky and Redman 1996) and released from muscle fibers during contraction (Cunha and Sebastiao 1993; Hellsten et al. 1998). Dystrophic muscle would be expected to contain high levels of extracellular ATP due mainly to fiber injury.

We propose now that in skeletal muscle, ATP is released upon contraction or electrical stimulation mainly through activation of pannexin 1 hemichannels. Any disturbance in either pannexin 1 channels or changes in P2 receptors expression or activity will have implications in skeletal muscle normal function. The possibility that this system is altered in muscular dystrophies raises new possibilities of therapeutic strategies in the treatment of diseases like DMD.

In addition to the structural role for dystrophin and its known associated proteins, there is clear evidence for signal transduction roles. The best studied signaling protein linked is the nNOS pathway. In DMD nNOS appears to be either drastically reduced or even absent (Niebroj-Dobosz and Hausmanowa-Petrusewicz 2005). It has been propose that part of muscle degeneration in DMD may result from the reduction in the production of nNOS/NO (Niebrój-Dobosz, 2005). Lately many additional signaling pathways have been demonstrated to be altered in dystrophy, such as: nuclear factor kappa-B (NF-kB), tumor necrosis factor (TNF)-alpha and interleukin (IL)-6 (Messina et al. 2011). The precise role of these signaling pathways remains mysterious, it is interesting to investigate whether the abnormal regulation of one (or more) of these pathways contributes to skeletal muscle pathogenesis in dystrophy.

To address the different pathways that could be altered in muscular dystrophy, many studies have compared gene expression profile between normal and dystrophic muscle based on microarray analysis. These analysis have been done in patients with DMD and in *mdx* mice. These studies include different types of muscle and in different times of the human disease (Chen et al. 2000) or in different life periods of *mdx* mice (Porter et al. 2003b; Lang et al. 2004; Porter et al. 2004; Dogra et al. 2008). In DMD patients biopsies that were individually analyzed, the upregulated genes are related with ECM and cytoskeleton, muscle structure and regeneration, immune response, signal transduction and cell-cell communication (Chen et al. 2000). In the mouse model there are many gene expression studies. The main muscles studied are diaphragm, extraocular muscles and leg muscle groups (Porter et al. 2003b; Lang et al. 2004; Dogra et al. 2008). Among the results, it is worth mentioning that the response to the lack of dystrophin varies in different muscle groups of human and *mdx* mice, and it was proposed that changes in gene expression could be related with the progression of the disease (Porter et al. 2003b; Lang et al. 2004; Porter et al. 2004; Dogra et al. 2008). Moreover, some groups studied the profile of gene expression in skeletal muscle implicated in specific pathways such as regeneration (Turk et al. 2005), inflammation (Evans et al. 2009a), immune system (Evans et al. 2009b) and specific transcription factors (Dogra et al. 2008). Also there are some studies that propose that expression of utrophin in the *mdx* mouse muscle results in a gene expression profile that is similar to that seen for the *wt* mouse (Baban and Davies 2008).

The analysis performed by Porter et al. (2002) established that numerous pathogenic pathways in *mdx* skeletal muscles are closely related and share features with DMD (Porter et al. 2002). Among the genes that were increased in *mdx* muscle is purinergic receptor P2X. The $P2X_4$ up regulation in dystrophic muscle has been attributed to vascular permeability changes and to inflammatory responses (Porter et al. 2002). Later, Yeung et al. (2004) demonstrated that P2X4 were expressed in infiltrating macrophages in dystrophic human and mouse muscle, and could be related with the inflammatory process (Yeung et al. 2004). Jiang et al. 2005 demonstrated that there is a differential expression of P2X receptors that change during the progression of the disease in both human and mouse dystrophic muscle (Jiang et al. 2005). They found that the $P2X_1$ and $P2X_6$ receptors are expressed during the process of regeneration in mouse muscular dystrophy, and the expression of $P2X_2$ is associated with type 1 fibers. Nevertheless, the work of Yeung et al. (2006) demonstrated that increase in P2X receptors increased the susceptibility of dystrophic myoblasts to extracellular ATP (Yeung et al. 2006). They proposed that changes in P2X will significant contribute to pathogenic Ca^{2+} entry.

Moreover, studies of Ryten et al. (2002, 2004) identified a role for ATP in the regulation of skeletal muscle formation, through inhibiting the proliferation and increase the rate of differentiation of satellite cells (Ryten et al. 2002; Ryten et al. 2004) Later, they show that the $P2X_2$, $P2X_5$ and $P2Y_1$ receptors were strongly expressed in *mdx* skeletal muscle and in the cells known to be important for muscle regeneration.

As previously described, P2 receptors have been implicated in the alteration on intracellular calcium. This could also be releated with some of the signaling pathways that are dependent on calcium homeostasis, like the activation of proteases. It has been demonstrated that changes in intracellular calcium can activate calpain and proteolytic damage to sarcomer proteins, like titin (Goll et al. 2003; Zhang et al. 2008).

The original sarcoglycan (SG) complex has four subunits and comprises a subcomplex of the dystrophin-associated protein complex (Hack et al. 2000). Gene defects in α-sarcoglycan also lead to a severe muscular dystrophy, type 2D limb-girdle muscular dystrophy (Roberds et al. 1994). The role of sarcoglycans in dystrophin complex function is not entirely understood. The α-sarcoglycan was described as an ecto-ATPase with distinctive enzymatic properties *in vitro* (Betto et al. 1999). Later on, α-sarcoglycan was demonstrated to significantly contribute to total ecto-nucleotidase activity of C2C12 myotubes and during the differentiation of this cell type (Sandona et al. 2004). As a result, mutations of the α-sarcoglycan gene causing the loss of its enzymatic function could represent an important mechanism to explain the pathogenesis mechanisms leading to dystrophy.

Taken these studies together, we can conclude that modifications in ATP signaling, due to changes in ATP release mechanism or receptors expression and availability, could be implicated in several mechanisms potentially involved in diseases. For these reasons ATP signaling has been considered as a good candidate for therapeutic targets for the treatment of muscle diseases

6. Gene expression in DMD

Microarrays analysis has been the basis of a number of publications in which dystrophic muscle is compared with unaffected muscle. Gene expression comparison of human biopsies from DMD and normal skeletal muscle has shown that many of the differentially expressed genes reflect in histo-pathology changes. For example, immune response signals and ECM genes are overexpressed in DMD muscle, an indication of the infiltration of inflammatory cells and connective tissue (Haslett et al. 2002). cDNA analysis of individual DMD patients have shown that genes related to immune response, sarcomere, ECM and signaling/cell growth were increased. Up-regulation of these genes accompanies dystrophic changes in DMD muscles such as myofiber necrosis, inflammation and muscle regeneration (Noguchi et al. 2003). Up-regulated inflammatory gene expression and activated immune cells are present in dystrophic muscle and play a critical role in muscle wasting (Evans et al. 2009b). The pro-inflammatory cytokines TNF-alpha, IL-1beta and IL-6 are up-regulated in Duchenne patients and *mdx* mice (Porreca et al. 1999; Porter et al. 2002; Kumar and Boriek 2003; Acharyya et al. 2007; Hnia et al. 2008). The fact that a number of chemokines are expressed directly by the muscle cell suggests that muscle tissue may contribute to chemotaxis process (Porter et al. 2003a). Using microarray technology we have shown that membrane depolarization induces expression and repression of a number of genes in both normal (RCMH) and DMD (RCDMD) human skeletal muscle cell lines. Importantly, modulated genes are mostly different for these two cell lines (Cárdenas et al. 2010). Nevertheless, the expression of only 44 of them is modified in both cell lines. The pattern of expression (up- or down-regulation) of these common genes is strikingly different between cell lines, and they appear to be regulated in opposite ways (Cárdenas et al. 2010).

Within these 44 genes we identified genes related to the immune response (HLA-DQB1), cytoskeleton/ECM proteins (ADD1, KRT1, and FBLN1), and signaling (NRG and POU2F2), among others. We found that 18 of these 44 genes are related to processes associated with Ca^{2+}, and 10 of them have been related in some way to dystrophy (Cárdenas et al. 2010).

Within the genes whose expression increases in RCDMD cells, particularly interesting in relation to muscle function and development, are those coding for the two isoforms of neuregulin (NGR1-β2 and NRG1-γ) and the POU2F2 gene (Cárdenas et al. 2010). NRG1 is a growth factor that potentiates myogenesis and may play an important role in differentiation of satellite cells in muscle regeneration (Hirata et al. 2007). Moreover, NRG stimulates Ca^{2+}-induced glucose transport during contraction (Canto et al. 2006) and is implicated in the metabolic and proliferative response of muscle to exercise (Lebrasseur et al. 2003). POU2F2 has been described as a transcription factor expressed in developing mouse skeletal muscle (Dominov and Miller 1996).

In addition, we found variations in the expression of ICEBERG, HLA-DQB1, ADD1, FBLN1 and TRIO genes that also have been associated with Ca^{2+} and dystrophy (Cárdenas et al. 2010). Considering that changes observed in DMD muscle biopsies have been related to elevation of intracellular Ca^{2+} concentration, which could activate Ca^{2+}-dependent degradation pathways, resulting in myofibril disruption and muscle necrosis (Turner et al. 1993). It will be interesting to analyze the roles described for the above mentioned genes. To our knowledge, there are no studies describing the role of membrane depolarization on the expression of these genes, and further studies are needed to explore the involvement of IP_3-mediated slow Ca^{2+} signals in the expression of some of these particular genes in skeletal muscle cells (Cárdenas et al. 2010).

Gene expression profiling at different stages in *mdx* models have also evidenced the highly dynamic process of the disease onset. These works, show that dystrophy in *mdx* models have an onset at 3 weeks of age, with a peak in pathology around 8 weeks. Interestingly, at this stage, there is a marked upregulation of almost 9 fold of the purinergic receptor $P2X_4$ (Porter et al. 2003b).

Although no therapy described to date can effectively slow or halt muscle degeneration in dystrophic patients (Kapsa et al. 2003), a promising pharmacological treatment for DMD aims to increase levels of utrophin and to identify molecules that modulate utrophin expression (regulatory pathways) by activation of its promoter (Dennis et al. 1996), in muscle fibers of affected patients to compensate for the absence of dystrophin (Miura and Jasmin 2006).

Indeed, utrophin is considered the autosomal homolog of dystrophin because it shares structural and functional motifs throughout the length of the molecule (Love et al. 1989; Khurana et al. 1990; Nguyen et al. 1991; Ohlendieck et al. 1991; Tinsley et al. 1992). It is capable of associating with members of the DAPs with similar affinity to dystrophin as well (Matsumura et al. 1992; Winder et al. 1995). Studies in the dystrophin-deficient *mdx* mice have established that the elevation of utrophin levels in dystrophic muscle fibers can restore sarcolemmal expression of DAPs members and alleviate the dystrophic pathology (Miura and Jasmin 2006). Direct evidence for the ability of utrophin to functionally substitute for dystrophin comes from experiments demonstrating that transgene-driven utrophin overexpression can effectively rescue dystrophin-deficient muscle in *mdx* mice (Tinsley et al. 1996; Deconinck et al. 1997; Tinsley et al. 1998).

6.1 Electrical stimulation induces calcium-dependent up-regulation of neuregulin-1β in dystrophic skeletal muscle cell lines

Neuregulin (NRG) is one of many factors that increase utrophin expression (Miura and Jasmin 2006). It belongs to a family of proteins structurally related to the epidermal growth factor (EGF) that are synthesized in and secreted from motoneurons and muscle (Falls 2003). Four members of NRG proteins, NRG-1 to NRG-4, have been identified. The best-studied and most characterized products are those encoded by NRG-1 gene.

Neuregulin-1 (NRG-1) was initially described as a neurotrophic factor involved in neuromuscular junction formation in skeletal muscle, but recently it has emerged as a myokine, with relevant effects on myogenesis, muscle metabolism and regeneration, and has been considered as a strong candidate to transduce muscle adaptation to chronic exercise (Lebrasseur et al. 2003; Guma et al. 2010).

Interestingly, NRG-1 treatment increases utrophin mRNA levels and transcriptional activity in mouse and human myotubes (Gramolini et al. 1999; Khurana et al. 1999). Moreover, Krag et al. (2004) described that intraperitoneal injection of a small peptide region of NRG-1 ectodomain increases utrophin expression in *mdx* mice (Krag et al. 2004). Observed increase was accompanied by a reduction in muscle degeneration and inflammation, and by decreased susceptibility to the damage induced by lengthening contractions. Improvement in muscle function was deemed to result specifically from the up-regulation of utrophin because NRG-1 administration has no beneficial effect in dystrophin/utrophin double-knockout animals (Krag et al. 2004).

However, regardless the evidences supporting such important roles for NRG-1 in skeletal muscle, the molecular mechanisms involved in its expression are still unclear.

When we investigated the effect of membrane depolarization on global gene expression in dystrophic RCDMD cells using microarrays technology, our data revealed that membrane potential changes, induced by electrical stimulation, resulted in significant up or down regulation of 150 genes after 4 h. Interestingly, two NRG-1 isoforms (β and γ) appear within the ten highest up-regulated genes (Cárdenas et al. 2010).

Taking into account the important biological effects of NRG-1 in the muscle and its potential clinical implication in DMD, we focused our study on the regulation of muscle NRG-1 expression, specifically on NRG-1β isoform, that displays a higher affinity for NRG receptor (Juretić et al. n.d.). NRG-1β increased expression was confirmed by quantitative PCR. We observed that electrical stimulation induces a significant increase of NRG-1β mRNA level in RCDMD cells, with a maximun at 4 h post-stimuli, but has no effect on NRG-1β expression in RCMH cells treated with the same procedure, suggesting that activation of molecular pathways involved in the regulation of NRG-1β gene expression are different in normal and dystrophic cells. Western blot analysis of stimulated RCDMD cells demonstrates that observed increase in NRG-1β mRNA levels was followed by actual enhancement of the corresponding protein (Juretić et al. n.d.).

Accumulating evidence suggests that integral dystrophin-DAPs complex components are also implicated in signaling in DMD, and that mutations in non-DAP protein encoding genes may lead to the muscular dystrophy phenotype, supporting the idea that more than one molecular pathway is implicated in the disease (Haslett et al. 2002). Thus, it is likely that the lack of DAP proteins in the cell membrane will somehow affect the regulation of Ca^{2+} transients and gene expression in dystrophic cells after electrical stimulation. In fact, Balghi et al. (2006) have demonstrated that IP_3 production after depolarization is significantly elevated in SolC1(-) dystrophin deficient myotubes and that the presence of mini-dystrophin under the membrane leads to reduced IP_3 production (Balghi et al. 2006b).

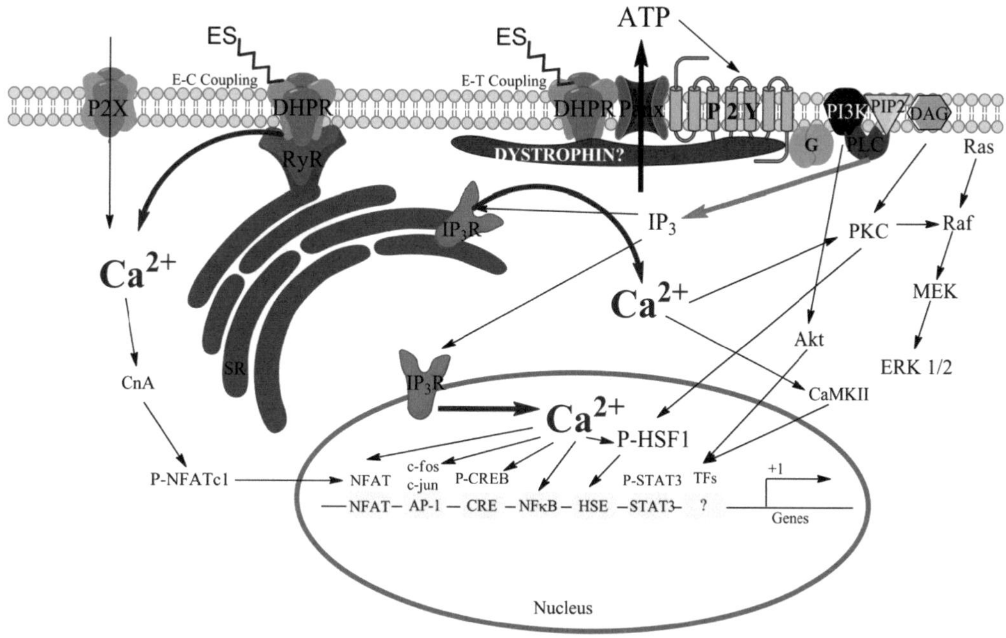

Fig. 1. **Diagram for the model for excitation-transcription coupling in skeletal muscle.** Two protein complexes are proposed to be present in the transverse tubule (T-T) membrane. The first one is the excitation-contraction (E-C) complex, comprising the voltage sensing dihydropyridine receptor (DHPR, Cav1.1) and the ryanodine receptor (RyR). We propose that purinergic P2X receptors also contribute to the fast calcium transient associated to E-C coupling. The excitation-transcription (E-T) coupling complex comprises also the DHPR, pannexin1 (Panx), the purinergic receptor P2Y linked to a G protein and possibly the phosphatidyl inositol 3 kinase (PI3K) and phospholipase C (PLC). It is likely that dystrophin is playing a role stabilizing this complex in the membrane. Upon electrical stimulation (ES), membrane depolarization will trigger a conformational change in DHPR which somehow will induce opening of Panx channel and ATP will be released. ATP acting on P2Y receptors will activate PI3K via G protein and in turn PLC will be recruited to the membrane producing inositol (1,4,5) trisphosphate (IP_3) and diacyl glycerol (DAG). IP_3R- mediated calcium signals will be responsible for activation of kinases (PKC, CaMK II, ERK½) and transcription factors leading finally to gene expression.

7. Final remarks

Results discussed here point out to the important role of slow Ca^{2+} transients evoked by electrical stimulation in the activation of the pathways that couple excitation to gene expression in dystrophin-deficient muscle cells (a putative role for dystrophin is schematized in Fig. 1). If we find ways to intervene such pathways in a manner that can compensate dystrophin dysfunction, the understanding of this new role of dystrophin will give new insights to the design of a therapeutic strategy in order to potentiate muscle survival and regeneration in DMD.

8. Acknowledgements

We thank Sonja Buvinic, Mariana Casas and Nora Riveros, whose work and ideas provided input to this chapter. This work was supported by FONDECYT 1110467, 11100267, FONDAP 15010006, and CONICYT AT-24100066 (FA) and AT-24110211 (DV).

9. References

Abbracchio, MP, Boeynaems, JM, Barnard, EA, Boyer, JL, Kennedy, C, Miras-Portugal, MT, King, BF, Gachet, C, Jacobson, KA, Weisman, GA & Burnstock, G (2003). Characterization of the UDP-glucose receptor (re-named here the P2Y14 receptor) adds diversity to the P2Y receptor family. *Trends Pharmacol Sci*, 24, 2, pp. 52-55.

Abbracchio, MP, Burnstock, G, Boeynaems, JM, Barnard, EA, Boyer, JL, Kennedy, C, Knight, GE, Fumagalli, M, Gachet, C, Jacobson, KA & Weisman, GA (2006). International Union of Pharmacology LVIII: update on the P2Y G protein-coupled nucleotide receptors: from molecular mechanisms and pathophysiology to therapy. *Pharmacol Rev*, 58, 3, pp. 281-341.

Acharyya, S, Villalta, SA, Bakkar, N, Bupha-Intr, T, Janssen, PM, Carathers, M, Li, ZW, Beg, AA, Ghosh, S, Sahenk, Z, Weinstein, M, Gardner, KL, Rafael-Fortney, JA, Karin, M, Tidball, JG, Baldwin, AS & Guttridge, DC (2007). Interplay of IKK/NF-kappaB signaling in macrophages and myofibers promotes muscle degeneration in Duchenne muscular dystrophy. *J Clin Invest*, 117, 4, pp. 889-901.

Ahn, AH & Kunkel, LM (1993). The structural and functional diversity of dystrophin. *Nat Genet*, 3, 4, pp. 283-291.

Alderton, JM & Steinhardt, RA (2000). How calcium influx through calcium leak channels is responsible for the elevated levels of calcium-dependent proteolysis in dystrophic myotubes. *Trends Cardiovasc Med*, 10, 6, pp. 268-272.

Allen, DG, Gervasio, OL, Yeung, EW & Whitehead, NP (2010). Calcium and the damage pathways in muscular dystrophy. *Can J Physiol Pharmacol*, 88, 2, pp. 83-91.

Araya, R, Liberona, JL, Cardenas, JC, Riveros, N, Estrada, M, Powell, JA, Carrasco, MA & Jaimovich, E (2003). Dihydropyridine receptors as voltage sensors for a depolarization-evoked, IP3R-mediated, slow calcium signal in skeletal muscle cells. *J Gen Physiol*, 121, 1, pp. 3-16.

Araya, R, Riquelme, MA, Brandan, E & Saez, JC (2004). The formation of skeletal muscle myotubes requires functional membrane receptors activated by extracellular ATP. *Brain Res Brain Res Rev*, 47, 1-3, pp. 174-188.

Baban, D & Davies, KE (2008). Microarray analysis of mdx mice expressing high levels of utrophin: therapeutic implications for dystrophin deficiency. *Neuromuscul Disord*, 18, 3, pp. 239-247.

Balghi, H, Sebille, S, Constantin, B, Patri, S, Thoreau, V, Mondin, L, Mok, E, Kitzis, A, Raymond, G & Cognard, C (2006a). Mini-dystrophin expression down-regulates overactivation of G protein-mediated IP3 signaling pathway in dystrophin-deficient muscle cells. *J Gen Physiol*, 127, 2, pp. 171-182.

Balghi, H, Sebille, S, Mondin, L, Cantereau, A, Constantin, B, Raymond, G & Cognard, C (2006b). Mini-dystrophin expression down-regulates IP3-mediated calcium release events in resting dystrophin-deficient muscle cells. *J Gen Physiol*, 128, 2, pp. 219-230.

Banachewicz, W, Suplat, D, Krzeminski, P, Pomorski, P & Baranska, J (2005). P2 nucleotide receptors on C2C12 satellite cells. *Purinergic Signal*, 1, 3, pp. 249-257.

Baranova, A, Ivanov, D, Petrash, N, Pestova, A, Skoblov, M, Kelmanson, I, Shagin, D, Nazarenko, S, Geraymovych, E, Litvin, O, Tiunova, A, Born, TL, Usman, N, Staroverov, D, Lukyanov, S & Panchin, Y (2004). The mammalian pannexin family is homologous to the invertebrate innexin gap junction proteins. *Genomics*, 83, 4, pp. 706-716.

Barbe, MT, Monyer, H & Bruzzone, R (2006). Cell-cell communication beyond connexins: the pannexin channels. *Physiology (Bethesda)*, 21, pp. 103-114.

Batchelor, CL & Winder, SJ (2006). Sparks, signals and shock absorbers: how dystrophin loss causes muscular dystrophy. *Trends Cell Biol*, 16, 4, pp. 198-205.

Berchtold, MW, Brinkmeier, H & Muntener, M (2000). Calcium ion in skeletal muscle: its crucial role for muscle function, plasticity, and disease. *Physiol Rev*, 80, 3, pp. 1215-1265.

Betto, R, Senter, L, Ceoldo, S, Tarricone, E, Biral, D & Salviati, G (1999). Ecto-ATPase activity of alpha-sarcoglycan (adhalin). *J Biol Chem*, 274, 12, pp. 7907-7912.

Blake, DJ, Weir, A, Newey, SE & Davies, KE (2002). Function and genetics of dystrophin and dystrophin-related proteins in muscle. *Physiol Rev*, 82, 2, pp. 291-329.

Boittin, FX, Petermann, O, Hirn, C, Mittaud, P, Dorchies, OM, Roulet, E & Ruegg, UT (2006). Ca2+-independent phospholipase A2 enhances store-operated Ca2+ entry in dystrophic skeletal muscle fibers. *J Cell Sci*, 119, Pt 18, pp. 3733-3742.

Bours, MJ, Swennen, EL, Di Virgilio, F, Cronstein, BN & Dagnelie, PC (2006). Adenosine 5'-triphosphate and adenosine as endogenous signaling molecules in immunity and inflammation. *Pharmacol Ther*, 112, 2, pp. 358-404.

Broch-Lips, M, Pedersen, TH & Nielsen, OB (2010). Effect of purinergic receptor activation on Na+-K+ pump activity, excitability, and function in depolarized skeletal muscle. *Am J Physiol Cell Physiol*, 298, 6, pp. C1438-1444.

Brunschweiger, A & Muller, CE (2006). P2 receptors activated by uracil nucleotides--an update. *Curr Med Chem*, 13, 3, pp. 289-312.

Burnstock, G (2004). Introduction: P2 receptors. *Curr Top Med Chem*, 4, 8, pp. 793-803.

Burnstock, G & Ulrich, H (2011). Purinergic signaling in embryonic and stem cell development. *Cell Mol Life Sci*, 68, 8, pp. 1369-1394.

Buvinic, S, Almarza, G, Bustamante, M, Casas, M, Lopez, J, Riquelme, M, Saez, JC, Huidobro-Toro, JP & Jaimovich, E (2009). ATP released by electrical stimuli elicits calcium transients and gene expression in skeletal muscle. *J Biol Chem*, 284, 50, pp. 34490-34505.

Campbell, L, Abulrob, AN, Kandalaft, LE, Plummer, S, Hollins, AJ, Gibbs, A & Gumbleton, M (2003). Constitutive expression of p-glycoprotein in normal lung alveolar epithelium and functionality in primary alveolar epithelial cultures. *J Pharmacol Exp Ther*, 304, 1, pp. 441-452.

Canto, C, Chibalin, AV, Barnes, BR, Glund, S, Suarez, E, Ryder, JW, Palacin, M, Zierath, JR, Zorzano, A & Guma, A (2006). Neuregulins mediate calcium-induced glucose transport during muscle contraction. *J Biol Chem*, 281, 31, pp. 21690-21697.

Capote, J, DiFranco, M & Vergara, JL (2010). Excitation-contraction coupling alterations in mdx and utrophin/dystrophin double knockout mice: a comparative study. *Am J Physiol Cell Physiol*, 298, 5, pp. C1077-1086.

Cárdenas, C, Juretic, N, Bevilacqua, J, García, N, Figueroa, R, Hartley, R, Taratuto, AL, Gejman, L, Riveros, N, Molgó, J & Jaimovich, E (2010). Abnormal distribution of inositol 1,4,5-trisphosphate receptors in human muscle can be related to altered calcium signals and gene expression in Duchenne dystrophy derived cells. *FASEB J*. 24, 9, pp. 3210-3221

Cardenas, C, Liberona, JL, Molgo, J, Colasante, C, Mignery, GA & Jaimovich, E (2005). Nuclear inositol 1,4,5-trisphosphate receptors regulate local Ca2+ transients and modulate cAMP response element binding protein phosphorylation. *J Cell Sci*, 118, Pt 14, pp. 3131-3140.

Carrasco, MA, Riveros, N, Rios, J, Muller, M, Torres, F, Pineda, J, Lantadilla, S & Jaimovich, E (2003). Depolarization-induced slow calcium transients activate early genes in skeletal muscle cells. *Am J Physiol Cell Physiol*, 284, 6, pp. C1438-1447.

Casas, M, Figueroa, R, Jorquera, G, Escobar, M, Molgo, J & Jaimovich, E (2010). IP(3)-dependent, post-tetanic calcium transients induced by electrostimulation of adult skeletal muscle fibers. *J Gen Physiol*, 136, 4, pp. 455-467.

Chen, YW, Zhao, P, Borup, R & Hoffman, EP (2000). Expression profiling in the muscular dystrophies: identification of novel aspects of molecular pathophysiology. *J Cell Biol*, 151, 6, pp. 1321-1336.

Cho, YR, Jang, HS, Kim, W, Park, SY & Sohn, UD (2010). P2X and P2Y Receptors Mediate Contraction Induced by Electrical Field Stimulation in Feline Esophageal Smooth Muscle. *Korean J Physiol Pharmacol*, 14, 5, pp. 311-316.

Corriden, R & Insel, PA (2010). Basal release of ATP: an autocrine-paracrine mechanism for cell regulation. *Sci Signal*, 3, 104, pp. re1.

Culligan, K, Banville, N, Dowling, P & Ohlendieck, K (2002). Drastic reduction of calsequestrin-like proteins and impaired calcium binding in dystrophic mdx muscle. *J Appl Physiol*, 92, 2, pp. 435-445.

Cunha, RA & Sebastiao, AM (1993). Adenosine and adenine nucleotides are independently released from both the nerve terminals and the muscle fibres upon electrical stimulation of the innervated skeletal muscle of the frog. *Pflugers Arch*, 424, 5-6, pp. 503-510.

D'Hondt, C, Ponsaerts, R, De Smedt, H, Vinken, M, De Vuyst, E, De Bock, M, Wang, N, Rogiers, V, Leybaert, L, Himpens, B & Bultynck, G (2011). Pannexin channels in

ATP release and beyond: an unexpected rendezvous at the endoplasmic reticulum. *Cell Signal*, 23, 2, pp. 305-316.

Deconinck, N, Tinsley, J, De Backer, F, Fisher, R, Kahn, D, Phelps, S, Davies, K & Gillis, JM (1997). Expression of truncated utrophin leads to major functional improvements in dystrophin-deficient muscles of mice. *Nat Med*, 3, 11, pp. 1216-1221.

Dennis, CL, Tinsley, JM, Deconinck, AE & Davies, KE (1996). Molecular and functional analysis of the utrophin promoter. *Nucleic Acids Res*, 24, 9, pp. 1646-1652.

Divet, A, Lompre, AM & Huchet-Cadiou, C (2005). Effect of cyclopiazonic acid, an inhibitor of the sarcoplasmic reticulum Ca-ATPase, on skeletal muscles from normal and mdx mice. *Acta Physiol Scand*, 184, 3, pp. 173-186.

Dogra, C, Srivastava, DS & Kumar, A (2008). Protein-DNA array-based identification of transcription factor activities differentially regulated in skeletal muscle of normal and dystrophin-deficient mdx mice. *Mol Cell Biochem*, 312, 1-2, pp. 17-24.

Dominov, JA & Miller, JB (1996). POU homeodomain genes and myogenesis. *Dev Genet*, 19, 2, pp. 108-118.

Dubyak, GR (2009). Both sides now: multiple interactions of ATP with pannexin-1 hemichannels. Focus on "A permeant regulating its permeation pore: inhibition of pannexin 1 channels by ATP". *Am J Physiol Cell Physiol*, 296, 2, pp. C235-241.

Edwards, JN, Friedrich, O, Cully, TR, von Wegner, F, Murphy, RM & Launikonis, BS (2010). Upregulation of store-operated Ca2+ entry in dystrophic mdx mouse muscle. *Am J Physiol Cell Physiol*, 299, 1, pp. C42-50.

Eltit, JM, Garcia, AA, Hidalgo, J, Liberona, JL, Chiong, M, Lavandero, S, Maldonado, E & Jaimovich, E (2006). Membrane electrical activity elicits inositol 1,4,5-trisphosphate-dependent slow Ca2+ signals through a Gbetagamma/phosphatidylinositol 3-kinase gamma pathway in skeletal myotubes. *J Biol Chem*, 281, 17, pp. 12143-12154.

Eltit, JM, Yang, T, Li, H, Molinski, TF, Pessah, IN, Allen, PD & Lopez, JR (2010). RyR1-mediated Ca2+ leak and Ca2+ entry determine resting intracellular Ca2+ in skeletal myotubes. *J Biol Chem*, 285, 18, pp. 13781-13787.

Estrada, M, Cardenas, C, Liberona, JL, Carrasco, MA, Mignery, GA, Allen, PD & Jaimovich, E (2001). Calcium transients in 1B5 myotubes lacking ryanodine receptors are related to inositol trisphosphate receptors. *J Biol Chem*, 276, 25, pp. 22868-22874.

Evans, NP, Misyak, SA, Robertson, JL, Bassaganya-Riera, J & Grange, RW (2009a). Dysregulated intracellular signaling and inflammatory gene expression during initial disease onset in Duchenne muscular dystrophy. *Am J Phys Med Rehabil*, 88, 6, pp. 502-522.

Evans, NP, Misyak, SA, Robertson, JL, Bassaganya-Riera, J & Grange, RW (2009b). Immune-mediated mechanisms potentially regulate the disease time-course of duchenne muscular dystrophy and provide targets for therapeutic intervention. *PM R*, 1, 8, pp. 755-768.

Falls, DL (2003). Neuregulins: functions, forms, and signaling strategies. *Exp Cell Res*, 284, 1, pp. 14-30.

Fitz, JG (2007). Regulation of cellular ATP release. *Trans Am Clin Climatol Assoc*, 118, pp. 199-208.

Gervasio, OL, Whitehead, NP, Yeung, EW, Phillips, WD & Allen, DG (2008). TRPC1 binds to caveolin-3 and is regulated by Src kinase - role in Duchenne muscular dystrophy. *J Cell Sci*, 121, Pt 13, pp. 2246-2255.

Goll, DE, Thompson, VF, Li, H, Wei, W & Cong, J (2003). The calpain system. *Physiol Rev*, 83, 3, pp. 731-801.

Goonasekera, SA, Lam, CK, Millay, DP, Sargent, MA, Hajjar, RJ, Kranias, EG & Molkentin, JD (2011). Mitigation of muscular dystrophy in mice by SERCA overexpression in skeletal muscle. *J Clin Invest*, 121, 3, pp. 1044-1052.

Gramolini, AO, Angus, LM, Schaeffer, L, Burton, EA, Tinsley, JM, Davies, KE, Changeux, JP & Jasmin, BJ (1999). Induction of utrophin gene expression by heregulin in skeletal muscle cells: role of the N-box motif and GA binding protein. *Proc Natl Acad Sci U S A*, 96, 6, pp. 3223-3227.

Grasa, L, Gil, V, Gallego, D, Martin, MT & Jimenez, M (2009). P2Y(1) receptors mediate inhibitory neuromuscular transmission in the rat colon. *Br J Pharmacol*, 158, 6, pp. 1641-1652.

Grishin, SN, Teplov, AY, Galkin, AV, Devyataev, AM, Zefirov, AL, Mukhamedyarov, MA, Ziganshin, AU, Burnstock, G & Palotas, A (2006). Different effects of ATP on the contractile activity of mice diaphragmatic and skeletal muscles. *Neurochem Int*, 49, 8, pp. 756-763.

Guma, A, Martinez-Redondo, V, Lopez-Soldado, I, Canto, C & Zorzano, A (2010). Emerging role of neuregulin as a modulator of muscle metabolism. *Am J Physiol Endocrinol Metab*, 298, 4, pp. E742-750.

Hack, AA, Groh, ME & McNally, EM (2000). Sarcoglycans in muscular dystrophy. *Microsc Res Tech*, 48, 3-4, pp. 167-180.

Haslett, JN, Sanoudou, D, Kho, AT, Bennett, RR, Greenberg, SA, Kohane, IS, Beggs, AH & Kunkel, LM (2002). Gene expression comparison of biopsies from Duchenne muscular dystrophy (DMD) and normal skeletal muscle. *Proc Natl Acad Sci U S A*, 99, 23, pp. 15000-15005.

Hellsten, Y, Maclean, D, Radegran, G, Saltin, B & Bangsbo, J (1998). Adenosine concentrations in the interstitium of resting and contracting human skeletal muscle. *Circulation*, 98, 1, pp. 6-8.

Hirata, M, Sakuma, K, Okajima, S, Fujiwara, H, Inashima, S, Yasuhara, M & Kubo, T (2007). Increased expression of neuregulin-1 in differentiating muscle satellite cells and in motoneurons during muscle regeneration. *Acta Neuropathol*, 113, 4, pp. 451-459.

Hnia, K, Gayraud, J, Hugon, G, Ramonatxo, M, De La Porte, S, Matecki, S & Mornet, D (2008). L-arginine decreases inflammation and modulates the nuclear factor-kappaB/matrix metalloproteinase cascade in mdx muscle fibers. *Am J Pathol*, 172, 6, pp. 1509-1519.

Hollingworth, S, Zeiger, U & Baylor, SM (2008). Comparison of the myoplasmic calcium transient elicited by an action potential in intact fibres of mdx and normal mice. *J Physiol*, 586, Pt 21, pp. 5063-5075.

Iwata, Y, Katanosaka, Y, Hisamitsu, T & Wakabayashi, S (2007). Enhanced Na+/H+ exchange activity contributes to the pathogenesis of muscular dystrophy via involvement of P2 receptors. *Am J Pathol*, 171, 5, pp. 1576-1587.

Jacobson, KA & Boeynaems, JM (2010). P2Y nucleotide receptors: promise of therapeutic applications. *Drug Discov Today*, 15, 13-14, pp. 570-578.

Jacobson, KA, Ivanov, AA, de Castro, S, Harden, TK & Ko, H (2009). Development of selective agonists and antagonists of P2Y receptors. *Purinergic Signal*, 5, 1, pp. 75-89.

Jaimovich, E, Reyes, R, Liberona, JL & Powell, JA (2000). IP(3) receptors, IP(3) transients, and nucleus-associated Ca(2+) signals in cultured skeletal muscle. *Am J Physiol Cell Physiol*, 278, 5, pp. C998-C1010.

Jarvis, MF & Khakh, BS (2009). ATP-gated P2X cation-channels. *Neuropharmacology*, 56, 1, pp. 208-215.

Jia, M, Li, MX, Fields, RD & Nelson, PG (2007). Extracellular ATP in activity-dependent remodeling of the neuromuscular junction. *Dev Neurobiol*, 67, 7, pp. 924-932.

Jiang, T, Yeung, D, Lien, CF & Gorecki, DC (2005). Localized expression of specific P2X receptors in dystrophin-deficient DMD and mdx muscle. *Neuromuscul Disord*, 15, 3, pp. 225-236.

Jorquera, G, Juretic, N, Jaimovich, E & Riveros, N (2009). Membrane depolarization induces calcium-dependent upregulation of Hsp70 and Hmox-1 in skeletal muscle cells. *Am J Physiol Cell Physiol*, 297, 3, pp. C581-590.

Juretić, N, Jorquera, G, Caviedes, P, Jaimovich, E & Riveros, N (n.d.). Electrical stimulation induces calcium-dependent up-regulation of neuregulin-1β in dystrophic skeletal muscle cell lines. Manuscript in preparation

Juretic, N, Garcia-Huidobro, P, Iturrieta, JA, Jaimovich, E & Riveros, N (2006). Depolarization-induced slow Ca2+ transients stimulate transcription of IL-6 gene in skeletal muscle cells. *Am J Physiol Cell Physiol*, 290, 5, pp. C1428-1436.

Juretic, N, Urzua, U, Munroe, DJ, Jaimovich, E & Riveros, N (2007). Differential gene expression in skeletal muscle cells after membrane depolarization. *J Cell Physiol*, 210, 3, pp. 819-830.

Kapsa, R, Kornberg, AJ & Byrne, E (2003). Novel therapies for Duchenne muscular dystrophy. *Lancet Neurol*, 2, 5, pp. 299-310.

Kargacin, ME & Kargacin, GJ (1996). The sarcoplasmic reticulum calcium pump is functionally altered in dystrophic muscle. *Biochim Biophys Acta*, 1290, 1, pp. 4-8.

Khurana, TS, Hoffman, EP & Kunkel, LM (1990). Identification of a chromosome 6-encoded dystrophin-related protein. *J Biol Chem*, 265, 28, pp. 16717-16720.

Khurana, TS, Rosmarin, AG, Shang, J, Krag, TO, Das, S & Gammeltoft, S (1999). Activation of utrophin promoter by heregulin via the ets-related transcription factor complex GA-binding protein alpha/beta. *Mol Biol Cell*, 10, 6, pp. 2075-2086.

Krag, TO, Bogdanovich, S, Jensen, CJ, Fischer, MD, Hansen-Schwartz, J, Javazon, EH, Flake, AW, Edvinsson, L & Khurana, TS (2004). Heregulin ameliorates the dystrophic phenotype in mdx mice. *Proc Natl Acad Sci U S A*, 101, 38, pp. 13856-13860.

Kumar, A & Boriek, AM (2003). Mechanical stress activates the nuclear factor-kappaB pathway in skeletal muscle fibers: a possible role in Duchenne muscular dystrophy. *FASEB J*, 17, 3, pp. 386-396.

Lang, JM, Esser, KA & Dupont-Versteegden, EE (2004). Altered activity of signaling pathways in diaphragm and tibialis anterior muscle of dystrophic mice. *Exp Biol Med (Maywood)*, 229, 6, pp. 503-511.

Lebrasseur, NK, Cote, GM, Miller, TA, Fielding, RA & Sawyer, DB (2003). Regulation of neuregulin/ErbB signaling by contractile activity in skeletal muscle. *Am J Physiol Cell Physiol*, 284, 5, pp. C1149-1155.

Liberona, JL, Powell, JA, Shenoi, S, Petherbridge, L, Caviedes, R & Jaimovich, E (1998). Differences in both inositol 1,4,5-trisphosphate mass and inositol 1,4,5-trisphosphate receptors between normal and dystrophic skeletal muscle cell lines. *Muscle Nerve*, 21, 7, pp. 902-909.

Liu, HT, Toychiev, AH, Takahashi, N, Sabirov, RZ & Okada, Y (2008). Maxi-anion channel as a candidate pathway for osmosensitive ATP release from mouse astrocytes in primary culture. *Cell Res*, 18, 5, pp. 558-565.

Lopez, JR, Briceno, LE, Sanchez, V & Horvart, D (1987). Myoplasmic (Ca2+) in Duchenne muscular dystrophy patients. *Acta Cient Venez*, 38, 4, pp. 503-504.

Love, DR, Hill, DF, Dickson, G, Spurr, NK, Byth, BC, Marsden, RF, Walsh, FS, Edwards, YH & Davies, KE (1989). An autosomal transcript in skeletal muscle with homology to dystrophin. *Nature*, 339, 6219, pp. 55-58.

Matsumura, K, Ervasti, JM, Ohlendieck, K, Kahl, SD & Campbell, KP (1992). Association of dystrophin-related protein with dystrophin-associated proteins in mdx mouse muscle. *Nature*, 360, 6404, pp. 588-591.

May, C, Weigl, L, Karel, A & Hohenegger, M (2006). Extracellular ATP activates ERK1/ERK2 via a metabotropic P2Y1 receptor in a Ca2+ independent manner in differentiated human skeletal muscle cells. *Biochem Pharmacol*, 71, 10, pp. 1497-1509.

Messina, S, Bitto, A, Aguennouz, M, Vita, GL, Polito, F, Irrera, N, Altavilla, D, Marini, H, Migliorato, A, Squadrito, F & Vita, G (2011). The soy isoflavone genistein blunts nuclear factor kappa-B, MAPKs and TNF-alpha activation and ameliorates muscle function and morphology in mdx mice. *Neuromuscul Disord*, 21, 8, pp. 579-589.

Millay, DP, Sargent, MA, Osinska, H, Baines, CP, Barton, ER, Vuagniaux, G, Sweeney, HL, Robbins, J & Molkentin, JD (2008). Genetic and pharmacologic inhibition of mitochondrial-dependent necrosis attenuates muscular dystrophy. *Nat Med*, 14, 4, pp. 442-447.

Miura, P & Jasmin, BJ (2006). Utrophin upregulation for treating Duchenne or Becker muscular dystrophy: how close are we? *Trends Mol Med*, 12, 3, pp. 122-129.

Mokri, B & Engel, AG (1998). Duchenne dystrophy: electron microscopic findings pointing to a basic or early abnormality in the plasma membrane of the muscle fiber. 1975. *Neurology*, 51, 1, pp. 1 and 10 pages following.

Morine, KJ, Sleeper, MM, Barton, ER & Sweeney, HL (2010). Overexpression of SERCA1a in the mdx diaphragm reduces susceptibility to contraction-induced damage. *Hum Gene Ther*, 21, 12, pp. 1735-1739.

Nakamura, T, Iwanaga, K, Murata, T, Hori, M & Ozaki, H (2011). ATP induces contraction mediated by the P2Y(2) receptor in rat intestinal subepithelial myofibroblasts. *Eur J Pharmacol*, 657, 1-3, pp. 152-158.

Nakata, H, Yoshioka, K & Kamiya, T (2004). Purinergic-receptor oligomerization: implications for neural functions in the central nervous system. *Neurotox Res*, 6, 4, pp. 291-297.

Nguyen, TM, Ellis, JM, Love, DR, Davies, KE, Gatter, KC, Dickson, G & Morris, GE (1991). Localization of the DMDL gene-encoded dystrophin-related protein using a panel of nineteen monoclonal antibodies: presence at neuromuscular junctions, in the sarcolemma of dystrophic skeletal muscle, in vascular and other smooth muscles, and in proliferating brain cell lines. *J Cell Biol*, 115, 6, pp. 1695-1700.

Niebroj-Dobosz, I & Hausmanowa-Petrusewicz, I (2005). The involvement of oxidative stress in determining the severity and progress of pathological processes in dystrophin-deficient muscles. *Acta Biochim Pol*, 52, 2, pp. 449-452.

Noguchi, S, Tsukahara, T, Fujita, M, Kurokawa, R, Tachikawa, M, Toda, T, Tsujimoto, A, Arahata, K & Nishino, I (2003). cDNA microarray analysis of individual Duchenne muscular dystrophy patients. *Hum Mol Genet*, 12, 6, pp. 595-600.

North, RA (2002). Molecular physiology of P2X receptors. *Physiol Rev*, 82, 4, pp. 1013-1067.

Ohlendieck, K, Ervasti, JM, Matsumura, K, Kahl, SD, Leveille, CJ & Campbell, KP (1991). Dystrophin-related protein is localized to neuromuscular junctions of adult skeletal muscle. *Neuron*, 7, 3, pp. 499-508.

Petrof, BJ, Shrager, JB, Stedman, HH, Kelly, AM & Sweeney, HL (1993). Dystrophin protects the sarcolemma from stresses developed during muscle contraction. *Proc Natl Acad Sci U S A*, 90, 8, pp. 3710-3714.

Porreca, E, Guglielmi, MD, Uncini, A, Di Gregorio, P, Angelini, A, Di Febbo, C, Pierdomenico, SD, Baccante, G & Cuccurullo, F (1999). Haemostatic abnormalities, cardiac involvement and serum tumor necrosis factor levels in X-linked dystrophic patients. *Thromb Haemost*, 81, 4, pp. 543-546.

Porter, JD, Guo, W, Merriam, AP, Khanna, S, Cheng, G, Zhou, X, Andrade, FH, Richmonds, C & Kaminski, HJ (2003a). Persistent over-expression of specific CC class chemokines correlates with macrophage and T-cell recruitment in mdx skeletal muscle. *Neuromuscul Disord*, 13, 3, pp. 223-235.

Porter, JD, Khanna, S, Kaminski, HJ, Rao, JS, Merriam, AP, Richmonds, CR, Leahy, P, Li, J, Guo, W & Andrade, FH (2002). A chronic inflammatory response dominates the skeletal muscle molecular signature in dystrophin-deficient mdx mice. *Hum Mol Genet*, 11, 3, pp. 263-272.

Porter, JD, Merriam, AP, Leahy, P, Gong, B, Feuerman, J, Cheng, G & Khanna, S (2004). Temporal gene expression profiling of dystrophin-deficient (mdx) mouse diaphragm identifies conserved and muscle group-specific mechanisms in the pathogenesis of muscular dystrophy. *Hum Mol Genet*, 13, 3, pp. 257-269.

Porter, JD, Merriam, AP, Leahy, P, Gong, B & Khanna, S (2003b). Dissection of temporal gene expression signatures of affected and spared muscle groups in dystrophin-deficient (mdx) mice. *Hum Mol Genet*, 12, 15, pp. 1813-1821.

Powell, JA, Carrasco, MA, Adams, DS, Drouet, B, Rios, J, Muller, M, Estrada, M & Jaimovich, E (2001). IP(3) receptor function and localization in myotubes: an unexplored Ca(2+) signaling pathway in skeletal muscle. *J Cell Sci*, 114, Pt 20, pp. 3673-3683.

Rando, TA (2001). The dystrophin-glycoprotein complex, cellular signaling, and the regulation of cell survival in the muscular dystrophies. *Muscle Nerve*, 24, 12, pp. 1575-1594.

Raqeeb, A, Sheng, J, Ao, N & Braun, AP (2011). Purinergic P2Y2 receptors mediate rapid Ca(2+) mobilization, membrane hyperpolarization and nitric oxide production in human vascular endothelial cells. *Cell Calcium*, 49, 4, pp. 240-248.

Roberds, SL, Leturcq, F, Allamand, V, Piccolo, F, Jeanpierre, M, Anderson, RD, Lim, LE, Lee, JC, Tome, FM, Romero, NB & et al. (1994). Missense mutations in the adhalin gene linked to autosomal recessive muscular dystrophy. *Cell*, 78, 4, pp. 625-633.

Robert, V, Massimino, ML, Tosello, V, Marsault, R, Cantini, M, Sorrentino, V & Pozzan, T (2001). Alteration in calcium handling at the subcellular level in mdx myotubes. *J Biol Chem*, 276, 7, pp. 4647-4651.

Ryten, M, Dunn, PM, Neary, JT & Burnstock, G (2002). ATP regulates the differentiation of mammalian skeletal muscle by activation of a P2X5 receptor on satellite cells. *J Cell Biol*, 158, 2, pp. 345-355.

Ryten, M, Yang, SY, Dunn, PM, Goldspink, G & Burnstock, G (2004). Purinoceptor expression in regenerating skeletal muscle in the mdx mouse model of muscular dystrophy and in satellite cell cultures. *FASEB J*, 18, 12, pp. 1404-1406.

Sabirov, RZ & Okada, Y (2005). ATP release via anion channels. *Purinergic Signal*, 1, 4, pp. 311-328.

Sandona, D, Danieli-Betto, D, Germinario, E, Biral, D, Martinello, T, Lioy, A, Tarricone, E, Gastaldello, S & Betto, R (2005). The T-tubule membrane ATP-operated P2X4 receptor influences contractility of skeletal muscle. *FASEB J*, 19, 9, pp. 1184-1186.

Sandona, D, Gastaldello, S, Martinello, T & Betto, R (2004). Characterization of the ATP-hydrolysing activity of alpha-sarcoglycan. *Biochem J*, 381, Pt 1, pp. 105-112.

Shestopalov, VI & Panchin, Y (2008). Pannexins and gap junction protein diversity. *Cell Mol Life Sci*, 65, 3, pp. 376-394.

Silinsky, EM & Redman, RS (1996). Synchronous release of ATP and neurotransmitter within milliseconds of a motor nerve impulse in the frog. *J Physiol*, 492 (Pt 3), pp. 815-822.

Smith, DO (1991). Sources of adenosine released during neuromuscular transmission in the rat. *J Physiol*, 432, pp. 343-354.

Spencer, MJ, Croall, DE & Tidball, JG (1995). Calpains are activated in necrotic fibers from mdx dystrophic mice. *J Biol Chem*, 270, 18, pp. 10909-10914.

Suadicani, SO, Brosnan, CF & Scemes, E (2006). P2X7 receptors mediate ATP release and amplification of astrocytic intercellular Ca2+ signaling. *J Neurosci*, 26, 5, pp. 1378-1385.

Surprenant, A & North, RA (2009). Signaling at purinergic P2X receptors. *Annu Rev Physiol*, 71, pp. 333-359.

Tinsley, J, Deconinck, N, Fisher, R, Kahn, D, Phelps, S, Gillis, JM & Davies, K (1998). Expression of full-length utrophin prevents muscular dystrophy in mdx mice. *Nat Med*, 4, 12, pp. 1441-1444.

Tinsley, JM, Blake, DJ, Roche, A, Fairbrother, U, Riss, J, Byth, BC, Knight, AE, Kendrick-Jones, J, Suthers, GK, Love, DR & et al. (1992). Primary structure of dystrophin-related protein. *Nature*, 360, 6404, pp. 591-593.

Tinsley, JM, Potter, AC, Phelps, SR, Fisher, R, Trickett, JI & Davies, KE (1996). Amelioration of the dystrophic phenotype of mdx mice using a truncated utrophin transgene. *Nature*, 384, 6607, pp. 349-353.

Turk, R, Sterrenburg, E, de Meijer, EJ, van Ommen, GJ, den Dunnen, JT & t Hoen, PA (2005). Muscle regeneration in dystrophin-deficient mdx mice studied by gene expression profiling. *BMC Genomics*, 6, pp. 98.

Turner, PR, Fong, PY, Denetclaw, WF & Steinhardt, RA (1991). Increased calcium influx in dystrophic muscle. *J Cell Biol*, 115, 6, pp. 1701-1712.

Turner, PR, Schultz, R, Ganguly, B & Steinhardt, RA (1993). Proteolysis results in altered leak channel kinetics and elevated free calcium in mdx muscle. *J Membr Biol*, 133, 3, pp. 243-251.

Turner, PR, Westwood, T, Regen, CM & Steinhardt, RA (1988). Increased protein degradation results from elevated free calcium levels found in muscle from mdx mice. *Nature*, 335, 6192, pp. 735-738.

Vandebrouck, A, Ducret, T, Basset, O, Sebille, S, Raymond, G, Ruegg, U, Gailly, P, Cognard, C & Constantin, B (2006). Regulation of store-operated calcium entries and mitochondrial uptake by minidystrophin expression in cultured myotubes. *FASEB J*, 20, 1, pp. 136-138.

Vandebrouck, C, Martin, D, Colson-Van Schoor, M, Debaix, H & Gailly, P (2002). Involvement of TRPC in the abnormal calcium influx observed in dystrophic (mdx) mouse skeletal muscle fibers. *J Cell Biol*, 158, 6, pp. 1089-1096.

Volonte, C & D'Ambrosi, N (2009). Membrane compartments and purinergic signalling: the purinome, a complex interplay among ligands, degrading enzymes, receptors and transporters. *FEBS J*, 276, 2, pp. 318-329.

von Kugelgen, I (2006). Pharmacological profiles of cloned mammalian P2Y-receptor subtypes. *Pharmacol Ther*, 110, 3, pp. 415-432.

Voss, AA (2009). Extracellular ATP inhibits chloride channels in mature mammalian skeletal muscle by activating P2Y1 receptors. *J Physiol*, 587, Pt 23, pp. 5739-5752.

Winder, SJ, Hemmings, L, Maciver, SK, Bolton, SJ, Tinsley, JM, Davies, KE, Critchley, DR & Kendrick-Jones, J (1995). Utrophin actin binding domain: analysis of actin binding and cellular targeting. *J Cell Sci*, 108 (Pt 1), pp. 63-71.

Woods, CE, Novo, D, DiFranco, M & Vergara, JL (2004). The action potential-evoked sarcoplasmic reticulum calcium release is impaired in mdx mouse muscle fibres. *J Physiol*, 557, Pt 1, pp. 59-75.

Yegutkin, GG (2008). Nucleotide- and nucleoside-converting ectoenzymes: Important modulators of purinergic signalling cascade. *Biochim Biophys Acta*, 1783, 5, pp. 673-694.

Yeung, D, Kharidia, R, Brown, SC & Gorecki, DC (2004). Enhanced expression of the P2X4 receptor in Duchenne muscular dystrophy correlates with macrophage invasion. *Neurobiol Dis*, 15, 2, pp. 212-220.

Yeung, D, Zablocki, K, Lien, CF, Jiang, T, Arkle, S, Brutkowski, W, Brown, J, Lochmuller, H, Simon, J, Barnard, EA & Gorecki, DC (2006). Increased susceptibility to ATP via alteration of P2X receptor function in dystrophic mdx mouse muscle cells. *FASEB J*, 20, 6, pp. 610-620.

Yeung, EW, Whitehead, NP, Suchyna, TM, Gottlieb, PA, Sachs, F & Allen, DG (2005). Effects of stretch-activated channel blockers on [Ca2+]i and muscle damage in the mdx mouse. *J Physiol*, 562, Pt 2, pp. 367-380.

Zhang, BT, Yeung, SS, Allen, DG, Qin, L & Yeung, EW (2008). Role of the calcium-calpain pathway in cytoskeletal damage after eccentric contractions. *J Appl Physiol*, 105, 1, pp. 352-357.

Section 3

Disease Diagnosis and Management

11

Effects of Dietary Phosphate on Ectopic Calcification and Muscle Function in mdx Mice

Eiji Wada, Namiko Kikkawa, Mizuko Yoshida,
Munehiro Date, Tetsuo Higashi and Ryoichi Matsuda
The University of Tokyo,
Japan

1. Introduction

Calcium deposits in extra-skeletal tissues are highly correlated with lifestyle diseases. The mechanisms and clinical effects of such deposition have been widely studied due to increase mortality rate. Vascular calcification is a major complication in a number of diseases, including chronic kidney disease (CKD) and diabetes (Giachelli, 2009). The number of regulation mechanisms affecting calcium precipitation in soft tissues remains underestimated, as many regulators are considered to be involved in this complex process (Hu et al., 2010; Kendrick et al., 2011). Elevated serum phosphate levels which leads hyperphosphatemia is one of the prevalent factors of vascular calcification in CKD (El-Abbadi et al., 2009). The kidneys play a central role in the regulation of phosphate homeostasis. In individuals with normal renal function, serum phosphate levels are strictly controlled through dietary intake, intestinal absorption, renal excretion, and bone metabolism. When the kidneys are either mechanically or functionally impaired, phosphate metabolism is imbalanced. Abnormalities of phosphate metabolism related to kidney malfunction may play a central role in the deposition of calcium and phosphate in extra-skeletal tissues. Ectopic calcification in skeletal muscle has been reported to occur in three Duchenne muscular dystrophy (DMD) animal models; mdx mice (Coulton et al., 1987; Kikkawa et al., 2009), dystrophic puppies (Nguyen et al., 2002), and hypertrophic muscular dystrophy cats (Gaschen et al., 1992). In this chapter, we review the mechanisms of ectopic calcification in mdx mice and report a new finding of effects of dietary phosphate intake on calcium deposits and muscle function in mdx mice.

2. Ectopic calcification in animal models of muscular dystrophy

The mdx mouse, dystrophic canine, and hypertrophic muscular dystrophy feline develop progressive muscle lesions and calcium deposits in skeletal muscle during muscle regeneration. The pathological features of dystrophic golden retriever puppies are particularly severe and are similar to those of DMD boys, who are characterized by progressive muscle necrosis that leads to early death. Nguyen et al. (2002) detected early ectopic calcification in muscles from 4-day-old and 2-month-old puppies. Thus calcium deposition in skeletal muscle appears to be an early event associated with muscle degeneration.

In mdx mice, the observed muscle pathology is relatively mild compared with DMD patients but calcifying lesions are commonly seen in the lower limbs and diaphragm of mice from approximately five weeks of age. Recently, ectopic calcification (Fig. 1) has been reported to be a characteristic feature of muscular pathology (Korff et al., 2006; Verma et al., 2010). For example, Korff et al. (2006) found that myocardial calcification commonly occurs in mice following necrosis induced by mechanical stresses and proposed that calcification in the heart is dependent upon genetic background. Verma et al. (2010) suggested that the absence of ectopic calcification in the diaphragm serves as a marker of amelioration of mdx pathology. In addition, one of the prednisone-induced side effects in a canine model of DMD is skeletal muscle calcification (Liu et al., 2004). However, a palliative glucocorticoid therapy using prednisone is a feasible and effective treatment approach for DMD despite of the serious potential side effects (Wong et al., 2002; Khan, 1993). Studies in these animals have revealed that the percentages of calcified myofibers in necrotic lesions increase dose dependently. It is speculated that calcium deposits in skeletal muscle are occurred as results of abnormal calcium and phosphate homeostasis and delayed muscle degeneration and regeneration cycle.

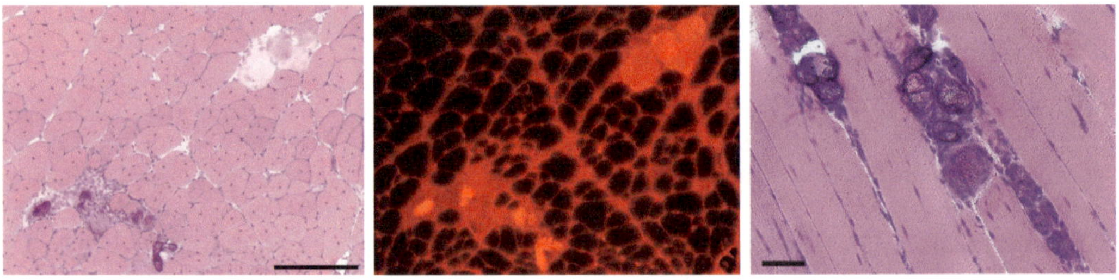

Fig. 1. Ectopic calcification in mdx mice (90 days old). Transverse (left and center) and longitudinal (right) sections, stained with H&E (left and right) and Evans blue (center). The bar represents 100 μm.

3. Identification of calcium deposits in mdx mice skeletal muscle

Our group is actively studying ectopic calcification in mdx mice skeletal muscle (Kikkawa et al., 2009). We performed experiments with 90-day-old mdx and control mice (C57BL/10: B10) fed a commercial standard chow (CE-2; Clea Japan, Tokyo, Japan) and water *ad libitum*. Following sacrificed of the mice, high-resolution X-ray micro-computed tomography (CT) imaging of the hind limbs of mdx and B10 mice using a SkyScan-1074 scanner (SkyScan, Kontich, Belgium) revealed that all mdx mice had muscle calcification in the hind limb, whereas no calcium precipitation was observed in the control mice (Fig. 2).

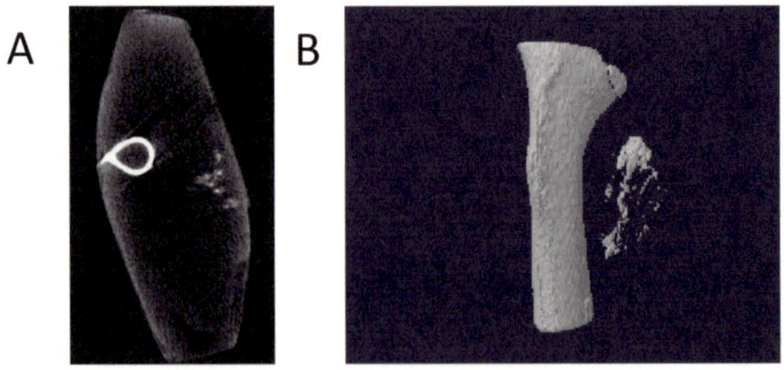

Fig. 2. Images of the hind limb of a two-month-old mdx mouse. X-ray-absorbing materials are shown as gray shadows and the femeur can be seen in the center of the X-ray image. (A) CT image. (B) Reconstructed 3D image. (Kikkawa et al., 2009)

The main composition of calcium deposits in the skeletal muscle was identified using an back-scattered electron imaging and energy-dispersive X-ray spectrometry (EDS) analysis by S-4500 SEM (Hitachi, Tokyo, Japan). In a cross-section of the muscle from an mdx mouse, spotty and bright crystals were observed. The EDS spectra obtained from the crystals indicated the presence of both calcium and phosphorus (Fig. 2A-B). To determine whether the composition of the deposits consisted of a calcium phosphate phase, muscle samples were analyzed using a JEM-2010 TEM (JEOL, Tokyo, Japan) equipped with an EDS detector. The electron diffraction pattern from an obtained TEM image of the specimen nearly was an identical match with a simulated diffraction pattern of hydroxyapatite ($Ca5(PO4)3OH$; HA) (Fig. 3C). Based on these results, we concluded that the calcification of mdx skeletal muscles is due to the precipitation of hydroxyapatite.

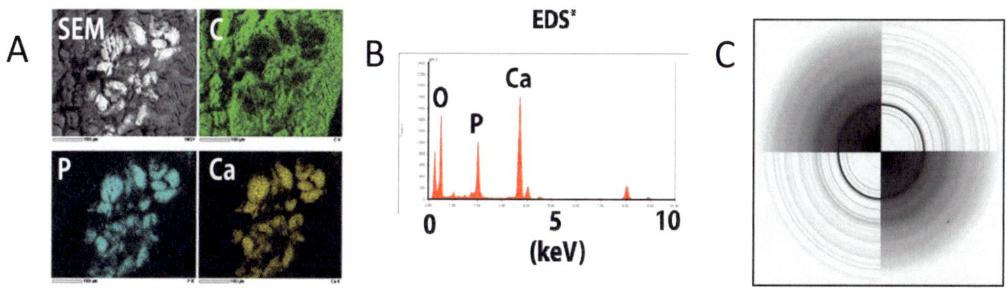

Fig. 3. SEM and TEM analyses of ectopic calcification in mdx mice skeletal muscle. (A) Electron probe microanalysis identified the particles as calcium phosphate. (B) Energy dispersive X-ray spectroscopy. (C) Identical match of X-ray diffraction of the particles and HA. (Kikkawa et al., 2009).

4. Serum biochemistry of mdx and B10 mice fed a commercial diet

As we determined that ectopic calcification is composed of HA, the main component of bones, we suspected that mdx mice have a metabolic disorder of calcium (Ca) and phosphate (Pi) homeostasis. To examine the levels of Ca and Pi in blood, serum samples were collected from two-month-old mdx and B10 mice fed a commercial diet (CE-2 containing 1.0 g/100 g Pi and 1.0 g/100 g Ca) and water *ad libitum*. The two minerals were measured using an automated clinical chemistry analyzer Fuji Dri-chem 4000 (Fujifilm, Tokyo, Japan). Comparison of the serum mineral components of mdx and B10 mice revealed that mdx mice had significantly higher serum Pi levels (1.41 fold; $P<0.05$) than the control mice, whereas no significant differences in serum Ca levels were detected. These results are supported by a previous study in mdx and B10 mice by Brazeau et al. (1992).

The concentrations of serum fibroblast growth factor-23 (FGF-23), which is an important regulator of phosphorus, were also measured using an FGF-23 ELISA kit (Kainos Laboratories, Tokyo, Japan). The serum level of FGF-23 of mdx mice was significantly higher (1.5 fold; $P<0.05$) than that of B10 mice.

Nearly all of the identified functions of FGF-23 are activated or operate through Klotho, a single transmembrane protein of the β-glycosidase family that is expressed in the distal kidney tubules and parathyroid gland (Kuro-o, 2010). Both FGF-23 and Klotho have emerged as responsible factors for mediating phosphate homeostasis. It has been reported that soft tissue calcification and hyperphosphatemia are observed in mice lacking either FGF-23 (Razzaque et al., 2006) or Klotho (Kuro-o et al., 1997). Klotho mutant mice also exhibit multiple age-associated disorders, such as arteriosclerosis, osteoporosis, short-life span, and ectopic calcification. However, as these phenotypes are rescued by the restriction of dietary phosphorus alone in male Klotho mice (Morishita et al., 2010) we predicted that the amount of dietary Pi intake influences the precipitation of calcium in mdx mice, and that the restriction of dietary Pi may improve mdx muscle pathology and function.

5. Influence of phosphate diet

Based on our findings that mdx mice have calcium deposits composed of HA and exhibit higher serum phosphate levels, we speculated that dietary phosphate intake might modulate ectopic calcification in mdx mice. To test this speculation, mdx mice and B10 mice were divided into three diet groups (n=30) from weaning (20 days old) that were fed diets with Pi contents of 2.0 g/100 g (high-Pi diet), 1.0 g/100 g (mid-Pi diet), and 0.7 g/100 g (low-Pi diet) manufactured by Oriental Yeast Company (Tokyo, Japan). Other ingredients, including calcium (1.2 g/100 g) in the diets were present in the same amounts among the groups. The experimental diets were based on the CE-2 and mid-Pi diet was a same composition with CE-2 diet which was fed to pregnant and nursing mice of both genotypes. All mice were housed in cages with pulp bedding (Palmas-μ; Material Research Center, Tokyo, Japan) in a controlled room with a 12-h light/dark cycle and a temperature of 25℃. The experimental chows and water were available *ad libitum*. Mice were either sacrificed with an overdose of diethylether at age 30, 60, or 90 days or used for measurements of muscular function at age 60 days. Twenty-four hours before euthanasia, mice were received an intraperitoneal injection of Evans blue dye (EBD, 100 mg/kg) which incorporates into regenerating myofibers with permeable membranes (Matsuda et al., 1995). All procedures were performed in accordance with the ethical guidelines of the University of Tokyo.

5.1 Changes in ectopic calcification in skeletal muscle

Changes in ectopic calcification in mdx mice skeletal muscle induced by dietary phosphate content were observed using a modified whole body double-staining method involving alizarin red S and alcian blue, which stain bones and cartilage respectively (Dingerkus et al., 1977; McLeod, 1980; Webb et al., 1994). Briefly, 90-day-old mice were sacrificed and fixed in 95% ethanol (EtOH) for 7 days after the skin and organs were removed. The EtOH was then replaced in acetone and the samples were further incubated for 3~4 days. After partial drying, samples were stained in a mixed solution of 0.3% alcian blue 8GX (Fluka, Germany) in 70% EtOH, 0.1% alizarin red S (WAKO, Osaka, Japan) in 95% EtOH, and 2.0% potassium hydrogen phthalate in 70% EtOH for 3 days. Each stained mouse was washed in distilled water and placed in 0.75% potassium hydroxide (KOH) in MilliQ water for 2 days to initiated maceration and clearing. Clearing was continued by adding increasing concentration of glycerol (20%, 50%, 70% and 100%) in 0.75% KOH to obtain a completely cleared specimen (Fig. 4A). Calcified regions were stained reddish violet, similar to appearance of stained bones.

Imaging of the stained and cleared samples showed that no bone-like red staining was present in the skeletal muscles of B10 mice fed any of the three phosphate diets (Fig. 4A-a). However, in mid-Pi fed mdx mice, striped and spotty red stained areas, particularly in the back, gluteus, and lower limbs muscles, were detected (Fig. 4A-b), while excessive calcification was clearly observed in the samples from high-Pi fed mdx mice (Fig. 4A-c, Fig. 4B). The staining revealed severe calcification, particularly in the diaphragm, back, gluteus, and lower limbs muscles, where severely degenerated muscle fibers were visible macroscopically by EBD staining (Fig. 4C). In contrast, bone-like red staining was rarely seen in the whole bodies of the low-Pi fed mdx mice (Fig. 4A-d, Fig. 4B).

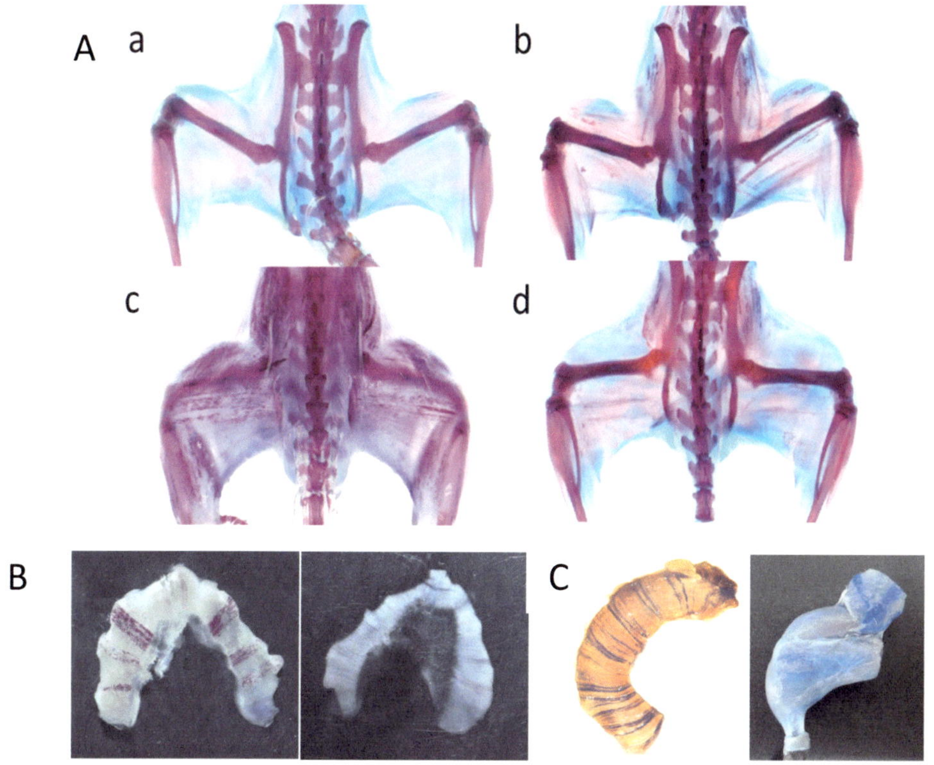

Fig. 4. Results of whole-body double staining of mdx and B10 mice, and Evans blue dye staining of mdx mice. (A) Images of the whole-body double staining of the lower body. (A-a) Lower body of a B10 mouse fed a high-Pi diet. The lower body of mdx mice (A-b) fed a mid-Pi diet, (A-c) high-Pi diet and (A-d) low-Pi diet. (B) Pictures of the whole body double staining of diaphragm. Diaphragm of an mdx mouse fed a high-Pi diet (left) and low-Pi diet (right). (C) Evans blue dye in the diaphragm (left) and lower limb (right) of an mdx mouse. Evans blue-positive lesions are seen in blue.

Quadriceps muscle samples from low-Pi, mid-Pi, and high-Pi fed mdx mice at 30, 60, and 90 days of age were sectioned at 8 μm thickness to determine the onset of calcifying lesions. Hematoxylin and eosin (H&E) and alizarin red S (1%) staining were used to observe pathology and detect calcification in the samples (Fig. 5). Histology showed early mineralization in degenerating myofibers in high-Pi fed mdx mice at 30 days of age (only fed a high-Pi diet only for 10 days), whereas no alizarin red-positive areas were present in either mid-Pi or low-Pi fed mdx mice of the same age. In addition, few calcium deposits were seen in mid-Pi fed mdx mice by the age of 60 days or in low-Pi fed mdx mice even by

90 days of age. Calcium deposits were extensive throughout the entire sections of high-Pi fed mdx mice at 90 days of age.

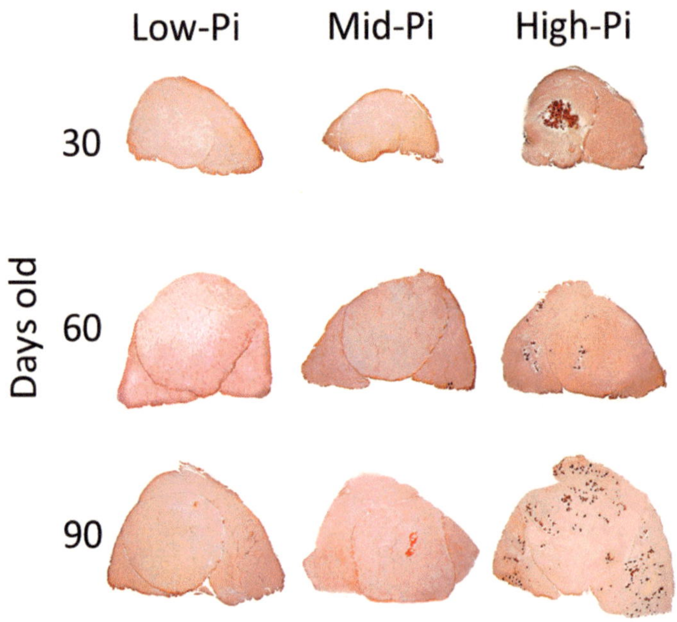

Fig. 5. Alizarin red S-stained cryosections of mdx mice quadriceps muscle. Calcium deposits are stained red.

5.2 Ectopic calcification in other tissues

Although the presence of calcification is rarely reported in organs of mdx mice other than skeletal muscle, including the heart and kidneys, these mice exhibit abnormal cardiac pathology and function (Zhang et al., 2008) and their myocardium is vulnerable (Costas et al., 2010). Rodent models of muscular dystrophies may have potential for sensitivity to myocardial calcification when challenged by mechanical or chemical stressors, because such calcification is commonly observed in the hamster model of muscular dystrophy (Burbach, 1987). For instance, Elsherif et al. (2008) found that dystrophin and β1 integrin double-knockout mice (β1KOmdx) show exacerbated myocardiopathy and extensive calcification in the heart, particularly under pregnancy-induced stress. Thus we predicted that high-Pi intake would also affect calcification in the myocardium of mdx mice.

Calcification in the heart was evaluated by 8 µm cryosections of samples from the three Pi-diet group mice. We found that high-Pi intake induced relatively few cases of myocardial calcification in mdx mice at both 60 and 90 days of age (4 of 30 samples). The form of the crystallization observed in the heart was similar to that of myofiber calcification, although the amount was considerably less (Fig. 6A, C). The incidence of calcification in the heart was absent in mdx fed mid-Pi or low-Pi diets. None of B10 mice fed any of the three types of phosphate diets exhibited myocardial calcification.

As previously described, klotho mutant mice display a number of age-related diseases, including soft tissue calcification. Morishita et al. (2010) reported that klotho mice fed a normal diet show kidney calcification, whereas mice fed a low-Pi diet have reduced precipitation of calcium in the kidneys. We found that a high-Pi intake results in slight ectopic calcification in kidneys of mdx mice (Fig. 6B, D) whereas mdx mice fed mid-Pi or low-Pi diets showed no evidence of calcium deposition in the kidneys. Similar to the findings in the heart, B10 mice under all phosphate diets also showed no calcification in the kidneys.

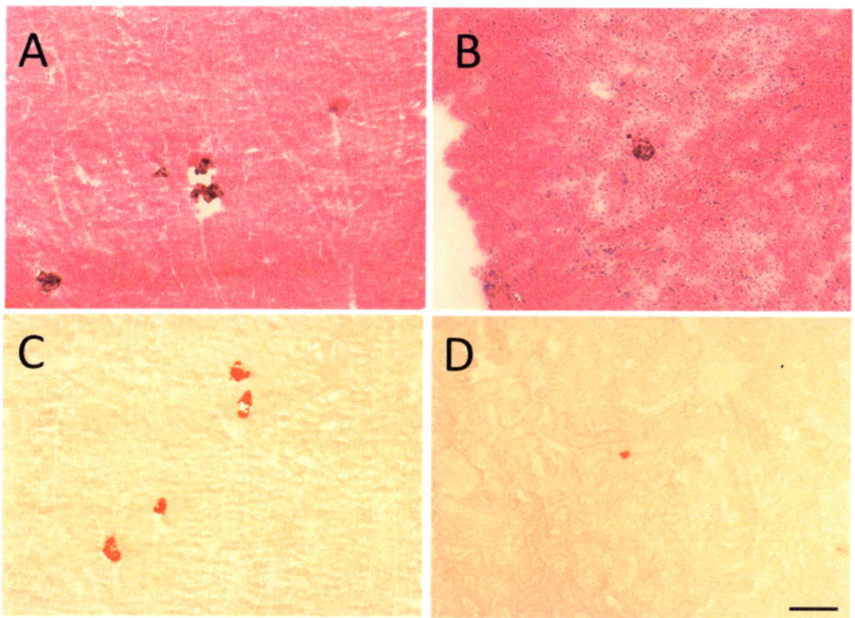

Fig. 6. H&E and alizarin red S-stained cryosections of the heart and kidneys of an mdx mouse fed a high-Pi diet. H&E-stained cryosections of the heart (A) and kidney (B). Alizarin red S-stained cryosections of the heart (C) and kidney (D). The bar represents 100 μm.

5.3 Changes in serum biochemistry

We also examined the serum calcium and phosphate concentrations of B10 and mdx mice fed the three types of Pi diets. The serum phosphate levels of high-Pi fed mdx mice were significantly higher than those of B10 mice fed the same diet, and mdx mice under mid-Pi and low-Pi diets (Fig. 7). However, no marked differences in serum calcium concentrations of mdx mice were detect in the different diet groups. Serum phosphate concentration is largely influenced by dietary intake, with the over-consumption of phosphate often resuting to cause hyperphosphatemia (Calvo et al., 1994), secondary hyperparathyroidism with bone re-sorption (Lutwak et al., 1975), and bone loss (Draper et al., 1979). It is likely that high phosphate intake leads to overworked kidneys and a reduced rate of calcium and phosphate filtration.

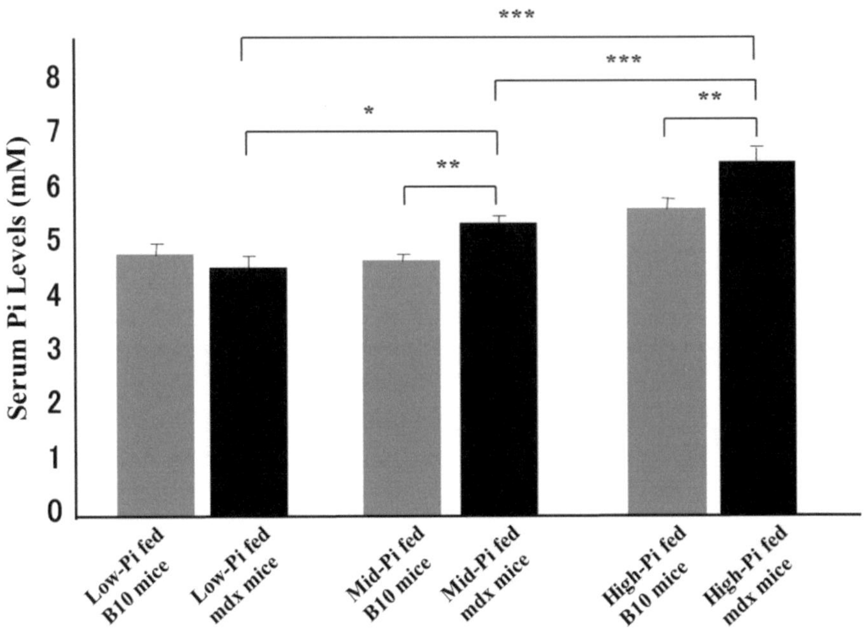

Fig. 7. Serum Pi levels of three-month-old B10 and mdx mice fed three types of Pi diets. Comparison of B10 and mdx mice fed the three Pi diets. (*: $p<0.05$; **: $p<0.01$; ***: $p<0.001$).

6. Effects of ectopic calcification on muscle function of mdx mice

High-Pi intake induced severe ectopic calcification throughout the skeletal muscle of mdx mice. The presence of ectopic calcification in muscles appeared to have a negative impact on the force output of skeletal muscle. To date, no studies have reported the pathophysiological effects of the accumulation of calcium phosphate in muscles. For this reason, we have investigated the effects of ectopic calcification on skeletal muscle contraction of mdx mice.

For muscle force measurements, *in situ* maximal isometric twitch force and tetanic force of right triceps surae muscle (TSM) were recorded. The isometric force recording system was custom-made and the experimental protocols were based on the design of Dorchies et al. (2006). Sixty-day-old B10 and mdx mice fed the three phosphate diets were lightly anesthetized by diethylether gas and then immobilized on a cork board by covering the bodies with Novix-II (Asahi Techno Glass, Chiba, Japan). A confined area of skin and myofasia of the right hindlimb was cut and exposed, and the sciatic nerve was dissected to induce the analgesic conditions. The knee joint was firmly immobilized by a needle that served as the fulcrum and the Achilles tendon of the leg was then severed and connected to a platinum electrode clip associated with a force transducer (DS2-50N Digital Force Gauge; Imada, Aichi, Japan). A second platinum electrode was directly inserted into the TSM. Experimental trials were started after the animals recovered from anesthesia. Using this procedure, we avoided negative effects (*i.e.* muscle relaxation) of the anesthetic regimen, which we previously confirmed and were able to collect real data without any disturbances. For the measurement of maximal single twitch, muscles were stimulated with a square wave pulse (0.5-msec duration) of stimulation voltage. Tetanic force was measured with 200-msec bursts of frequency set to 100 Hz. Muscle length and weight of TSM were measured to estimate the cross-sectional area

(CSA) of the muscle (in mm^2). The specific twitch and tetanic force were normalized by dividing the measured force by the CSA. Using manual settings of the optimal muscle length, maximal twitch contractions were measured within trials up to 20 contractions and all tetanic force measurements were made at locations where the single twitch force was the greatest.

6.1 Results of maximal single force (MSF) and maximal tetanic force (MTF) measurements

Pre-tests results revealed that B10 mice fed the normal CE-2 diet had significantly stronger maximal single force in response to single-pulse stimulation than that of mdx mice (data not shown). This result is consistent with a previous study by Dorchies et al. (2006). Furthermore, although mdx mice have a heavier body weight and muscle mass of the TSM, they exhibited weaker muscle force compared with the control mice. This finding was also consisted with that reported previously (Quinlan et al., 1992), although the muscle mass of anterior tibial muscle was compared, rather than TSM. Therefore, we are confident that our isometric force recording system can be used to evaluate and compare muscle forces between B10 and mdx mice fed the different phosphate diets (Table 1).

We did not detect any significant differences in twitch force between B10 mice of the three phosphate diets groups. However, the high-Pi diet mdx mice had significantly lower ($p<0.001$) single force than that of mdx mice fed a mid-Pi diet (Fig. 8A), while maximal single force was significantly higher in mdx mice fed a low-Pi diet compared with mid-Pi diet mdx mice. Notably, however, this value was still lower (25% less) than the corresponding value of B10 mice fed a low-Pi diet.

The maximal tetanic force in response to burst stimulation was also measured for all mice. Similar to the results of twitch force, B10 mice had significantly higher tetanic force than mdx mice for all three phosphate diets, whereas no marked differences were detected among B10 mice. Mdx mice fed a high-Pi diet produced significantly less ($p<0.001$) tetanic force than the other mdx mice (Fig. 8B). Based on these findings, we conclude that high-Pi diet has a greater influence on generating the tetanic force in mdx mice than producing twitch force. These results strongly suggest that calcium deposits in muscles interfere with muscle function. The improvement of muscle forces was likely due to the reduction of ectopic calcification because low Pi-diet did not have a positive effect on force generation in B10 mice, which have no ectopic calcification. However, it is also likely that other factors related to dietary phosphate restriction also contribute to improving muscle function.

Mouse	#	Weight (g)	MSF (mN/mm^2)	MTF (mN/mm^2)
Low-Pi B10	7	23.1±1.0	102.5±4.6	344.8±15.2
Low-Pi mdx	7	23.8±1.4	74.2±2.4	254.9±14.6
Mid-Pi B10	7	22.3±0.7	100.0±4.1	341.0±11.1
Mid-Pi mdx	7	25.2±0.5	66.8±1.5	246.4±7.2
High-Pi B10	7	22.8±0.7	101.0±3.3	335.6±6.3
High-Pi mdx	7	23.6±0.7	59.6±2.0	193.9±9.6

Table 1. Results of MSF and MTFmeasurements of B10 and mdx mice for the three Pi diet conditions.

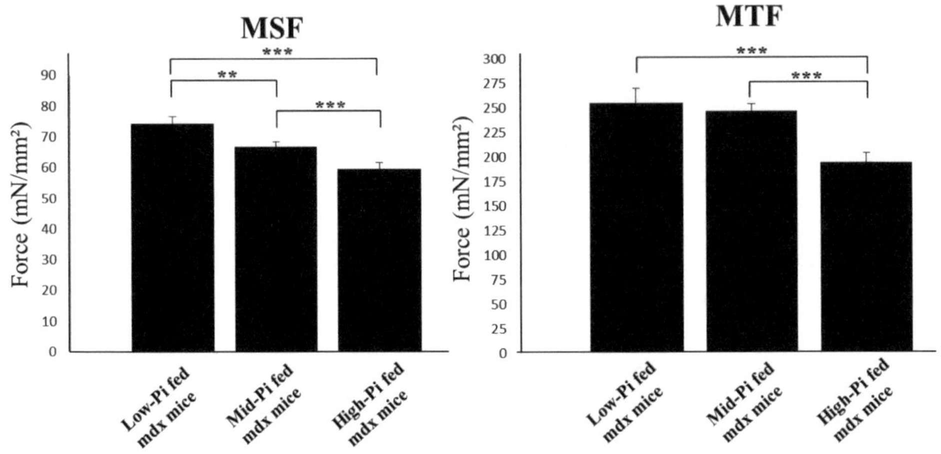

Fig. 8. MSF and MTF measurements of mdx mice for the three Pi diet conditions. (A) Results of MSF. (B) Results of MTF (**: $p<0.01$; ***: $p<0.001$).

7. Reduced calcification by low Pi diet in a longitudinal study

Although the influence of dietary phosphate intake on the precipitation of calcium in mdx mice skeletal muscles has been clarified, the effects of phosphate restriction on severe ectopic calcification remained unclear. To understand the impact of phosphate restriction on the deposition of calcium, a longitudinal study was conducted for four mdx mice raised on high-Pi diet from weaning to 60 days of age. At age of 60 days, whole-body images of the mdx mice were taken by noninvasive CT scanning using a Latheta LTC-200 X-ray micro CT scanner (Hitachi Aloka Medical, Tokyo, Japan) (Fig. 9). The mdx mice were then divided into two groups, a continuously fed high-Pi diet group and a low-Pi diet group, until the age of 90 days, at which point whole-body images of the mice were taken again. The whole-body images and volume density of ectopic calcification in the lower body (from the top of os coxae to ankle joint) were compared (Fig. 10). Mice fed a high-Pi diet displayed an increased volume (0.066 cm^3) of ectopic calcification from 60 to 90 days of age, whereas mdx mice fed a low-Pi diet had a reduced (-0.007 cm^3). Thus, it was concluded that the restriction the restriction of dietary phosphate from the age of 60 days reduced the pre-formed ectopic calcification within one month, while continuously feeding the mice a high-Pi diet led to more severe calcium deposits.

8. Mechanisms of calcification

The complete mechanism underlying progressive muscle degeneration due to dystrophin deficit is unclear. Dystrophin-deficient muscles are highly susceptible to the oxidative stress that results from the early onset of muscle degeneration. Muscle necrosis actively occurs following the degeneration, leading to fibrosis and calcification of muscle fibers (Vercherat et al., 2009). It has been suggested that vascular calcification is actively regulated by osteogenic gene expression in vascular smooth muscle cells (Giachelli, 1999). Attention has been focused on inorganic phosphate as one of the potential factors regulating the observed cellular phenotypic changes, as smooth muscle cells *in vitro* cultured under high-Pi conditions undergo osteogenesis and form calcium deposits (Jono et al., 2000). As skeletal muscle satellite cells possess multilineage potential (Asakura et al., 2001; Wada et al., 2002), they might also undergo osteogenic differentiation under high-Pi conditions.

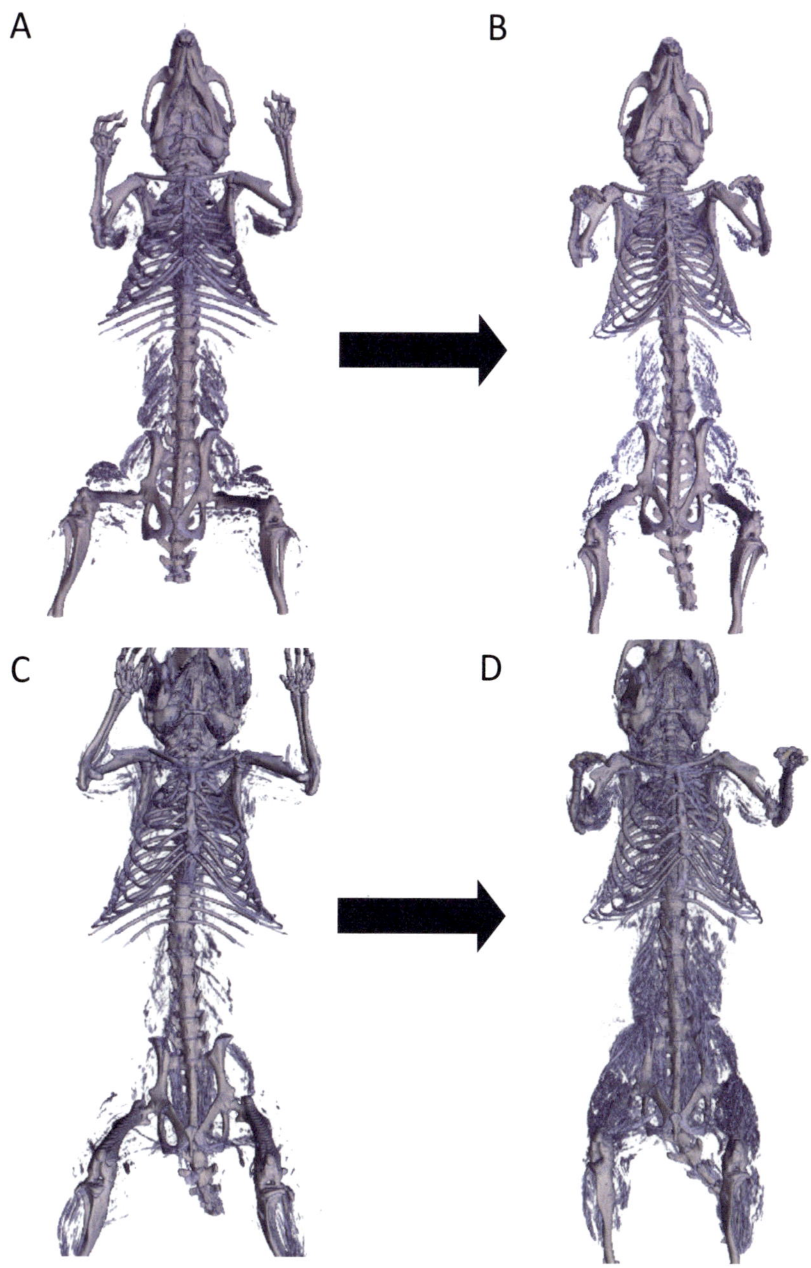

Fig. 9. 3D images of 60-day-old mdx mice fed a high-Pi diet (left) and the images of the same mice after 30 days (A,C) Sixty-day-old mdx mice fed a high-Pi diet. (B) The same mdx mice (90-day-old) fed a low-Pi diet for 30 days. (D) The same mdx mice (90-day-old) fed a high-Pi diet for 30 days. Bones are shown in grey and ectopic calcification is in light blue.

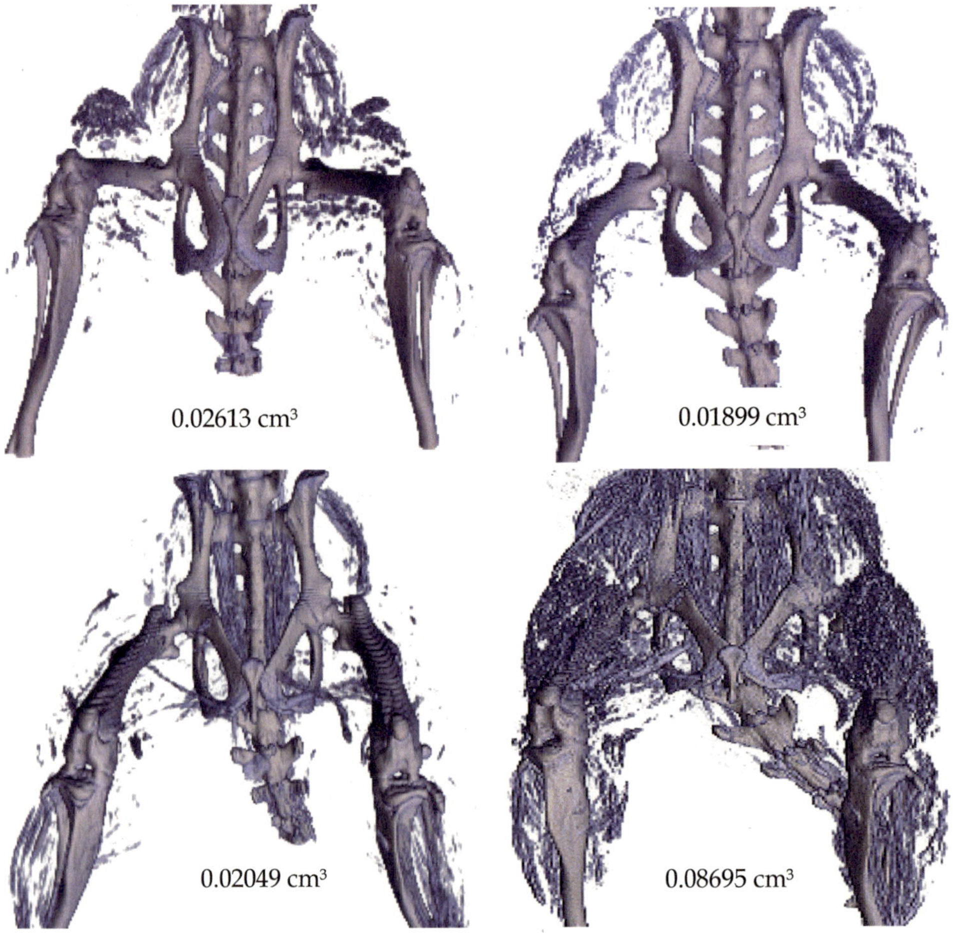

Fig. 10. Enlarged 3D images of the lower limbs of mdx mice fed a high-Pi diet (left) and the images of the same mice fed either low-Pi (top right) or high-Pi diets (bottom right) for 30 days. The numbers represent the volume densities of ectopic calcification in the lower body (from the top of os coxae to ankle joint).

8.1 Pi-induced osteogenesis and reduced myogenesis in C2C12 cells

To study the effects of Pi on muscle cell differentiation, murine myoblast-derived C2C12 cells were cultured for four days under various Pi concentrations and then immunostained for the presence of myogenic (myosin heavy chain; MyHC) and osteogenic (Matrix Gla Protein; MGP) markers. When cultured in normal differentiation medium (Pi=1 mM), the cells underwent muscle differentiation and formed myotubes. Myogenesis proceeded until the Pi concentration of the differentiation medium reached 5 mM, while myotube formation was strongly suppressed at 7 mM. (Fig. 11).

The expression of Runx2, a transcription factor of osteogenesis, increased with the rise of the Pi concentration (Fig. 12A). The retardation of myogenesis caused by the high Pi concentration was also evident by the decrease in both the fusion index and myogenin expression (Fig. 12A). It was notable that in medium containing 5 mM Pi, myogenesis was not inhibited and the C2C12 cells differentiated into myotubes, while the expression Runx2 was augmented (Fig. 12B). Further observation revealed that myogenin and Runx2 did not colocalize in the nuclei of myotubes, rather, Runx2 was localized in the cytoplasm. This finding suggests that Runx2 is inactive in myogenic cells, as it has been reported that Runx2 activity is regulated by translocation between the nucleus and cytoplasm (Zaidi et al., 2001). Upregulation of Runx2 expression was observed by Western blotting not only when the C2C12 cells were cultured under high-Pi conditions, but also when cultured in the presence of calcium deposits, which were generated by the addition of sodium phosphate and calcium chloride to the medium (Fig. 12C). Osteocalcin, another osteogenic marker which is a secreted protein whose expression is regulated by Runx2, was also examined (Fig 12D). RT-PCR was performed with RNA samples prepared from C2C12 cells cultured under the various Pi concentrations for four days. Osteocalcin expression was undetectable when the cells were cultured with 1 mM Pi, but increased with the elevation of the Pi concentration. We also measured calcium deposition in C2C12 cells cultured under the various Pi concentrations and found that although the cells did not deposit calcium under normal Pi conditions, cells cultured in medium containing 3 mM Pi or higher deposited calcium (alizarin red S-positive cells; Fig. 12E). The amount of calcium deposits increased significantly at higher Pi concentrations.

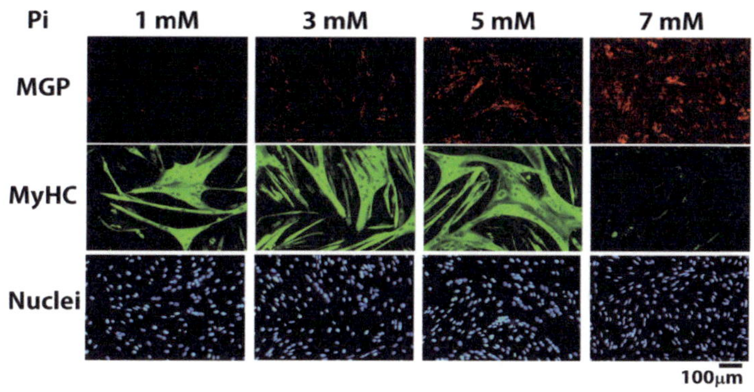

Fig. 11. Immunocytochemistry of C2C12 cells cultured under various Pi concentrations. Cells were immunostained for MyHC (green), MGP (red), and nuclei (blue).

8.2 Pi-induced calcification in primary cultures of skeletal muscle cells

Cells isolated from mdx skeletal muscle tissue were cultured in normal Pi (1.3 mM) to high-Pi (5 mM) medium to study the effects of Pi in primary culture cells. The cells formed myotubes when cultured in normal medium, whereas myotube formation was strongly inhibited under high-Pi conditions. The results of both alizarin red S and von Kossa staining revealed that numerous calcium deposits were present in cells after ten days of culture in high-Pi medium, but none detected in cells cultured in normal medium (Fig. 13). Therefore, Pi induces osteogenesis in myoblasts, resulting in calcification while inhibiting myogenesis. We conclude that the calcification of skeletal muscle is mainly due to the elevation of intracellular Pi levels.

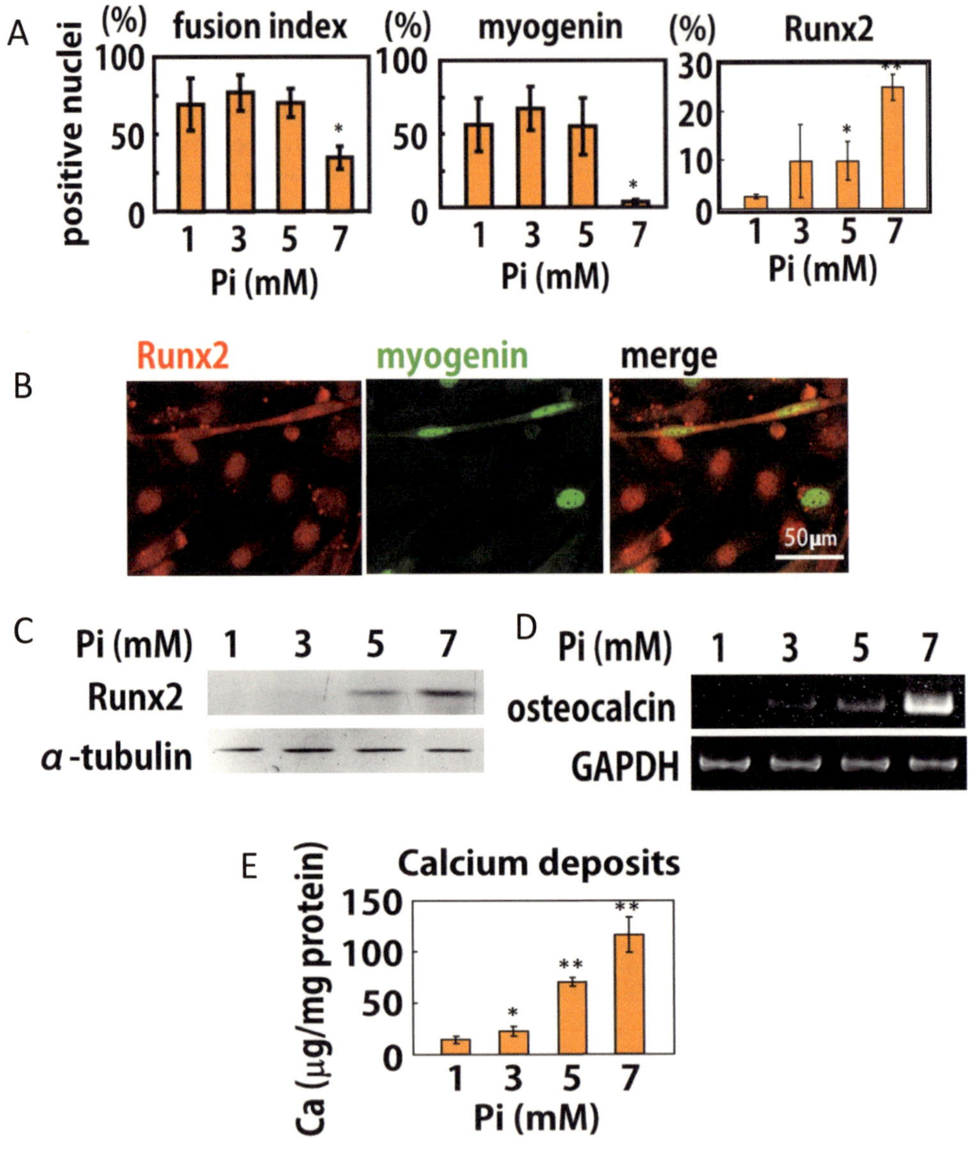

Fig. 12. Immunocytochemistry and RT-PCR of C2C12 cells cultured under various Pi concentrations (1, 3, 5, and 7 m). (A) The fusion index, myogenin expression, and expression of Runx2 were quantified. The fusion index and ratio of nuclei expressing myogenin decreased, while the ratio of Runx2-expressing nuclei increased with increasing Pi concentration. (B) Close observation of cells cultured in medium containing 5 mM Pi by staining with Hoechst 33258 to show the nuclei, or immunostained for myogenin or Runx2. (C) Western blotting of C2C12 cells cultured under increased Pi or Ca concentrations. (D) RT-PCR for osteocalcin in C2C12 cells cultured under various Pi concentrations. (E) Quantification of calcium deposites generated by C2C12 cells cultured under various Pi concentrations. (*: $p<0.05$; **: $p<0.01$).

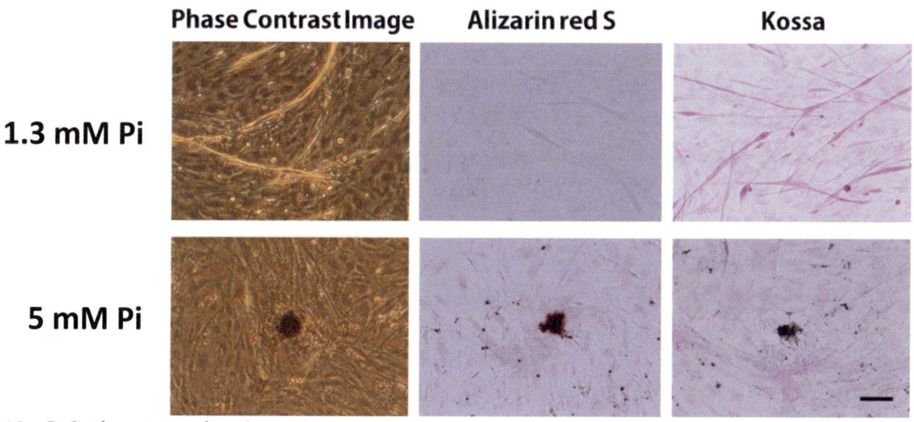

Fig. 13. Calcification of mdx mouse muscle-derived primary culture cells. Calcium deposits were stained red or black with alizarin red S and von Kossa staining, respectively. No calcification was observed when cells were cultured in normal medium containing 1.3 mM Pi. The von Kossa-stained samples were counterstained with nuclear fast red, and myotubes appear pink. The bar represents 100μm.

9. Conclusion

In this study, we reviewed the mechanisms underlying calcification in skeletal muscle cells following the elevation of intracellular Pi concentrations and revealed the effects of dietary phosphate intake on ectopic calcification in mdx mice. Both *in vivo* and *in vitro*, high-Pi conditions lead to the precipitation of calcium in mdx mice. We have demonstrated that the presence of ectopic calcification in skeletal muscle exacerbates the impaired muscle function of mdx mice, which represents a novel finding. The main goal of our studies is to understand the effects and efficacy of nutritional components on muscular dystrophy as a prior therapy. The effects of dietary phosphate intake on muscle pathology and kidney function need to further elucidated in future studies. Furthermore, the therapeutic potential of nutrition, particularly phosphate intake, should be considered when treating patients with DMD.

10. Acknowledgement

This work has been supported by Health and Labour Sciences Research Grant (19A-020) for Research on Psychiatric and Neurological Diseases and Mental Health, Intramural Research Grant(23-5) for Neurological and Psychiatric Disorders of NCNP and a Research Grant for Nervous and Mental Disorders [20B-13] from the Ministry of Health, Labour and Welfare, Japan.

11. References

Asakura, A.; Komaki, M. & Rudnicki, M. (2001). Muscle Satellite Cells are Multipotential Stem Cells that Exhibit Myogenic, Osteogenic, and Adipogenic Differentiation. Differentiation, Vol.68, pp.245-253.

Burbach, J. (1987). Ultrastructure of Cardiocyte Degeneration and Myocardial Calcification in the Dystrophic Hamster. *The American Journal of Anatomy*, Vol.179, pp.291-307.

Calvo, M. (1994). The Effects of High Phosphoru Intake on Calcium Homeostasis. *Advances in Nutritional Researches*, Vol.9, pp.183-207.

Costas, J.; Nye, D.; Henley, J. & Plochocki, J. (2010). Voluntary Exercise Induces Structural Remodeling in the Hearts of Dystrophin-deficient Mice. *Muscle Nerve*, Vol.42, pp.881-885.

Coulton, G.; Morgan, J.; Partridge, T. & Sloper, J. (1988). The mdx Mouse Skeletal Muscle Myopathy: I. A Histological, Morphometric and Biochemical Investigation. *Neuropathology and Applies Neurobiology*, Vol.14, pp.53-70.

Dingerkus, G. & Uhler, L. (1977). Enzyme Clearing of Alcian Blue Stained Whole Small Vertebrates for Demonstration of Cartilage. *Biotechnic & Histochemistry*, Vol.52, pp.229-232.

Dorchies, O.; Wagner, S.; Vuadens, O.; Waldhauser, K.; Buetler, T.; Kucera, P. & Ruegg, U. (2006). Green Tea Extract and Its Major Polyphenol(-)-epigallocatechin Gallate Improve Muscle Function in a Mouse Model of Duchenne Muscular Dystrophy. *American Journal of Physiology. Cell Physiology*, Vol.290, pp.616-625.

Draper, H. & Bell, R. (1979). Nutrition and Osteoporosis. *Advances in Nutritional Researches*, Vol.145, pp.389-391.

El-Abbadi, M.; Pai, A.; Leaf, E.; Yang, H.; Bartley, B.; Quan, K.; Ingalls, C.; Liao, H. & Giachelli, C. (2009). Phosphate Feeding Induces Arterial Medial Calcification in Uremic Mice: Role of Serum Phosphorus, Fibroblast Growth Factor-23, and Osteopontin. *Kidney International*, Vol.75, pp.1297-1307.

Elsherif, L.; Huang, M.; Shai, S.; Yang, Y.; Li, R.; Chun, J.; Mekany, M.; Chu, A.; Kaufman, S. & Ross, R. (2008). Combined Deficiency of Dystrophin and β1 Integrin in Cardiac Myocyte Causes Myocardial Dysfunction, Fibrosis and Calcification. *Circulation Research*, Vol.102, pp.1109-1117.

Gaschen, F.; Hoffman, E.; Gorospe, J.; Uhl, E.; Senior, D.; Cardinet, G. & Pearce, L. (1992). Dystrophin Deficiency Causes Lethal Muscle Hypertrophy in Cats. *Journal of the Neurological Sciences*, Vol.110, pp.149-159.

Giachelli, C. (2009). The Emerging Role of Phosphate in Vascular Calcification. Kidney International, V0l75, pp.890-897.

Hu, M.; Kuro-o,M. & Moe, O. (2010). Klotho and Kidney Disease. *Journal of Nephrology*, Vol.16, pp.136-144.

Kendrick, J.; Kestenbaum, B. & Chonchol, M. (2011). Phosphate and Cardiovascular Disease. *Advances in Chronic Kidney Disease*, Vol.18, pp.113-119.

Khan, M. (1993). Corticosteroid Therapy in Duchenne Muscular Dystrophy. *Journal of the Neurological Sciences*, V0l.120, pp.8-14.

Kikkawa, M.; Ohno, T.; Nagata, Y.; Shiozuka, M.; Kogure, T. & Matsuda, R. (2009). Ectopic Calcification is Caused by Elevated Levels of Serum Inorganic Phosphate in Mdx Mice. *Cell Structure and Function*, Vol.34, pp.77-88.

Korff, S.; Riechert, N.; Schoensiegel, F.; Weichenhan, D.; Autschbach, F.; Katus, H. & Ivandic, B. (2006). Calcification of Myocardial Necrosis is Common in Mice. *Virchows Archiv*, Vol.448, pp.630-638.

Kuro-o. (2010). Overview of the FGF-23-Klotho Axis. *Pediatric Nephrology*, Vol.25, pp.583-590.

Kuro-o, M.; Matsumura, Y.; Aizawa, H.; Kawaguchi, H.; Suga, T.; Utsugi, T.; Ohyama, Y.; Kurabayashi, M.; Kaname, T.; Kume, E.; Iwasaki, H.; Iida, A.; Shiraki-Iida, T.; Nishikawa, S.; Nagai, R. & Nabeshima, Y. (1997). Mutation of the Mouse *Klotho* Gene Leads to a Syndrome Resembling Ageing. *Nature*, Vol.309, pp.45-51.

Liu, J.; Okamura, C.; Bogan, D.; Bogan, J.; Childers, M. & Kornegay. J. (2004). Effects of Prednisone in Canine Muscular Dystrophy. *Muscle Nerve*, Vol.30, pp.767-773.

Lutwak, L. (1975). Metabolic and Biochemical Considerations of Bone. *Annals of Clinical and Laboratory Science*, Vol.5, pp.185-194.

Matsuda, R.; Nishikawa, A. & Tanaka, H. (1995). Visualization of Dystrophic Muscle Fibers in Mdx Mouse by Vital Staining with Evans Blue: Evidence of Apoptosis in Dystrophin-Deficient Muscle. *Journal of Biochemistry*, Vol.118, pp.959-964.

McLeod, M. (1980). Differential Staining of Cartilage and Bone in Whole Mouse Fetuses by Alcian Blue and Alizarin Red S. *Teratology*, Vol.22, pp.229-301.

Morishita, K.; Shirai, A.; Kubota, M.; Katakura, Y.; Nabeshima, Y.; Takeshige, K. & Kamiya, T. (2010). The Progression of Aging in *Klotho* Mutant Mice Can Be Modified by Dietary Phosphorus and Zinc. *The Journal of Nutrition*, Vol.131, pp.3182-3188.

Nguyen, F.; Cherel, L.; Guigand, I.; Goubault-Leroux & Myers, M. (2002). Muscle Lesions Associated with Dystrophin Deficiency in Neonatal Golden Retriver Puppies. *Journal of Comparative Pathology*, Vol.126, pp.100-108.

Quinlan, J.; Johnson, S.; McKee, M. & Lyden, S. (1992). Twitch and Tetanus in mdx Mouse Muscle. *Muscle Nerve*, Vol.15, pp.837-842.

Razzaque, M.; Sitara, D.; Taguchi, T.; St-Arnaud, R. & Lanske, B. (2006). Premature Aging-like Phenotype in Fibroblast Growth Factor 23 Null Mice is a Vitamin D Mediated Process. *The FASEB Journal*, Vol.20, pp.720-722.

Vercherat, C.; Chung, T.; Yalcin, S.; Gulbagci, N.; Gopinadhan, S.; Ghaffari, S. & Taneja, R. (2009). Stra13 Regulates Oxidative Stress Mediated Skeletal Muscle Degeneration. *Human Molecular Genetics*, Vol.18, pp.4304-4316.

Verma, M.; Asakura, Y.; Hirai, H.; Watanabe, S.; Tastad, C.; Fong, G.; Ema, M.; Call, J.; Lowe, D. & Asakura, A. (2010). *Fit-1* Haploinsufficiency Ameliorates Muscular Dystrophy Phenotype by Developmentally Increased Vasculature in Mdx Mice. *Human Molecular Genetics*, Vol.19, pp.4145-4159.

Wada, M.; Inagawa-Ogashiwa, M.; Shimizu, S.; Yasumoto, S. & Hashimoto, N. (2002). Generation of Different Fates from Multipotent Muscle Stem Cells. *Development*, Vol.129, pp.2987-2995.

Webb, G. & Byrd, R. (1994). Simultaneous Differential Staining of Cartilage and Bone in Rodent Fetuses: an Alcian Blue and Alizarin Red S Procedure Without Glacial Acetic Acid. *Biotechnic and Histochemistry*, Vol.64, pp.181-185.

Wong, B. & Christopher, C. (2002). Corticosteroids in Duchenne Muscular Dystrophy: a Reappraisal. *Journal of Child Neurology*, Vol.17, pp.183-190.

Zaidi, S.; Javed, A.; Choi, J.; van Wijnen, A.; Stein, J.; Lian, J. & Stein, G. (2001). A Specific Targeting Signal Directs Runx2/Cbfa1 to Subnuclear Domains and Contributes to Transactivation of the Osteocalcin Gene. *Journal of Cell Sciences*, Vol.114, pp.3093-3102.

Zhang, W.; Hove, M.; Schneider, J.; Stuckey, D.; Sebag-Montefiore, L.; Bia, B.; Radda, G.; Davis, K.; Neubauer, S. & Clarke, K. (2008). Abnormal Cardiac Morphology, Function and Energy Metabolism in the Dystrophic mdx Mouse: An MRI and MRS Study. *Journal of Molecular and Cellular Cardiology*, Vol.45, pp.754-760.

12

Rehabilitation in Muscular Dystrophies: Changing Approach

Imelda J.M. de Groot, Nicoline B.M. Voet,
Merel Jansen and Lenie van den Engel-Hoek
Radboud University Nijmegen Medical Centre
The Netherlands

1. Introduction

Life expectancy is increasing in muscular dystrophies: as an example due to technical medical interventions like spine surgery and home ventilation, boys with Duchenne muscular dystrophy become men. Increasing evidence concerning retarding drugs becomes available for muscular dystrophies. Cardiac symptoms can effectively be treated with drugs and also cardioprotective drugs are tested. New retarding treatments, like exon skipping, stem cell treatment or vector-gene transfer, are in the phase of animal studies or already in randomized clinical trials. Together these treatments are changing the course of the muscular dystrophies.

In line with these developments rehabilitation management is also changing. In the past the treatment was focused on maintaining walking abilities as long as possible with physiotherapy, stretching, and with or without braces. However, due to the slower progression of the disorder and the technical possibilities of home ventilation the focus is changing to arm- and hand-function. There are good technical solutions for the loss of ambulation as there are many type of electrical wheelchairs. All kind of technical and electronic supports are available to operate telephone, television, radio etc. However, in all kind of daily activities a certain ability of the arm and hand is necessary. Training and support of these functions in muscular dystrophies come into prominence.

New symptoms or symptoms not noticed in the past are becoming more apparent. This can be due to the increasing age that they are now identified or augment during the longer course of the disease, such as feeding and swallowing problems, gastrointestinal and urogenital problems.

Already known symptoms like osteoporosis in muscular dystrophies also increase if corticosteroids are used. For example vertebral fractures are more seen in boys with Duchenne muscular dystrophy. The question is whether we can retard osteoporosis by means of supported physical activities with weight load on the bones. In the light of increasing life expectancy and the possibilities to use sophisticated orthoses or exoskeletons, it is important to maintain the physical capacities with balanced training.

Also due to increasing life expectancy an unforeseen population emerges who want to participate in social life in broad sense: education, jobs, friends, relationships, marriage, children. This desire is in slight contrast to adults who received the diagnosis muscular dystrophy in adulthood, they are attempting to maintain their participation in social life. Possibilities to live independent with supportive devices need to be established, robotics as support in daily activities will develop, and with the possibilities of the world wide web and computer technology education and jobs become available.

In this chapter we will not describe the established rehabilitation managements, but will describe the new focuses on training, the new or less noticed symptoms, and the development of new devices.

2. Training

2.1 Physical training for children with a muscular dystrophy

2.1.1 Disuse

Muscular dystrophies in children comprise a heterogeneous group of myopathies that appear during childhood. The most common muscular dystrophy in children is Duchenne Muscular Dystrophy (DMD) affecting 1/4200 life-born boys. Other muscular dsytrophies are Myotonic Dystrophy (MD), Becker Muscular Dystrophy (BMD), Limb Girdle Muscular Dystrophy (LGMD) and FacioScapuloHumeral muscular Dystrophy (FSHD). All muscular dystrophies are characterized by progressive loss of muscle function and only symptomatic treatments (such as corticosteroids and assisted mechanical ventilation) are currently available. An important aim in the management of muscular dystrophies is to delay the loss of functional abilities and to maintain independency. Physical training could retard the loss of physical abilities as a result of disuse.

Children with a muscular dystrophy are less physically active compared to age-matched healthy controls in their daily life (McDonald et al 2005). The more sedentary lifestyle can be explained primarily by the disease, but also by disuse(McDonald 2002, Bar-or and Rowland 2004). Disuse can be defined a discrepancy between children's capacity and performance, and gradually causes a secondary reduction of physical activity. Indeed, the increasing amount of energy a certain activity costs, and the fear of falls with the need for help to stand up, make children move less. An early decline of the physical activity level enhances the loss of functional abilities. This appears from the loss of arm functions that occurs fast after the onset of wheelchair-dependency(McDonald et al. 1995). An electric wheelchair limits arm functions (like lifting and reaching), since a top blade and a central operating joystick force children to function within the outlines of the wheelchair. Another example is the high number of children with DMD (20-40%) that loses the ability to walk as a result of a fracture of the lower extremity(Vestergaard et al , 2001). From this perspective, the saying "use it or lose it" is certainly applicable to children with a muscular dystrophy and encourages physical training.

2.1.2 Evidence for training

The number of studies that investigated the effects of physical training in children with a muscular dystrophy is limited (Voet et al. 2010). None of them were performed in a randomized controlled setting and most studies focused on DMD. Furthermore, clinical trials in children only investigated the effect of resistance exercises. This is remarkable, as recent studies in adults with BMD and the mdx mice (a mouse model for DMD) encourage aerobic exercises.

Previous clinical trials among boys with DMD showed that (sub)maximal resistance exercises have limited positive effects on muscle strength and time functional tests (such as the time it takes to walk 10m) but, importantly, are not harmful. In a study by Vignos et al. (1966), the effects of a one-year maximum resistance exercise program (i.e. the maximum load that could be lifted through ten repetitions) were examined(Vignos, Jr. and Watkins, 1966). Fourteen ambulatory children with DMD exercised their legs, arms and abdominal muscles and were compared with a control group of children with DMD who did not exercise. Results from this study showed that muscle strength decreased in control group, while strength was maintained during the training period in the exercise group. However, children were not randomly allocated to the exercise or non-exercise (natural cohort) group. Another study by De Lateur et al. (1979) showed that a six-month submaximal isokinetic exercise program could be of limited value in increasing strength in DMD (de Lateur and Giaconi, 1979). In this study, four ambulatory children with DMD performed quadriceps exercises with one leg (4 to 5 days per week), while the other leg was not trained at all. Finally, Scott et al. (1981) investigated the effects of six months manually applied resistance exercises and "free exercises" in eighteen boys with DMD(Scott et al., 1981). At six months, no statistically differences were found between the two groups at the level of muscle strength, locomotor abilities and functional abilities. No evidence for training-induced physical deterioration was found.

With respect to aerobic exercises, recent studies in mdx mice (an animal model for DMD) showed that voluntary wheel running had positive effects on muscle strength and fatigue resistance and non-weight bearing exercises (such as swimming) had no detrimental effects 1998; Hayes and Williams 1996). Dynamic exercises (bicycle training) improved endurance and muscles strength in adult BMD patients as well(Sveen et al. 2008) . In this study of Sveen et al. (2008), eleven ambulatory BMD patients, and seven healthy age-matched controls, participated in a 12-weeks cycling training. Participants cycled thirty minutes at 65% of their maximal oxygen uptake (VO_{2max}). At 12 weeks, workload and VO_{2max} were improved without an increase in CK level. Although this study was conducted among adults, the results of this study might be applicable for children with a muscular dystrophy as well.

Results of recently published clinical trial protocols, such as the protocol of the randomized controlled trials No Use is Disuse (NUD)(Jansen et al. 2010), will increase insight into what type of physical training (type, intensity, frequency, duration) should be recommended to children with a muscular dystrophy. The NUD study investigates whether an assisted bicycle training is beneficial and does not cause any harm for boys with DMD. Motor-assistance allowed cycling with the legs and arms (arm cranking) even when muscle strength was insufficient to achieve fully active movements. In another part of the study, the effect of an arm training with arm support is investigated. Both ambulatory and wheelchair-dependent children participate in this study. Preliminary data show that assisted training is effective in boys with DMD in maintaining functional capacities.

2.1.3 Training mechanisms

The mechanism by which training could oppose the physical deterioration in children with a muscular dystrophy is still unclear. Muscle fibers in muscular dystrophy patients are abnormally vulnerable to contraction-induced injury due to the absence, or lack, of mechanical reinforcement of the sarcolemmal membrane(Petrof 1998). Eccentric exercises should therefore be avoided(Lim et al 2004). Conversely, a recently published review by Markert et al. (2011) described that enhancing myofiber repair, decreasing muscle fibrosis and the production of antioxidants against oxidative damage are potential explainable factors for exercise-induced improvements(Markert et al. 2011). Work-induced damage could enhance muscle regeneration and repair(Okano et al. 2005), and low-stress exercise may produce beneficial effects on myofiber contractility and energetic efficiency(Petrof 1998).

2.1.4 International training guidelines

International training guidelines for children with a muscular dystrophy are preferably disease-specific and should be adapted to the individual child(Edouard et al. 2007). Based on the currently available evidence, guidelines for ambulatory boys with DMD recommend voluntary active exercises (such as swimming) and to avoid eccentric exercises(Eagle 2002). For wheelchair-dependent children, passive or actively-assisted mobilizing exercises to maintain comfort and symmetry are advised(Eagle 2002). A cardiomyopathy could be a contraindication to participate in any physical training programs(Edouard et al. 2007). It is suggested that the training intensity could be based on children's perceived exertion instead of maximum heart rate when performance is predominantly limited by the peripheral capacity instead of the oxygen transport(Jansen et al. 2010).

To conclude, physical training could delay the physical deterioration as a result of disuse in children with a muscular dystrophy. Disuse enhances the loss of functional abilities, whereas physical training could be beneficial. Currently available evidence is limited to uncontrolled clinical trials and further research is required to develop specific training prescriptions. At this moment, international guidelines recommend voluntary (dynamic) exercises to maintain comfort and symmetry, and to avoid eccentric exercises.

2.2 Training and fatigue in adult muscular dystrophies

2.2.1 Physical exercise

In a study by McDonald the three problems most frequently cited as "very significant" by patients with slowly progressive neuromuscular disease were muscle weakness (57%), difficulty exercising (43%) and fatigue (40%) {McDonald 2002}. Two main types of fatigue can be distinguished. Physiological fatigue, or muscle fatigue, has been defined as a reduction in maximal voluntary muscle force (MVC) during exercise. Experienced fatigue, on the other hand, is the subjective feeling of fatigue. Muscle fatigue is not necessarily accompanied by experienced fatigue, or vice versa. Distinguishing experienced fatigue from muscle weakness, the key feature in muscular dystrophy, may be difficult. In a study by Kalkman 61% of patients with facioscapulohumeral dystrophy (FSHD) (n = 139) and 74% of patients with myotonic dystrophy (MD) (n = 322) were "severely fatigued" {Kalkman et al, 2005 }. Patients with MD had higher scores for experienced fatigue, reported greater problems with concentration and had more difficulties with initiative and planning than patients with FSHD. In FSHD patients and MD patients, social functioning was related to fatigue severity. Apparently, fatigue is not only a frequent, but also a relevant problem in muscular dystrophy. In a subsequent longitudinal study Kalkman built a model of perpetuating factors, which contribute to the continuation of experienced fatigue {Kalkman et al, 2007 }. In FSHD, the level of physical (in)activity has a central place in the model. Due to fatigue, patients often alter their lifestyles and reduce their activities. Low physical activity levels may lead to even greater weakness and atrophy of skeletal muscles, which causes a vicious circle of disuse and weakness. Physical inactivity in turn can lead to chronic cardiovascular and muscle deconditioning and increased cardiovascular health risks {McDonald, 2002 }. In addition, pain complaints influence levels of experienced fatigue both directly and indirectly by decreasing physical activity (see figure below). In MD, physical activity and pain did not significantly contribute to experienced fatigue. Yet, sleep disturbances lead to higher levels of experienced fatigue in both FSHD and MD patients. The observed patterns of perpetuating factors can be used as a basis to develop evidence-based interventions to reduce fatigue. Specific attention should be paid to sleep disturbances in both patient groups. Specifically in FSHD, treatment of fatigue should also be directed at increasing physical activity and reducing pain complaints. Irrespective of its cause, physical inactivity should be discouraged in muscular dystrophy patients because of an increasing risk of cardiovascular disease and muscle deconditioning.

In the past, many patients with muscular dystrophy were advised not to exercise because of the belief that too much exercise might lead to overuse weakness {Johnson, 1971;Johnson, 1971;Carter, 1995;Fowler, 1984;Petrof, 1998}. Yet, in their Cochrane review on muscle strength training and aerobic exercise training for patients with muscle diseases, Voet concluded that moderate-intensity strength training in MD and FSHD appeared not to be harmful, although there was insufficient evidence to establish its benefit {Voet et al , 2010}. This conclusion was based on merely two randomised clinical trials {Lindeman et al , 1995;van der Kooi et al, 2004}. For this reason, Cup reviewed not only randomised clinical trials, but also controlled clinical trials and other designs of sufficient quality {Cup et al, 2007}. All types of exercise therapy and other physical therapy modalities were included for patients with muscular dystrophy, among which were patients with FSHD, LGMD, MD and DMD. Cup *et al.* also concluded that exercise training is not harmful in muscular dystrophies. However, based on the reviewed studies, there was insufficient evidence for the effectiveness of muscle strengthening exercises, although there were some indications that aerobic exercises may have a positive effect on body functions, as well as on activities and participation. Because of the weakness of the muscle membrane there is concern about the potentially damaging effects of eccentric and high-intensity muscle contractions during strength training. In animal models of muscular dystrophy, there is evidence that eccentric contractions, known to stress muscle fibers, cause greater cell injury to these dystrophic muscle fibers. Although transferring results from animal studies to humans must be done with caution, eccentric training studies in muscular dystrophy patients are so far being avoided.

To conclude, although the current scientific evidence is scarce, aerobic exercise training appears not to be harmful in muscular dystrophies and could have a positive effect on functioning, activities and participation, but the number of high-quality studies is low. When prescribing exercise training, the recommendations from the ACSM Position Stand can be used as requirements to achieve an effective, safe and individualised exercise prescription {1998}.

2.2.2 Alternative training

Muscular dystrophies have a large impact on psychosocial functioning as patients must continuously adapt to their progressive illness. Illness cognitions and coping styles influence the level of physical activity and, consequently, experienced fatigue and health status. Hence, changing illness cognitions and coping style may lead to a better quality of life. A cognitive behaviour approach has been proven successful in the chronic fatigue syndrome {Prins et al, 2001;Chambers et al, 2006} and for post-cancer fatigue {Gielissen et al, 2007;Gielissen et al, 2006} and may be effective in patients with muscular dystrophy as well.

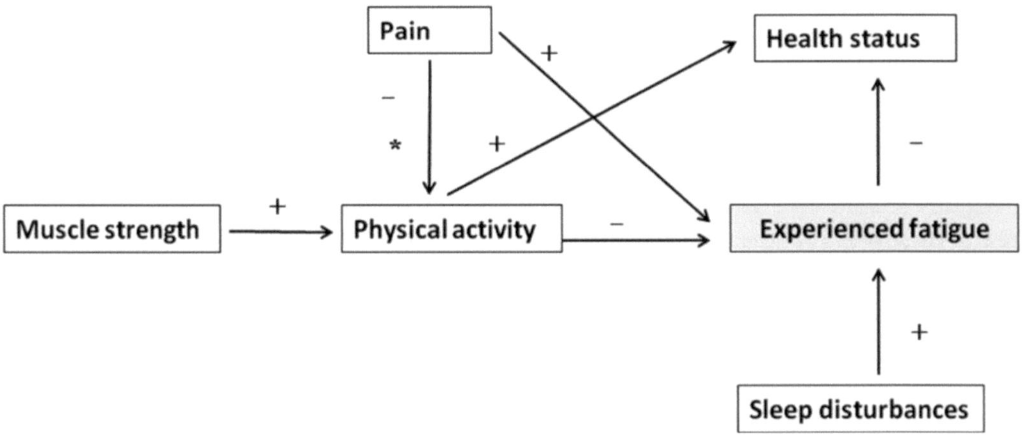

Fig. 1. Cognitive behaviour therapy in FSHD should, for instance, be focused on the known perpetuating factors of experienced fatigue as described by Kalkman i.e. sleep disturbances, pain complaints and physical inactivity (Della et al. 49-53;Kalkman et al. 571-79). Therapy should be adapted to the life of each individual, resulting in an individualised treatment approach. Altogether, cognitive behaviour therapy seems a rational, promising treatment for fatigue in muscular dystrophies.

3. Feeding problems and dysphagia

3.1 Swallowing

Swallowing is a complex sensorimotor process that depends on information from multiple levels of the central and peripheral nervous system. Descending excitatory and inhibitory signals from the cortex and subcortex and ascending signals from the oropharyngeal area trigger the central pattern generator (CPG) in the bulbar reticular formation (Jean 2001, Leopold 2010). This network of premotor neurons and interneurons drives the motor neurons of swallowing in cranial nerves (CN) V, VII, IX, X and XII. Muscles of lips, submental muscle group, tongue, palate, larynx, pharynx and esophagus, innervated by these CNs, are excited and inhibited sequentially, when a person forms a bolus and swallows (Ertekin 2003). The oral phase and the initiation of the pharyngeal phase are under voluntary neural control, whereas the completion of the pharyngeal phase and the esophageal phase are under involuntary neural control (Miller 2008). In dysphagia, problems may occur in the oral, pharyngeal, esophageal phase, or in more than one phase (Arvedson 2008). In children with neurologic etiologies from different origins, dysphagia is often reported with variable signs and symptoms. The dysphagia of children with CP is characterized by oral motor problems and frequent aspiration of thin liquid with no observable response (silent aspiration) (Rogers 1994). In neuromuscular disorders (NMD), weakness of the muscles is due to damage along the course of the peripheral nerve (lower motor neuron) or the muscle itself (Dubowitz 2000). Feeding and swallowing problems are not uncommon in muscular dystrophies, which can lead to dehydration, malnutrition or aspiration pneumonia.In patients with chronic muscle disease a prevalence of 35% of feeding problems and dysphagia was reported (Kumin 1994).

3.2 Problems in the oral phase

In NMD chewing problems and the need to multiple swallows to clear the oral cavity (piecemeal deglutition) are the main problems in the oral phase of swallowing. Reduced bite force and weakness of the masticatory muscles (Morel-Verdebout 2007) causes chewing problems and the inability to eat solid or firm food. The reduced range of mandibular motion, reported in SMA type II (Van Bruggen 2011) and DMD (Botteron 2009) may reduce the quality of chewing and results in a hampered food comminution, inadequate food bolus formation, and oral transport. Moreover, the limited mandibular range of motion has an impact on oral hygiene and dental care. Facial muscle weakness can lead to craniofacial and dental malocclusion (Kumin 1994; Pane 2006) which aggravates the chewing problems.

Reduced strength of the tongue muscles causes piecemeal deglutition, especially with thick liquid and solid food (van den Engel-Hoek 2009). This results in prolonged oral transit time and oral residue after swallowing.

3.3 Problems in the pharyngeal phase

The initiation of the pharyngeal phase is typically normal in patients with NMD, but problems with solid food and residue after swallow are reported in patients with SMA type II (van den Engel-Hoek 2009), DMD (Aloysius 2008;Shinonaga 2008), in MD (Leonard 2001) and congenital myopathies (Mehta 2006;de Swart 2002). In all patient groups the problems occurred more in advanced stages. Dysphagia and feeding problems were also reported in nemaline myopathy, but more in the neonatal period and infancy than in adults (Bagnall 2006). Residue after swallow is caused a combination of reduced strength of the tongue and submental muscle group, and reduced opening of the upper esophageal sphincter. In patients with oculopharyngeal muscular dystrophy (OPMD) the dysphagia was aggravated by the retroflexion of the head, caused by ptosis (de Swart 2002). In patients with SMA II a retracted position of the head, due to a lumbar lordosis and a diminished head balance, caused reduced movement of the submental muscle group resulting in more post swallow residue with thick liquid and solid food than with thin liquid. The post swallow residue places patients at risk for aspiration the airway reopens (Arvedson 1998)

3.4 Swallowing assessments

A videofluroscopic swallow study (VFSS) is generally considered as the gold standard method for diagnosing dysphagia in adults (Logemann 2000) and children (Hiorns 2006), especially to detect aspiration. However, a VFSS was not considered as additional benefit to a careful feeding history in patients with DMD (Aloysius 2008). Other assessments are available to describe oral structures and biomechanical oral functions needed for feeding and swallowing to better understand the nature and clinical course of dysphagia in NMD. Surface EMG (sEMG) of the submental muscle group, tongue pressure, ultrasonographic and manometric assessments during swallowing can be used to understand the nature and clinical course of dysphagia in NMD.

Patients are not always mentioning swallowing difficulties (Leonard 2001;Stubgen 2008). They should also always be carefully interviewed for symptoms of swallowing difficulties that may require a swallowing assessment and a careful observation of oral motor abilities during mealtime (Messina 2008; Manzur 2008).

3.5 Recommendations

To improve their quality of life and nutritional state, NMD patients with swallowing difficulties benefit from dietetic and swallowing recommendations. This can be nutritional, related to consistencies, safe swallowing techniques or advices about postural management and feeding aids . The dysphagia in NMD show different patterns in flaccid bulbar paresis like NMD than in neuromuscular disorders. In contrast to the usual advice for thickening the food, in NMD more liquid food is advised or alternating thick with thin consistencies. Strategies are recommended to reduce problems in chewing and oral and pharyngeal post swallow residue. Careful chewing and bolus preparation to a liquid consistency, effortful swallowing and double swallows can reduce problems of reduced pharyngeal clearing. In case of post swallow residue it is also advised to clear the oral and pharyngeal cavity with water after mealtime. Positioning of the head in sitting position can also be important to prevent residue. In case of a retracted head position, like in SMA II (van den Engel 2009) a more flexed head position prevented laryngeal post swallow residue. Also in patients with OPMD a slightly flexed head improved swallowing (de Swart 2002).

4. Gastrointestinal problems

If swallowing and chewing gets more difficult, eating takes too much time or energy, enteral tube feeding is a possibility. The percutaneous gastrostomy is quite regular, although there are also complications described during (re)placement. In myotonic dystrophy impairment of gastrointestinal motility is known and seems to be gradual worsening(Bellini et al 2006), probably related to gastrointestinal symptoms like regurgitation, dyspepsia, abodominal pain, bloating, and changes in bowl habits. Although there is only a low correlation between the degree of skeletal muscle involvement and the presence and severity of gastrointestinal disturbances it is a positive correlation (Bellini et al 2006). Also in boys with Duchenne and Becker muscular dystrophy abnormalities in gastric motility are seen and the possibility of progressive failure in neuromuscular function is put forward (Borelli et al 2005). Promotility agents are advised as are good diet, stool softeners, and hydration (Bellini et al 2006, Wagner et al 2007). There is little evidence on the benefits of exercise and chronic constipation (Leung et al 2011), but practical experience often reported is that doing exercise or standing in a standing table or frame does seem to help. This would be in line with the former recommendations for exercise.

5. Urogenital problems in muscular dystrophies

Lower urinary tract symptoms are described in boys with Duchenne muscular dystrophy and seem not to be rare (van Wijk et al 2009). Nearly 85 % of the boys/men with Duchenne muscular dystrophy reported lower urinary tract symptoms, and 51 % had more than 3 problems. The main problems were post micturation dribble, straining, (urge) incontinence, and feeling of incomplete emptying. There is a very low correlation between age and functional abilities and lower urinary tract problems; these problems seem not to worsen with disease progression. In 42 % the boys/men mentioned that the complaints influenced their social life, and 25 % reported a decrease in quality of life. Also in myotonic dystrophy urinary tract symptoms are reported but only anecdotal. This is probably an underreported symptom and should have attention in the management.

It is recommended to ask for lower urinary tract symptoms, use a micturation questionnaire if there are concerns, and register for several days the pattern. Up till now no pathophysiological studies are available, the possibility of a bladder-sphincter dys-synergy is suggested, and the symptoms are treated symptomatically by medication.

6. Technical possibilities

New very sophisticated devices are being developed like exoskeletons, robot arms and motion controlled orthoses (see for example websites of www.Flextension.nl and www.FocalMeditech.nl). Not only can these devices support a natural function, but they can also simulate a natural movement. It is possible that with an exoskeleton a person with severe paresis can still move in a rather natural way. In an earlier stage these devices can also be used for assisted training and it is theoretically possible that by regular use one can prevent contractures. Robotica can potentially reduce the extent of personal help needed, thus making an adjusted independent life possible and making participation in social life possible.

7. References

1998, American College of Sports Medicine Position Stand. The recommended quantity and quality of exercise for developing and maintaining cardiorespiratory and muscular fitness, and flexibility in healthy adults: Med.Sci.Sports Exerc., v. 30, no. 6, p. 975-991.

Aloysius A., P. Born, M. Kinali, T. Davis, M. Pane, E. Mercuri, 2008, Swallowing difficulties in Duchenne muscular dystrophy: indications for feeding assessment and outcome of videofluroscopic swallow studies, Eur. J. Paediatr. Neurol., v.12, n. 3, p. 239-45.

Arvedson J.C., M.A. Lefton-Greif, 1998, Pediatric videofluoroscopic swallow studies: a professional manual with caregiver guidelines, San Antonio, Texas: Communication Skill Builders, Psychological Corporation.

Arvedson J.C., 2008, Assessment of pediatric dysphagia and feeding disorders: clinical and instrumental approaches. Dev Disabil Res Rev, v. 12, no. 2, p. 118-27.

Bagnall A.K., M.A. Al-Mahaizea, A.Y. Manzur, 2006, Feeding and speech difficulties in typical congenital Nemaline myopathy, Advances in Speech-Language Pathology, v. 8, n. 1, p. 7-16.

Bellini M., S. Biagi, C. Stasi, F. Costa, M.G. Mumolo, A. Ricchiutti, S. Marchi, 2006, Gastrointestinal manifestations in myotonic dystrophy, World J Gastroenterol v. 28, n.12, p.1821-1828

Borrelli O., G. Salvi, V. Mancini, L. Santoro, F. Tagliente, E.F. Romeo, S. Cucchiara, 2005, Evolution of gastric electrical features and gastric emptying in children with Duchenne and Becker Muscular Dystrophy, Am.J.Gastroenterol, v. 100, p. 695-702

Botteron S., C.M. Verbout, P.Y. Jeannet, S. Kiliaridis, 2009, Orofacial dysfunction in Duchenne muscular dystrophy, Arch. Oral. Biol., v. 54, n. 1, p. 26-31

Carter, G. T., M. A. Wineinger, S. A. Walsh, S. J. Horasek, R. T. Abresch, and W. M. Fowler, Jr., 1995, Effect of voluntary wheel-running exercise on muscles of the mdx mouse: Neuromuscul.Disord., v. 5, no. 4, p. 323-332.

Chambers, D., A. M. Bagnall, S. Hempel, and C. Forbes, 2006, Interventions for the treatment, management and rehabilitation of patients with chronic fatigue syndrome/myalgic encephalomyelitis: an updated systematic review: J.R.Soc.Med., v. 99, no. 10, p. 506-520.

Cup, E. H., A. J. Pieterse, J. M. Ten Broek-Pastoor, M. Munneke, B. G. van Engelen, H. T. Hendricks, G. J. van der Wilt, and R. A. Oostendorp, 2007, Exercise therapy and other types of physical therapy for patients with neuromuscular diseases: a systematic review: Arch.Phys.Med.Rehabil., v. 88, no. 11, p. 1452-1464.

De Lateur B.J., R.M. Giaconi. 1979. Effect on maximal strength of submaxiaml exercise in Duchenne muscular dystrophy. Am J Phys Med 58 (1): 26-36

Della, M. G. et al., 2007, Sleep quality in Facioscapulohumeral muscular dystrophy: J.Neurol.Sci., v. 263, no. 1-2, p. 49-53.

De Swart B.J., G. W. Padberg, B.G. van Engelen, 2002, Less is more: treatment of aggravating behaviour in myasthenia gravis patients with dysphagia, Eur. J. Neurol., v. 9, n. 6, p. 688-9.

Dubowitz V., 2000, Muscle disorders in childhood. London: W.B.Saunders Company LTD.

Dupont-Versteegden E.E., R.J. McCarter, M.S. Katz. 1994. Voluntary exercise decreases progression of muscular dystrophy in diaphragm of mdx mice. J Appl Physiol 77 (4): 1736-41

Eagle M. 2002. Report on the muscular dystrophy campaign workshop: exercise in neuromuscular diseases. Neuromuscul Disord 12 (10): 975-83

Edouard P, et a;. 2007. Training programs for children: literature review. Ann Readapt Med Phys 50 (6): 510-09.

Ertekin C, I. Aydogdu, 2003, Neurophysiology of swallowing, Clin Neurophysio, v. 114, no. 12, p. 2226-44

Fowler, W. M., Jr., 1984, Importance of overwork weakness: Muscle Nerve, v. 7, no. 6, p. 496-499.

Gielissen, M. F., C. A. Verhagen, and G. Bleijenberg, 2007, Cognitive behaviour therapy for fatigued cancer survivors: long-term follow-up: Br.J.Cancer, v. 97, no. 5, p. 612-618.

Gielissen, M. F., S. Verhagen, F. Witjes, and G. Bleijenberg, 2006, Effects of cognitive behavior therapy in severely fatigued disease-free cancer patients compared with patients waiting for cognitive behavior therapy: a randomized controlled trial: J.Clin.Oncol., v. 24, no. 30, p. 4882-4887.

Hayes A, D.A. Williams. 1996. Beneficial effects of voluntary wheel running on the properties of dystrophic mouse muscle. J Appl Physiol 80 (2): 670-79

Hayes A et al 1998. Contractile function and low-intensity exercise effects of old dystrophic (mdx) mice. Am J Physiol 274 (4): C1138-C1144.

Hiorns M.P., M.M. Ryan, 2006, Current practice in paediatric videofluoroscopy, Pediatr. Radiol., v. 36, n. 9, p. 911-9.

Janssen M. I.J.M. de Groot, N. van Alfen, A.C.H. Geurts. 2010 Physical training in boys with Duchenne Muscular Dystrophy: the protocol of the No Use is Disuse study. BMC Pediatr. 10: 55

Jean A, 2001, Brain stem control of swallowing: neuronal network and cellular mechanisms, Physiol. Rev., v 81, no 2, p. 929-69

Johnson, E. W., and R. Braddom, 1971, Over-work weakness in facioscapulohuumeral muscular dystrophy: Arch.Phys.Med.Rehabil., v. 52, no. 7, p. 333-336.

Kalkman, J. S., M. L. Schillings, S. P. van der Werf, G. W. Padberg, M. J. Zwarts, B. G. van Engelen, and G. Bleijenberg, 2005, Experienced fatigue in facioscapulohumeral dystrophy, myotonic dystrophy, and HMSN-I: J.Neurol.Neurosurg.Psychiatry, v. 76, no. 10, p. 1406-1409.

Kalkman, J. S., M. L. Schillings, M. J. Zwarts, B. G. van Engelen, and G. Bleijenberg, 2007, The development of a model of fatigue in neuromuscular disorders: a longitudinal study: J.Psychosom.Res., v. 62, no. 5, p. 571-579.

Kumin L., 1994, Intelligibility of speech in children with Down syndrome in natural settings: parents' perspective, Percept Mot Skills, v.78, n. 1, p. 307-13

Leopold N.A, S.K. Daniels, 2010, Supranuclear control of swallowing., Dyspahgia, v. 25, no. 3, p. 250-7.

Leonard R.J., K.A. Kendall, R. Johnson, S. McKenzie, 2001, Swallowing in myotonic muscular dystrophy: a videofluoroscopic study, Arch. Phys. Med. Rehabil., v. 82, n. 7, p. 979-85.

Leung L., T. Riutta, J. Kotecha, W. Rosser, 2011, Chronic constipation: an evidence-based review, J.Am.Board Fa,. Med., v. 24, no.4, p. 436-451

Lim, J.H., D.Y Kim, M.S. Bang, 2004, Effects of exercise and steroid on skeletal muscle apoptosis in the mdx mouse. Muscle Nerve 30, no 4, p 456-62

Lindeman, E., P. Leffers, F. Spaans, J. Drukker, J. Reulen, M. Kerckhoffs, and A. Koke, 1995, Strength training in patients with myotonic dystrophy and hereditary motor and sensory neuropathy: a randomized clinical trial: Arch.Phys.Med.Rehabil., v. 76, no. 7, p. 612-620.

Logemann J.A., B.R. Pauloski, A.W. Rademaker, L.A. Colangelo, P.J. Kahrilas, C.H. Smith, 2000, Temporal and biomechanical characteristics of oropharyngeal swallow in younger and older men, J. Speech Lang. Hear. Res., v, 43, n. 5, p. 1264-74.

Manzur A.Y., M. Kinali, F. Muntoni, 2008, Update on the management of Duchenne muscular dystrophy, Arch. Dis. Child., v.93, n. 11, p. 986-90.

Markert, C.D. et al , 2011Exercise and Duchenne muscular dystrophy: toward evidence-based exercise prescription, Muscle Nerve 43, no 4, p 464-78

McDonald, C.M., et al , 1995, Profiles on neuromuscular diseases. Duchenne muscular dystrophy. Am. J. Phys Med. Rehabil. 74, no 5 suppl, p S70-92

McDonald, C. M., 2002, Physical activity, health impairments, and disability in neuromuscular disease: Am.J.Phys.Med.Rehabil., v. 81, no. 11 Suppl, p. S108-S120.

Mehta S.G., G. D. Watts, B. McGillivray, S. Mumm, S.J. Hamilton, S. Ramdeen, D. Novack, C. Briggs, M.P. Whyte, V.E. Kimonis, 2006, Manifestations in a family with autosomal dominant bone fragility and limb-girdle myopathy, Am. J. Med. Genet., v. 140, n. 4, p. 322-30.

Messina S., M. Pane, P.D. Rose, I. Vasta, D. Sorleti, A.Aloysius, F. Sciarra, F. Mangiola, M. Kinali, E. Bertini, E. Mercuri, 2008, Feeding problems and malnutrition in spinal muscular atrophy type II, Neuromuscul. Disord., v. 18, n.5, p. 389-93.

Miller A.J., 2008, The neurobiology of swallowing and dysphagia. Dev Disabil Res Rev, v. 14, no. 2, p. 77-86.

Morel-Verdebout c., S. Botteron, S. Killiaridis, 2007, Dentofacial characteristics of growing patients with Duchenne muscular dystrophy: a morphological study, Eur. J. Orthod., v. 29, n. 5, p. 500-7.

Okano, T, et al , 2005, Chronic exercise accelerates the degeneration-regeneration cycle and down regulates insulin-like growth factor-1 in muscle of mdx mice. Muscle Nerver 32, no 2, p 1991-99.

Pane M., I. Vaste, S. Messina, D. Sorletti, A. Aloysius, F. Sciarra, F. Mangiola, M. Kinali, E. Ricci, E. Mercuri, 2006, Feeding problems and weight gain in Duchenne muscular dystrophy, Eur. J. Paediatr. Neurol., v. 10, n. 5-6, p. 231-6.

Petrof, B. J., 1998, The molecular basis of activity-induced muscle injury in Duchenne muscular dystrophy: Mol.Cell Biochem., v. 179, no. 1-2, p. 111-123.

Prins, J. B., G. Bleijenberg, E. Bazelmans, L. D. Elving, T. M. de Boo, J. L. Severens, G. J. van der Wilt, P. Spinhoven, and J. W. van der Meer, 2001, Cognitive behaviour therapy for chronic fatigue syndrome: a multicentre randomised controlled trial: Lancet, v. 357, no. 9259, p. 841-847.

Rogers B, J. Arvedson, G. Buck, P. Smart, M. Msall, 1994, Characteristics of dysphagia in children with cerebral palsy, Dysphagia, v. 9, n.1, p. 69-73.

Scott, O. M., et al. , 1981, Effect of exercise in Duchenne muscular dystrophy, Physiotherapy, 67, no 6, p174-76.

Shinonaga C., M. Fukuda, Y. Suzuki, T. Higaki, Y. Ischida, E. Ischii, M. Hyodo, T. Morimoto, N. Sano, 2008, Evaluations of swallowing function in Duchenne muscular dystrophy, Dev. Med. Child Neurol., v. 50, n. 6, p. 478-80.

Stubgen J.P., 2008, Facioscapulohumeral muscular dystrophy: a radiologic and manometric study of the pharynz and esophagus, Dysphagia, v. 23, n. 4, p. 341-7.

Sveen, M.L. et al ,2008, Endurance training improves fitness and strength in patients with Becker muscular dystrophy, Brain, 131, pt 11, p 2824-31.

Van Bruggen H.W., L. van den Engel-Hoek, W.L. van der Pol, A. de Weier, I.J.M. de Groot, M.H. Steenks, 2011, Impaired mandibular function in Spinal Muscular Atrophy type II: need for early recognition, J. Child Neurol., e-pud ahead

van den Engel-Hoek L., C.E. .Erasmus, H.W. van Bruggen, B.J.M. de Swart,L.T. Sie, M.H. Steenks, I.J.M. de Groot IJM, 2009, Dysphagia in spinal muscular atrophy type II, more than a bulbar problem?, Neurology; v. 73, p.1787-1791

van der Kooi, E. L., O. J. Vogels, R. J. van Asseldonk, E. Lindeman, J. C. Hendriks, M. Wohlgemuth, S. M. van der Maarel, and G. W. Padberg, 2004, Strength training and albuterol in facioscapulohumeral muscular dystrophy: Neurology, v. 63, no. 4, p. 702-708.

Van Wijk E., B.J. Messelink, L. Heijnen, I.J.M. de Groot, 2009, Prevalence and psychosocial impact of lower urinary tract symptoms in patients with Duchenne muscular dystrophy, Neuromusc.Disord, v. 19, p.754-758

Vestergaard, P, et al , 2001, Fracture risk in patients with muscular dystrophy and spinal muscular atrophy, J. Rehabil. Med, 33, no 4, p. 150-55

Vignos P.J., M.P. Watkins, 1966, The effect of exercise in muscular dystrophy, JAMA, 197, no 11, p. 843-48

Voet, N. B., E. L. van der Kooi, I. I. Riphagen, E. Lindeman, B. G. van Engelen, and A. C. Geurts, 2010, Strength training and aerobic exercise training for muscle disease: Cochrane.Database.Syst.Rev., no. 1, p. CD003907.

Wagner K.R., N. Lechtzin, D.P. Judge, 2007, Current treatment of adult Duchenne muscular dystrophy, Bioch.Biophys.Acta, v. 1772, p.229-237

13

Database of Wards for Patients with Muscular Dystrophy in Japan

Toshio Saito[1] and Katsunori Tatara[2]
[1]*Division of Neurology, National Hospital Organization Toneyama National Hospital,*
[2]*Division of Pediatrics, National Hospital Organization Tokushima National Hospital,*
Japan

1. Introduction

Twenty-seven hospitals in Japan specialize in treatment of muscular dystrophy patients, including inpatient care, of which 26 belong to the National Hospital Organization, and the other is the National Center of Neurology and Psychiatry. Since 1999, Japanese muscular dystrophy research groups investigating nervous and mental disorder have been developing a database of cases treated at these 27 institutions. In that regard, we conducted a survey of inpatients with muscular dystrophy and other neuromuscular disorders based on data collected by the National Hospital Organization and National Center of Neurology and Psychiatry. Herein, we examined data obtained between 1999 and 2010 in order to evaluate the medical condition of inpatients with muscular dystrophy in Japan.

2. Subjects and methods

The database includes numbers of inpatients, gender, age, diagnosis, respiratory condition, nutritional state, number of death cases, causes of death, and other relevant findings from data collected annually on October 1 every year since 1999. We examined these data using longitudinal and horizontal analyses.

3. Sequential changes in total numbers of inpatients treated at muscular dystrophy wards of National Hospital Organization and National Center of Neurology and Psychiatry

The total numbers of inpatients treated at the muscular dystrophy wards of the National Hospital Organization and National Center of Neurology and Psychiatry were quite consistent during the examination period. The lowest number of inpatients was 2066 in 2007 and the highest was 2193 in 2003 (Fig. 1).

3.1 Details regarding number of inpatients

The number of inpatients with Duchenne muscular dystrophy gradually decreased (882~770) every year (Fig. 2), whereas that of those with myotonic dystrophy gradually increased (327~411) (Fig. 3). The numbers of inpatients with other types of muscular dystrophy, such

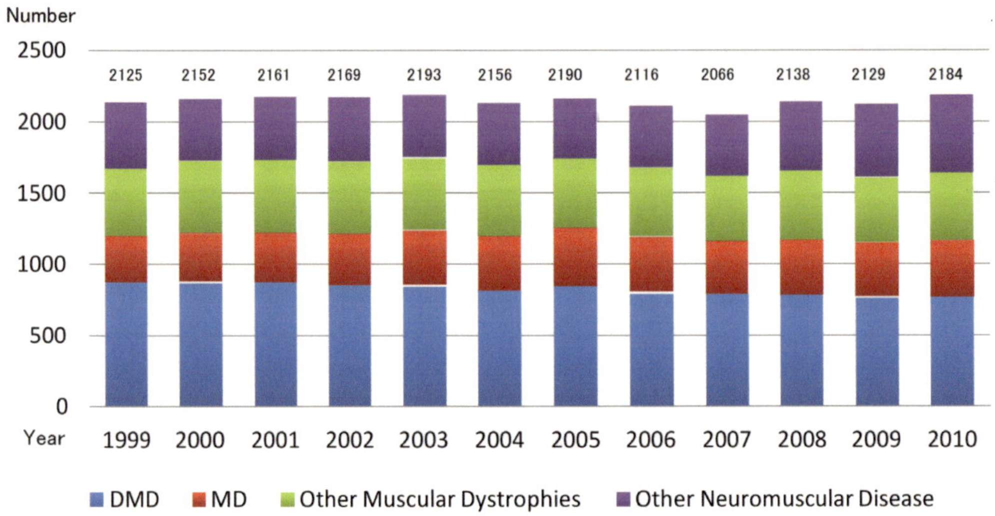

"Other muscular dystrophies" includes Becker muscular dystrophy, Fukuyama congenital muscular dystrophy, limb-girdle muscular dystrophy, facio-scapulo-humeral muscular dystrophy, Ullrich muscular dystrophy, and others.
"Other neuromuscular disease" includes amyotrophic lateral sclerosis, spinal muscular atrophy, hereditary sensory motor neuropathy, congenital myopathy, and others.
DMD, Duchenne muscular dystrophy; MD, myotonic dystrophy

Fig. 1. Total numbers of inpatients in muscular dystrophy wards of National Hospital Organization and National Center of Neurology and Psychiatry.

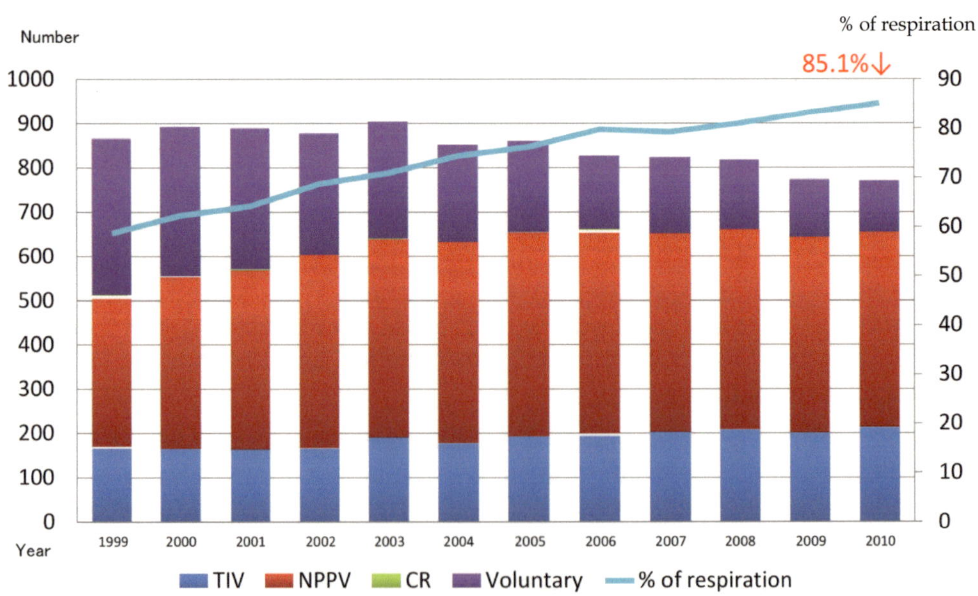

The number with Duchenne muscular dystrophy has gradually decreased every year.
TIV,tracheostomy intermittent ventilation; NPPV, non-invasive positive pressure ventilation

Fig. 2. Sequential changes in number of inpatients with Duchenne muscular dystrophy and rate of mechanical ventilation dependence.

as Becker muscular dystrophy (94~105), Fukuyama congenital muscular dystrophy (50~64), limb-girdle type muscular dystrophy (185~216), and facio-scapulo-humeral muscular dystrophy (64~72) showed some fluctuations. Inpatients with spinal muscular atrophy showed a gradual decreasing tendency from 73 in 1999 to 56 in 2010, while those with amyotrophic lateral sclerosis increased every year from 29 to 132 (Fig. 4). Other diseases encountered in these patients included congenital metabolic disease, mitochondrial disease, various types of myopathy, peripheral nerve disease, bone disease, chromosomal abnormalities, spinocerebellar ataxia, neonatal period disease sequelae, infectious diseases, and others, though their numbers were small and equalled around 10% of all diseases.

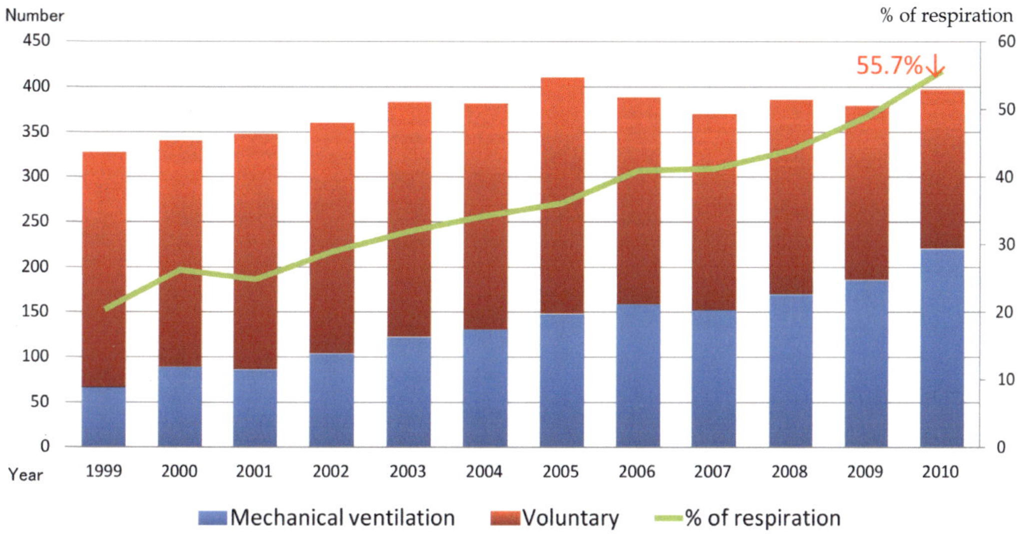

The number with myotonic dystrophy has gradually increased every year.

Fig. 3. Sequential changes in number of inpatients with myotonic dystrophy and rate of mechanical ventilation dependence.

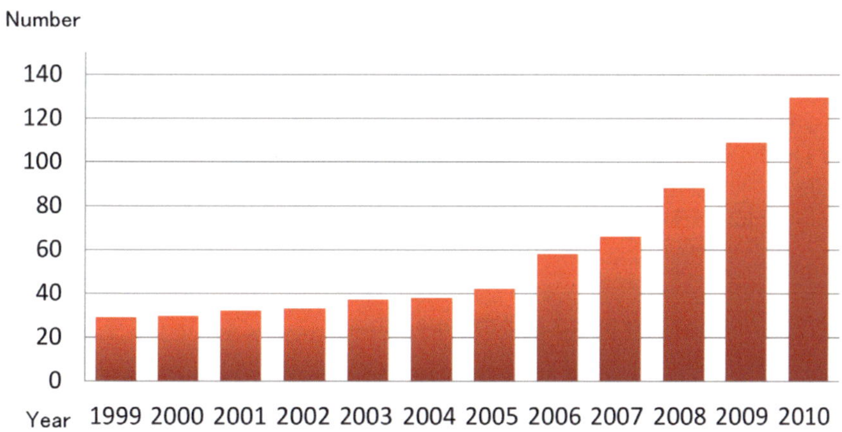

The number with amyotrophic lateral sclerosis has gradually increased every year.

Fig. 4. Sequential changes in number of inpatients with amyotrophic lateral sclerosis.

3.2 Sequential changes in respiratory care for inpatients and rate of mechanical ventilation dependence

The rate of mechanical ventilation use in 1999 was 37.9%, which gradually increased to 62.9% in 2010 (Fig. 5), while that for Duchenne muscular dystrophy patients in 1999 was 58.7% and gradually increased to 85.1% in 2010 (Fig. 2). Although the total number of inpatients with Duchenne muscular dystrophy gradually decreased, cases of non-invasive ventilation gradually increased and tracheostomy cases were also slightly increased. The rate of mechanical ventilation use for myotonic dystrophy patients in 1999 was 20.3%, which gradually increased to 55.7% in 2010 (Fig. 3).

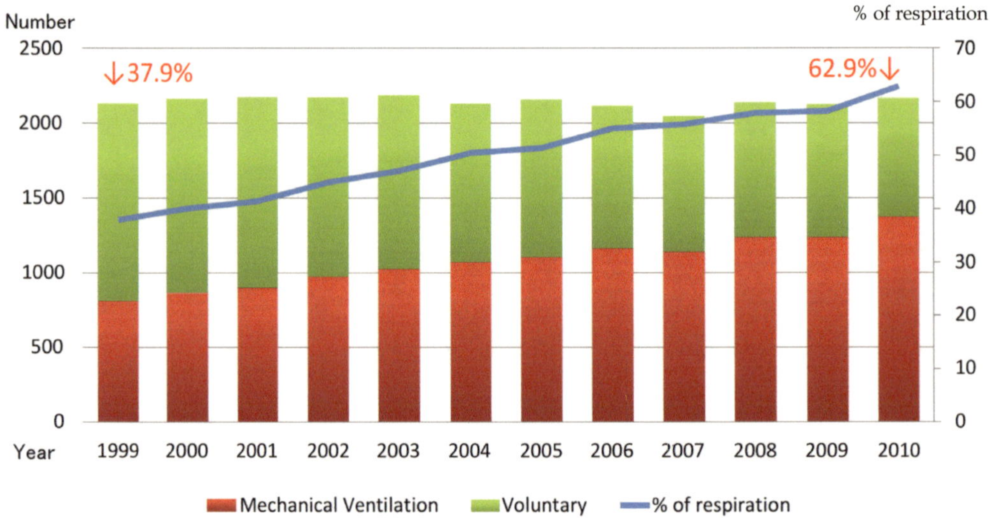

The rate of mechanical ventilation use in 1999 was 37.9%, which gradually increased to 62.9% in 2010.

Fig. 5. Sequential changes in respiratory care for inpatients and rate of mechanical ventilation dependence.

3.3 Analysis of mean age of inpatients

3.3.1 Changes in age distribution of inpatients in muscular dystrophy wards

The age distribution of inpatients in muscular dystrophy wards in 1999 showed 2 peaks. Those with Duchenne muscular dystrophy largely constituted the younger age peak in the 20s, while those with myotonic dystrophy larger constituted the older age peak in the 50s. These age peaks shifted to a higher range and became slightly flattened in 2009 (Fig. 6).

3.3.2 Sequential changes in mean age of inpatients

The mean age of the inpatients in 1999 was 36.6 years old, which gradually increased to 45.3 years old in 2010. That of Duchenne muscular dystrophy patients in 1999 was 23.6 years old, which gradually increased to 29.4 years old in 2010, while that of myotonic dystrophy patients changed only slightly from 51.4 years old in 1999 to 53.6 years old in 2010 (Fig. 7).

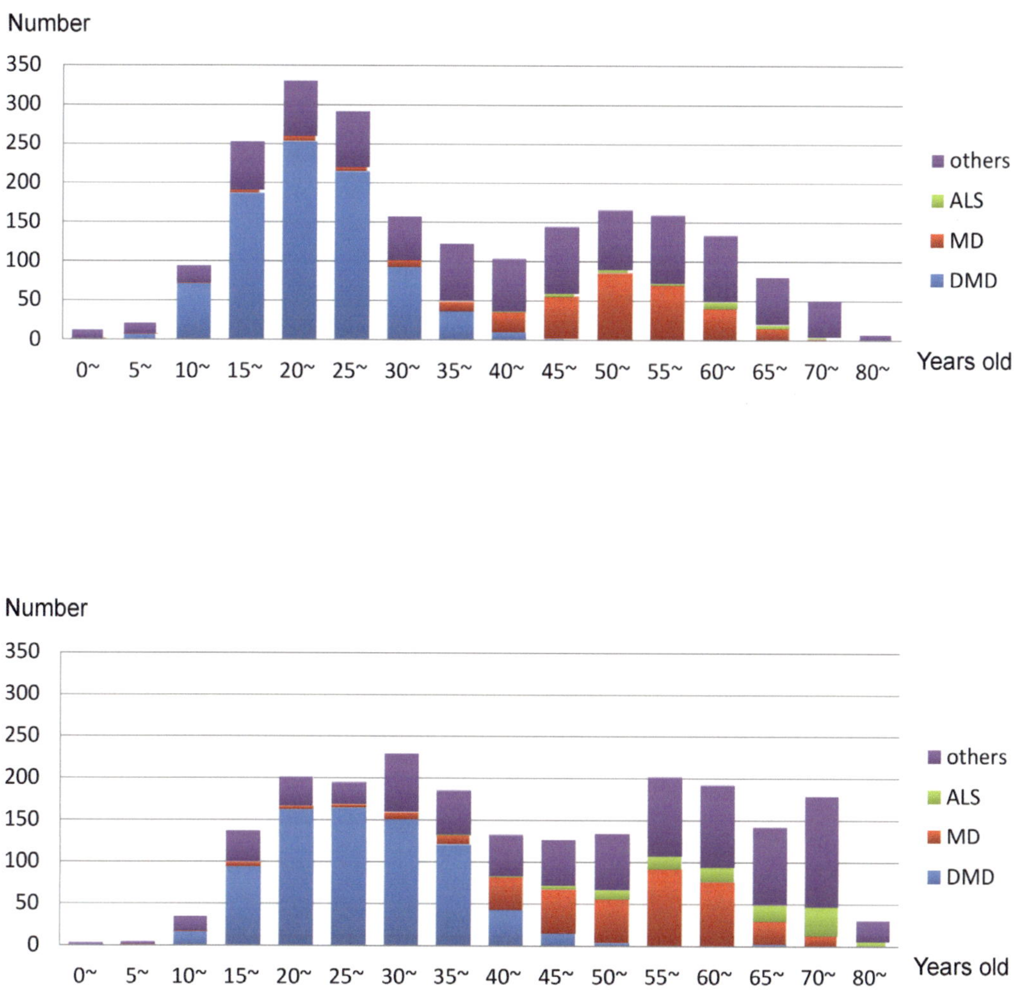

Upper: 1999. Lower: 2009. The age distribution of inpatients in muscular dystrophy wards shifted to a higher range over time.

Fig. 6. Changes in age distribution of inpatients in muscular dystrophy wards.

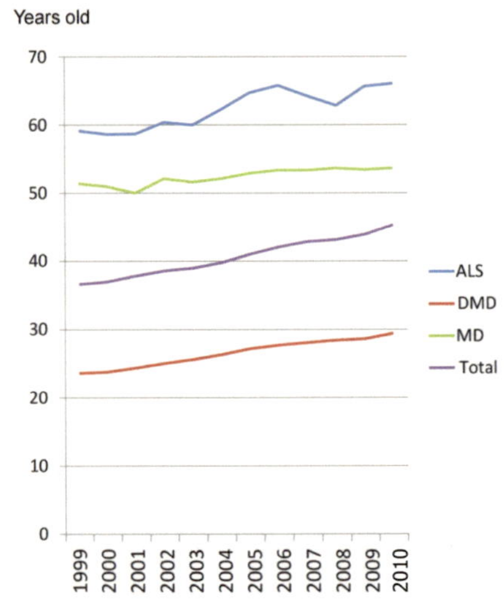

The mean age of the inpatients was gradually increased. DMD, Duchenne muscular dystrophy; MD, myotonic dystrophy; ALS, amyotrophic lateral sclerosis

Fig. 7. Sequential changes in mean age of inpatients.

Gradual changes in age distribution of inpatients with Duchenne muscular dystrophy was observed. The age peak in 1999 shifted to a higher range and became slightly flattened in 2009 (Fig. 8).

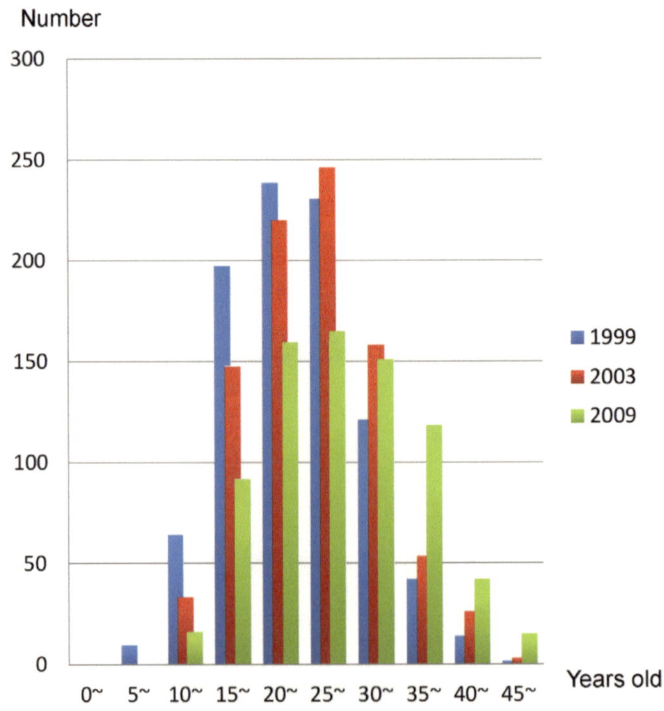

Fig. 8. Changes in age distribution of inpatients with Duchenne muscular dystrophy.

3.4 Sequential changes in numbers of patients receiving oral nutrition and those with Duchenne muscular dystrophy who underwent a percutaneous endoscopic gastrostomy

The proportion of patients with Duchenne muscular dystrophy receiving oral nutrition in 1999 was 95.1%, which gradually decreased to 70.6% in 2010. In contrast, the number who required tube feeding, including a nasal nutrition tube and undergoing a percutaneous endoscopic gastrostomy, gradually increased to 107 in 2010.

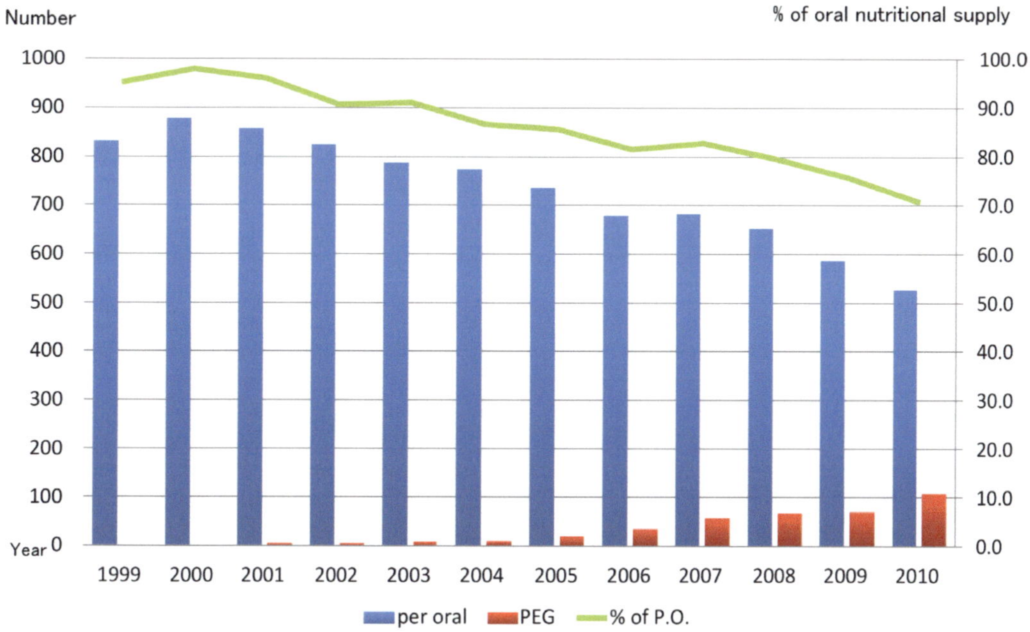

PEG, percutaneous endoscopic gastrostomy

Fig. 9. Sequential changes in numbers of Duchenne muscular dystrophy patients and those who underwent an endoscopic gastrostomy patients receiving oral nutrition.

3.5 Death case analysis

The total number of deaths reported from 2000 to 2010 was 1307, which ranged from 95-174 annually in a variable pattern (Fig. 10). The number of Duchenne muscular dystrophy patients who died was 409, while that of myotonic dystrophy patients was 363.

The mean age of death among Duchenne muscular dystrophy patients was 26.7 years old in 2000, which gradually increased to 35.1 years old by 2010. On the other hand, the mean age of death for myotonic dystrophy patients was 59.0 years old in 2000 and 59.1 years old in 2010, which was not significantly different (Fig. 10).

The most frequent cause of death among Duchenne muscular dystrophy patients was heart failure, accounting for 47%. As for myotonic dystrophy patients, the most frequent cause was respiratory disorders, such as respiratory failure and respiratory tract infection, which accounted for 64% (Fig. 11).

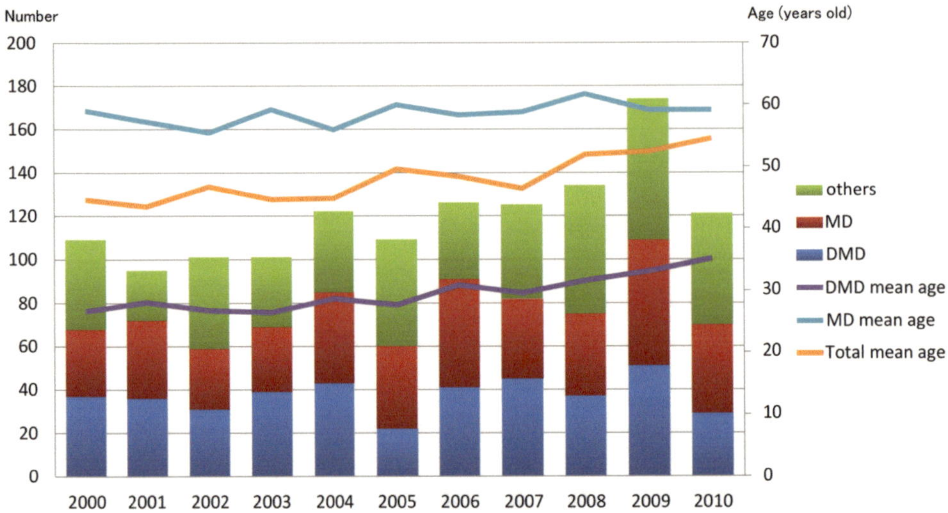

DMD, Duchenne muscular dystrophy; MD, myotonic dystrophy

Fig. 10. Sequential numbers of deaths and mean age at death reported to the database.

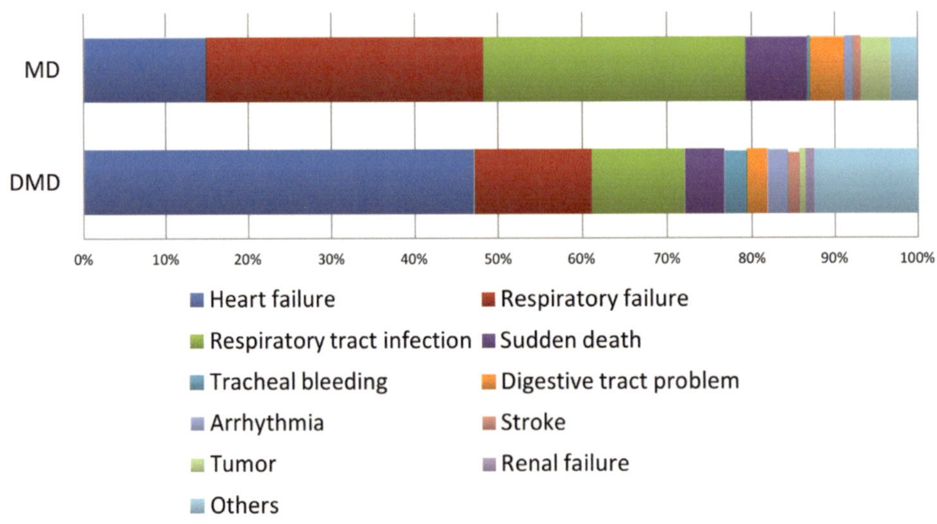

The most frequent cause of death among Duchenne muscular dystrophy patients was heart failure. In contrast, that of myotonic dystrophy patients was respiratory disorder.
DMD, Duchenne muscular dystrophy; MD, myotonic dystrophy

Fig. 11. Causes of death among Duchenne muscular dystrophy and myotonic dystrophy patients (2000~2010).

3.6 Proportional changes in numbers of inpatients in muscular dystrophy wards of each institution

Twenty-seven hospitals in Japan specialize in treatment of muscular dystrophy patients are not same in terms of types of muscular dystrophy of inpatient, disease severity, and actual care. Fig. 12 shows the proportion of inpatients by each institution. The upper figure, which shows the proportion in 1999, is arranged according to rate of Duchenne muscular dystrophy inpatients. There were significant differences in regard to the proportion of inpatients among the institutions in 1999, which changed over time. In 2009, the proportion of inpatients with amyotrophic lateral sclerosis was notable.

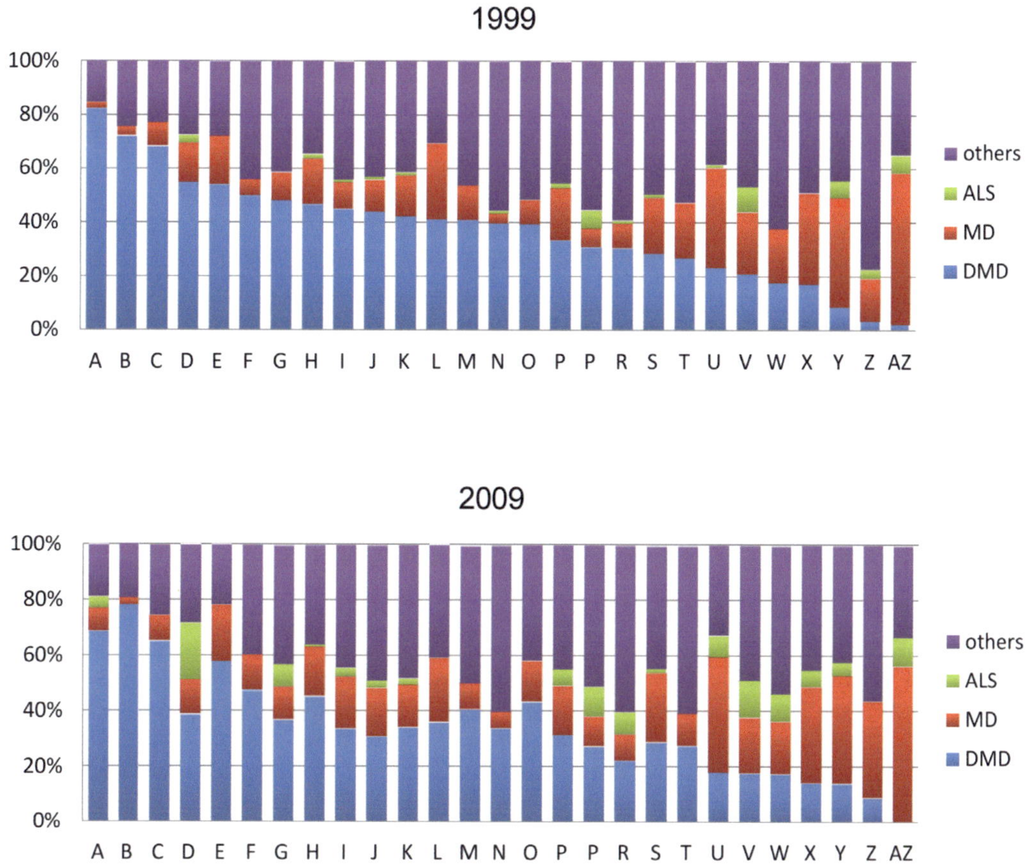

Upper: 1999. Lower: 2009. A~AZ represent the individual institution. Institute AZ, which had lowest rate of DMD patients among institutions in 1999, has no DMD patient in 2009.
DMD, Duchenne muscular dystrophy; MD, myotonic dystrophy; ALS, amyotrophic lateral sclerosis

Fig. 12. Changes in proportions of inpatients in muscular dystrophy wards of each institution

3.7 Sequential changes in respiratory conditions of Duchenne muscular dystrophy patients at each institution (1999~2009).

The total number of Duchenne muscular dystrophy patients treated from 1999 to 2009 was 1427. The changes in motor function of the patients were nearly uniform, whereas the therapeutic respiratory conditions varied among the institutions.

Figure 13 presents the respiratory conditions of the patients for the 11-year period from 1999 to 2009. In the 10s, almost patients keep voluntary respiratory function. In the 20s, various respiratory patterns are observed, which seem not to be different among the institutions. In more than 30s, there were apparent differences among the institutions. Some institutes have no tracheostomy older patients, which generation is generally supposed not to be compensated by non-invasive positive pressure ventilation and use tracheotomy ventilation.

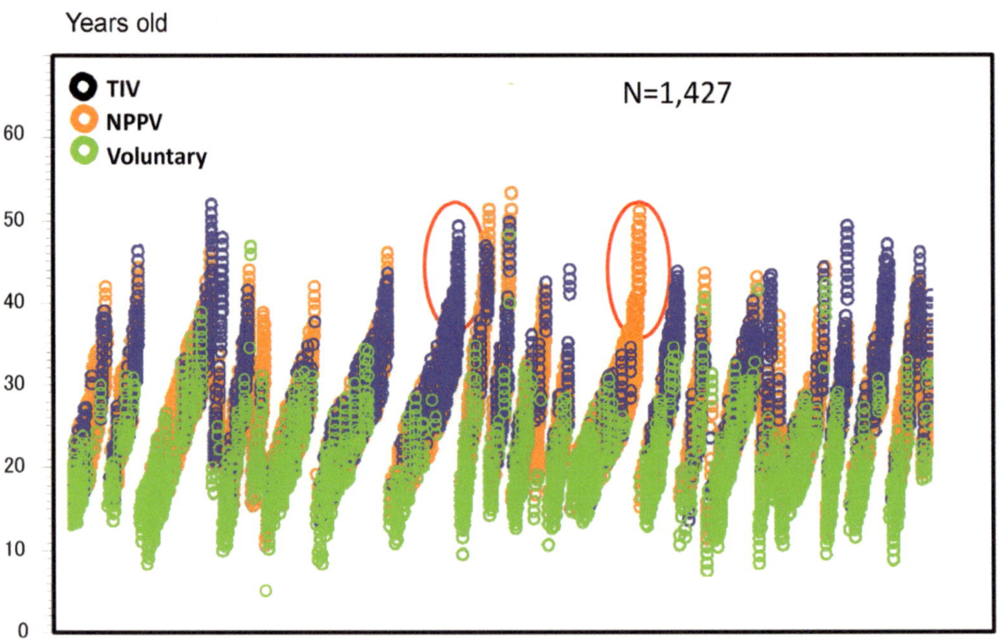

Each cluster indicates a single institution. The vertical axis indicates the course of a single Duchenne muscular dystrophy patient. The respiratory conditions of older patients differed among the institutions. For example, the left oval indicates a tracheostomy case and the right oval a non-invasive positive pressure ventilation case.
TIV,tracheostomy intermittent ventilation; NPPV, non-invasive positive pressure ventilation

Fig. 13. Sequential changes in respiratory conditions of Duchenne muscular dystrophy patients treated at each institution (1999~2009).

4. Conclusion

Wards for patients with muscular dystrophy were originally established in Japan in 1964 and then gradually expanded throughout the country. As a result, approximate 2500 beds are now provided among 27 institutions. In the early days, many of the patients were boys with Duchenne muscular dystrophy, who received education in schools near the hospital where they received care. However, over time, regular public elementary and junior high schools began to accept disabled children, and such patients were then able to receive an education at schools in their home town. Thus, cases of admission for the purpose of education gradually decreased.

On the other hand, progress in therapeutic strategies for respiratory failure (American Thoracic Society Documents, 2004), heart failure (Ishikawa, 1999; Matsumura, 2010) and other complications associated with muscular dystrophy prolonged the life span of affected individuals (Bushby 2010a, b). Now, most inpatients admitted to a muscular dystrophy ward have a severe general condition and many are assisted by mechanical ventilation (Tatara, 2008). In addition, in terms of nutritional control (American Thoracic Society Documents, 2004; Bushby 2010b), the number of percutaneous endoscopic gastrostomy patients with Duchenne muscular dystrophy has gradually increased.

Thus, the age and disease severity of inpatients have been gradually progressed with this changing environment. And social welfare systems related to muscular dystrophy wards in Japan also have been changing during this research. The social role of wards for inpatients with muscular dystrophy has been changing. The gradual increase of number of inpatients with amyotrophic lateral sclerosis means that the ward for patients with muscular dystrophy is no longer only for patients with muscular dystrophy. Present wards have purpose for care and treatment for severe disabilities, not limited to patients with muscular dystrophy.

There are some reports concerned with prognosis of patients with Duchenne muscular dystrophy from single institution belonging to the National Hospital Organization (Ishikawa, 2011; Matsumura, 2011). Just as these reports, we showed the increasing mean age of death among Duchenne muscular dystrophy patients. Although the most frequent cause of death among Duchenne muscular dystrophy patients was heart failure, the progression for cardioprotection therapy to cardiomyopathy (Ishikawa, 1999; Matsumura, 2010) improved the prognosis.

However, the present findings showed that there are apparent differences in regard to the proportion of inpatients and therapeutic conditions among institutions. Hereafter, these differences will be more remarkable. So far almost same therapy has been offered among the National Hospital Organization and National Center of Neurology and Psychiatry. However, these conditions will not continue and may influence the prognosis of patients with muscular dystrophy in Japan.

Social role of wards for patients with muscular dystrophy at establishment, offering patients with muscular dystrophy opportunities of education and treatment, has changed into offering severe disabilities care and treatment. We should consider how to manage these conditions.

5. Acknowledgments

This study was supported by a Research Grant for Nervous and Mental Disorders from the Ministry of Health, Labour and Welfare of Japan.

We are grateful to Dr. Mitsuru Kawai for the kind advice, as well as the members of the FUKUNAGA (1999-2005) and SHINNO (2006-2011) muscular dystrophy research groups of the National Hospital Organization for the data collection.

Institutions specializing in muscular dystrophy treatment in Japan (Fig.14)

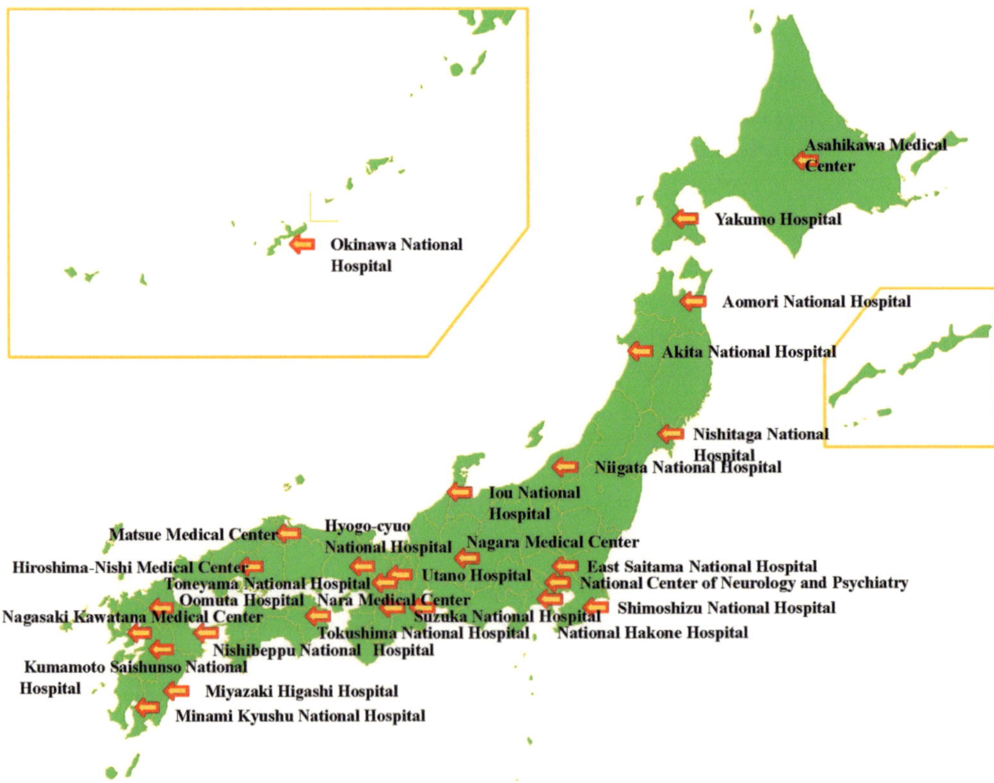

Fig. 14. Institutions specializing in muscular dystrophy treatment in Japan

National Hospital Organization:

- Asahikawa Medical Center, Yakumo Hospital, Aomori National Hospital,
- Akita National Hospital, Nishitaga National Hospital, East Saitama National Hospital,
- Shimoshizu National Hospital, National Hakone Hospital, Niigata National Hospital,
- Iou National Hospital, Nagara Medical Center, Suzuka National Hospital,
- Nara Medical Center, Utano Hospital, Toneyama National Hospital,
- Hyogo-cyuo National Hospital, Hiroshima-Nishi Medical Center, Matsue Medical Center,
- Tokushima National Hospital, Oomuta Hospital, Nagasaki Kawatana Medical Center,
- Kumamoto Saishunso National Hospital, Nishibeppu National Hospital,
- Miyazaki Higashi Hospital, Minami Kyushu National Hospital, Okinawa National Hospital

National Center of Neurology and Psychiatry

6. References

American Thoracic Society Documents (2004). Respiratory Care of the Patient with Duchenne Muscular Dystrophy. ATS Consensus Statement · *American Journal of Respiratory and Critical Care Medicine*, Vol 170, pp 456–465.

Bushby K, Finkel R, Birnkrant DJ, Case LE, Clemens PR, Cripe L, Kaul A, Kinnett K, McDonald C, Pandya S, Poysky J, Shapiro F, Tomezsko J, Constantin C, for the DMD care considerations working group (2010a). Diagnosis and management of Duchenne muscular dystrophy, part 1: diagnosis, and pharmacological and psychosocial management. *The Lancet Neurology,* Vol.9, pp 77-93.

Bushby K, Finkel R, Birnkrant DJ, Case LE, Clemens PR, Cripe L, Kaul A, Kinnett K, McDonald C, Pandya S, Poysky J, Shapiro F, Tomezsko J, Constantin C, for the DMD care considerations working group (2010b). Diagnosis and management of Duchenne muscular dystrophy, part 2: implementation of multidisciplinary care. *The Lancet Neurology*, Vol.9, pp 177–189.

Ishikawa Y, Bach JR, Minami R (1999). Cardioprotection for Duchenne's muscular dystrophy.*American Heart Journal* Vol.137, pp 895–902.

Ishikawa Y, Miura T, Ishikawa Y, Aoyagi T, Ogata H, Hamada S, Minami R (2011). Duchenne muscular dystrophy: Survival by cardio-respiratory interventions. *Neuromuscular Disorders* Vol. 21, pp 47–51.

Matsumura T, Tamura T, Kuru S, Kikuchi Y, Kawai M (2010) · Carvedilol can prevent cardiac events in Duchenne muscular dystrophy. *Internal Medicine* Vol. 49, pp 1357-1363.

Matsumura T, Saito T, Fujimura H, Shinno S, Sakoda S (2011). A longitudinal cause-of-death analysis of patients with Duchenne muscular dystrophy.*Rinsho-shinkeigaku* Vol. 51, pp743-750.

Tatara K, Shinno S (2008). Management of mechanical ventilation and prognosis in Duchenne muscular dystrophy. *IRYO*, Vol. 62, pp 566–571.

14

Diagnosis of the Muscular Dystrophies

Leigh B. Waddell, Frances J. Evesson, Kathryn N. North,
Sandra T. Cooper and Nigel F. Clarke
*Institute for Neuroscience and Muscle Research,
Children's Hospital at Westmead and Discipline of Paediatrics & Child Health,
University of Sydney,
Australia*

1. Introduction

The diagnosis of muscular dystrophies (MDs) has advanced considerably since these disorders were first described in the 1800s, due to characterisation of phenotypes and advances in biochemical and molecular analyses. Over the last ten years in particular, there has been a rapid expansion in the list of genes that are known to cause MD. Providing a specific genetic diagnosis to a patient is important for many reasons. It resolves many uncertainties for families, enables accurate genetic counselling and options for prevention and prenatal diagnosis, and provides doctors and families with information about prognosis, which allows medical care to be individualised. In some cases, a genetic diagnosis prompts the clinician to begin surveillance and/or interventions that may be life-saving, such as aggressive cardiac surveillance in disorders associated with cardiac arrhythmias or cardiomyopathy. In addition, knowledge of the primary genetic cause will be an essential prerequisite to prescribe specific gene-based or biochemical therapies when they are developed in the future. Making a genetic diagnosis should now be the universal goal for all patients with MD.

Diagnosis of the three most common forms of MD, Duchenne muscular dystrophy (DMD), myotonic dystrophy and Facioscapulohumeral muscular dystrophy (FSHD) MD, is now straightforward in most patients, as clinical features guide the appropriate genetic tests to be requested. However, establishing the specific diagnosis in many patients with other forms of MD remains difficult. The main reasons are the large number of potential genetic causes in several subgroups of MD, a lack of specific features to guide diagnosis and the wide range of phenotypes that are possible with many genetic forms. These combine to make it a challenge for the clinician to predict the correct genetic cause from the patient's clinical presentation and history, or from standard clinical tests alone. Laboratory investigations, including muscle histopathology and protein analysis (immunohistochemistry and Western blotting), are useful to guide genetic testing in many situations. However, even in well-resourced diagnostic services, the genetic cause remains unknown in a large proportion of MD patients. It is likely that many of these patients have as yet undiscovered genetic forms of MD.

This chapter summarises the most important clinical and laboratory information to consider when diagnosing MDs, and the approach to diagnosing the different forms. This includes an appreciation of clinical presentations, the use of specialised muscle imaging, muscle histopathology, laboratory protein analysis and specific genetic tests. We also discuss the challenges when diagnosing many rare forms of MD, and how new technologies may aid this process.

2. The different forms of muscular dystrophy

The MDs are a genetically and phenotypically diverse group of disorders. In children, the most common form of MD is Duchenne MD (DMD), caused by mutations in the *DMD* gene that encodes dystrophin, with an estimated prevalence of 1 in 3000 males (Jones and North 1997). Most affected boys lose ambulation around 10 years of age and die from respiratory or cardiac complications in the third or fourth decades of life. Becker MD (BMD) is a less severe condition associated with a later age of onset and slower disease progression that is also caused by mutations in the dystrophin protein.

In adults, the most common forms of MD are myotonic dystrophy type 1 (DM1) and facioscapulohumeral MD (FSHD). The average estimated prevalence of DM1 is ~1 in 10,000 (Norwood, Harling et al. 2009; Turner and Hilton-Jones 2010) and for FSHD it is 1 in 20,000 (Norwood, Harling et al. 2009; Statland and Tawil 2011). DM1 is a multi-system disorder caused by a trinucleotide repeat expansion (CTG) in the *DMPK* gene on chromosome 19 and there is a wide range of severity that partially correlates with the size of the repeat expansion (McNally and Pytel 2007; Turner and Hilton-Jones 2010). The classical form of DM1 is characterised by progressive muscle weakness that begins in the muscles of the face, ankle, hands and neck and myotonia, a delayed relaxation of muscles after contraction. Patients also have an increased risk of cardiac conduction defects, cataracts, type 2 diabetes, daytime somnolence and balding (males especially). Congenital onset DM1 is strongly associated with respiratory difficulties at birth and intellectual disabililty (Turner and Hilton-Jones 2010). A second form of myotonic dystrophy (DM2) is due to mutations in the *ZNF9* gene, does not have a congenital onset form, and is probably less common. FSHD is characterised by weakness of the facial, scapular, ankle and upper arm muscles and is caused by deletions of large D4Z4 DNA repeats in the sub-telomeric region of chromosome 4q (McNally and Pytel 2007; Pandya, King et al. 2008).

Disease	Gene	Chromosome	Protein	Year Identified
FSHD	*DUX4*	4q35	Double homeobox 4	1990 [1]
Myotonic Dystrophy (DM1)	*DMPK*	19q13	*Expansion of non-coding triplet (CTG) repeat*	1992 [2,3]
Myotonic Dystrophy (DM2)	*ZNF9*	3q21	*Expansion of non-coding quadruplet (CCTG) repeat*	2001 [4,5]
Oculopharyngeal MD	*PABPN1*	14q11.2-q13	Poly(A) binding protein, nuclear 1	1998 [6-8]
MD with Lipodystrophy	*PTRF*	17q21-23	Cavin-1	2009 [9]
DMD/BMD	*DMD*	Xp21.2	Dystrophin	1986/87 [10-14]

Disease	Gene	Chromosome	Protein	Year Identified
EDMD	*EMD*	Xq28	Emerin	1994 [15]
	FHL1	Xq27.2	Four and a half LIM domain 1	2009 [16]
	LMNA	1q21.2	Lamin A/C	1999 [17]
	SYNE1	6q25	Nesprin-1	2007 [18]
	SYNE2	14q23	Nesprin-2	2007 [18]
LGMD1A	*MYOT*	5q31	Myotilin	2000 [19]
LGMD1B	*LMNA*	1q22	Lamin A/C	2000 [20]
LGMD1C	*CAV3*	3p25	Caveolin-3	1998 [21,22]
LGMD1D	*	7q36.3		[23]
LGMD1E	*	6q23		[24]
LGMD1F	*	7q32		[25]
LGMD1G	*	4q21		[26]
LGMD2A	*CAPN3*	15q15.1	Calpain-3	1995 [27,28]
LGMD2B	*DYSF*	2p13	Dysferlin	1998 [29,30]
LGMD2C	*SGCG*	13q12	γ-sarcoglycan	1995 [31]
LGMD2D	*SGCA*	17q12-21.33	α-sarcoglycan	1994 [32]
LGMD2E	*SGCB*	4q12	β-sarcoglycan	1996 [33]
LGMD2F	*SGCD*	5q33	δ-sarcoglycan	1996 [34]
LGMD2G	*TCAP*	17q12	Telethonin	2000 [35]
LGMD2H	*TRIM32*	9q31-34	Tripartite motif-containing 32	2002 [36,37]
LGMD2I	*FKRP*	19q13.3	Fukutin related protein	2001 [38,39]
LGMD2J	*TTN*	2q31	Titin	2002 [40]
LGMD2K	*POMT1*	9q34	Protein O-mannosyl-transferase 1	2005 [41]
LGMD2L	*ANO5*	11p14.3	Anoctamin 5	2010 [42]
LGMD2M	*FKTN*	9q31-33	Fukutin	2006 [43,44]
LGMD2N	*POMT2*	14q24	Protein O-mannosyl-transferase 2	2007 [45]
LGMD2O	*POMGnT1*	1p34	Protein O-linked mannose beta 1,2-N-acetylglucosaminyl transferase 1	2007 [46]
MDC1A	*LAMA2*	6q2	Laminin α2 chain of merosin	1995 [47-49]
MDC1B	*	1q42		[50]
MDC1C	*FKRP*	19q13	Fukutin related protein	2001 [51]
MDC1D	*LARGE*	22q12	Like-glycosyltransferase	2003 [52]
FCMD	*FCMD*	9q31-33	Fukutin	1998 [53,54]
WWS	*FCMD*	9q31-33	Fukutin	2003 [55]
	POMT1	9q34	Protein O-mannosyl-transferase 1	2002 [56]
	POMT2	14q24.3	Protein O-mannosyl-transferase 2	2005 [57]
	FKRP	19q13	Fukutin related protein	2005 [58]
	POMGnT1	1p3	Protein O-linked mannose beta 1,2-N-acetylglucosaminyl transferase 1	2003 [59]

Disease	Gene	Chromosome	Protein	Year Identified
MEB	*POMGnT1*	1p3	Protein O-linked mannose beta 1,2-N-acetylglucosaminyl transferase 1	2001 [60]
	FKRP	19q13	Fukutin related protein	2005 [58]
	POMT2	14q24.3	Protein O-mannosyl-transferase 2	2006 [61]
Rigid Spine Syndrome	*SEPN1*	1p36	Selenoprotein N1	2001 [62,63]
UCMD	*COL6A1*	21q22.3	Collagen VI, subunit α1	2003 [64,65]
	COL6A2	21q22.3	Collagen VI, subunit α2	2001 [66,67]
	COL6A3	2q37	Collagen VI, subunit α3	2002 [68]
Bethlem myopathy	*COL6A1*	21q22.3	Collagen VI, subunit α1	1996 [69]
	COL6A2	21q22.3	Collagen VI, subunit α2	1996 [69]
	COL6A3	2q37	Collagen VI, subunit α3	1998 [70,71]
CMD integrin defect	*ITGA7*	12q13	Integrin α7	1998 [72]
CMD dynamin 2 defect	*DNM2*	19p13.2	Dynamin 2	2008 [73]
CMD joint hyperlaxity	*	3p23-21		[74]

Adapted from the NMD Gene Table 2011 (Kaplan 2010). * = no gene discovered yet. **Abbreviations:** FSHD: Facio-scapulo-humeral MD, MD: muscular dystrophy, DMD: Duchenne MD, BMD: Becker MD, EDMD: Emery-Dreifuss MD, LGMD: limb-girdle MD, MDC: MD congenital, FCMD: Fukuyama congenital MD, WWS: Walker-Warburg Syndrome, MEB: Muscle-eye-brain disease, UCMD: Ullrich congenital MD and CMD: congenital MD. References: 1(Wijmenga, Frants et al. 1990), 2(Brook, McCurrach et al. 1992), 3(Renwick, Bundey et al. 1971), 4(Liquori, Ricker et al. 2001), 5(Ranum, Rasmussen et al. 1998), 6(Brais, Bouchard et al. 1998), 7(Brais, Xie et al. 1995), 8(Robinson, Hammans et al. 2005), 9(Hayashi, Matsuda et al. 2009), 10(Burghes, Logan et al. 1987), 11(Hoffman, Brown et al. 1987), 12(Koenig, Hoffman et al. 1987), 13(Koenig, Monaco et al. 1988), 14(Monaco, Neve et al. 1986), 15(Bione, Maestrini et al. 1994), 16(Gueneau, Bertrand et al. 2009), 17(Bonne, Di Barletta et al. 1999), 18(Zhang, Bethmann et al. 2007), 19(Hauser, Horrigan et al. 2000), 20(Muchir, Bonne et al. 2000), 21(McNally, de Sa Moreira et al. 1998), 22(Minetti, Sotgia et al. 1998), 23(Speer, Vance et al. 1999), 24(Messina, Speer et al. 1997), 25(Palenzuela, Andreu et al. 2003), 26(Starling, Kok et al. 2004), 27(Richard, Brenguier et al. 1997), 28(Richard, Broux et al. 1995), 29(Bashir, Britton et al. 1998), 30(Liu, Aoki et al. 1998), 31(Noguchi, McNally et al. 1995), 32(Roberds, Leturcq et al. 1994), 33(Bonnemann, Passos-Bueno et al. 1996), 34(Nigro, de Sa Moreira et al. 1996), 35(Moreira, Wiltshire et al. 2000), 36(Frosk, Weiler et al. 2002), 37(Weiler, Greenberg et al. 1998), 38(Brockington, Blake et al. 2001), 39(Driss, Amouri et al. 2000), 40(Hackman, Vihola et al. 2002), 41(Balci, Uyanik et al. 2005), 42(Bolduc, Marlow et al. 2010), 43(Godfrey, Escolar et al. 2006), 44(Murakami, Hayashi et al. 2006), 45(Biancheri, Falace et al. 2007), 46(Godfrey, Clement et al. 2007), 47(Helbling-Leclerc, Zhang et al. 1995), 48(Hillaire, Leclerc et al. 1994), 49(Tome, Evangelista et al. 1994), 50(Brockington, Sewry et al. 2000), 51(Brockington, Blake et al. 2001), 52(Longman, Brockington et al. 2003), 53(Kobayashi, Nakahori et al. 1998), 54(Toda, Segawa et al. 1993), 55(de Bernabe, van Bokhoven et al. 2003), 56(Beltran-Valero de Bernabe, Currier et al. 2002), 57(van Reeuwijk, Janssen et al. 2005), 58(Beltran-Valero de Bernabe, Voit et al. 2004), 59(Taniguchi, Kobayashi et al. 2003), 60(Yoshida, Kobayashi et al. 2001), 61(Mercuri, D'Amico et al. 2006), 62(Moghadaszadeh, Desguerre et al. 1998), 63(Moghadaszadeh, Petit et al. 2001), 64(Giusti, Lucarini et al. 2005), 65(Pan, Zhang et al. 2003), 66(Camacho Vanegas, Bertini et al. 2001), 67(Higuchi, Shiraishi et al. 2001), 68(Demir, Sabatelli et al. 2002), 69(Jobsis, Keizers et al. 1996), 70(Pan, Zhang et al. 1998), 71(Speer, Tandan et al. 1996), 72(Hayashi, Chou et al. 1998), 73(Susman, Quijano-Roy et al. 2010), 74(Tetreault, Duquette et al. 2006) and 75(Kaplan 2010).

Table 1. Table of muscular dystrophy genes and proteins.

The other major forms of MD are grouped by age of onset or clinical phenotype (see Table 1). Each specific genetic form of MD has a characteristic pattern of disease onset, severity, clinical course and involvement of particular muscle groups, although there is marked overlap between phenotypes (see Table 2). The congenital MDs (CMD) are characterised by onset of muscle weakness within the first year of life (often at birth) and usually have a slowly progressive disease course. In the limb girdle MDs (LGMD), patients can present during childhood or adulthood with weakness that is most prominent in proximal limb or shoulder and/or pelvic girdle muscles. They are subdivided based on mode of inheritance into LGMD type 1 (autosomal dominant) and LGMD type 2 (autosomal recessive); DMD and BMD can be considered as X-linked forms of LGMD. Emery Dreifuss MD (EDMD) is a clinical syndrome with several possible genetic causes characterised by prominent weakness in the upper arm and ankle dorsiflexor muscles, early contractures of the elbows, ankles and neck and cardiac involvement. Other forms of MD with notable phenotypes are oculopharyngeal MD, where mainly the muscles of the eye and throat are affected, and the distal myopathies which mainly affect the muscles of the hands and feet.

In addition to the different forms of MD listed so far, a wide range of muscle conditions have clinical and histological features that overlap with the MDs and these should be kept in mind whenever a diagnosis of a MD is considered. The most important differential diagnoses are the myofibrillar myopathies (characterised by desmin-positive inclusions in muscle fibres, prominent distal limb muscle involvement, cardiomyopathy and peripheral neuropathy) and some severe forms of congenital myopathy (especially those due to *RYR1* and *DNM2* mutations).

3. Overview of the approach to diagnosis

A diagnosis of MD usually begins with a patient presenting with muscle weakness, muscle pain, reduced stamina; or in children, delayed motor development. Occasionally a raised serum creatine kinase (CK) level is the first sign of a MD and an incidental finding during investigation of other symptoms. A detailed clinical history and examination can provide important clues about the diagnosis and the most appropriate path of investigation. Muscle imaging is a non-invasive option that may be helpful in particular situations. A muscle biopsy is still required for the diagnosis of many types of MD. In most children and some adults a skin biopsy is taken for fibroblast cell culture at this time. Standard muscle histopathology provides information about muscle architecture and frozen portions of the muscle biopsy can be used for a range of protein analyses. Information from all of these sources is used to direct genetic testing, which usually provides the definitive diagnosis. This process is outlined in Figure 1.

3.1 Clinical information

Clinical information remains of paramount importance in the diagnostic process, even with recent advances in genetics (Bushby, Norwood et al. 2007; Norwood, de Visser et al. 2007; Guglieri and Bushby 2008). Each MD has a characteristic clinical pattern in terms of age of onset, rate of progression, severity and range of muscles involved. In some forms of MD, the pattern of clinical features is sufficiently distinct for a relatively accurate provisional

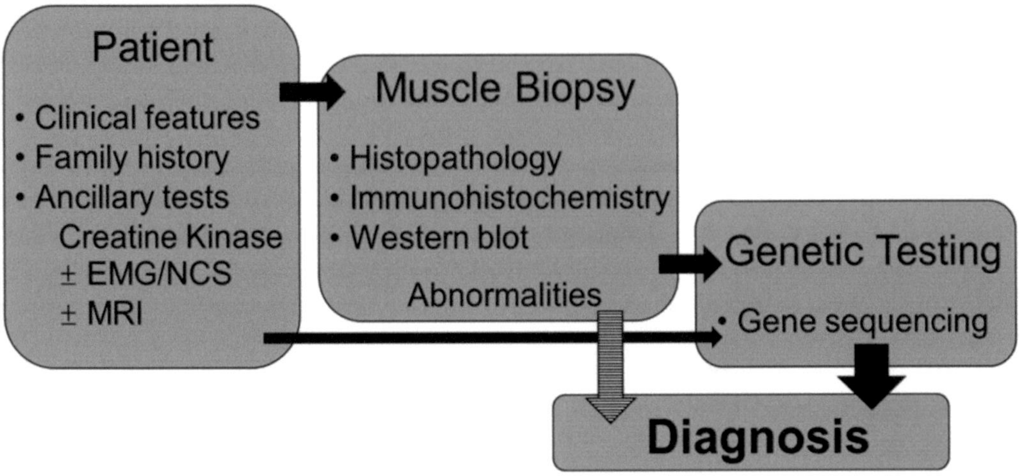

Abbreviations: EMG: Electromyography, NCS: nerve conduction studies, MRI: magnetic resonance imaging.

Fig. 1. Overview of MD diagnostic process.

diagnosis to be made on the basis of clinical history, examination and some basic clinical tests. This is the case for the three most common forms of MD - myotonic dystrophy, FSHD and DMD. It is recommended that clinician spends time familiarising themselves with these three disorders in particular, as they are the most common conditions encountered. Genetic testing is widely available for these conditions and many patients no longer require a muscle biopsy, so long as the clinician can make an accurate provisional diagnosis from clinical features.

Age of disease onset is a key feature that is used to classify major subgroups of MD. The congenital muscular dystrohies (CMDs) present in the first two years of life, most often at birth. The limb girdle MDs (LGMDs) begin after age 2 years. Onset can vary between the first decade of life to old age depending on the specific form of LGMD and its severity.

The pattern of weakness may also provide clues to the MD subtype. For example while LGMDs are characterised by proximal weakness, some subtypes may also have significant involvement of scapular stabilisers or distal limb muscles (see Table 2). Other important variables include the presence or absence of brain, cardiac or respiratory muscle involvement, calf muscle hypertrophy, contractures and skin abnormalities (see Table 2).

The level of creatine kinase (CK) in blood, which is thought to be a marker of ongoing muscle necrosis or damage, can also help to differentiate between forms of MD. While some fluctuation in CK levels from day to day occurs and there is a tendency for CK levels to drop with disease progression, categorising CK results into broad ranges such as normal, mildly raised, moderately raised and markedly elevated is useful.

Disease	Gene	Prevalence*	Age of onset (yrs)	CK	Distal	Cardiac	Respiratory	Muscle hypertrophy	Spine	Contractures	Useful diagnostic information	References
FSHD	*DUX4*	Common	10-50	↑-↑↑							CE, FHx, GT	1,2
Myotonic Dystrophy (DM1)	*DMPK*	Common	0-80	↑-↑↑	✓	✓	✓				CE, FHx, EMG, GT	3
Myotonic Dystrophy (DM2)	*ZNF9*	Probably uncommon	10-60	↑-↑↑	✓	✓		✓			CE, FHx, EMG, GT	3
DMD-BMD	*DMD*	Common	DMD: 2-6 BMD:>5	↑↑-↑↑↑		✓	✓	✓	✓	✓	CE, FHx, IHC, WB, GT, SEQ	4,5
EDMD	*EMD*	Uncommon	>3	↑-↑↑		✓		✓	✓	✓✓	IHC, WB, SEQ	6,7
	FHL1	Rare	4-48	N-↑↑		✓			✓	✓	SEQ	8
	LMNA	Uncommon	>3	N-↑↑		✓✓			✓	✓✓	SEQ	
LGMD1A	*MYOT*	Rare	>25	↑-↑↑	✓	✓					SEQ	9
LGMD1B	*LMNA*	Uncommon	>3	↑-↑↑	✓	✓✓			✓		SEQ	10
LGMD1C	*CAV3*	Uncommon	>4	↑↑-↑↑↑				✓			IHC, WB, SEQ	11
LGMD2A	*CAPN3*	Common	2-40	↑-↑↑↑			✓		✓	✓	± WB, SEQ	12,13
LGMD2B	*DYSF*	Moderately common^	12-25	↑↑↑	✓						IHC, WB, SEQ	14-16
LGMD2C	*SGCG*	Rare	>3	↑↑-↑↑↑		✓	✓	✓	✓	✓	IHC, WB, SEQ	17-21
LGMD2D	*SGCA*	Rare	>3	↑↑-↑↑↑		✓	✓	✓	✓	✓	IHC, WB, SEQ	17-21
LGMD2E	*SGCB*	Rare	>3	↑↑-↑↑↑		✓	✓	✓	✓	✓	IHC, WB, SEQ	17-21
LGMD2F	*SGCD*	Rare	>3	↑↑-↑↑↑		✓	✓	✓	✓	✓	IHC, WB, SEQ	17-21
LGMD2G	*TCAP*	Rare	9-20	↑-↑↑↑	✓	?		✓	✓		IHC, SEQ	22,23
LGMD2H	*TRIM32*	Rare‡	8-30	↑↑-↑↑↑				✓			SEQ	24
LGMD2I	*FKRP*	Common	2-40	↑↑-↑↑↑		✓	✓	✓	✓	✓	IHC$^+$, WB$^+$, SEQ	25
LGMD2J	*TTN*	Rare	8-30	N-↑	✓						MRI, (SEQ)	26
LGMD2L	*ANO5*	Common	>17	↑↑↑	✓			✓			SEQ	27,28
MDC1A	*LAMA2*	Common	0	↑↑-↑↑↑			✓		✓	✓	IHC, WB, SEQ	29-32
MDC1C	*FKRP*	Rare	0	↑↑↑		✓	✓	✓	✓	✓	IHC$^+$, WB$^+$, SEQ	33
FCMD	*FKTN*	Common†	0	↑↑-↑↑↑		✓	✓	✓	✓	✓	IHC$^+$,	34

Disease	Gene	Prevalence*	Age of onset (yrs)	CK	Distal	Cardiac	Respiratory	Muscle hypertrophy	Spine	Contractures	Useful diagnostic information	References
											WB^{+}, SEQ	
Rigid Spine Syndrome	*SEPN1*	Uncommon	0-2	N-↑			✓✓		✓✓		SEQ	35
UCMD	*COL6A1-3*	Common	0	N-↑↑			✓		✓	✓✓	IHC, FIBS, SEQ	36-38
Bethlem myopathy	*COL6A1-3*	Common	2-20	N-↑↑			✓		✓	✓✓	FIBS, SEQ	36,38

This table does not include the rarest forms of muscular dystrophy. Brain involvement can be seen in congenital myotonic dystrophy (DM1), DMD, the α-dystroglycanopathies and MDC1A. * = Prevalence varies for some disorders in different populations. Distal = prominent distal limb muscle involvement. CK = creatine kinase. Spine = prominent scoliosis or spinal rigidity. N = CK within normal range, ↑ = CK level 1 to 4 times upper limit of normal, ↑↑ = CK 4 to 15 times upper limit of normal, ↑↑↑ = CK > 15 times upper limit of normal. ✓= commonly associated, ✓✓= key feature for diagnosis and/or management. ^ = in Indian subcontinent especially, ‡ = mainly reported in Manitoba Hutterites, † = mainly reported in Japanese. CE = important clinical examination findings, FHx = clues from family history, GT = specific genetic test (other tthan full gene sequencing), EMG = Electromyography, IHC = immunohistochemistry, WB = Western blot, SEQ = direct gene sequencing, MRI = magnetic resonance imaging, FIBS = fibroblast culture, $^{+}$ = protein studies assess levels of glycolsylated α-dystroglycan. References: 1(Statland and Tawil 2011), 2(Sorrel-Dejerine and Fardeau 1982), 3(Turner and Hilton-Jones 2010), 4(Bushby, Finkel et al. 2010), 5(Jones and North 1997), 6(Bonne, Mercuri et al. 2000), 7(Emery 1989), 8(Gueneau, Bertrand et al. 2009), 9(Hauser, Horrigan et al. 2000), 10(van der Kooi, van Meegen et al. 1997), 11(Minetti, Sotgia et al. 1998), 12(Fardeau, Hillaire et al. 1996), 13(Piluso, Politano et al. 2005), 14(Bushby, Bashir et al. 1996), 15(Guglieri, Magri et al. 2008), 16(Zatz, de Paula et al. 2003), 17(Azibi, Bachner et al. 1993), 18(Bonnemann, Passos-Bueno et al. 1996), 19(Jones, Kim et al. 1998), 20(Lim, Duclos et al. 1995), 21(Passos-Bueno, Moreira et al. 1996), 22(Moreira, Vainzof et al. 1997), 23(Moreira, Wiltshire et al. 2000), 24(Borg, Stucka et al. 2009), 25(Brockington, Yuva et al. 2001), 26(Udd, Partanen et al. 1993), 27(Bolduc, Marlow et al. 2010), 28(Hicks, Sarkozy et al. 2011), 29(Allamand and Guicheney 2002), 30(Jones, Morgan et al. 2001), 31(North, Specht et al. 1996), 32(Tome 1999), 33(Brockington, Blake et al. 2001), 34(Toda and Kobayashi 1999), 35(Moghadaszadeh, Petit et al. 2001), 36(Bertini and Pepe 2002), 37(Nadeau, Kinali et al. 2009),and 38(Peat, Smith et al. 2008).

Table 2. Discriminating clinical features in genetically characterised muscular dystrophies.

3.2 Muscle pathology

The MDs are characterised by the presence of 'dystrophic' changes on muscle biopsy and one should be cautious about making a diagnosis of a MD if these are not present. The specific pathological features that in combination signify a dystrophy include variation in fibre size, increased internal nuclei, increased connective and adipose tissue, (Norwood, de Visser et al. 2007) and the presence of regenerating and degenerating fibres (see Figure 2). In addition, fibre splitting and inflammatory cell infiltrates are sometimes seen in MDs but are less specific for these disorders. These histological features likely arise from recurrent episodes of muscle fibres necrosis and regeneration that occur because fibres are more prone to damage than normal during muscle contraction (Jones and North 1997; Voit 2001). The relative prominence of different dystrophic features varies depending on the specific type of dystrophy, the age of the patient and the muscle biopsied (since the degree of involvement varies among different muscle groups in different dystrophies).

It is rarely possible to define the genetic cause of a MD from biopsy features alone but the pattern of dystrophic features can provide clues about the diagnosis. For example, dystrophic changes are often mild in the caveolinopathies (Minetti, Sotgia et al. 1998; Waddell, Lemckert et al. 2011), and the laminopathies (Quijano-Roy, Mbieleu et al. 2008; Rankin, Auer-Grumbach et al. 2008) compared to the dystrophinopathies and sarcoglycanopathies (Bonnemann, Passos-Bueno et al. 1996; Eymard, Romero et al. 1997). LGMD2B (dysferlin) (Norwood, de Visser et al. 2007) and LGMD2L (anoctamin-5) (Hicks, Sarkozy et al. 2011) often have an infiltration of inflammatory cells as an additional feature, and patients can be initially misdiagnosed with polymyositis (Norwood, de Visser et al. 2007). Young patients with Ullrich congenital muscular dystrophy (UCMD) (collagen VI) may only show non-specific myopathic changes or congenital fibre type disproportion (CFTD) (Peat, Smith et al. 2008; Schessl, Goemans et al. 2008). Mutations in *SEPN1* can cause various changes on muscle pathology including those resembling CMD, multiminicore disease or CFTD (Ferreiro, Quijano-Roy et al. 2002; Clarke, Kidson et al. 2006). The presence of other pathological abnormalities can be a clue to specific disorders, such as rimmed vacuoles which are associated with LGMD2G (telethonin) (Moreira, Vainzof et al. 1997) and LGMD2J (Udd, Partanen et al. 1993).

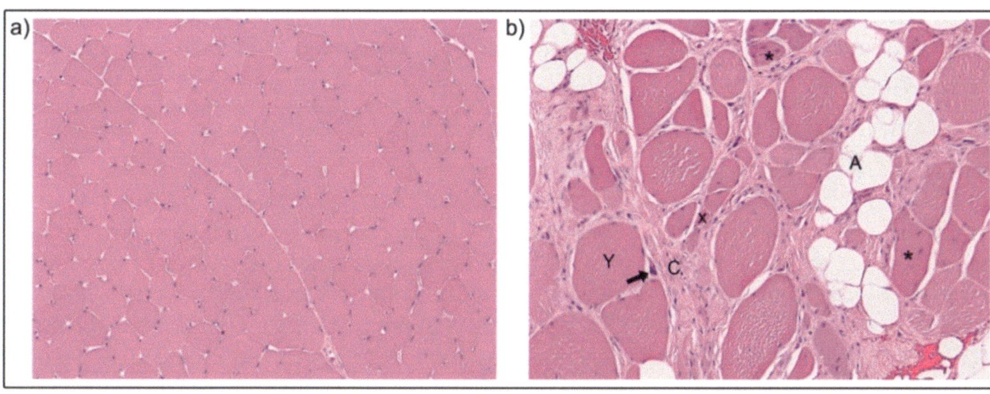

Human muscle in cross section stained with Haematoxylin and Eosin. a) Normal muscle. b) Dystrophic muscle showing a large variation in fibre size with both atrophic (X) and hypertrophic (Y) fibres, increased internal nuclei (*), increased connective (C) and adipose tissue (A) and the presence of regenerating and degenerating fibres (arrow pointing to likely degenerating fibre).

Fig. 2. Healthy and dystrophic human muscle.

3.3 Muscle imaging – MRI and ultrasound

Muscle magnetic resonance imaging has long been used as an adjunct to the diagnosis of inflammatory myopathies, but its usefulness in other neuromuscular disorders is increasingly recognized (Himmrich, Popov et al.). MRI is able to define the pattern of muscle involvement more precisely than clinical examination. Some dystrophies are associated with consistent and relatively specific patterns of abnormality on T1-weighted MRI scans of the thighs, calves and pelvis. For example, muscle MRI of patients with LGMD2I (*FKRP*) and LGMD2A (calpain-3) show marked signal changes in the adductor muscles, posterior thigh muscles and posterior calf muscles, with additional signal changes of medial gastrocnemius and soleus muscles in LGMD2A patients, differentiating these disorders from the other forms of LGMD (Fischer, Walter et al. 2005). Muscle MRI in combination with detailed clinical information and biochemical analysis is now being used increasingly to guide genetic investigations (Mercuri, Pichiecchio et al. 2002; Mercuri, Jungbluth et al. 2005).

Relatively distinct patterns of muscle involvement have also been described for the dystrophinopathies (Lamminen 1990; Lamminen, Tanttu et al. 1990), the sarcoglycanopathies (α, β and γ) (Eymard, Romero et al. 1997; Lodi, Muntoni et al. 1997), dysferlinopathy (Meola, Sansone et al. 1996; Cupler, Bohlega et al. 1998; Suzuki, Aoki et al. 2004; Paradas, Llauger et al. 2010), Bethlem myopathy (Mercuri, Cini et al. 2002; Mercuri, Cini et al. 2003; Mercuri, Lampe et al. 2005), and for mutations in *ANO5* (Hicks, Sarkozy et al. 2011), *LMNA*, *EMD* (Mercuri, Counsell et al. 2002), and *TTN* (Udd, Vihola et al. 2005).

Muscle MRI has been used to direct investigations in older patients with CMD, since distinctive patterns of muscle involvement are described for Ullrich CMD (Mercuri, Cini et al. 2002; Mercuri, Cini et al. 2003; Mercuri, Lampe et al. 2005) and *SEPN1*-related myopathies (Flanigan, Kerr et al. 2000; Mercuri, Talim et al. 2002; Mercuri, Clements et al. 2010). The need for a general anaesthetic to perform an MRI scan on patients less than age 5 years makes it a less attractive investigation for young patients.

Muscle MRI can also assist in choosing an appropriate muscle to biopsy, so that muscles that are affected by the disease process but not completely atrophied are targeted (Norwood, de Visser et al. 2007).

3.4 Protein analysis

While the specific type of MD can rarely be defined from routine histological stains, immunohistochemistry (IHC) and Western blot (WB) analysis of the expression of several MD proteins can be extremely useful to identify the likely genetic cause (Vogel and Zamecnik 2005; Bushby, Norwood et al. 2007). It is important that these studies are performed in a laboratory with expertise in these techniques (Norwood, de Visser et al. 2007). IHC is used to identify whether the protein is present or absent and whether it is normally localised. WB is generally more sensitive to reductions in protein expression but is technically more challenging. IHC has well-established roles in the diagnosis of the CMDs (Peat, Smith et al. 2008), the dystrophinopathies (Bonilla, Samitt et al. 1988; Hoffman, Fischbeck et al. 1988; Jones, Kim et al. 1998) and the sarcoglycanopathies (Vainzof, Passos-Bueno et al. 1996; Bonnemann, Wong et al. 2002) in particular. However, IHC is not helpful in all forms of MD. For example, in some dominant LGMDs such as LGMD1B, lamin A/C staining usually appears normal by IHC (Lo, Cooper et al. 2008). Mild to moderate 'secondary' staining abnormalities can arise in association with a primary abnormality in another protein or due to the disease process itself. Therefore the results of a single stain should always be considered in the context of other IHC results, the clinical situation and ideally protein quantification on Western blot (Ohlendieck, Matsumura et al. 1993; Mizuno, Yoshida et al. 1994; Vainzof, Passos-Bueno et al. 1996; Jones, Kim et al. 1998 (Lo, Cooper et al. 2008). For example, absence of dystrophin in DMD often results in partial loss of staining of other components of the dystrophin-associated protein complex (e.g. the sarcoglycans) and merosin. Reduced or abnormal localisation of dysferlin by IHC occurs in ~45% of all dystrophic muscle biopsies (Lo, Cooper et al. 2008), and it is only the absence of dysferlin by IHC and WB that indicates a primary dysferlinopathy.

Obtaining a muscle biopsy from a patient is an invasive procedure and biopsies are precious resources for both diagnosis and research. The single section WB technique (Cooper, Lo et al. 2003) has been an important advance on traditional methods by significantly reducing the amount of muscle biopsy used for each blot, from 20 - 100 mg down to one 8 μm cryosection. WB analysis has been found to be more effective for diagnosis than IHC for several forms of LGMD, such as LGMD2B (dysferlin) (Vainzof, Anderson et al. 2001; Nguyen, Bassez et al. 2005; Lo, Cooper et al. 2008), LGMD1C (caveolin-3) (Minetti, Sotgia et al. 1998; Carbone, Bruno et al. 2000; Herrmann, Straub et al. 2000; Lo, Cooper et al. 2008) , Becker MD (dystrophin) (Voit, Stuettgen et al. 1991) and arguably the alpha-dystroglycanopathies (Peat, Smith et al. 2008). However the sensitivity and specificity of WB is relatively poor for LGMD2A (calpain-3) (Fanin, Fulizio et al. 2004; Saenz, Leturcq et al. 2005; Groen, Charlton et al. 2007; Lo, Cooper et al. 2008) and the laminopathies (Menezes et al. 2011).

3.5 Genetic analysis

A provisional diagnosis can often be made by considering the clinical information, muscle pathology and protein studies, which can then be confirmed by direct gene sequencing (Bushby, Norwood et al. 2007; Norwood, de Visser et al. 2007). Even with recent advances, it is often difficult to correctly predict the correct LGMD sub-type and several genes may need to be tested before a definitive diagnosis is made. If genetic testing identifies mutations previously published or listed in on-line databases, a firm diagnosis can be made. However, if previously unreported genetic changes are found, then further functional protein studies may be useful to differentiate pathogenic mutations from rare harmless sequence variants.

Even in the best diagnostic centres, establishing a genetic cause for MD is only possible in around 90% of patients. Likely reasons are that the full phenotypic spectrum of many known genes is still being clarified and many MD genes likely remain unidentified. Whole exome or whole genome sequencing and other techniques that capitalise on recent advances in gene sequencing are likely to provide new opportunities to diagnose patients with MD. These approaches also have the capacity to identify new MD disease genes, which may account for many of the currently undiagnosed patients worldwide.

4. Diagnosis in specific forms of muscular dystrophy

4.1 Myotonic dystrophy

Myotonic dystrophy can usually be suspected from clinical examination and family history (see Section 2) and the clinician should have a low threshold for requesting genetic testing for DM1 since it is so common. Electromyography (EMG) is useful for showing characteristic myotonic discharges although these may not be present in young children with DM1 and in the occasional adult patient with DM2. Both DM1 and DM2 are multi-system disorders and involve predisposition to cataracts, cardiac conduction defects, cardiomyopathy, testicular failure and diabetes, as well as myotonia and muscle weakness. In myotonic dystrophy, muscle biopsy histopathology lacks specific diagnostic features but common features include smallness of a particular fibre type (type 1 atrophy in DM1 and type 2 atrophy in DM2), prominent internal nuclei and mild dystrophic changes. Genetic testing for DM1 is widely available and involves assessment of the size of a triplet repeat (CTG) in the *DMPK* gene (normal 5-34 repeats, asymptomatic/premutation 35-49 repeats, mild DM1 phenotype 50-~150, classical DM1 ~100-1000, congenital DM1 > 2000 repeats), (2000; Turner and Hilton-Jones 2010). Repeat numbers correlate only approximately with the severity of the phenotype and a normal genetic test excludes this condition. There is a tendency for the disease severity of DM1 to worsen when inherited by descendents due to further expansion in the size of the *DMPK* gene CTG repeat, a phenomenon called *anticipation*.

DM2 should be considered as a diagnosis if there are strong clinical clues for DM1 in an adult but genetic testing for DM1 is normal. In DM2, proximal limb weakness is more prominent than in DM1, weakness of facial and ankle dorsiflexor muscles may be less prominent and a congenital-onset form has not been described (Turner and Hilton-Jones 2010). Genetic testing for DM2, which is caused by an expansion of a quadruplet repeat (CCTG) the *ZNF9* gene, is technically more challenging and is less widely performed.

4.2 Facioscapulohumeral MD (FSHD)

A diagnosis of FSHD should be suspected when there is prominent (often asymmetric) weakness of muscles of the face, scapular stabilisers, upper arms and ankle dorsiflexor muscles that begins in late childhood to young adulthood on clinical examination (Sorrel-Dejerine and Fardeau 1982). With disease progression many other muscle groups become involved such as neck extensors, abdominal and pelvic muscles. Although FSHD follows an autosomal dominant pattern of inheritance, a negative family history does not exclude the condition as reduced penetrance (~10% especially in women) and *de novo* mutations (~20%) are relatively common. If a diagnosis of FSHD is considered possible on the basis of a clinical examination, genetic testing is the first investigation of choice since muscle biopsy usually shows non-specific dystrophic abnormalities and no protein studies are helpful. FSHD has a complex genetic cause that is not yet fully understood, but is associated with reduced numbers of large scale D4Z4 repeats in the subtelomeric region of chromosome 4. Genetic testing for the 4q deletion is technically challenging and is only 95% sensitive for the condition with the possibility of intermediate results, which are often difficult to interpret. As a result, testing is best conducted in an experienced laboratory, and family studies and the input of a clinical geneticist may assist when results are unclear.

4.3 Duchenne muscular dystrophy (DMD)

The diagnosis of DMD can usually be suspected on the basis of family history, age of onset, and clinical examination. DMD is an X-linked disorder that usually only affects males. Serum CK levels are markedly elevated in all male patients from birth. DMD gene testing using multiplex ligation-dependent probe amplification (MLPA) is a useful preliminary test that detects exon deletions or duplications and is diagnostic in about 75% of DMD patients (and in around 90% of BMD patients). If MLPA is negative, a muscle biopsy is often requested for protein studies. Marked dystrophic features are usually present and absence of dystrophin protein using IHC and/or WB is also diagnostic for DMD (Figure 3). These methods can also be used to detect reduced protein levels or the presence of a truncated protein product in patients with the milder form of the condition, Becker MD (BMD). Dystrophin sequencing may be required to determine point mutations that cannot be detected with MLPA. Around two-thirds of women who have a son with DMD are carriers of the mutation and gonadal mosaicism is relatively common in women who test negative for the mutation in DNA from blood leukocytes. Identifying the mutation causing DMD in

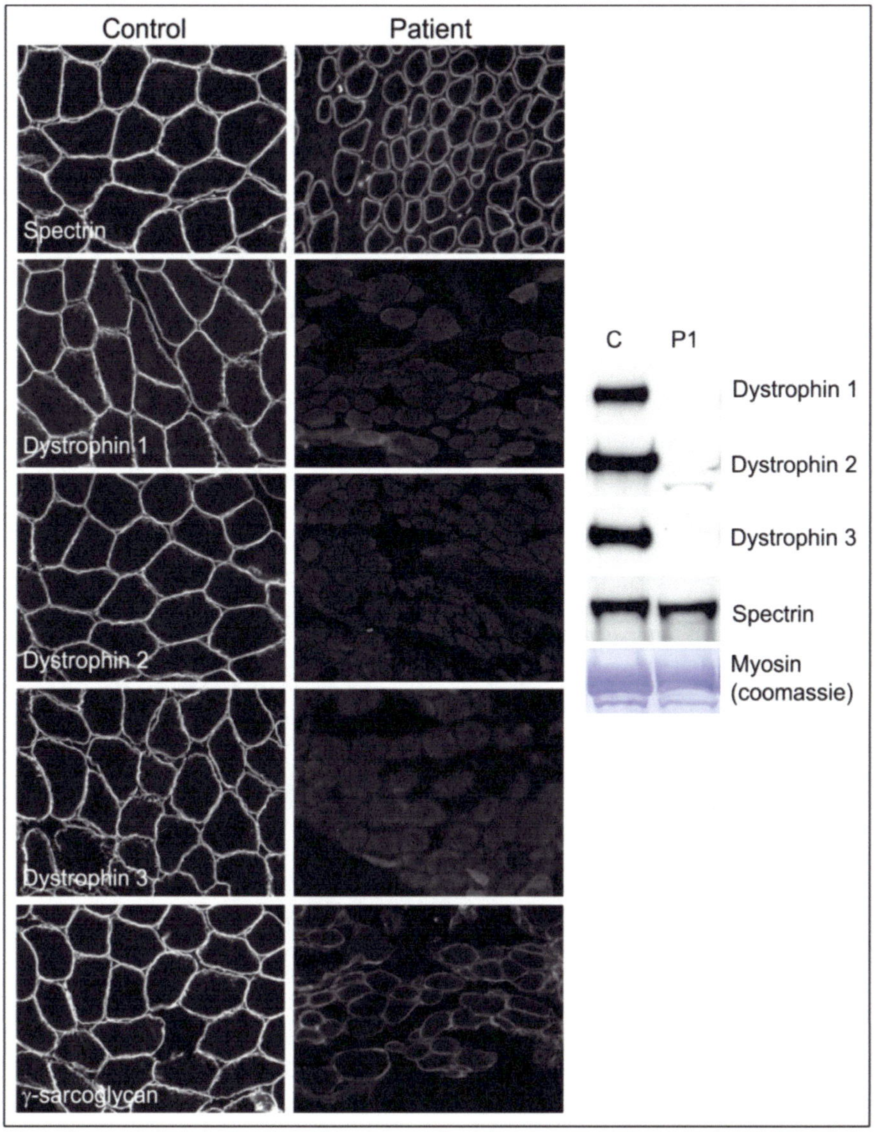

IHC and WB confirm dystrophin-deficiency in a patient with suspected DMD (P1). All patient muscle is stained with spectrin (NCL-SPEC1, Leica Microsystems, Wetzlar, Germany) as a control for membrane integrity. Three antibodies raised to different epitopes spanning the large dystrophin protein are used to help distinguish between total absence of dystrophin (DMD) and reduction or truncation of dystrophin (BMD) (NCL-Dys1, 2 & 3, Leica Microsystems, Wetzlar, Germany). Primary loss of dystrophin can result in secondary reductions in other members of the dystrophin-protein complex (sarcoglycans, dystroglycans) as shown here by a secondary reduction in γ-sarcoglycan (NCL-γ SARC, Leica Microsystems, Wetzlar, Germany), compared to control muscle. Western blot confirms absence of dystrophin protein when probed with the three dystrophin antibodies, strongly suggesting a primary abnormality in dystrophin which was confirmed by DMD gene analysis. Coomassie staining of myosin is used to show that equal amounts of protein are loaded for both patient and control in the WB.

Fig. 3. Immunohistochemistry and Western blot analysis of dystrophin and γ-sarcoglycan in the diagnosis of a patient with DMD.

each family is extremely useful so that highly accurate genetic testing is available for other women in the family who may be at risk of having affected sons. Approximately 10% of females with *DMD* gene mutations will show signs of muscle weakness (manifesting carriers) due to skewing of their ratio of X-chromosome inactivation, but most only become symptomatic during adulthood with mild muscle weakness and/or cardiomyopathy.

4.4 LGMD2B (dysferlinopathy)

A diagnosis of LGMD2B, due to autosomal recessive mutations in the *DYSF* gene, should be considered in patients with muscle weakness that begins in the late teenage years or early adulthood. It is common for *DYSF* patients to present with early involvement of calf muscles (also called Miyoshi myopathy) and difficulty standing on tip-toes. However, some *DYSF* patients present with a classical LGMD pattern of weakness involving the hip and shoulder girdles. Early calf wasting markedly raised serum CK levels (often 5000 - 20 000 U/ml) are distinguishing features of a primary dysferlinopathy, in contrast to many other forms of MD with calf hypertrophy. *DYSF* patient biopsy samples often display a prominent inflammatory cell infiltrate, sometimes leading to misdiagnosis of polymyositis. A range of abnormal dysferlin staining patterns are seen in many types of MD as non-specific secondary abnormalities (see Figure 4b), but complete absence of staining by IHC and WB (Figure 4a) is specific for LGMD2B.

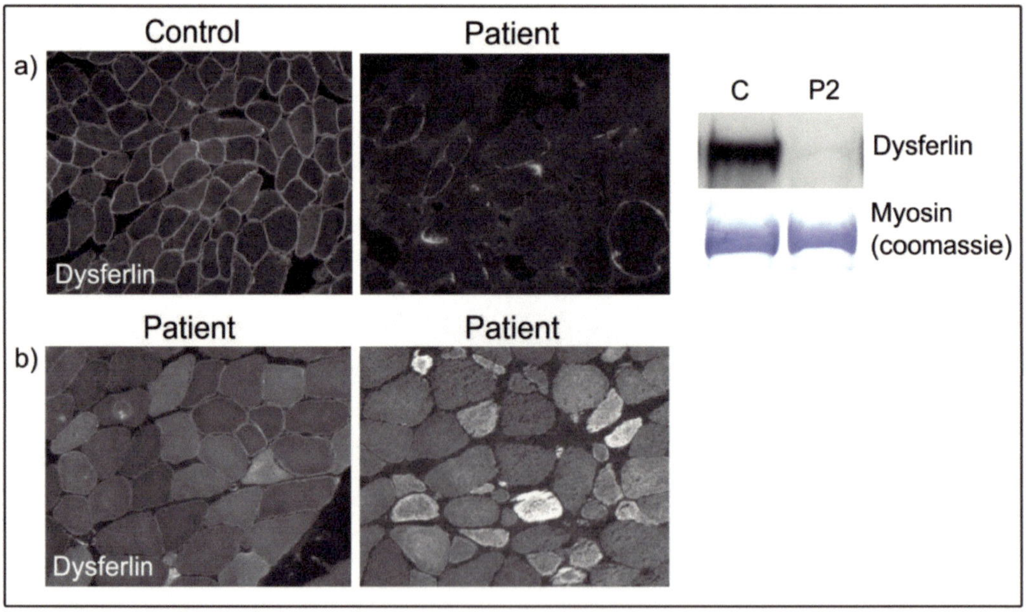

a) IHC of LGMD2B patient muscle shows a severe reduction in dysferlin (NCL-Hamlet, Leica Microsystems) staining at the muscle membrane compared to control muscle, and a corresponding loss of dysferlin by WB (P2). Genetic analysis of this patient confirmed mutations in the *DYSF* gene.
b) Secondary reductions and abnormal dysferlin protein localisation by IHC occur commonly as secondary abnormalities in many dystrophies but absence on WB is specific to dysferlinopathies.

Fig. 4. Immunohistochemistry and Western blot analysis of dysferlin in the diagnosis of LGMD2B.

4.5 LGMD2I

Patients with LGMD2I, due to autosomal recessive mutations in *FKRP*, usually present with a classical LGMD pattern of weakness, often with greater involvement of the lower limbs, and calf hypertrophy. Some patients also have macroglossia (an enlarged tongue) and ankle contractures. α-dystroglycan staining by IHC is usually reduced in LGMD2I patients (see Figure 5), although the reduction may be subtle and is rarely absent. WB can be used to look for reduction of glycosylated α-dystroglycan, which usually appears as a smeared band at ~156 kDa due to variable glycosylation of the core protein which results in a range of final molecular weights (Figure 5). Almost all LGMD2I patients have at least one copy of the c.826C>A (L276I) mutation, a founder mutation that is particularly common in Northern European populations (Walter, Petersen et al. 2004). Severe reductions in α-dystroglycan by IHC and WB can also be associated with other mutations in *FKRP*, or with mutations in the other 'alpha-dystroglycanopathy' genes encoding glycosylation enzymes that result in CMD, WWS or MEB phenotypes (see Table 1).

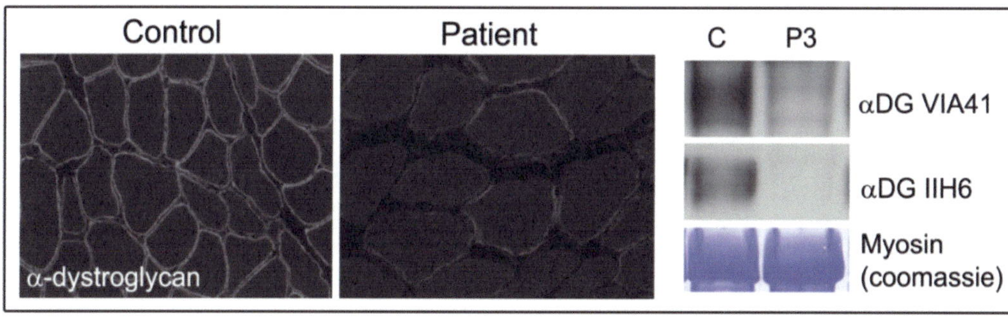

α-dystroglycan levels are reduced by IHC and WB (using both VIA41 (Millipore, CA, USA) and IIH6 (kind gift from Dr Kevin Campbell) antibodies that recognize glycosylated α-dystroglycan, in a number of glycosyltransferase disorders. Specific genetic testing is required to determine the particular genetic cause. In this case the patient was found to have recessive mutations in the *FKRP* gene, causing LGMD2I.

Fig. 5. Immunohistochemistry and Western blot analysis of α-dystroglycan in a patient with LGMD2I.

4.6 Emery-Dreifuss muscular dystrophy (EDMD)

EDMD should be suspected in patients who develop early joint contractures, particularly of the elbows, neck extensors and tendo-Achilles. Patients present with progressive muscle weakness and wasting particularly of the upper arm and ankle dorsiflexor muscles, and often develop cardiac abnormalities (heart block, arrhythmias or cardiomyopathy). Mutations in three genes are associated with this phenotype, *LMNA* (which follows autosomal dominant inheritance), *EMD* and *FHL1* (both X-linked genes), but further genetic causes are likely. IHC for emerin in skeletal muscle shows from the nuclear envelope in X-linked EDMD due to *EMD* mutations and is specific for this condition (see Figure 6). Emerin is also completely absent by WB in these patients (Figure 6). Finding mutations on *EMD* gene sequencing confirms the diagnosis and allows for carrier testing of at-risk females. There are no robust protein-based screening tests for *LMNA* mutations and direct sequencing is required to exclude the diagnosis. Clinicians should have a low threshold for testing both the *EMD* and *LMNA* genes if a diagnosis of EDMD is possible, due to the risk of developing potentially lethal cardic arrhythmias. Early diagnosis allows for introduction of close cardiac surveillance by electrocardiogram (ECG), Holter ambulatory ECG monitoring, echocardiography and the early use of implantable cardiac defibrillators to reduce morbidity and mortality.

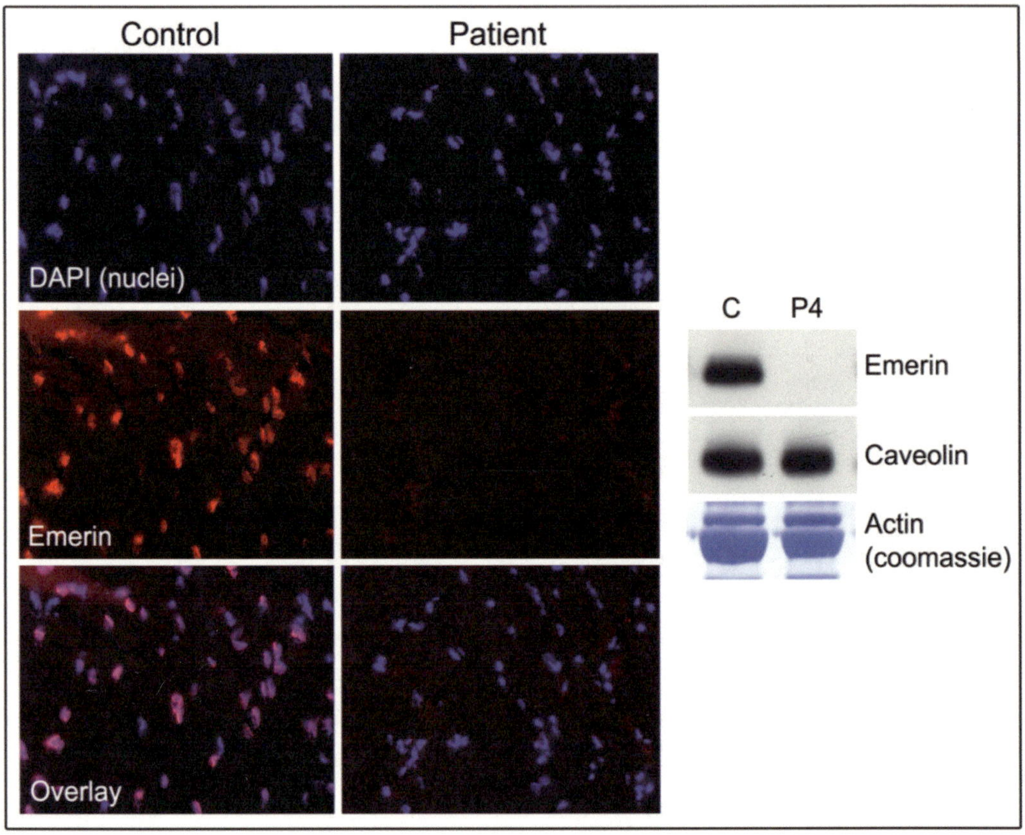

Examples of Emerin immunostaining is absent from the nuclear envelope in muscle from a patient with X-linked EDMD (nuclei are stained by DAPI (4',6-diamidino-2-phenylindole, dihydrochloride), Invitrogen, CA, USA). WB analysis shows absent staining for emerin (P4), and a genetic mutation (c.651_655dupGGGCC) was later identified. Immunoblot for caveolin-3 and coomassie staining of actin are used to show equal protein loading.

Fig. 6. Immunohistochemistry and Western blot analysis of emerin in the diagnosis of EDMD.

4.7 Ullrich congenital muscular dystrophy (UCMD) and Bethlem myopathy

Patients with UCMD usually present with generalised muscle weakness, wasting, hypotonia and marked distal laxity from birth (Nonaka, Une et al. 1981; De Paillette, Aicardi et al. 1989; Mercuri, Yuva et al. 2002). Clinically, patients often have a distinctive sandpaper-like skin rash, congenital hip dislocation, scoliosis, a high arched palate and prominent heels. IHC is a useful diagnostic test, and staining of muscle sections with collagen VI in combination with a muscle membrane marker, e.g. perlecan or collagen IV, can highlight a characteristic loss of collagen VI at the muscle membranes even though collagen VI staining may be retained in connective tissue between fibres (Figure 7). Reduced secretion of collagen VI by cultured

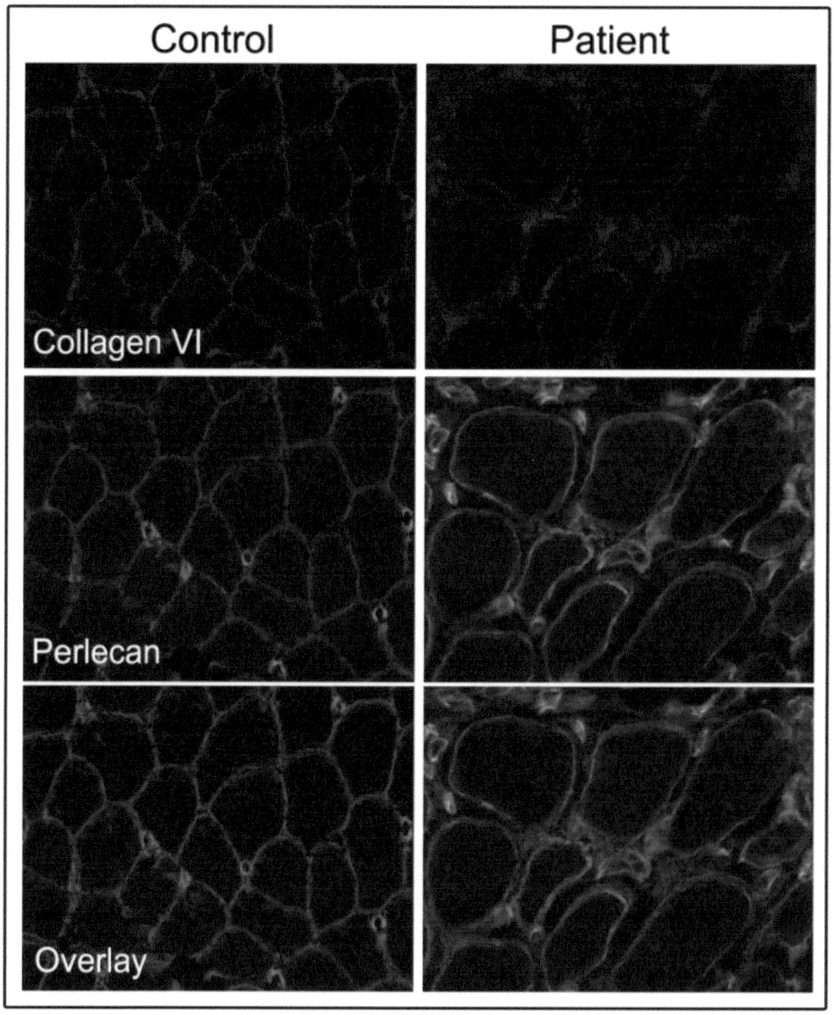

In UCMD and Bethlem myopathy, collagen VI is reduced or lost at the plasma membrane of muscle fibres but may be present in interstitial connective tissue. After carefully optimising conditions to achieve equal intensity of collagen VI (70-XR95, Fitzgerald Industries International Inc, MA, USA) and perlecan (A7L6, MAB1948, Miilipore, CA, USA) staining in control muscle, an overlay image can identify a reduction in collagen VI, relative to perlecan, at the muscle sarcolemmal membrane. In this example, an overlay image from control muscle appears mostly yellow/orange, with broadly equal intensities of perlecan (green) and collagen VI (red) staining. In contrast, an overlay image from a UCMD patient, reveals a dominance of perlecan (green labelling), indicating a relative deficiency of collagen VI (red label) at the muscle membrane. These results are consistent with a primary collagenopathy, and a dominant mutation was identified in the *COL6A2* gene.

Fig. 7. Immunohistochemistry analysis of collagen VI in the diagnosis of UCMD.

patient fibroblasts strongly supports a diagnosis of UCMD or Bethlem myopathy but genetic testing of the three genes that code for collagen VI chains (see Table 1) is required to confirm the diagnosis. Collagen VI gene mutations that do not result in severe protein abnormalities usually present in childhood with a less severe phenotype called Bethlem myopathy.

Progressive joint contractures are major sources of morbidity in both UCMD and Bethlem myopathy and close monitoring for scoliosis and respiratory insufficiency is important, particularly in UCMD.

5. Frequency of diagnosis of less common types of MD

The frequency of some forms of MD varies widely in different parts of the world, which can influence the most appropriate diagnostic approach to follow in different countries.

LGMD2A accounted for 50% of all LGMD patients in a Turkish study (Dincer, Leturcq et al. 1997), around 25% of patients in Italy (Guglieri, Magri et al. 2008; Fanin, Nascimbeni et al. 2009) and the United Kingdom (UK) (Norwood, Harling et al. 2009) but only 5-8% in American (Moore, Shilling et al. 2006), Brazilian (Vainzof, Passos-Bueno et al. 1999) and Australian (Lo, Cooper et al. 2008) studies. Although different diagnostic techniques may account for some of the variability, this finding points to major regional differences in the frequency of *CAPN3* gene mutations in different populations. Similarly LGMD2I seems particularly prevalent in Scandinavia (Sveen, Schwartz et al. 2006) and the UK (Norwood, Harling et al. 2009) compared with other populations (see Table 3). High rates of known genetic forms of LGMD likely contribute to a high overall rate of LGMD diagnosis in Turkey (Dincer, Leturcq et al. 1997), the UK (Norwood, Harling et al. 2009) and Denmark (Sveen, Schwartz et al. 2006). The rates identified for many forms of LGMD are similar in Australia (Lo, Cooper et al. 2008) to the USA (Moore, Shilling et al. 2006) and it is interesting that both populations are comprised of a mixture of ethnicities.

	LGMD								Total Diagnosis
	1A	1B	1C	2A	2B	2C,D,E,F	2G	2I	
Denmark [1]	NA	NA	NA	12%	2%	22%	NA	37%	73%
Turkey [2]	NA	NA	NA	50%	5%	20%	NA	NA	75%
Italy [3]	0%	0%	1.3%	28%	19%	18%	0%	6%	73%
Northern England [4]		9%		26%	6%	12%		19%	72%
USA [5]	0.6%	7%	0%	9%	3%	19%	NA	7%	46%
Italy [6]	NA	1%	1.5%	19%	8%	11%	NA	3%	43%
Brazil [7]	NA	NA	NA	5%	3%	17%	NA	NA	24%
Australia [8]	NA	1%	2.6%	8%	5%	2.6%	NA	2.6%	23%
Brazil [9]	NA	NA	NA	32%	22%	32%	3%	11%	N/A

LGMD = limb-girdle muscular dystrophy. NA = not assessed, N/A = retrospective review, no total diagnosis stated. References: 1(Sveen, Schwartz et al. 2006), 2(Dincer, Leturcq et al. 1997), 3(Guglieri, Magri et al. 2008), 4(Norwood, Harling et al. 2009), 5(Moore, Shilling et al. 2006), 6(Fanin, Nascimbeni et al. 2009), 7(Vainzof, Passos-Bueno et al. 1999), 8(Lo, Cooper et al. 2008) and 9(Zatz, de Paula et al. 2003).

Table 3. Diagnoses in LGMD cohort studies.

As for LGMD, the proportions of some forms of CMD have varied widely between studies in different countries. A Brazilian study diagnosed merosin-deficiency in around 40% of CMD patients (Ferreira, Marie et al. 2005), while this diagnosis accounted for only 8% of CMD patients in an Australian study (Peat, Smith et al. 2008). Differences in CMD ascertainment criteria may be partly responsible but it is likely there are true differences in disease incidence in different populations. Similarly, different rates of collagen VI diagnoses have been observed, ranging from 8% in Australia (Peat, Smith et al. 2008) to 1.7% in Brazil (Ferreira, Marie et al. 2005).

6. Future directions

In the past, genetic testing for MD has involved the sequencing of individual genes that were considered likely causes based on clinical presentation and screening tests. The large number of possible genetic causes with overlapping phenotypes has made it difficult to predict the correct genetic cause in many MD patients and consequently, finding the causative mutation in many families has often been a prolonged, expensive exercise. Recent advances in gene sequencing are likely to have a major impact on the diagnosis of MD in the near future. It is now possible to sequence multiple muscle disease genes and even the whole genome relatively cheaply in a single experiment (Metzker 2010). Next generation sequencing technologies will also facilitate the discovery of new MD genes, leading to increased rates of patient diagnosis. As thesetechnologies become more routinely used and costs reduce, the approach to diagnosing forms of MD such as, LGMD, that have many possible genetic causes is likely to move from the sequencing of individual candidate genes towards a multi-gene or genome-wide sequencing approach. Some diagnostic centres worldwide are already implementing this technology for the diagnosis of MDs. These methods bring new challenges, such as distinguishing genetic sequence variants that are the primary cause of the disease from variants that modify a phenotype or are harmless polymorphisms. It is likely that there will always be a need for centres with expertise in clinical phenotyping and protein studies to clarify the diagnosis when genetic analysis alone cannot confirm whether a sequence variant in a gene is truly disease-causing or not.

7. Glossary

BMD	Becker muscular dystrophy
CK	Creatine kinase
CMD	Congenital muscular dystrophy
DMD	Duchenne muscular dystrophy
DM	Myotonic dystrophy (DM1 Type 1, DM2 Type 2)
ECG	Electrocardiogram
EDMD	Emery Dreifuss muscular dystrophy
FCMD	Fukuyama congenital muscular dystrophy
FSHD	Facioscapulohumeral muscular dystrophy
IHC	Immunohistochemistry
LGMD	Limb girdle muscular dystrophy (Type 1 dominant, Type 2 recessive)
MD	Muscular dystrophy
MEB	Muscle-eye-brain disease
MLPA	Multiplex Ligation-dependent Probe Amplification
MRI	Magnetic resonance imaging
UCMD	Ullrich congenital muscular dystrophy
UK	United Kingdom
WB	Western blot
WWS	Walker-Warburg Syndrome

8. References

(2000). "New nomenclature and DNA testing guidelines for myotonic dystrophy type 1 (DM1). The International Myotonic Dystrophy Consortium (IDMC)." *Neurology* 54(6): 1218-1221.

Allamand, V. and P. Guicheney (2002). "Merosin-deficient congenital muscular dystrophy, autosomal recessive (MDC1A, MIM#156225, LAMA2 gene coding for alpha2 chain of laminin)." *Eur J Hum Genet* 10(2): 91-94.

Azibi, K., L. Bachner, et al. (1993). "Severe childhood autosomal recessive muscular dystrophy with the deficiency of the 50 kDa dystrophin-associated glycoprotein maps to chromosome 13q12." *Hum Mol Genet* 2(9): 1423-1428.

Balci, B., G. Uyanik, et al. (2005). "An autosomal recessive limb girdle muscular dystrophy (LGMD2) with mild mental retardation is allelic to Walker-Warburg syndrome (WWS) caused by a mutation in the POMT1 gene." *Neuromuscul Disord* 15(4): 271-275.

Bashir, R., S. Britton, et al. (1998). "A gene related to Caenorhabditis elegans spermatogenesis factor fer-1 is mutated in limb-girdle muscular dystrophy type 2B." *Nat Genet* 20(1): 37-42.

Beltran-Valero de Bernabe, D., S. Currier, et al. (2002). "Mutations in the O-mannosyltransferase gene POMT1 give rise to the severe neuronal migration disorder Walker-Warburg syndrome." *Am J Hum Genet* 71(5): 1033-1043.

Beltran-Valero de Bernabe, D., T. Voit, et al. (2004). "Mutations in the FKRP gene can cause muscle-eye-brain disease and Walker-Warburg syndrome." *J Med Genet* 41(5): e61.

Bertini, E. and G. Pepe (2002). "Collagen type VI and related disorders: Bethlem myopathy and Ullrich scleroatonic muscular dystrophy." *Eur J Paediatr Neurol* 6(4): 193-198.

Biancheri, R., A. Falace, et al. (2007). "POMT2 gene mutation in limb-girdle muscular dystrophy with inflammatory changes." *Biochem Biophys Res Commun* 363(4): 1033-1037.

Bione, S., E. Maestrini, et al. (1994). "Identification of a novel X-linked gene responsible for Emery-Dreifuss muscular dystrophy." *Nat Genet* 8(4): 323-327.

Bolduc, V., G. Marlow, et al. (2010). "Recessive mutations in the putative calcium-activated chloride channel Anoctamin 5 cause proximal LGMD2L and distal MMD3 muscular dystrophies." *Am J Hum Genet* 86(2): 213-221.

Bonilla, E., C. E. Samitt, et al. (1988). "Duchenne muscular dystrophy: deficiency of dystrophin at the muscle cell surface." *Cell* 54(4): 447-452.

Bonne, G., M. R. Di Barletta, et al. (1999). "Mutations in the gene encoding lamin A/C cause autosomal dominant Emery-Dreifuss muscular dystrophy." *Nat Genet* 21(3): 285-288.

Bonne, G., E. Mercuri, et al. (2000). "Clinical and molecular genetic spectrum of autosomal dominant Emery-Dreifuss muscular dystrophy due to mutations of the lamin A/C gene." *Ann Neurol* 48(2): 170-180.

Bonnemann, C. G., M. R. Passos-Bueno, et al. (1996). "Genomic screening for beta-sarcoglycan gene mutations: missense mutations may cause severe limb-girdle muscular dystrophy type 2E (LGMD 2E)." *Hum Mol Genet* 5(12): 1953-1961.

Bonnemann, C. G., J. Wong, et al. (2002). "Primary gamma-sarcoglycanopathy (LGMD 2C): broadening of the mutational spectrum guided by the immunohistochemical profile." *Neuromuscul Disord* 12(3): 273-280.

Borg, K., R. Stucka, et al. (2009). "Intragenic deletion of TRIM32 in compound heterozygotes with sarcotubular myopathy/LGMD2H." *Hum Mutat.*

Brais, B., J. P. Bouchard, et al. (1998). "Short GCG expansions in the PABP2 gene cause oculopharyngeal muscular dystrophy." *Nat Genet* 18(2): 164-167.

Brais, B., Y. G. Xie, et al. (1995). "The oculopharyngeal muscular dystrophy locus maps to the region of the cardiac alpha and beta myosin heavy chain genes on chromosome 14q11.2-q13." *Hum Mol Genet* 4(3): 429-434.

Brockington, M., D. J. Blake, et al. (2001). "Mutations in the fukutin-related protein gene (FKRP) cause a form of congenital muscular dystrophy with secondary laminin alpha2 deficiency and abnormal glycosylation of alpha-dystroglycan." *Am J Hum Genet* 69(6): 1198-1209.

Brockington, M., C. A. Sewry, et al. (2000). "Assignment of a form of congenital muscular dystrophy with secondary merosin deficiency to chromosome 1q42." *Am J Hum Genet* 66(2): 428-435.

Brockington, M., Y. Yuva, et al. (2001). "Mutations in the fukutin-related protein gene (FKRP) identify limb girdle muscular dystrophy 2I as a milder allelic variant of congenital muscular dystrophy MDC1C." *Hum Mol Genet* 10(25): 2851-2859.

Brook, J. D., M. E. McCurrach, et al. (1992). "Molecular basis of myotonic dystrophy: expansion of a trinucleotide (CTG) repeat at the 3' end of a transcript encoding a protein kinase family member." *Cell* 68(4): 799-808.

Burghes, A. H., C. Logan, et al. (1987). "A cDNA clone from the Duchenne/Becker muscular dystrophy gene." *Nature* 328(6129): 434-437.

Bushby, K., R. Bashir, et al. (1996). "The molecular biology of LGMD2B--towards the identification of the LGMD gene on chromosome 2p13." *Neuromuscul Disord* 6(6): 491-492.

Bushby, K., R. Finkel, et al. (2010). "Diagnosis and management of Duchenne muscular dystrophy, part 1: diagnosis, and pharmacological and psychosocial management." *Lancet Neurol* 9(1): 77-93.

Bushby, K., F. Norwood, et al. (2007). "The limb-girdle muscular dystrophies--diagnostic strategies." *Biochim Biophys Acta* 1772(2): 238-242.

Camacho Vanegas, O., E. Bertini, et al. (2001). "Ullrich scleroatonic muscular dystrophy is caused by recessive mutations in collagen type VI." *Proc Natl Acad Sci U S A* 98(13): 7516-7521.

Carbone, I., C. Bruno, et al. (2000). "Mutation in the CAV3 gene causes partial caveolin-3 deficiency and hyperCKemia." *Neurology* 54(6): 1373-1376.

Clarke, N. F., W. Kidson, et al. (2006). "SEPN1: associated with congenital fiber-type disproportion and insulin resistance." *Ann Neurol* 59(3): 546-552.

Cooper, S. T., H. P. Lo, et al. (2003). "Single section Western blot: improving the molecular diagnosis of the muscular dystrophies." *Neurology* 61(1): 93-97.

Cupler, E. J., S. Bohlega, et al. (1998). "Miyoshi myopathy in Saudi Arabia: clinical, electrophysiological, histopathological and radiological features." *Neuromuscul Disord* 8(5): 321-326.

de Bernabe, D. B., H. van Bokhoven, et al. (2003). "A homozygous nonsense mutation in the fukutin gene causes a Walker-Warburg syndrome phenotype." *J Med Genet* 40(11): 845-848.

De Paillette, L., J. Aicardi, et al. (1989). "Ullrich's congenital atonic sclerotic muscular dystrophy. A case report." *J Neurol* 236(2): 108-110.

Demir, E., P. Sabatelli, et al. (2002). "Mutations in COL6A3 cause severe and mild phenotypes of Ullrich congenital muscular dystrophy." *Am J Hum Genet* 70(6): 1446-1458.

Dincer, P., F. Leturcq, et al. (1997). "A biochemical, genetic, and clinical survey of autosomal recessive limb girdle muscular dystrophies in Turkey." *Ann Neurol* 42(2): 222-229.

Driss, A., R. Amouri, et al. (2000). "A new locus for autosomal recessive limb-girdle muscular dystrophy in a large consanguineous Tunisian family maps to chromosome 19q13.3." *Neuromuscul Disord* 10(4-5): 240-246.

Emery, A. E. (1989). "Emery-Dreifuss syndrome." *J Med Genet* 26(10): 637-641.

Eymard, B., N. B. Romero, et al. (1997). "Primary adhalinopathy (alpha-sarcoglycanopathy): clinical, pathologic, and genetic correlation in 20 patients with autosomal recessive muscular dystrophy." *Neurology* 48(5): 1227-1234.

Fanin, M., L. Fulizio, et al. (2004). "Molecular diagnosis in LGMD2A: mutation analysis or protein testing?" *Hum Mutat* 24(1): 52-62.

Fanin, M., A. C. Nascimbeni, et al. (2009). "Frequency of LGMD gene mutations in Italian patients with distinct clinical phenotypes." *Neurology* 72(16): 1432-1435.

Fardeau, M., D. Hillaire, et al. (1996). "Juvenile limb-girdle muscular dystrophy. Clinical, histopathological and genetic data from a small community living in the Reunion Island." *Brain* 119 (Pt 1): 295-308.

Ferreira, L. G., S. K. Marie, et al. (2005). "Dystrophin-glycoproteins associated in congenital muscular dystrophy: immunohistochemical analysis of 59 Brazilian cases." *Arq Neuropsiquiatr* 63(3B): 791-800.

Ferreiro, A., S. Quijano-Roy, et al. (2002). "Mutations of the selenoprotein N gene, which is implicated in rigid spine muscular dystrophy, cause the classical phenotype of multiminicore disease: reassessing the nosology of early-onset myopathies." *Am J Hum Genet* 71(4): 739-749.

Fischer, D., M. C. Walter, et al. (2005). "Diagnostic value of muscle MRI in differentiating LGMD2I from other LGMDs." *J Neurol* 252(5): 538-547.

Flanigan, K. M., L. Kerr, et al. (2000). "Congenital muscular dystrophy with rigid spine syndrome: a clinical, pathological, radiological, and genetic study." *Ann Neurol* 47(2): 152-161.

Frosk, P., T. Weiler, et al. (2002). "Limb-girdle muscular dystrophy type 2H associated with mutation in TRIM32, a putative E3-ubiquitin-ligase gene." *Am J Hum Genet* 70(3): 663-672.

Giusti, B., L. Lucarini, et al. (2005). "Dominant and recessive COL6A1 mutations in Ullrich scleroatonic muscular dystrophy." *Ann Neurol* 58(3): 400-410.

Godfrey, C., E. Clement, et al. (2007). "Refining genotype phenotype correlations in muscular dystrophies with defective glycosylation of dystroglycan." *Brain* 130(Pt 10): 2725-2735.

Godfrey, C., D. Escolar, et al. (2006). "Fukutin gene mutations in steroid-responsive limb girdle muscular dystrophy." *Ann Neurol* 60(5): 603-610.

Groen, E. J., R. Charlton, et al. (2007). "Analysis of the UK diagnostic strategy for limb girdle muscular dystrophy 2A." *Brain* 130(Pt 12): 3237-3249.

Gueneau, L., A. T. Bertrand, et al. (2009). "Mutations of the FHL1 gene cause Emery-Dreifuss muscular dystrophy." *Am J Hum Genet* 85(3): 338-353.

Guglieri, M. and K. Bushby (2008). "How to go about diagnosing and managing the limb-girdle muscular dystrophies." *Neurol India* 56(3): 271-280.

Guglieri, M., F. Magri, et al. (2008). "Clinical, molecular, and protein correlations in a large sample of genetically diagnosed Italian limb girdle muscular dystrophy patients." *Hum Mutat* 29(2): 258-266.

Hackman, P., A. Vihola, et al. (2002). "Tibial muscular dystrophy is a titinopathy caused by mutations in TTN, the gene encoding the giant skeletal-muscle protein titin." *Am J Hum Genet* 71(3): 492-500.

Hauser, M. A., S. K. Horrigan, et al. (2000). "Myotilin is mutated in limb girdle muscular dystrophy 1A." *Hum Mol Genet* 9(14): 2141-2147.

Hayashi, Y. K., F. L. Chou, et al. (1998). "Mutations in the integrin alpha7 gene cause congenital myopathy." *Nat Genet* 19(1): 94-97.

Hayashi, Y. K., C. Matsuda, et al. (2009). "Human PTRF mutations cause secondary deficiency of caveolins resulting in muscular dystrophy with generalized lipodystrophy." *J Clin Invest* 119(9): 2623-2633.

Helbling-Leclerc, A., X. Zhang, et al. (1995). "Mutations in the laminin alpha 2-chain gene (LAMA2) cause merosin-deficient congenital muscular dystrophy." *Nat Genet* 11(2): 216-218.

Herrmann, R., V. Straub, et al. (2000). "Dissociation of the dystroglycan complex in caveolin-3-deficient limb girdle muscular dystrophy." *Hum Mol Genet* 9(15): 2335-2340.

Hicks, D., A. Sarkozy, et al. (2011). "A founder mutation in Anoctamin 5 is a major cause of limb-girdle muscular dystrophy." *Brain* 134(Pt 1): 171-182.

Higuchi, I., T. Shiraishi, et al. (2001). "Frameshift mutation in the collagen VI gene causes Ullrich's disease." *Ann Neurol* 50(2): 261-265.

Hillaire, D., A. Leclerc, et al. (1994). "Localization of merosin-negative congenital muscular dystrophy to chromosome 6q2 by homozygosity mapping." *Hum Mol Genet* 3(9): 1657-1661.

Himmrich, E., S. Popov, et al. (2000). "[Hidden intracardiac conduction disturbances and their spontaneous course in patients with progressive muscular dystrophy]." *Z Kardiol* 89(7): 592-598.

Hoffman, E. P., R. H. Brown, Jr., et al. (1987). "Dystrophin: the protein product of the Duchenne muscular dystrophy locus." *Cell* 51(6): 919-928.

Hoffman, E. P., K. H. Fischbeck, et al. (1988). "Characterization of dystrophin in muscle-biopsy specimens from patients with Duchenne's or Becker's muscular dystrophy." *N Engl J Med* 318(21): 1363-1368.

Jobsis, G. J., H. Keizers, et al. (1996). "Type VI collagen mutations in Bethlem myopathy, an autosomal dominant myopathy with contractures." *Nat Genet* 14(1): 113-115.

Jones, K. J., S. S. Kim, et al. (1998). "Abnormalities of dystrophin, the sarcoglycans, and laminin alpha2 in the muscular dystrophies." *J Med Genet* 35(5): 379-386.

Jones, K. J., G. Morgan, et al. (2001). "The expanding phenotype of laminin alpha2 chain (merosin) abnormalities: case series and review." *J Med Genet* 38(10): 649-657.

Jones, K. J. and K. N. North (1997). "Recent advances in diagnosis of the childhood muscular dystrophies." *J Paediatr Child Health* 33(3): 195-201.

Kaplan, J. C. (2010). "The 2011 version of the gene table of neuromuscular disorders." *Neuromuscul Disord* 20(12): 852-873.

Kobayashi, K., Y. Nakahori, et al. (1998). "An ancient retrotransposal insertion causes Fukuyama-type congenital muscular dystrophy." *Nature* 394(6691): 388-392.

Koenig, M., E. P. Hoffman, et al. (1987). "Complete cloning of the Duchenne muscular dystrophy (DMD) cDNA and preliminary genomic organization of the DMD gene in normal and affected individuals." *Cell* 50(3): 509-517.

Koenig, M., A. P. Monaco, et al. (1988). "The complete sequence of dystrophin predicts a rod-shaped cytoskeletal protein." *Cell* 53(2): 219-228.

Lamminen, A. E. (1990). "Magnetic resonance imaging of primary skeletal muscle diseases: patterns of distribution and severity of involvement." *Br J Radiol* 63(756): 946-950.

Lamminen, A. E., J. I. Tanttu, et al. (1990). "Magnetic resonance of diseased skeletal muscle: combined T1 measurement and chemical shift imaging." *Br J Radiol* 63(752): 591-596.

Lim, L. E., F. Duclos, et al. (1995). "Beta-sarcoglycan: characterization and role in limb-girdle muscular dystrophy linked to 4q12." *Nat Genet* 11(3): 257-265.

Liquori, C. L., K. Ricker, et al. (2001). "Myotonic dystrophy type 2 caused by a CCTG expansion in intron 1 of ZNF9." *Science* 293(5531): 864-867.

Liu, J., M. Aoki, et al. (1998). "Dysferlin, a novel skeletal muscle gene, is mutated in Miyoshi myopathy and limb girdle muscular dystrophy." *Nat Genet* 20(1): 31-36.

Lo, H. P., S. T. Cooper, et al. (2008). "Limb-girdle muscular dystrophy: diagnostic evaluation, frequency and clues to pathogenesis." *Neuromuscul Disord* 18(1): 34-44.

Lodi, R., F. Muntoni, et al. (1997). "Correlative MR imaging and 31P-MR spectroscopy study in sarcoglycan deficient limb girdle muscular dystrophy." *Neuromuscul Disord* 7(8): 505-511.

Longman, C., M. Brockington, et al. (2003). "Mutations in the human LARGE gene cause MDC1D, a novel form of congenital muscular dystrophy with severe mental retardation and abnormal glycosylation of alpha-dystroglycan." *Hum Mol Genet* 12(21): 2853-2861.

McNally, E. M., E. de Sa Moreira, et al. (1998). "Caveolin-3 in muscular dystrophy." *Hum Mol Genet* 7(5): 871-877.

McNally, E. M. and P. Pytel (2007). "Muscle diseases: the muscular dystrophies." *Annu Rev Pathol* 2: 87-109.

Menezes, M.P., L.B. Waddell, et al. (2011) "The importance and challenge of making an early diagnosis in LMNA-related muscular dystrophy." *Neurol.* (Accepted 14th Dec 2011).

Meola, G., V. Sansone, et al. (1996). "Computerized tomography and magnetic resonance muscle imaging in Miyoshi's myopathy." *Muscle Nerve* 19(11): 1476-1480.

Mercuri, E., C. Cini, et al. (2002). "Muscle MRI findings in a three-generation family affected by Bethlem myopathy." *Eur J Paediatr Neurol* 6(6): 309-314.

Mercuri, E., C. Cini, et al. (2003). "Muscle magnetic resonance imaging in patients with congenital muscular dystrophy and Ullrich phenotype." *Neuromuscul Disord* 13(7-8): 554-558.

Mercuri, E., E. Clements, et al. (2010). "Muscle magnetic resonance imaging involvement in muscular dystrophies with rigidity of the spine." *Ann Neurol* 67(2): 201-208.

Mercuri, E., S. Counsell, et al. (2002). "Selective muscle involvement on magnetic resonance imaging in autosomal dominant Emery-Dreifuss muscular dystrophy." *Neuropediatrics* 33(1): 10-14.

Mercuri, E., A. D'Amico, et al. (2006). "POMT2 mutation in a patient with 'MEB-like' phenotype." *Neuromuscul Disord* 16(7): 446-448.

Mercuri, E., H. Jungbluth, et al. (2005). "Muscle imaging in clinical practice: diagnostic value of muscle magnetic resonance imaging in inherited neuromuscular disorders." *Curr Opin Neurol* 18(5): 526-537.

Mercuri, E., A. Lampe, et al. (2005). "Muscle MRI in Ullrich congenital muscular dystrophy and Bethlem myopathy." *Neuromuscul Disord* 15(4): 303-310.

Mercuri, E., A. Pichiecchio, et al. (2002). "A short protocol for muscle MRI in children with muscular dystrophies." *Eur J Paediatr Neurol* 6(6): 305-307.

Mercuri, E., B. Talim, et al. (2002). "Clinical and imaging findings in six cases of congenital muscular dystrophy with rigid spine syndrome linked to chromosome 1p (RSMD1)." *Neuromuscul Disord* 12(7-8): 631-638.
Mercuri, E., Y. Yuva, et al. (2002). "Collagen VI involvement in Ullrich syndrome: a clinical, genetic, and immunohistochemical study." *Neurology* 58(9): 1354-1359.
Messina, D. N., M. C. Speer, et al. (1997). "Linkage of familial dilated cardiomyopathy with conduction defect and muscular dystrophy to chromosome 6q23." *Am J Hum Genet* 61(4): 909-917.
Metzker, M. L. (2010). "Sequencing technologies - the next generation." *Nat Rev Genet* 11(1): 31-46.
Minetti, C., F. Sotgia, et al. (1998). "Mutations in the caveolin-3 gene cause autosomal dominant limb-girdle muscular dystrophy." *Nat Genet* 18(4): 365-368.
Moghadaszadeh, B., I. Desguerre, et al. (1998). "Identification of a new locus for a peculiar form of congenital muscular dystrophy with early rigidity of the spine, on chromosome 1p35-36." *Am J Hum Genet* 62(6): 1439-1445.
Moghadaszadeh, B., N. Petit, et al. (2001). "Mutations in SEPN1 cause congenital muscular dystrophy with spinal rigidity and restrictive respiratory syndrome." *Nat Genet* 29(1): 17-18.
Monaco, A. P., R. L. Neve, et al. (1986). "Isolation of candidate cDNAs for portions of the Duchenne muscular dystrophy gene." *Nature* 323(6089): 646-650.
Moore, S. A., C. J. Shilling, et al. (2006). "Limb-girdle muscular dystrophy in the United States." *J Neuropathol Exp Neurol* 65(10): 995-1003.
Moreira, E. S., M. Vainzof, et al. (1997). "The seventh form of autosomal recessive limb-girdle muscular dystrophy is mapped to 17q11-12." *Am J Hum Genet* 61(1): 151-159.
Moreira, E. S., T. J. Wiltshire, et al. (2000). "Limb-girdle muscular dystrophy type 2G is caused by mutations in the gene encoding the sarcomeric protein telethonin." *Nat Genet* 24(2): 163-166.
Muchir, A., G. Bonne, et al. (2000). "Identification of mutations in the gene encoding lamins A/C in autosomal dominant limb girdle muscular dystrophy with atrioventricular conduction disturbances (LGMD1B)." *Hum Mol Genet* 9(9): 1453-1459.
Murakami, T., Y. K. Hayashi, et al. (2006). "Fukutin gene mutations cause dilated cardiomyopathy with minimal muscle weakness." *Ann Neurol* 60(5): 597-602.
Nadeau, A., M. Kinali, et al. (2009). "Natural history of Ullrich congenital muscular dystrophy." *Neurology* 73(1): 25-31.
Nguyen, K., G. Bassez, et al. (2005). "Dysferlin mutations in LGMD2B, Miyoshi myopathy, and atypical dysferlinopathies." *Hum Mutat* 26(2): 165.
Nigro, V., E. de Sa Moreira, et al. (1996). "Autosomal recessive limb-girdle muscular dystrophy, LGMD2F, is caused by a mutation in the delta-sarcoglycan gene." *Nat Genet* 14(2): 195-198.
Noguchi, S., E. M. McNally, et al. (1995). "Mutations in the dystrophin-associated protein gamma-sarcoglycan in chromosome 13 muscular dystrophy." *Science* 270(5237): 819-822.
Nonaka, I., Y. Une, et al. (1981). "A clinical and histological study of Ullrich's disease (congenital atonic-sclerotic muscular dystrophy)." *Neuropediatrics* 12(3): 197-208.
North, K. N., L. A. Specht, et al. (1996). "Congenital muscular dystrophy associated with merosin deficiency." *J Child Neurol* 11(4): 291-295.

Norwood, F., M. de Visser, et al. (2007). "EFNS guideline on diagnosis and management of limb girdle muscular dystrophies." *Eur J Neurol* 14(12): 1305-1312.

Norwood, F. L., C. Harling, et al. (2009). "Prevalence of genetic muscle disease in Northern England: in-depth analysis of a muscle clinic population." *Brain* 132(Pt 11): 3175-3186.

Palenzuela, L., A. L. Andreu, et al. (2003). "A novel autosomal dominant limb-girdle muscular dystrophy (LGMD 1F) maps to 7q32.1-32.2." *Neurology* 61(3): 404-406.

Pan, T. C., R. Z. Zhang, et al. (1998). "CA repeat polymorphism of the COL6A3 gene on chromosome 2q37." *Hum Hered* 48(4): 235-236.

Pan, T. C., R. Z. Zhang, et al. (2003). "New molecular mechanism for Ullrich congenital muscular dystrophy: a heterozygous in-frame deletion in the COL6A1 gene causes a severe phenotype." *Am J Hum Genet* 73(2): 355-369.

Pandya, S., W. M. King, et al. (2008). "Facioscapulohumeral dystrophy." *Phys Ther* 88(1): 105-113.

Paradas, C., J. Llauger, et al. (2010). "Redefining dysferlinopathy phenotypes based on clinical findings and muscle imaging studies." *Neurology* 75(4): 316-323.

Passos-Bueno, M. R., E. S. Moreira, et al. (1996). "Linkage analysis in autosomal recessive limb-girdle muscular dystrophy (AR LGMD) maps a sixth form to 5q33-34 (LGMD2F) and indicates that there is at least one more subtype of AR LGMD." *Hum Mol Genet* 5(6): 815-820.

Peat, R. A., J. M. Smith, et al. (2008). "Diagnosis and etiology of congenital muscular dystrophy." *Neurology* 71(5): 312-321.

Piluso, G., L. Politano, et al. (2005). "Extensive scanning of the calpain-3 gene broadens the spectrum of LGMD2A phenotypes." *J Med Genet* 42(9): 686-693.

Quijano-Roy, S., B. Mbieleu, et al. (2008). "De novo LMNA mutations cause a new form of congenital muscular dystrophy." *Ann Neurol* 64(2): 177-186.

Rankin, J., M. Auer-Grumbach, et al. (2008). "Extreme phenotypic diversity and nonpenetrance in families with the LMNA gene mutation R644C." *Am J Med Genet A* 146A(12): 1530-1542.

Ranum, L. P., P. F. Rasmussen, et al. (1998). "Genetic mapping of a second myotonic dystrophy locus." *Nat Genet* 19(2): 196-198.

Renwick, J. H., S. E. Bundey, et al. (1971). "Confirmation of linkage of the loci for myotonic dystrophy and ABH secretion." *J Med Genet* 8(4): 407-416.

Richard, I., L. Brenguier, et al. (1997). "Multiple independent molecular etiology for limb-girdle muscular dystrophy type 2A patients from various geographical origins." *Am J Hum Genet* 60(5): 1128-1138.

Richard, I., O. Broux, et al. (1995). "Mutations in the proteolytic enzyme calpain 3 cause limb-girdle muscular dystrophy type 2A." *Cell* 81(1): 27-40.

Roberds, S. L., F. Leturcq, et al. (1994). "Missense mutations in the adhalin gene linked to autosomal recessive muscular dystrophy." *Cell* 78(4): 625-633.

Robinson, D. O., S. R. Hammans, et al. (2005). "Oculopharyngeal muscular dystrophy (OPMD): analysis of the PABPN1 gene expansion sequence in 86 patients reveals 13 different expansion types and further evidence for unequal recombination as the mutational mechanism." *Hum Genet* 116(4): 267-271.

Saenz, A., F. Leturcq, et al. (2005). "LGMD2A: genotype-phenotype correlations based on a large mutational survey on the calpain 3 gene." *Brain* 128(Pt 4): 732-742.

Schessl, J., N. M. Goemans, et al. (2008). "Predominant fiber atrophy and fiber type disproportion in early ullrich disease." *Muscle Nerve* 38(3): 1184-1191.

Sorrel-Dejerine, Y. and M. Fardeau (1982). "[Birth and metamorphosis of Landouzy-Dejerine progressive atrophic myopathy]." *Rev Neurol (Paris)* 138(12): 1041-1051.

Speer, M. C., R. Tandan, et al. (1996). "Evidence for locus heterogeneity in the Bethlem myopathy and linkage to 2q37." *Hum Mol Genet* 5(7): 1043-1046.

Speer, M. C., J. M. Vance, et al. (1999). "Identification of a new autosomal dominant limb-girdle muscular dystrophy locus on chromosome 7." *Am J Hum Genet* 64(2): 556-562.

Starling, A., F. Kok, et al. (2004). "A new form of autosomal dominant limb-girdle muscular dystrophy (LGMD1G) with progressive fingers and toes flexion limitation maps to chromosome 4p21." *Eur J Hum Genet* 12(12): 1033-1040.

Statland, J. M. and R. Tawil (2011). "Facioscapulohumeral muscular dystrophy: molecular pathological advances and future directions." *Curr Opin Neurol.*

Susman, R. D., S. Quijano-Roy, et al. (2010). "Expanding the clinical, pathological and MRI phenotype of DNM2-related centronuclear myopathy." *Neuromuscul Disord* 20(4): 229-237.

Suzuki, N., M. Aoki, et al. (2004). "Novel dysferlin mutations and characteristic muscle atrophy in late-onset Miyoshi myopathy." *Muscle Nerve* 29(5): 721-723.

Sveen, M. L., M. Schwartz, et al. (2006). "High prevalence and phenotype-genotype correlations of limb girdle muscular dystrophy type 2I in Denmark." *Ann Neurol* 59(5): 808-815.

Taniguchi, K., K. Kobayashi, et al. (2003). "Worldwide distribution and broader clinical spectrum of muscle-eye-brain disease." *Hum Mol Genet* 12(5): 527-534.

Tetreault, M., A. Duquette, et al. (2006). "A new form of congenital muscular dystrophy with joint hyperlaxity maps to 3p23-21." *Brain* 129(Pt 8): 2077-2084.

Toda, T. and K. Kobayashi (1999). "Fukuyama-type congenital muscular dystrophy: the first human disease to be caused by an ancient retrotransposal integration." *J Mol Med* 77(12): 816-823.

Toda, T., M. Segawa, et al. (1993). "Localization of a gene for Fukuyama type congenital muscular dystrophy to chromosome 9q31-33." *Nat Genet* 5(3): 283-286.

Tome, F. M. (1999). "The Peter Emil Becker Award lecture 1998. The saga of congenital muscular dystrophy." *Neuropediatrics* 30(2): 55-65.

Tome, F. M., T. Evangelista, et al. (1994). "Congenital muscular dystrophy with merosin deficiency." *C R Acad Sci III* 317(4): 351-357.

Turner, C. and D. Hilton-Jones (2010). "The myotonic dystrophies: diagnosis and management." *J Neurol Neurosurg Psychiatry* 81(4): 358-367.

Udd, B., J. Partanen, et al. (1993). "Tibial muscular dystrophy. Late adult-onset distal myopathy in 66 Finnish patients." *Arch Neurol* 50(6): 604-608.

Udd, B., A. Vihola, et al. (2005). "Titinopathies and extension of the M-line mutation phenotype beyond distal myopathy and LGMD2J." *Neurology* 64(4): 636-642.

Vainzof, M., L. V. Anderson, et al. (2001). "Dysferlin protein analysis in limb-girdle muscular dystrophies." *J Mol Neurosci* 17(1): 71-80.

Vainzof, M., M. R. Passos-Bueno, et al. (1996). "The sarcoglycan complex in the six autosomal recessive limb-girdle muscular dystrophies." *Hum Mol Genet* 5(12): 1963-1969.

Vainzof, M., M. R. Passos-Bueno, et al. (1999). "Sarcoglycanopathies are responsible for 68% of severe autosomal recessive limb-girdle muscular dystrophy in the Brazilian population." *J Neurol Sci* 164(1): 44-49.

van der Kooi, A. J., M. van Meegen, et al. (1997). "Genetic localization of a newly recognized autosomal dominant limb-girdle muscular dystrophy with cardiac involvement (LGMD1B) to chromosome 1q11-21." *Am J Hum Genet* 60(4): 891-895.

van Reeuwijk, J., M. Janssen, et al. (2005). "POMT2 mutations cause alpha-dystroglycan hypoglycosylation and Walker-Warburg syndrome." *J Med Genet* 42(12): 907-912.

Vogel, H. and J. Zamecnik (2005). "Diagnostic immunohistology of muscle diseases." *J Neuropathol Exp Neurol* 64(3): 181-193.

Voit, T. (2001). Congenital Muscular Dystrophies. *Disorders of voluntary muscle.* H.-J. D. Karpati G, Griggs RC. Cambridge, UK, Press Syndicate of the University of Cambridge: 503-524.

Voit, T., P. Stuettgen, et al. (1991). "Dystrophin as a diagnostic marker in Duchenne and Becker muscular dystrophy. Correlation of immunofluorescence and western blot." *Neuropediatrics* 22(3): 152-162.

Waddell, L. B., F. A. Lemckert, et al. (2011). "Dysferlin, annexin A1, and mitsugumin 53 are upregulated in muscular dystrophy and localize to longitudinal tubules of the T-system with stretch." *J Neuropathol Exp Neurol* 70(4): 302-313.

Walter, M. C., J. A. Petersen, et al. (2004). "FKRP (826C>A) frequently causes limb-girdle muscular dystrophy in German patients." *J Med Genet* 41(4): e50.

Weiler, T., C. R. Greenberg, et al. (1998). "A gene for autosomal recessive limb-girdle muscular dystrophy in Manitoba Hutterites maps to chromosome region 9q31-q33: evidence for another limb-girdle muscular dystrophy locus." *Am J Hum Genet* 63(1): 140-147.

Wijmenga, C., R. R. Frants, et al. (1990). "Location of facioscapulohumeral muscular dystrophy gene on chromosome 4." *Lancet* 336(8716): 651-653.

Yoshida, A., K. Kobayashi, et al. (2001). "Muscular dystrophy and neuronal migration disorder caused by mutations in a glycosyltransferase, POMGnT1." *Dev Cell* 1(5): 717-724.

Zatz, M., F. de Paula, et al. (2003). "The 10 autosomal recessive limb-girdle muscular dystrophies." *Neuromuscul Disord* 13(7-8): 532-544.

Zhang, Q., C. Bethmann, et al. (2007). "Nesprin-1 and -2 are involved in the pathogenesis of Emery Dreifuss muscular dystrophy and are critical for nuclear envelope integrity." *Hum Mol Genet* 16(23): 2816-2833.

15

Advances in Molecular Analysis of Muscular Dystrophies

Arunkanth Ankala and Madhuri R. Hegde
Emory University
USA

1. Introduction

Molecular genetic testing began in the mid-1980's in research laboratories which involved linkage analysis to aid disease gene discovery (Petersen 2000; Ensenauer, Michels et al. 2005). With the identification of novel disease causing genes, genetic tests became available and were launched in clinical testing laboratories in both academic and commercial settings. Unlike complex diseases such as cardiovascular diseases and cancers, diagnostic assays for monogenic Mendelian genetic disorders are relatively easy to design and use in a clinical diagnostic setting. Muscular dystrophies which affect muscles are mostly monogenic diseases and are either dominantly or recessively inherited. However, due to overlapping phenotype or similar clinical presentations of several disorders caused by closely associated genes, the diagnosis may often be elusive. Muscular dystrophies (MD) are a group of genetically and clinically heterogeneous hereditary myopathies characterized by hypotonia, skeletal muscle weakness, contractures, and delayed motor development. They are broadly classified into nine different types including Duchenne (DMD), Becker (BMD), limb girdle (LGMD), congenital (CMD), facioscapulohumeral (FCMD), myotonic (MD), oculopharyngeal (OPMD), distal and Emery-Dreifuss (EMD), some of which have several subtypes based on the gene involved. The clinical manifestations and severity of the various types and subtypes of muscular dystrophies vary widely, ranging from mild myopathy to even cardiac failure. Because of the heterogeneity and overlapping phenotype the patients often face a diagnostic odyssey before receiving the appropriate clinical and molecular diagnosis (Mendell, Sahenk et al. 1995; Mendell 2001). Given the recent improvement of molecular technologies, the classification of MDs in specific, has significantly changed from phenotype driven towards a more molecular based categorization. Therefore it is of pivotal importance to diagnose the molecular basis for the disease which includes determination of the gene and the genotype involved. Molecular diagnosis of the disease is important not only for subsequent patient follow-up but also for choosing the appropriate personalized therapy. Single gene sequencing is considered effective when a single missing protein is identified by a muscle biopsy and loss of that protein fits the phenotype. However, a comprehensive gene sequencing panel is necessary when ambiguous results arise or when muscle biopsies are difficult to obtain. Recent technological advances in sequencing using next generation sequencing and microarrays has made it possible to screen a large number of genes for causative mutations at a fairly low cost and in a reasonably less time. In this book chapter we will discuss the various technological advancements in the molecular diagnosis of various muscular dystrophies and its impact in the clinical world.

2. Mutation spectrum in genes associated with MD

As discussed in other chapters in this book, each type and subtype of MD is caused by mutations in different genes associated with muscle structure and function. Therefore identifying the gene is critical to diagnosis and treatment. Molecular approach to disease diagnosis is highly dependent on the mutation spectrum of the disease causing gene. For example, while *DMD* associated with Duchenne and Becker dystrophies has a high frequency of intragenic deletions (65%), mutation spectrum of *CAPN3* involved in LGMD2A shows a high frequency of point mutations (76%) (Figure 1). Based on these mutation spectrums, deletion-duplication analysis is suggested prior to sequencing analysis for *DMD* while the inverse is suggested for *CAPN3*.

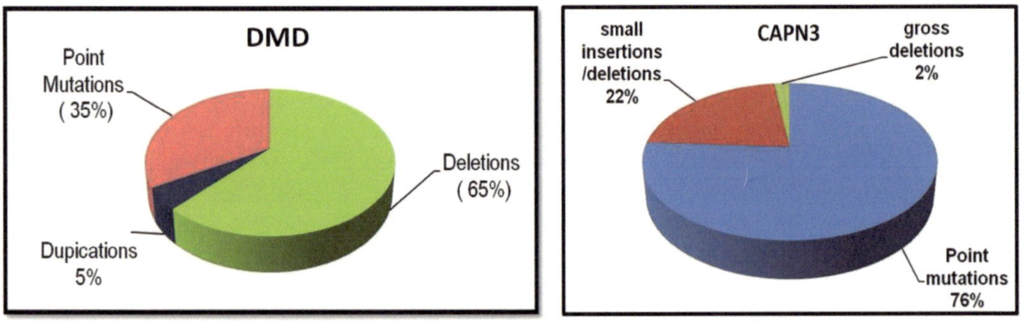

Fig. 1. Mutation spectrum of *DMD* and *CAPN3*

3. Traditional methods used for molecular diagnosis

Since the early practice of genetic testing for diseases that started in mid-1980, several DNA and protein based diagnostic methods have been developed. These traditional methods of diagnosis for muscular dystrophies include linkage analysis, multiplex PCR, Multiplex ligation-dependent probe amplification (MLPA), quantitative PCR, Southern blotting, Immunoblotting (IB) and Immunohistochemical (IHC) analysis. While MLPA, PCR and southern blotting involve DNA analysis, IHC and IB involve protein expression and require muscle biopsies. However, since performing a muscle biopsy is highly invasive it is not preferred both by the patients as well as physicians. Recent advances in molecular analysis for mutation detection have revolutionized the approach to diagnosing these patients (Witkowski 1989; Gangopadhyay, Sherratt et al. 1992; Whittock, Roberts et al. 1997; Ginjaar, Kneppers et al. 2000; Beroud, Carrie et al. 2004).

3.1 Immunohistochemistry

Prior to the development of gene based mutation-detection analysis, disease diagnosis for various MDs was through conventional screening of affected individuals by clinical examination which involved assessment of creatine phosphokinase (CPK) levels and immuno-histological examination of muscle tissue obtained only through an invasive biopsy (Love and Davies 1989; Love, Forrest et al. 1989). As can be seen in the figure below, dystrophic muscle fibers can be easily distinguished from control or normal fibers. These distinguishable characteristics include the high variation in the fiber size and shape, high frequency of internal nuclei, increased connective and adipose tissue in between fibers, as well as presence of large number of regenerating and degenerating fibers in dystrophic musculature (Norwood, de Visser et al. 2007). However these pathological findings vary widely based on the protein involved or disease associated and age of the patient during biopsy. Though immuno-histochemical findings may lead a way to the confirmation of muscular dystrophy, identifying the exact protein (or gene) involved and therefore the specific subtype of muscular dystrophy may always be elusive. This is because of the secondary reduction in protein levels of other closely integrated proteins (Hack, Ly et al. 1998). For example, a mutation in one sarcoglycan can often lead to reduced expression of other sarcoglycans as well (Hack, Ly et al. 1998). Therefore, molecular diagnosis is highly recommended for confirmation of the involved gene and therefore the specific subtype of MD.

Shown in the figure below, are the immunological findings of an individual with mutations in calpain3 (*CAPN3*) which causes LGMD2A (Figure 2). Though calpain3 analysis is not shown here, it can be observed that there is a secondary reduction in β-sarcoglycan. Moreover, in the same patient, Immunoblotting analysis showed occasional reduction of dysferlin protein levels as well. This suggests the importance of molecular diagnosis through DNA analysis, for proper management and therapy.

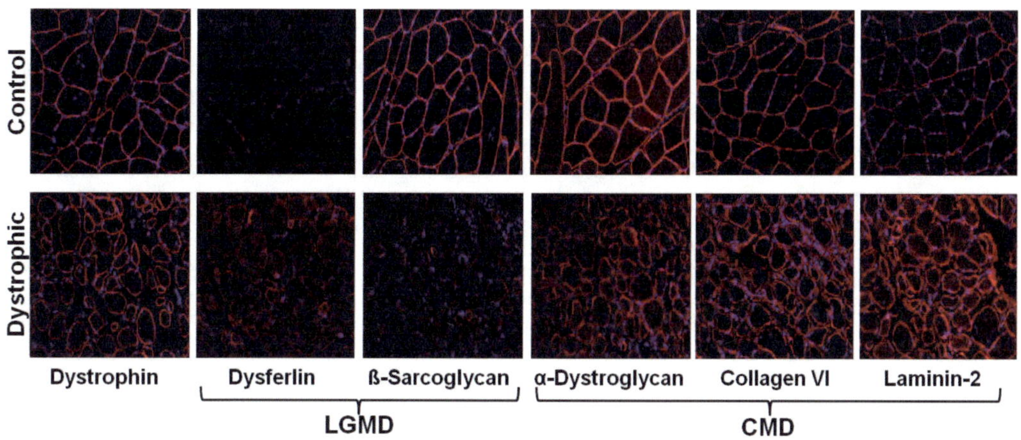

Fig. 2. Immunohistochemical findings in healthy and dystrophic muscle tissue

3.2 Multiplex western blotting

Immunoblotting or western blotting provides an alternative to IHC. IB provides more information regarding the expression and mutation of the protein compared to IHC. Skeletal muscle proteins such as dystrophin, dystroglycans, sarcoglycans and laminin-2 that are associated with Duchenne/Becker muscular dystrophies and different LGMDs as well as CMDs, physically interact and integrate to provide structural stability to the muscle fiber cells. Therefore mutation in one protein may result in altered expressions or stability of these closely associated proteins leading to overlapping phenotypes. Hence, looking at the expression levels of all proteins simultaneously may help better diagnose the disease. Instead of analyzing each protein individually as in IHC and regular IB, a multiplex WB using a cocktail of antibodies can be adopted (Anderson and Davison 1999). This is facilitated by the difference in the molecular sizes of the different proteins. In our laboratory, a variety of antibodies covering different domains of the proteins have been selected to avoid any variability in the hybridization and analyzed as shown (Figure 3).

In the figure below (Figure 3A), at least seven different proteins involved in various MDs were simultaneously analyzed in a set of clinically diagnosed dystrophic patients. Two different cocktails, each made of a set of antibodies targeting different proteins have been optimized for such diagnosis in our laboratory. As can be seen in the figure below, controls (lanes to the left) significantly express dystrophin while no detectable levels could be observed in the patients (lanes to the right). Though there appears to be a secondary reduction in the sarcoglycans as previously described, the complete absence of dystrophin strongly indicates that the causative protein (or gene) is perhaps dystrophin. Further molecular analysis involving deletion-duplication analysis or sequencing of the entire gene is required to confirm the exact mutation. Similarly, carrier and disease status can be inferred by immunoblotting analysis for other MDs like the limb girdle muscular dystrophy type 2 B (LGMD2B) by comparison of dysferlin protein expression (Figure 3B and C). The low expression of dysferlin protein in lane 2 (figure 3B) indicates probable carrier status while the relatively smaller bands in lane 2 (Figure 3C) indicates a probable functional dysferlin protein with a deletion. Both these findings were later confirmed by sequencing analysis.

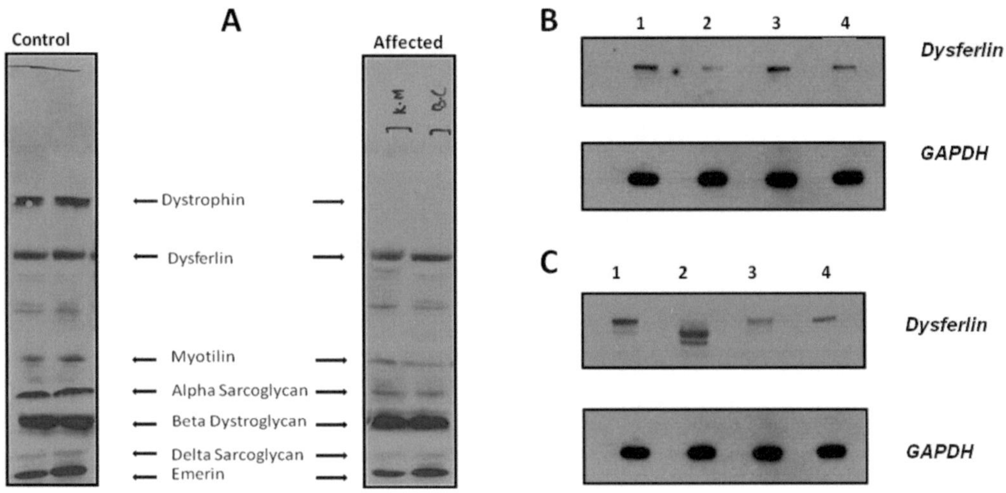

Fig. 3. Immunoblotting analysis of MD proteins. A) A multiplex immunoblot showing the differential expression of various muscle proteins with a clear indication of absence of dystrophin expression in the affected individual when compared to the control. B) Comparison of dysferlin expression in controls and unknowns for carrier and disease status. Lane 1, control healthy individual; lane 2-4 were unknowns C) Comparison of dysferlin expression in controls and unknowns for carrier and disease status. Lane 1, control healthy individual; lane 2-4 were unknowns.

3.3 Multiplex PCR

Multiplex PCR amplification of genomic DNA is a conventional and cost-effective method for identifying deletions in hot spot regions of the gene in affected individuals and involves visualization of bands through regular agarose gels stained with ethidium bromide. Using a combination of several primer pairs in 2-3 reactions, most of the exons including hot-spot regions for *DMD* would be tested for, at a reasonable expense (Beggs, Koenig et al. 1990). However dosage analysis is required for carrier females and is performed through quantitative PCR (qPCR) in which the copy number of the target sequence is directly proportional to the fluorescence of SYBR Green dye during the logarithmic phase. Both deletions and duplications can be identified by qPCR. For example, there would be no amplification of the target product in a male individual with deletion, while in carriers, the amount of product amplified would be half the amount observed in normals carrying two copies of the target sequence to start with. Similarly, in case of a duplication carrier, this ratio would be 3:2 compared to normal. Though these PCR based tools were useful for Duchenne and Becker muscular dystrophies where a majority (70-75%) of disease causing mutations were either deletions or duplications, they were not preferred for other muscular dystrophies.

3.4 Southern blotting

Southern blotting is an alternative technique for screening deletions and duplications in large genes like *DMD*. It involves gel electrophoresis combined with transfer of separated fragments on to membrane and subsequent target fragment detection by hybridization to known probes. It is used in clinical laboratories to confirm deletion and duplication mutations identified by multiplex PCR as well as to determine the extent of the deletion/duplication. Dosage analysis of copy number can also be performed through southern blotting by subsequent densitometry but can be challenging for carrier females (Medori, Brooke et al. 1989).

3.5 MLPA

Multiplex ligation-dependent probe amplification is a variation of conventional PCR and a significant advancement over the multiplex PCR method that permits multiple different targets to be amplified with only a single primer pair (Schouten, McElgunn et al. 2002). Clinically applicable MLPA based simultaneous screening of all 79 exons of DMD gene for deletions and duplications in Duchenne and Becker muscular dystrophy patients was developed around year 2005 and is widely used till date in several clinical laboratories around the world (Schwartz and Duno 2004; Janssen, Hartmann et al. 2005; Lalic, Vossen et al. 2005). It does not require costly equipments and is a very cost-effective method and has therefore been widely accepted by several diagnostic labs. In addition to deletions and duplications it may also identify point mutations. Since MLPA is highly dependant on hybridization of a single probe false positive results can occur in presence of a variation (single nucleotide, deletion or insertion) in the sequence hybridizing to the probe. For this reason single exon deletion need to be investigated further. The presence of variation may also hinder the precise definition of end points of deletions.

3.6 Sequencing

While most of the above mentioned DNA based methods are effective for deletion and duplication detection, they are not preferred for analysis of point mutations. As discussed earlier, majority of the smaller genes associated with MDs have a high frequency of point mutations than for deletions and duplications. Only *DMD* has a high frequency of deletions and duplications while point mutations still account for atleast 35%. Therefore thorough diagnosis of such MDs requires sequence analysis of the exonic regions. PCR amplification of each exon of the suspected gene with exon-specific primer pairs followed by Sanger sequencing is therefore practiced. Patient sequences obtained thus, are then compared to reference sequences and sequence variations as fine as single base-pair change (point mutations) and small indels are efficiently identified (Figure 4).

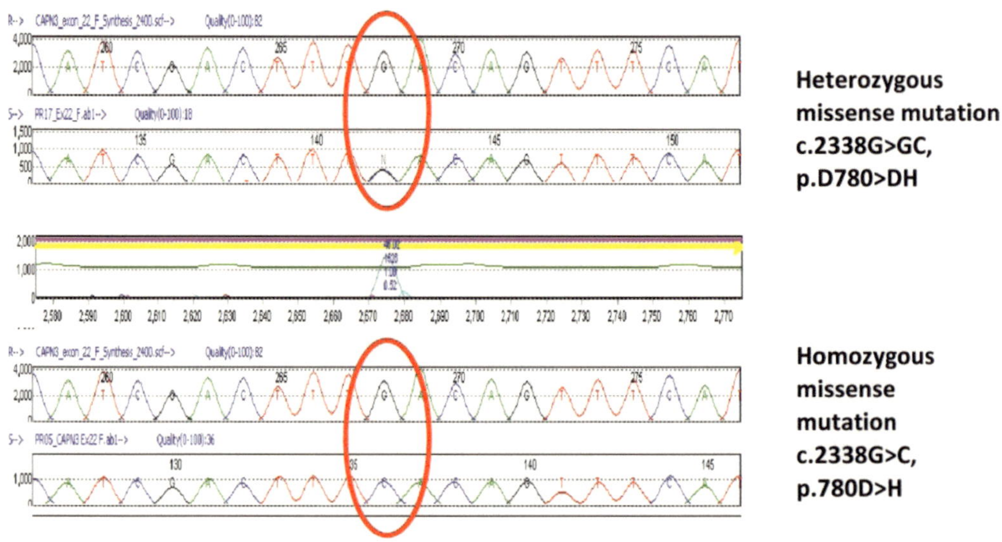

Fig. 4. Detection of Point mutations by Sanger sequencing. The upper half of the figure shows a heterozygous point mutation (missense mutation) as detected by a double peak at the corresponding nucleotide when sequenced by Sanger sequencing. The lower half of the figure shows the same point mutation to be present on both alleles making it a homozygous missense mutation.

However, such PCR amplification and sequence analysis may be feasible for small genes that have only few exons. Further, thorough characterization of the clinical presentations need to be performed to narrow down the possible causative gene. Overlapping clinical phenotype and heterogeneity of MDs leads to a suspicion of more than one gene. In such scenario, analysis of more than one gene, some of which have a large number of exons (79 in *DMD*, 55 in *DYSF*, 24 in *CAPN3*) may be very tedious and expensive for clinical diagnosis. Therefore high-throughput, cost effective methods for disease diagnosis have always been in demand.

4. New technological advances in molecular diagnosis

The completion of human genome project has revolutionized the field of human genetics and more specifically human medical genetics (Venter, Adams et al. 2001). High-throughput mutation detection methods such as comparative genomic hybridization arrays (aCGH) and target capture based next generation sequencing panels have been developed. This topic will focus on the various rapidly emerging comprehensive technologies and their advantages over traditional methods. This will include detailed discussion of the microarray based gene panels and next generation sequencing.

4.1 Application of microarrays to detect copy number variation in MD genes

Microarray based comparative genomic hybridization (aCGH), also called molecular karyotyping, is a recently developed technique that enables high-resolution, genome-wide analysis of genomic copy number variations (CNVs). The assay has become a powerful routine clinical diagnostic tool and its increasing resolution and accuracy is gradually replacing traditional cytogenetic approaches for CNV determination. Earlier, the detection potential of genomic imbalances was limited to >5-10Mb with even the highest quality G-banded chromosome analysis. However, with the advent of aCGH, deletions and duplications, as small as 50-100 kb in size are now routinely detected throughout the genome (Stankiewicz, Pursley et al. 2010). The wide-spread application of aCGH has also facilitated the identification of various recurrent CNVs and eventual characterization of several microdeletion and microduplication syndromes.

In a typical aCGH measurement, total genomic DNA is isolated from test (patient) and reference cell populations (or biological sample such as blood or saliva), differentially labeled and hybridized to oligonucleotide arrays. The relative hybridization intensity which is ideally proportional to the relative copy number of target sequence regions is then measured and calculated. The reference genome being normal, any increases and decreases in the intensity ratio directly indicate DNA copy-number variations (deletions or duplications) in the test or patient genome. The intensity data is typically normalized so that the modal ratio for the reference genome is set to a standard value of 0.0, and any decrease is inferred as deletion while an increase in signal in the test genome is inferred as duplication (Figure 5).

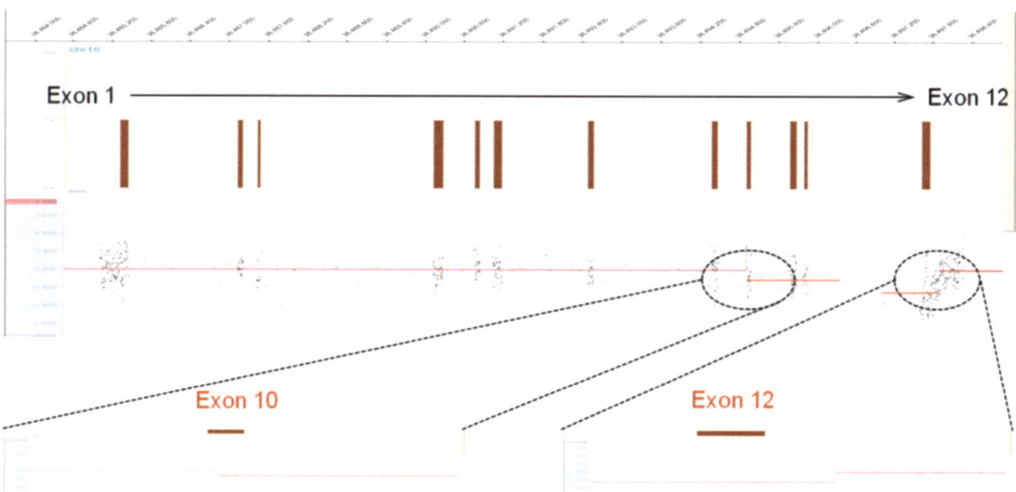

Fig. 5. The figure shows aCGH data for *IVD* gene locus (chr15:40,697,686-40,713,512) using a custom-designed 385K high-density array from NimbleGen. The zoomed in view of the corresponding array highlights the breakpoints for a patient with a deletion mutation encompassing exon 10 to exon 12 with breakpoints in intron 9 and the 3′ UTR. As can be seen in the above figure, the target sequence with normal copy number normalizes to value 0.0, while the deleted regions of exon 10 and exon 12 fall below 0.0 inferrring a loss of a copy number (deletion) compared to reference genome.

In our laboratory, gene-targeted high-resolution oligonucleotide CGH array was custom designed on a NimbleGen 385K platform (till June 2010) or OGT 44K platform (July 2010 onwards) to detect deletions and duplications in 450 genes associated with various genetic disorders. The NimbleGen 385K platform used long oligonucleotides (45–60 mer) to achieve isothermal *Tm* across the array, with repeat sequence masking implemented to ensure greater sensitivity and specificity. The OGT 44K platform has 44,000 unique sequence probes tiled on the array. Both arrays were designed with average spacing of 10 bp within coding regions and 25 bp within promoter, intronic regions, and 3' UTR, with repeat sequence masking. Use of intronic oligonucleotide probes allows robust detection of dosage changes of the gene within the entire genomic region, as well as determination of approximate breakpoints. The breakpoints for various deletions and duplications detected by the high-resolution aCGH analysis were as close as 500bp to the exact breakpoint determined by conventional sanger sequencing (Ankala, Kohn et al. 2012). Shown below is a figure with aCGH data for several patients with DMD (Figure 6). Deletion-duplication analysis for the entire *DMD* gene by aCGH shows the various intragenic regions that were found deleted in the patients. The zoomed in view of the data also shows the specific exons that were found deleted in these patients thus confirming the molecular diagnosis.

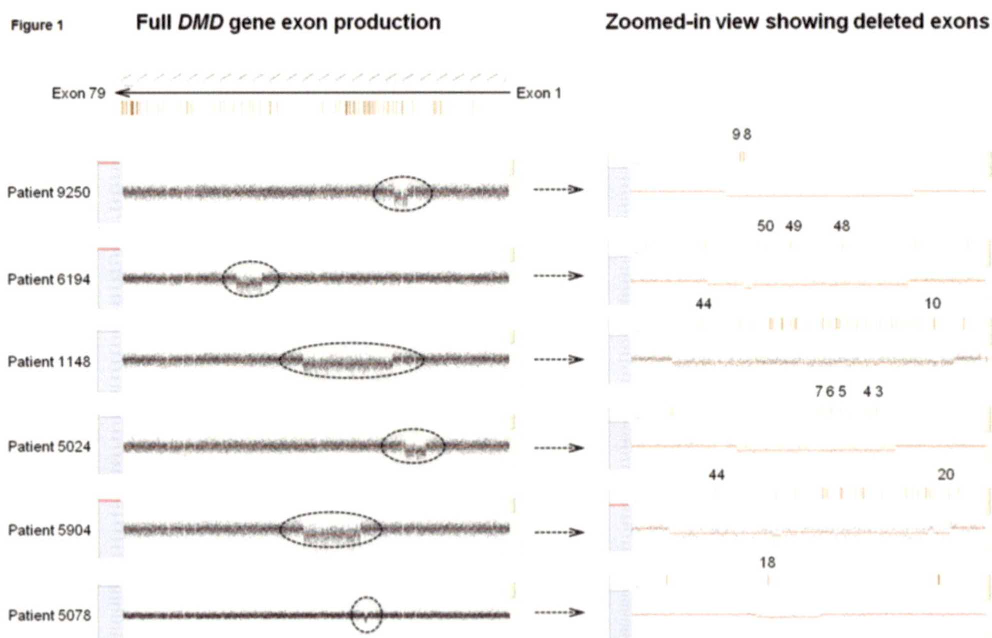

Fig. 6. The column on the left shows comparative genomic hybridization data for DMD gene locus (chrX:31,137,345-33,229,673) for six patient's DNA, using a custom-designed 385K high-density array from NimbleGen. Right column shows the zoomed in view of the corresponding array on the left, with the deleted exons highlighted in red. Each row refers to a patient.

Such a robust, diagnostic test capable of determining disease causing copy number variations (deletions or duplications) in one single assay makes clinical diagnosis rapid and economic. Almost all known MD associated genes can be analyzed simultaneously for mutations through one single affordable test which proves useful especially when the clinical phenotype is very overlapping and narrowing down of genes seems difficult.

4.2 Panel based approach for mutation detection in MDs for example CMD and LGMD

As subtypes of MD caused by different genes share similar clinical presentations simultaneous sequencing of all associated genes as a panel reduces costs and provides quick diagnosis. Several such sequencing panels of different MDs are currently offered in clinical diagnostic laboratories for molecular diagnosis. At least four different sequencing panels are offered at Emory Genetics Laboratory (EGL), which include LGMD, CMD and DMD. Table 1 summarizes the different genes involved in LGMD and the different number of exons in each of these genes.

4.3 Application of next generation sequencing to molecular diagnosis

The high demand for low-cost sequencing has instigated the development of high-throughput sequencing technologies that parallelize the sequence process, producing several thousands of reads or sequences simultaneously in a single reaction (Church 2006; Hall 2007). These high-throughput sequencing technologies have lowered the cost of DNA sequencing beyond what has been possible with the standard sanger sequencing methods (Mardis 2008; Mardis 2008; Schuster 2008). A variety of technologies called next-generation sequencing technologies emerged, each with a unique biochemical strategy (Brenner, Johnson et al. 2000; Church 2006; Mardis 2008; Valouev, Ichikawa et al. 2008; Drmanac, Sparks et al. 2010; Porreca 2010). In general, most of these approaches use an *in vitro* clonal amplification or PCR step to amplify the DNA molecules present in the sample. Illumina or Solexa sequencing, Applied Biosystem's SOLiD sequencing and Ion semiconductor sequencing developed by Ion Torrent Systems Inc are most recent and popular next generation sequencing techniques that are currently being used in clinical laboratories for molecular diagnosis. The sensitivity and specificity of these sequences or the next generation sequencing method is further improved by target capturing the regions of genomic interest from a biological sample or DNA. Particularly when specific regions of the genome need to be targeted or when the gene of interest has been narrowed down to a specific region of the chromosome, then target enrichment methods may be used to enrich the samples in these genomic regions and processed for further analysis of variants or mutations by next generations sequencing. Several capture technologies namely microarray based capture for DMD, RainDance (ten Bosch and Grody 2008) and Fluidigm PCR based capture, Agilent SureSelect and Nimblegen Sequence capture (ten Bosch and Grody 2008) are available in the market. Our comprehensive and comparative analysis of these capture technologies has suggested that RainDance and Fluidigm PCR- based strategies are ideal for clinical panels as they are robust and give a coverage of ~100X whereas in-solution sequence capture protocols from Agilent and Nimblegen are ideal for research based approaches to identify novel genes due to the ability to capture a large number of genes (exome) in a single experiment (Bainbridge, Wang et al. ; Cirulli, Singh et al.).

These target enrichment methods are used both in research and clinical laboratories. In research laboratories, this allows for new gene discovery when CNVs in a particular genomic region correlate with a recurrent clinical phenotype. However, clinical laboratories have a different application where a certain set of disease genes (such as those discussed in

Subtype	Gene Location	Inheritance mode	Gene	Protein	No. of exons
LGMD1A	5q31	AD	MYOT	Myotilin	10
LGMD1B	1q21.2-21.3	AD	LMNA	Progerin, lamin A/C	12
LGMD1C	3p25	AD	CAV3	Caveolin 3	2
LGMD2A	15q15	AR	CAPN3	Calpain 3	24
LGMD2B	2p13	AR	DYSF	Dysferlin	55
LGMD2C	13q12	AR	SGCG	Gamma Sarcoglycan	8
LGMD2D	17q21	AR	SGCA	Alpha Sarcoglycan	10
LGMD2E	4q12	AR	SGCB	Beta Sarcoglycan	6
LGMD2F	5q33	AR	SGCD	Delta Sarcoglycan	8
LGMD2G	17q12	AR	TCAP	telethonin, Titin Cap	2
LGMD2H	9q33.1	AR	TRIM32	TAT-interactive protein, tipartite motif containing 32	2
LGMD2I	19q13.33	AR	FKRP	Fukutin-related protein	4
LGMD2J	2q31	AR	TTN	titin	312
LGMD2K	9q34.1	AR	POMT1	protein-O-mannosyl transferase 1	20
LGMD2L	11p14.3	AR	ANO5	anoctamin 5	22
LGMD2M	9q31-33	AR	FKTN	Fukutin	10
LGMD2N	14Q24.3	AR	POMT2	protein O-mannosyltransferase 2	21
LGMD2O	1p34.1	AR	POMGNT1	protein-O-mannose B1,2-N-acetylglucosaminyl transferase 1	22

Table 1. **Known LGMD subtypes and causative genes.** Shown are the various subtypes of LGMDs and causative genes that have been found to be associated with each of these types of limb girdle muscular dystrophies. Also listed are the number of exons that make up each of these genes to give an overview of the number of sequencing reactions that may be required to sequence and analyze the entire list of genes. Titin alone has 312 exons, and combined with all other genes the number of exons total 550 which may require more than 550 PCR reactions to sequence amplification considering that some exons may be too long for one single sequencing reaction.

gene panels above) are targeted for mutation detection in patient sample. For example, in our clinical laboratory at Emory Genetics Laboratories, target enrichment is performed for a set of 91 genes associated with X-linked Intellectual Disability (XLID) to identify the causative gene and mutation in XLID patients. These two technologies in combination stand the most successful and economic diagnostic tool currently in use both in research and clinical laboratories.

4.4 Whole exome and whole genome sequencing

Whole genome sequencing refers to re-sequencing of the entire genome of the individual while whole exome sequencing refers to selective sequencing of only the coding regions of the genome namely exons. Both strategies may be applied to identifying causal genes and associated mutations for any genetic disorder. However, routine whole genome sequencing is still not feasible due to the high cost associated with the technology. On the other hand, whole exome sequencing is quite affordable as it involves targeted sequencing of all the exons (around 300,000) accounting for only about 1% (36.5 Mb) of the entire human genome (Senapathy, Bhasi et al. 2010). Since it is estimated that these protein coding regions of the human genome account for at least 85% of the disease-causing mutations, the technology is highly appreciable (Choi, Scholl et al. 2009). Currently, whole exome sequencing is being used in research labs for identification of new genes associated with diseases. It involves extensive data mining, validation and confirmation analysis which makes it quite expensive for clinical applications. Whole exome sequencing for mutation detection is currently offered in only one or two clinical labs.

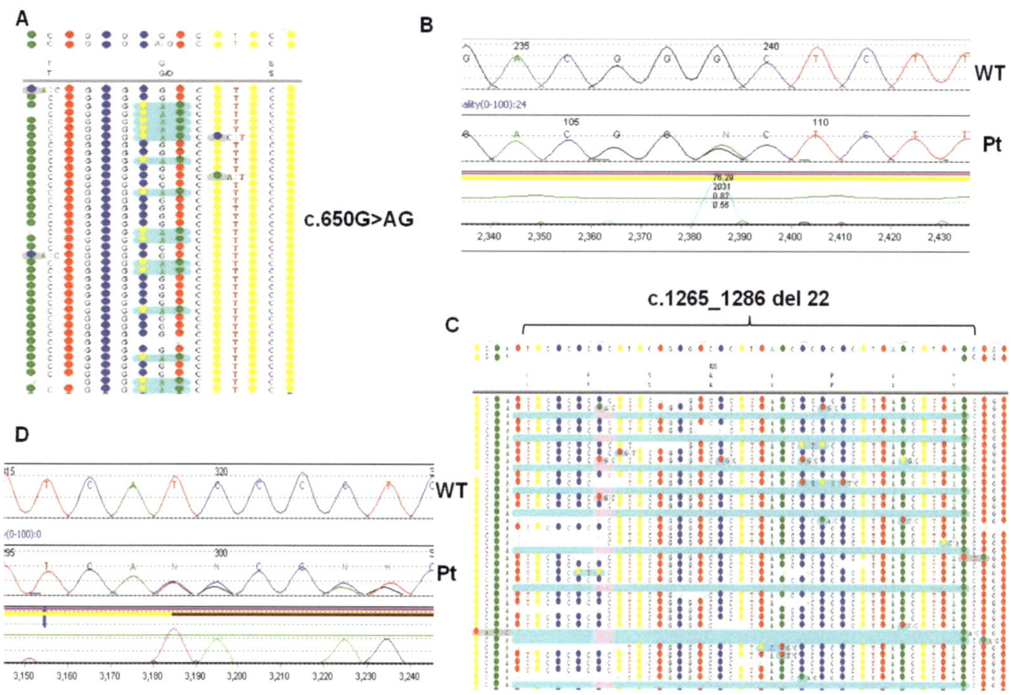

Fig. 7. Sequencing analysis and variant detection A) Next-generation sequencing analysis showing the sequence variants B) Sanger sequence analysis by mutation surveyor software showing the sequence variants and possible pathogenic mutations in the coding region of the gene C) Next-generation sequencing analysis showing a 22bp deletion D) Corresponding sanger sequence analysis by mutation surveyor software showing the start site of the 22bp deletion.

Using whole exome sequencing new candidate genes for several Mendelian disorders have been identified, demonstrating its potential (Ng, Turner et al. 2009; Jones, Ng et al. 2012). To demonstrate the potential of whole exome sequencing, we discuss a patient case that we analyzed through whole exome sequencing and identified pathogenic mutations in a novel gene. This particular patient was tested for all known genes associated with his clinical presentations but was found negative for any pathogenic mutations. We then performed whole exome analysis which gave a large number of variants. Using several filters such as score, coverage and allele percentages we narrowed down the variants. We found two novel mutations that were later confirmed through sanger sequencing (Figure 7).

5. Summary and future directions

We believe whole exome sequencing will become more feasible in the near future and will allow easy identification of disease associated genes and mutations. This definitely needs more sophisticated algorithms to filter the false-positives leaving fewer variants for confirmation and validation. Further, studies involving genotype-phenotype correlation will be very useful and will allow teasing out the various subtypes of the disease (Straub, Rafael et al. 1997; Culligan, Mackey et al. 1998; Gullberg, Tiger et al. 1999; Yurchenco, Cheng et al. 2004; Vainzof, Ayub-Guerrieri et al. 2008). This may be achieved through an integrated approach involving gene expression studies (geneST arrays) and protein antibody arrays. GeneST arrays are expected to give global muscle expression profile and indicate the variability in gene expression by identifying the up and down regulated genes (Vachon, Loechel et al. 1996; Tsao and Mendell 1999; Yamamoto, Kato et al. 2004; Wakayama, Inoue et al. 2008). Also active patient registries should be maintained for each disease type to provide ready access to a pool of information including clinical presentations and causative mutations. This will allow better understanding of the genotype-phenotype correlation and provide more focused approach for molecular diagnosis of the disease.

6. References

Anderson, L. V. and K. Davison (1999). "Multiplex Western blotting system for the analysis of muscular dystrophy proteins." *Am J Pathol* 154(4): 1017-1022.

Ankala, A., J. N. Kohn, et al. (2012). "Aberrant firing of replication origins potentially explains intragenic nonrecurrent rearrangements within genes, including the human DMD gene." *Genome Res* 22(1): 25-34.

Bainbridge, M. N., M. Wang, et al. "Whole exome capture in solution with 3 Gbp of data." *Genome Biol* 11(6): R62.

Beggs, A. H., M. Koenig, et al. (1990). "Detection of 98% of DMD/BMD gene deletions by polymerase chain reaction." *Hum Genet* 86(1): 45-48.

Beroud, C., A. Carrie, et al. (2004). "Dystrophinopathy caused by mid-intronic substitutions activating cryptic exons in the DMD gene." *Neuromuscul Disord* 14(1): 10-18.

Brenner, S., M. Johnson, et al. (2000). "Gene expression analysis by massively parallel signature sequencing (MPSS) on microbead arrays." *Nat Biotechnol* 18(6): 630-634.

Choi, M., U. I. Scholl, et al. (2009). "Genetic diagnosis by whole exome capture and massively parallel DNA sequencing." *Proc Natl Acad Sci U S A* 106(45): 19096-19101.

Church, G. M. (2006). "Genomes for all." *Sci Am* 294(1): 46-54.

Cirulli, E. T., A. Singh, et al. "Screening the human exome: a comparison of whole genome and whole transcriptome sequencing." *Genome Biol* 11(5): R57.

Culligan, K. G., A. J. Mackey, et al. (1998). "Role of dystrophin isoforms and associated proteins in muscular dystrophy (review)." *Int J Mol Med* 2(6): 639-648.

Drmanac, R., A. B. Sparks, et al. (2010). "Human genome sequencing using unchained base reads on self-assembling DNA nanoarrays." *Science* 327(5961): 78-81.

Ensenauer, R. E., V. V. Michels, et al. (2005). "Genetic testing: practical, ethical, and counseling considerations." *Mayo Clin Proc* 80(1): 63-73.

Gangopadhyay, S. B., T. G. Sherratt, et al. (1992). "Dystrophin in frameshift deletion patients with Becker muscular dystrophy." *Am J Hum Genet* 51(3): 562-570.

Ginjaar, I. B., A. L. Kneppers, et al. (2000). "Dystrophin nonsense mutation induces different levels of exon 29 skipping and leads to variable phenotypes within one BMD family." *Eur J Hum Genet* 8(10): 793-796.

Gullberg, D., C. F. Tiger, et al. (1999). "Laminins during muscle development and in muscular dystrophies." *Cell Mol Life Sci* 56(5-6): 442-460.

Hack, A. A., C. T. Ly, et al. (1998). "Gamma-sarcoglycan deficiency leads to muscle membrane defects and apoptosis independent of dystrophin." *J Cell Biol* 142(5): 1279-1287.

Hall, N. (2007). "Advanced sequencing technologies and their wider impact in microbiology." *J Exp Biol* 210(Pt 9): 1518-1525.

Janssen, B., C. Hartmann, et al. (2005). "MLPA analysis for the detection of deletions, duplications and complex rearrangements in the dystrophin gene: potential and pitfalls." *Neurogenetics* 6(1): 29-35.

Jones, M. A., B. G. Ng, et al. (2012). "DDOST Mutations Identified by Whole-Exome Sequencing Are Implicated in Congenital Disorders of Glycosylation." *Am J Hum Genet*.

Lalic, T., R. H. Vossen, et al. (2005). "Deletion and duplication screening in the DMD gene using MLPA." *Eur J Hum Genet* 13(11): 1231-1234.

Love, D. R. and K. E. Davies (1989). "Duchenne muscular dystrophy: the gene and the protein." *Mol Biol Med* 6(1): 7-17.

Love, D. R., S. M. Forrest, et al. (1989). "Molecular analysis of Duchenne and Becker muscular dystrophies." *Br Med Bull* 45(3): 659-680.

Mardis, E. R. (2008). "The impact of next-generation sequencing technology on genetics." *Trends Genet* 24(3): 133-141.

Mardis, E. R. (2008). "Next-generation DNA sequencing methods." *Annu Rev Genomics Hum Genet* 9: 387-402.

Medori, R., M. H. Brooke, et al. (1989). "Genetic abnormalities in Duchenne and Becker dystrophies: clinical correlations." *Neurology* 39(4): 461-465.

Mendell, J. R. (2001). "Congenital muscular dystrophy: searching for a definition after 98 years." *Neurology* 56(8): 993-994.

Mendell, J. R., Z. Sahenk, et al. (1995). "The childhood muscular dystrophies: diseases sharing a common pathogenesis of membrane instability." *J Child Neurol* 10(2): 150-159.

Ng, S. B., E. H. Turner, et al. (2009). "Targeted capture and massively parallel sequencing of 12 human exomes." *Nature* 461(7261): 272-276.

Norwood, F., M. de Visser, et al. (2007). "EFNS guideline on diagnosis and management of limb girdle muscular dystrophies." *Eur J Neurol* 14(12): 1305-1312.

Petersen, G. M. (2000). "Genetic testing." *Hematol Oncol Clin North Am* 14(4): 939-952.

Porreca, G. J. (2010). "Genome sequencing on nanoballs." *Nat Biotechnol* 28(1): 43-44.

Schouten, J. P., C. J. McElgunn, et al. (2002). "Relative quantification of 40 nucleic acid sequences by multiplex ligation-dependent probe amplification." *Nucleic Acids Res* 30(12): e57.

Schuster, S. C. (2008). "Next-generation sequencing transforms today's biology." *Nat Methods* 5(1): 16-18.

Schwartz, M. and M. Duno (2004). "Improved molecular diagnosis of dystrophin gene mutations using the multiplex ligation-dependent probe amplification method." *Genet Test* 8(4): 361-367.

Senapathy, P., A. Bhasi, et al. (2010). "Targeted genome-wide enrichment of functional regions." *PLoS One* 5(6): e11138.

Stankiewicz, P., A. N. Pursley, et al. (2010). "Challenges in clinical interpretation of microduplications detected by array CGH analysis." *Am J Med Genet A* 152A(5): 1089-1100.

Straub, V., J. A. Rafael, et al. (1997). "Animal models for muscular dystrophy show different patterns of sarcolemmal disruption." *J Cell Biol* 139(2): 375-385.

ten Bosch, J. R. and W. W. Grody (2008). "Keeping up with the next generation: massively parallel sequencing in clinical diagnostics." *J Mol Diagn* 10(6): 484-492.

Tsao, C. Y. and J. R. Mendell (1999). "The childhood muscular dystrophies: making order out of chaos." *Semin Neurol* 19(1): 9-23.

Vachon, P. H., F. Loechel, et al. (1996). "Merosin and laminin in myogenesis; specific requirement for merosin in myotube stability and survival." *J Cell Biol* 134(6): 1483-1497.

Vainzof, M., D. Ayub-Guerrieri, et al. (2008). "Animal models for genetic neuromuscular diseases." *J Mol Neurosci* 34(3): 241-248.

Valouev, A., J. Ichikawa, et al. (2008). "A high-resolution, nucleosome position map of C. elegans reveals a lack of universal sequence-dictated positioning." *Genome Res* 18(7): 1051-1063.

Venter, J. C., M. D. Adams, et al. (2001). "The sequence of the human genome." *Science* 291(5507): 1304-1351.

Wakayama, Y., M. Inoue, et al. (2008). "Reduced expression of sarcospan in muscles of Fukuyama congenital muscular dystrophy." *Histol Histopathol* 23(12): 1425-1438.

Whittock, N. V., R. G. Roberts, et al. (1997). "Dystrophin point mutation screening using a multiplexed protein truncation test." *Genet Test* 1(2): 115-123.

Witkowski, J. A. (1989). "Dystrophin-related muscular dystrophies." *J Child Neurol* 4(4): 251-271.

Yamamoto, T., Y. Kato, et al. (2004). "Expression of genes related to muscular dystrophy with lissencephaly." *Pediatr Neurol* 31(3): 183-190.

Yurchenco, P. D., Y. S. Cheng, et al. (2004). "Loss of basement membrane, receptor and cytoskeletal lattices in a laminin-deficient muscular dystrophy." *J Cell Sci* 117(Pt 5): 735-742.

16

Motor Function Measure Scale (MFM): New Instrument for Follow-Up Brazilian Patients with Neuromuscular Disease

Cristina Iwabe[1], Anamarli Nucci[2],
Beatriz Helena Miranda Pfeilsticker[3] and Luis Alberto Magna[4]
[1]*Faculty of Medical Sciences (FCM), Campinas State University (UNICAMP)*
[2]*Department of Neurology, FCM UNICAMP,*
[3]*Department of Neurology, FCM UNICAMP,*
[4]*Department of Medical Genetics, FCM UNICAMP,*
Brazil

1. Introduction

Neuromuscular disorders include a variety of conditions that affect motor neurons (spinal muscular atrophy), peripheral nerves (neuropathy), neuromuscular junction (myasthenia gravis) or muscle fibers (myopathy) (1).

Myopathy is characterized by primary and generally irreversible skeletal muscle tissue degeneration, including genetic, inflammatory, metabolic or endocrine disorders and the different are charaterized by the muscle fibre type affected, mode of inheritance, age of onset and course of evolution (2,3,4).

The term muscular dystrophy has been used in cases of rapidly progressive myopathy as well as of slow progressive degeneration of muscle, such as myotonic dystrophy (2).

Myotonic Dystrophy (MD) is defined as the most common inherited myopathy in adults, with multisystemic involvement (cardiovascular, respiratory, nervous, visual, endocrine), autossomal dominant pattern and distinct clinical manifestations (2,5,6). Depending on the genetic trait, MD is classified as type 1 (MD-1), type 2 (MD-2) (7), or type 3 (8); being the type 1 the most common and the type 3, very rare.

The MD-1, described by Steinert in 1909, is caused by expansion of CTG nucleotides repeat in the region of the gene for dystrophy myotonic protein kinase (DMPK) on chromosome 19; over 35 and ranging from 80 to more than 4,000 repetitions in the affected individuals. This abnormal protein is responsible for the disability of muscle, cardiac and nervous cells, involving several systems (9).

This disease can be classified in: congenital, infantile, classic (age of onset between 10 to 50 years) and with minimal involvement (10). Usually the earlier the onset of symptoms, the greater the number of repetitions of the nucleotides (7,11).

The muscle involvement is the main clinical feature with variations in the degree of weakness (facial, neck and distal muscles of limbs), as well as myotonia. In the congenital form, the deficit is prominent at birth without myotonia. In the infantile form, weakness is relatively mild, and in adults form there is slowly progression of the symptoms (11).

In contrast to muscular dystrophy, the congenital myopathy is described as non-progressive or slowly progressive and rarely fatal disease. Among them is included the Congenital Fibre Type Disproportion (CFTD) (12). The CFTD is a congenital myopathy described by Brooke (13) as having generalized weakness, hypotonia at birth and slow progression of symptoms associated with abnormal histological predominance of type 1 muscle fibres, and smaller size of at least 12% than type 2. The patients have abnormalities such as congenital hip dislocation, foot deformities, kyphoscoliosis, ligament laxity, high palate and underweight (14,15,16,17).

The CFTD pattern suggests a autossomal dominant trait although sporadic recessive cases has been described (18,19,20,21). Distinct mutations in the gene that codes the α-skeletal muscle actin (ACTA1), selenoprotein N (SEPN1) and α-tropomyosin (TPM3) proteins were identified in some cases, but the molecular mechanisms that cause the disparity of the fibres are still unknown (22,23).

Individuals with CFTD show different degrees of weakness, more severe in the early stages of development, especially in the lower limbs (20). Generally they have a good prognosis, but in some cases they may be associated with respiratory (14,20) or cardiac (16,21) failures.

Considering the CFTD and MD-1, both have weakness as the main physical limitation (17,24,25) and the individuals become more and more dependent to achieve their routine activities. Rehabilitation programs must measure and maximize patients motor skills and optimizing their functionality.

Now a days, several therapeutic techniques and other health professionals assessment tools can be used for patient selection, therapeutic monitoring and to establish prognosis for recovery (26).

Generally, the evaluations are qualitative test, not allowing for the individual assessment of the recovery of the better patients (27). Currently, Medical Research Council scale (MRC) for measuring muscle strength is being used for clinical examination and patient follow-up however, it does not reflect the real abilities of each individual (28)There are several scales to measure function in neuromuscular diseases, including the Barthel Index (BI), Vignos scale and Motor Function Measure (MFM) (28).

The MFM have been developed and validated for neuromuscular diseases by the research group of the Department of Pediatric Reeducation L'Escale, Lyon, France.This is a more comprehensive, specific and functional scale, analyzing the function of the head, trunk, proximal and distal segments in several neuromuscular diseases (28).

The scale comprises 32 items, including static and dynamic evaluations, divided into three dimensions:

- Dimension 1 (D1): a standing position and transfers, with 13 items
- Dimension 2 (D2): axial and proximal motor function, with 12 items.

- Dimension 3 (D3): distal motor function, with seven items, six of which are related to the upper limbs.

Each item is graduated on a 4-point scale (scores 0 to 3), with the instructions detailed in the scoring manual, specific to each item. Score 0 - can not start the requested task or can not keep the starting position. Score 1 – initializes the item. Score 2 - partially performs the requested movement or fully realized, but imperfectly. Score 3 - completes the item, with controlled movement (normal).

In cases of tendon retraction or joint limitation, the individual is graduated as not presenting adequate strength to perform the movement, preventing them from receiving the maximum degree. The total score and each dimension are expressed in percentages relative to maximum score (96 points).

In 2008, Iwabe et al. (29) demonstrated the reliability of the Portuguese version's MFM (P-MFM), showing a high correlation intra and inter examiner results.

The aim of this chapter is to describe the validation of the P-MFM and its applicability to evaluate the motor function in muscular myopathy and dystrophy individuals.

2. P-MFM Validation

The population comprised a total of 65 patients, 37 male and 28 female, average 33.09 years (8-60 years), with laboratory findings confirming clinical diagnosis of congenital muscular dystrophy (n = 7), Duchenne (n = 5), Becker (n = 4), limb girdle (n = 4), facioscapulohumeral (n = 8), distal myopathy (n = 4), mitochondrial (n = 3), centrocore (n = 6), congenital fibre types disproportion (n = 1), myotonic dystrophy (n = 21) and spinal muscular atrophy (n = 2); outcome in the Neuromuscular Diseases Clinic of the Faculty of Medical Sciences, Campinas State University (UNICAMP).

Patients were evaluated according to the P-MFM, BI and Vignos scales. All evaluations were performed by the same examiner and BI questions were answered by the patient, or in some cases with the help of their parents.

Statistical analysis - the total scores and each of the three dimensions of P-MFM were correlated with Vignos scale and BI by the Spearman correlation coefficient, with significance level of 5% ($p < 0.05$).

It was observed that in P-MFM scale, both its three dimensions and total score, were correlated negatively and significantly with the Vignos scale, and correlated positively and significantly with the BI (Table 1).

P-MFM	Vignos scale	BI
Dimension 1	-0,858*	0,946*
Dimension 2	-0,852*	0,871*
Dimension 3	-0,671*	0,736*
Total	-0,894*	0,980*

* - p < 0,001

Table 1. Correlation between P-MFM, Vignos scale and BI.

Validation is defined as the ability of an instrument to measure a particular aspect, and for this it is necessary the correlation with other validate scales, and similar characteristics (30). Miller et al. (31) defined some factors for the scale's development and validation. The instrument must represent the function at the moment, following the patient's evolution over the time, and each individual serving as his own control.

The MFM was developed for this purpose, containing items easily implementable and understandable by patients from different age groups (6-60 years). This scale has the capacity of analyze the most important motor functions and deficiency in several neuromuscular diseases. It can measure the activity of the proximal and distal segments members; as well as the standing position and transfering at the moment and over time (28).

The capacity of MFM scale to analyze the various body segments and their mobility in all neuromuscular diseases, empathizes its use in research and clinical. To be applied in Brazil, it was necessary perform the validation process of the Portuguese version, considering that the scale item was approved in reproducibility and reliability (29).

In Brazil, there are only two assessment instruments validated for patients with dystrophy (32).

The P-MFM validation study used two functional scales, the BI and Vignos scale (33,34,35,36). BI and Vignos scale are clinical instruments often used to assess the level of functionality in neuromuscular diseases (35). These two scales were used in the study by Nair et al. (37), with Duchenne muscular dystrophy, showing to be a valid instrument for assessing the functional limitations in this patients.

Previous validation studies about functional neuromuscular diseases using the BI and Vignos scale (28,38,39) demonstrated the correlation between them. Studies analyzing the functionality of individuals with neuromuscular diseases after clinical or surgical treatment, or correlating it to other parameters, such as muscle strength using these same scales (40,41,42,43,44) established them as easy to use instruments.

In this study, we found a high significant correlation among the P-MFM, Vignos scale and BI, allowing for validation of the Portuguese version of MFM.

3. Applicability of P-MFM in family with CFTD, associated muscle magnetic ressonance

We studied members of a family with clinical and laboratory CFTD. They were evaluated for muscle strength (MRC scale) and motor function by the scale P-MFM (29) and were previously examined in the Neuromuscular Diseases Clinic through physical examination, serological and neurophysiological tests and muscle biopsy. One sample was taken from the biceps muscle from the father in a family. The obtained sample was fixed in isopentane and frozen in liquid nitrogen. Sections were stained with hematoxylin-eosin (H & E), Gomori trichrome modified (TRI) or oil red O and analyzed by histochemical techniques for nicotinamide adenine dinucleotide phosphatase, nicotinamide dehydrogenase tetrazolium reductase (NADH-TR), succinate dehydrogenase (SDH) and immunohistochemistry for slow and fast myosin, desmin and alpha B crystalline.

Muscle magnetic resonance imaging (mMRI) was performed in magnetic field of 2.0 Tesla, T1-weighted images in axial plane for the leg muscles from each patient, according to De Cauwer et al. (45).

Image data were analyzed quantitatively according to the degree proposed by Mercuri et al. (46) and modified by Nucci (47).

0 = normal appearance
1 = slight appearance of "moth-food", with sporadic areas of hyperintensity.
2 = moderate appearance of "moth-food" with related areas of hyperintense spaced, comprising less than 30% of muscle volume.
= 2.5 appearance of "moth-food" with moderate hyper spaced areas, comprising 30 to 60% of muscle volume.
3 = severe appearance of "moth-food", with numerous areas of confluence of hyperintense with muscle still present in the periphery.
4 = complete fatty degeneration, with replacement of muscle by connective tissue and fat.

The family pedigree is shown in Figure 1. It was not possible to examine patient´s mother (I-1) and patient´s uncle (I-2). Throughout the family´s history, the patient´s mother was indicated as asymptomatic, and the uncle as having the phenotype very similar with myopathy aspects.. Thus, I-2 was marked as affected in the pedigree.

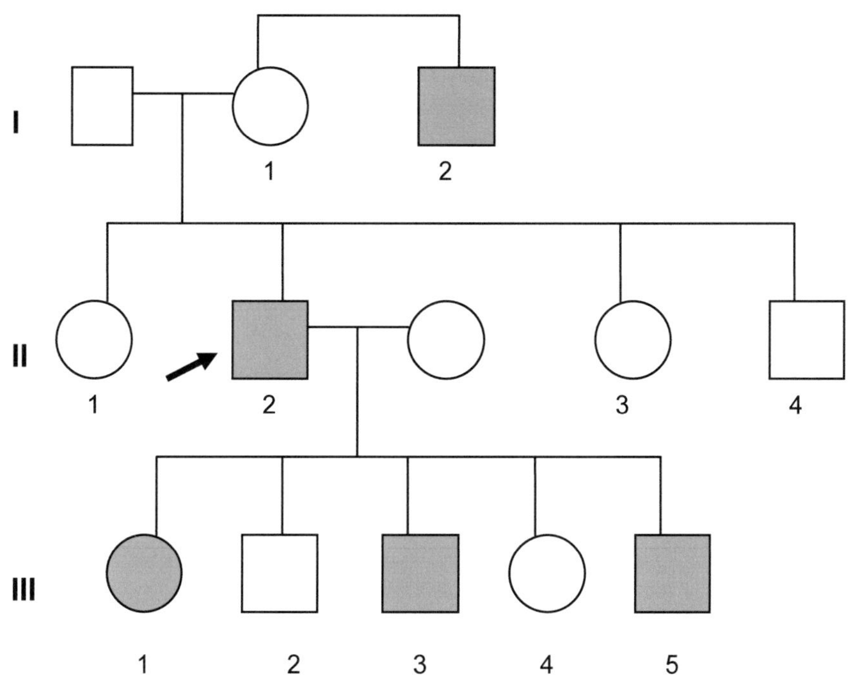

Fig. 1. Family pedigree. The grey figures are the affects cases. The white figures are the normal cases

CASE II -2 Male, 48-year-old with consanguineous parents, complaining about muscle weakness since childhood, considered a "sick child" due to limitations in physical activities and difficulty in gaining weight. The acquisition of motor milestones was delayed, just being able to walk around 5 years old. The initial clinical examination showed a collaborative and lanky patient (1.78 meters, 48 kg), with severe scoliosis dextro-convex compensate cervical, and high palate. A complex gait was observed due to the misalignment of the spinal cord and the tendency to walk with his feet fallen. The muscles stretch reflexes were hypoactive, but the cranial nerves, the cognition and sensibility were normal. The laboratory findings for creatine kinase (CK) showed 181 U / L (normal values below 170), and the study for motor and sensory nerves conduction were within normal limits. Electromyography (EMG) of the deltoid and biceps brachii showed the most potential of motor units with respect polyphasic, low amplitude and short duration, myopathy indicative,, despite the present right quadriceps were relatively normal. The electrocardiogram (ECG) and routine laboratory tests showed no abnormalities. The main morphologic abnormality in biopsy was a disproportion of the fibre types with small type 1

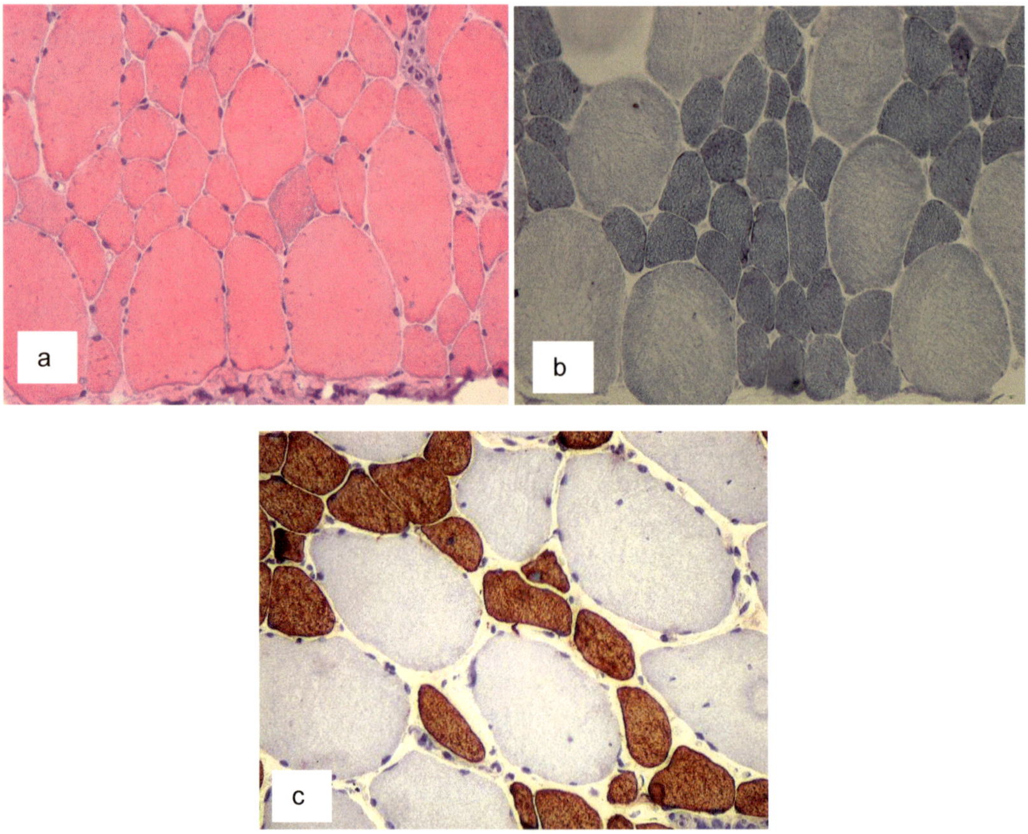

Fig. 2. a - H & E staining showing two populations of muscle fibres with different diameters average. b - NADH-TR staining where small diameter fibres show a higher oxidative activity (type 1) than the large fibres (type 2). c - Immunohistochemistry for myosin slow - small diameter fibres are positively stained for slow myosin fibres (type 1), in contrast to the larger fibres that are unmarked (type 2).

fibres (Figures 10 a-c). The electron microscopy showed neither central focus, minifocus, nemaline bodies nor mitochondrial alterations, also no protein deposits were observed.

The most significant data from the biceps muscle biopsy from case II-2 is illustrated in figure 2 c.

CASE III - 1 Female, 13 years old, daughter of the Case II-2, non-consanguineous parents. She was born at 40 weeks gestational age, 50 cm height, 2.670g weight, cesarean delivery for fetal distress, and a history of reduced fetal movements. The child presented a congenital hypotonia and delayed motor development, acquiring the standing posture approximately at 19 months of age with a clumsy posture. She did not gain weight like a normal child and physical activities were restricted. Like her father, she showed progressive deviation of the spine, and recently complained with pain in the dorsal region, especially during physical activity. On examination, the patient was a tall and thin child, with marked kyphoscoliosis, long face, high palate, atrophy muscle and global hypoactive muscle stretch reflexes. There were no motor deficits in the face or external ophthalmoparesis. CK values were between 65 to 73 U / L (normal below 145 U / L). Glucose, IgA, IgG and IgM, transaminases, and electrolytes were normal, but with a TSH value of 7.23 IU / ml (normal 4.5) and FT4 of 1.68 ng / dl (normal range). Sensory nerve conduction velocity (median, ulnar, radial and sural) and motor nerves (median, ulnar, peroneal and tibial) were within normal limits. EMG of deltoid, biceps, rectus femoris, tibialis anterior and gastrocnemius showed myopathic changes. The patient was doing physical therapy in 50-minute sessions per week in pediatric neurology ambulatory UNICAMP. At 15 years old she had an episode of severe pneumonia which complicated by fatal septicemia.

CASE III - 3. Male, 10 years old, third son of the case II -2. He was born at 38 weeks gestational age with cesarean delivery, and had a history of reduced fetal movements. The child presented a congenital hypotonia and delayed motor development to roll, sit and crawl, acquiring the standing posture around 11 months age, and unsteady gait around 2 years old. According to his parents, he used to present recurrent episodes of urinary tract infection, pneumonia and ear infections during childhood. In the first consultation, there was a decreased in motor performance, diffused muscle hypotrophy, scoliosis, high palate and hypoactivity of muscle stretch reflexes. There was no facial weakness or external ophthalmoparesis. Sensibility and cognition were preserved. Values of CK, glucose, IgA, IgG and IgM, transaminases, electrolytes, vitamin B12 and TSH were normal. The EMG test was not performed at the request of his father.

CASE III - 5. Male, 9 months of age, born after 38 weeks of pregnancy, cesarean delivery, and with a history of reduced fetal movements. He had a slight delay in motor development, and at clinical examination an evident hypotonia, with preserved muscle stretch reflexes. Laboratory findings revealed mild microcytic hypochromic anemia, CK of 89 U / L (normal 170 U / L) and TSH and T4 L-us normal. Clinical monitoring was suggested by over time. He was re-evaluated at 2 years and 6 months of age. At this time he was walking without support, with mild myopathic patterns. The muscle stretch reflexes were hypoactive, hypotonia clearly present and dextro-convex scoliosis and lumbar cord. For treatment physiotherapy was indicated. We did not evaluate him using the scale P-MFM due to this method is recommended for patients over 6 years.

Figure 3 a-c illustrate the data from the mMRI for cases II-2, III-1 and III3.

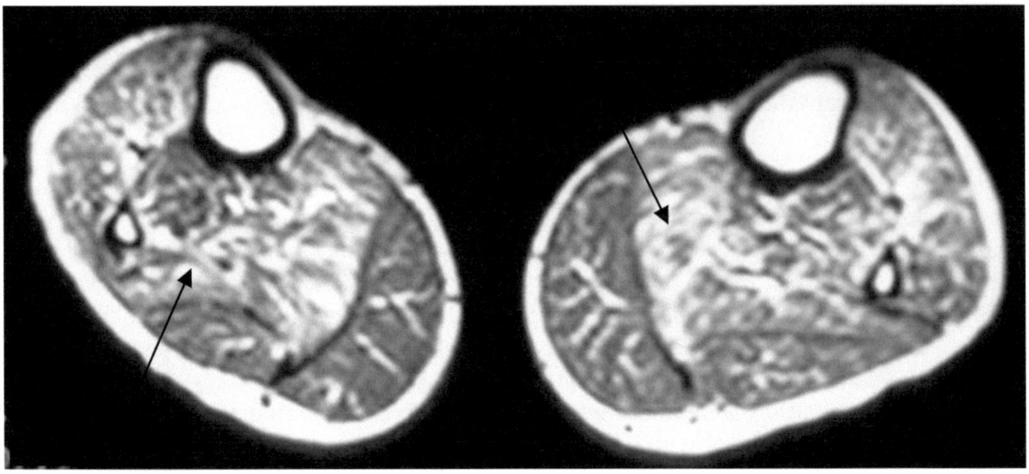

Fig. 3.a - Case II-2. mMRI, T1-weighted images and axial sections showing fatty infiltration of muscle compartments of the anterior, posterior deep and superficial leg, with greater involvement of the anterior and deep posterior compartment.

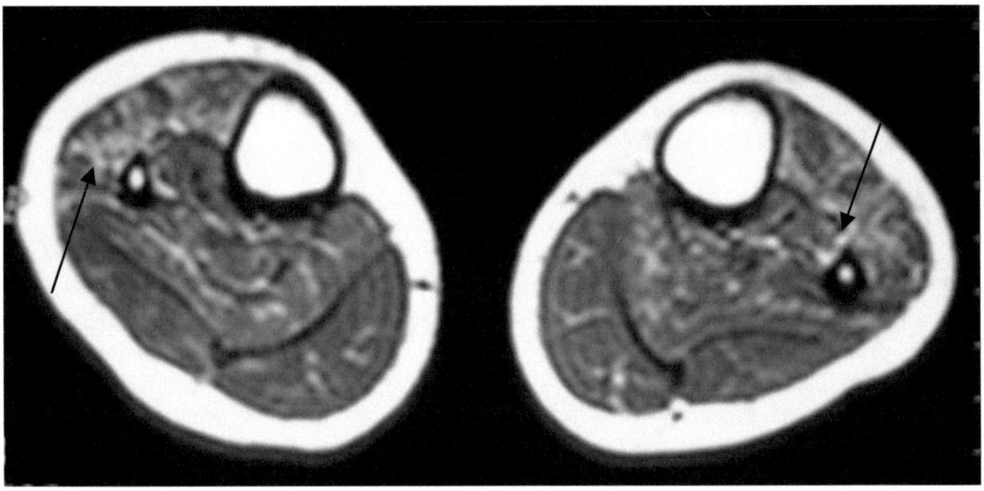

Fig. 3.b - Case III-1. mMRI, T1-weighted images and axial sections showing fatty infiltration of muscle compartments of the anterior, posterior deep and superficial leg with less alteration of the superficial posterior compartment. Note the symmetry condition.

Figure 4 represents the scores of each dimension and the total score of P-MFM in cases II - 2, III - 1 and III - 3, at different ages.

Different types of muscle fibres are present in the muscles of normal adults in a typical mosaic pattern, with ratio of approximately 1 / 3 of fibre type 1 (Figures 2a and 2b). The differentiation of the fibres occurs between the 22° week of gestation and the first year of life. At birth, the child had about 40% of type 1 fibre. The percentage of these fibres increased up to 60% in the first year of life and remained unchanged until adulthood. The sizes of type 1 and 2 fibres are almost equal in childhood, with little variability in relation to adults (75).

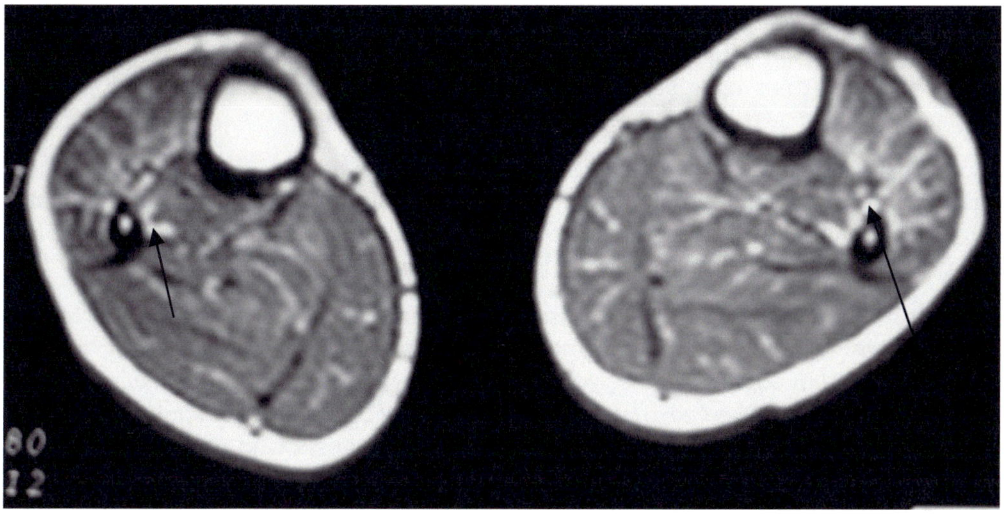

Fig. 3.c - Case III-3. mMRI, T1-weighted images and axial sections showing fatty infiltration of muscle compartments of the anterior, posterior deep and superficial leg with less alteration of the superficial posterior compartment. Note the relative preservation of muscle compared with the previous cases.

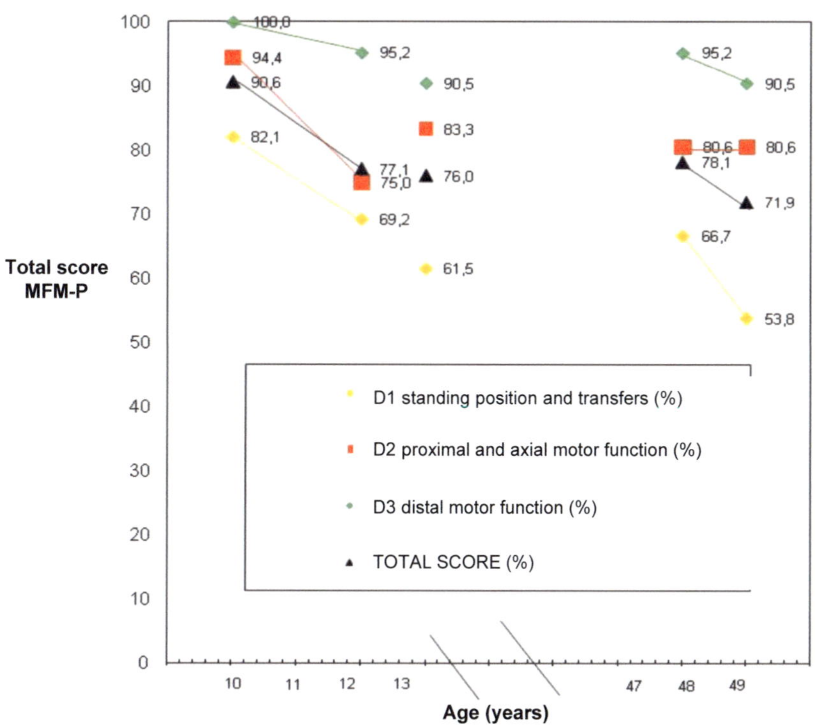

Fig. 4. Distribution of scores for each dimension and total score of the P-MFM from each patient. The evaluation at 10 and 12 years refers to case III-3, the evaluation at 13 years refers to the case III-1, and evaluation at 48 and 49 years to case II-2.

The mutation in the genes ACTA1 (22), SEPN1 (48) or TPM3 (23) express the morphological and histochemical alteration in CFTD (49). Since the first description of this disease, approximately 67 cases have been described (16), but just a few cases originally in Brazil (50).

Clinical characteristics of patients in the study were similar to those described in previously works, such as congenital hypotonia, delayed motor skills, kyphoscoliosis and high palate. Also data for additional tests as EMG myopathic pattern and CK levels are normal or slightly altered according to the literature (14,17,51,52,53,54).

The natural course of CFTD is in most cases characterized by slow progression of weakness, affecting mainly the lower limbs beginning at the proximal muscles and progressing to distal. However, in some patients weakness is widespread (16,17). The deterioration of muscle strength was observed in our patients, with difficulties to standing, walking and running. During assessment of motor function, all patients showed greater difficulties in activities related to standing position and transfers (Dimension 1) due to loss of muscle strength.

All the seven cases described by Sobrado et al. (17) had difficulty in activities like those described in our study (raising themselves from a chair or from the floor, walking or running on heels), in addition to muscle weakness in lower limbs (grade 3 to 4). These data agree with descriptions of Linssen et al. (55) in which cases presenting degree of muscle strength equal to 4, have functional limitations.

Some patients with CFTD have severe respiratory complications, as with the patient in the case III - 1. This condition could happen due to hypotrophy of type 1 fibres found in the respiratory muscles, including the diaphragm (14,16,20,22,48,49) or as a result of severe kyphoscoliosis, which progressively diminished lung capacity. Thus, it is important that patients be monitored for maintenance of a postural alignment and breathing function.

The mMRI is proposed as a useful method to study congenital and metabolic myopathy (56), although there are few publications using this technique in CFTD (17). In the current study, it was possible to qualitatively observe intense changes in distal segments of the lower limbs in all images of affected patients. These changes correspond to an increased leg muscle weakness with difficulties in performing activities according to the P-MFM scale.

The evaluation of muscle function by P-MFM associated with the examination of mMRI led to a full characterization and motor phenotype evaluation in these patients. The first evaluation using the P-MFM in family's members showed a co-occurrence of more intense abnormalities in the mMRI with the worst scores in standing position and transfer. There was also a correlation between the age and severity of the mMRI and P-MFM score.

4. Correlation between muscle strength and P-MFM in myotonic dystrophy

The study included a total of 21 patients, 10 males and 11 females, from 20 to 60 years old, with an average of 38.14 years, and with clinical-laboratory diagnosis of MD-1, outcoming the Neuromuscular Diseases Clinic Clinical Hospital of UNICAMP.

Patients were evaluated by MFM-P (29) and submitted to examination of muscle strength by MRC scale (1976) that includes 14 muscle groups of upper limbs (UL), 14 groups in the cervical muscles and lower limbs, trunk flexors and extensors. Muscles were grouped according to the segment's function.

Statistical analysis - The correlation of each of the three dimensions and the total score P-MFM, with the degrees obtained by the MRC scale in the muscle groups studied was made using Pearson's correlation coefficient.

Patients showed a variation in the degree of muscle strength from 2 to 4. In the distal muscle groups, such as flexors, extensors of the fingers and wrist extensors, the degrees of force were grade 2-4. And the proximal muscles strength varied from 3 to 4.

In the lower limbs, muscle strength ranged from grade 2 to 5. In distal muscles the strength varied from 2 to 4 and the proximal muscles strength ranged from grade 3 to 5. Also the evaluation of axial muscles showed strength ranged varying from grade 2 to 4.

The deficits found in patients were symmetrical in both the axial region and in the upper and lower segments.

To analyze the distribution of the total score and each dimension of the P-MFM scale values were arbitrarily classified as: mild (100 to 70%, independent patient), moderate (69.9 to 50%, partially dependent) and severe (<50%, dependent).

A higher number of patients presented lower scores (<50%) in activities related to P-MFM Dimension 1 (standing position and transfers) (Table 2).

Score	**Dimension (score)**			
	D1	**D2**	**D3**	**Total score**
Mild (100– 70%)	4 (89,74 – 76,92)	18 (100 – 80,56)	20 (100 – 71,43)	12 (95,83 – 72,92)
Moderate (69,9– 50%)	7 (69,23 – 53,85)	3 (63,89 – 58,33)	01 (57,14)	09 (66,67 – 54,17)
Severe (< 50%)	10 (48,72 – 25-64)	----	---	---

Table 2. Number of patients according to scores obtained in each dimension and total score of P-MFM

Analyzing the correlations between the degrees of upper limb strength in each dimension and total score P-MFM, we observed a significantly positive correlation between the proximal muscles and Dimension1 and Dimension 2, and correlation between the distal muscles and Dimension 3.

Similarly for lower limbs, we observed a significantly positive correlation between the plantar flexors and extensors of the hips strength with the scores of D1; and also between the finger extensors and dorsiflexors of the ankles strength with the scores of D2. The strength values of the finger extensors, dorsiflexors, ankle inverters and eversion were significantly positive correlated with the score of D3; and the plantar flexors, dorsiflexors, eversion ankles, and hip extensors strength were significantly positive correlated with the total score of P-MFM.

Analyzing the correlations between the neck and trunk strength, with each dimension and the total score of P-MFM, we observed a significantly correlation between the neck and abdominal flexor with D1; between neck flexors with the D3; and between neck flexors and abdominal flexor with total score.

The assessment of functional capacity and degree of muscle strength in patients with neuromuscular disease are essential aspects for their diagnosis and follow-up. Assistance in clinical decisions, treatment, prevention of any complications (like respiratory failure or retractions), indication of the type and intensity of exercise are important aspects to be considered (57,58).

The MD-1 shows a pattern of muscle weakness primarily affecting the facial muscles, neck flexors, and dorsiflexors of fingers. The proximal muscles may not show deficits or mild clinical signs (2,59,60). Lindeman et al. (59,61) showed that in MD-1 there is a great variability in degrees of strength in the affected muscle groups (62.63). The symmetric and progressive muscular weakness involves proximal muscles (64). The deficit predominantly distal and axial deficits, as well as the later weakness proximal segments was also demonstrated in studies by Whittaker et al. (60), Lindeman and Drukker (65) and Lindeman et al. (66). Similar topography of motor impairment was observed in this study, in patients with MD-1.

The strength graduated in 4 on the MRC scale, defined as the ability of active muscle contraction against moderate resistance, was correlated with a negative impact on the ability to perform functions like running, climbing stairs and walking (55,59,67,68,69,70,71,72).

In this study, we found a great variability in the degree of muscle strength with greater involvement in distal segments of the lower limbs, and motor skills assessed by the P-MFM and a greater activity limitation in the standing position and transfers. The positive correlations obtained between muscle groups and the dimensions of P-MFM were restricted, noting that the most significant one occurred between the groups with lower degree of strength of the distal segment (hand and foot) and D3.

According to Whittaker et al. (60) the weakness of flexors and extensors of fingers and wrist is the major cause of disability in DM-1. This early involvement of distal muscles allowed the correlation of these groups, especially with the D3. The proximal and axial body segments act as posture stabilizer factors to provide a stable basis for the distal movement (73). Considering that during the measurement of the scale items the subjects had trunk and limbs supported, they did not need an effective action from the muscles of the trunk and proximal limbs. So, it was possible to correlate specifically the strength of distal muscles with their respective activities.

Poor limitations in proximal muscle groups (extensors of the hip and shoulder) were observed in few activities (Dimensions 1 and 2) limiting other activities (60,65,66) in late stage of this disease.

The proximal muscular deficit can influence the performance function (64, 74, 75, 76.77, 78). According to Galassi et al. (79) and Linssen et al. (55) even when the weakness is predominantly in the distal limb segments, there is a bilateral proximal atrophy area in the computer tomography scans from patients with muscular dystrophy, also demonstrating the involvement of bilateral and proximal muscles, even when there is a clear manifestation of symptoms.

Lindeman et al. (59,61,76)and Aldehag et al. (80) correlated a specific muscle with a particular activity (like the quadriceps strength and standing up from a chair) in patients with DM-1, and found a positive correlation between strength and function. However Dawes et al. (81) found no correlation between muscle strength and function, when these activities were more complex.

Besides strength, other variables may be influencing the individual's functional ability, such as age (82), gender and weight (83). In our cases these variables were not considered because they were not included in the objectives.

So, it is important to analyze a large number of myotonic dystrophy patients to observe any correlation between strength and motor function.

5. Final considerations

The use of MFM proved to be an interesting tool in the study of the congenital myopathies as CFTD; although we were limited by time and sample size. The correlation of severe myopathy and mMRI data for smaller scale scores P-MFM, enables the use of a non-invasive diagnostic tool to study the course of myopathy diseases. They also indicate that both methods could be used in to analyse the results of pharmacological interventions and rehabilitation in these diseases.

The P-MFM has a high reliability and validity to be used as a tool for clinical diagnosis and monitoring of neuromuscular diseases, allowing the inclusion of Brazilian patients in international clinical trials. Thus, we can mention that:

1. The positive correlations between the BI, Vignos scale and P-MFM allowed the validation of P-MFM in Brazil.
2. The application of P-MFM could demonstrate the progressive dysfunction in two of the three members of a family with CFTD. The muscle magnetic resonance showed that the more severe the motor function, the worse were the changes in the image worst severe functional motor, the worst change images.
3. The application of P-MFM in MD-1 showed the predominance of distal myopathy, expressed by the lower scores of muscle strength correlating positively with the scores mainly in D3.

6. References

[1] Jensen MP, Abresch RT, Carter GT. The reliability and validity of a self report version of the FIM instrument in persons with neuromuscular disease and chronic pain. Arch Phys Med Rehabil. 2005; 86: 116-22.
[2] Harper PS. Myotonic dystrophy London: WB Saunders; 2001.436p.
[3] Otsuka MA, Boffa CFB, Vieira ABAM. Distrofias Musculares: Fisioterapia aplicada. Rio de Janeiro: Ed Revinter; 2005. p.2-28.
[4] Beenakker EAC, Maurits NM, Fock JM, Brouwer OF, Van der Hoeven J. Functional ability and muscle force in healthy children and ambulant Duchenne muscular dystrophy patients. Eur J Paediatr Neurol. 2005; 9: 387-93.

[5] Giorgio A, Dotti MT, Battaglini M, Marino S, Mortilla M, Stromillo ML et al. Cortical damage in brains of patients with adult-form of myotonic dystrophy type 1 and no or minimal MRI abnormalities. J Neurol. 2006; 253: 1471-7.

[6] Angeard N, Gargiulo M, Jacquette A, Radvanyi H, Eymard B, Heron D. Cognitive profile in childhood myotonic dystrophy type I: is there a global impairment? Neuromuscul Disord. 2007; 17: 451-8.

[7] Schara U, Schoser, BGH. Myotonic dystrophies type 1 and 2: a summary on current aspects. Semin Pediatr Neurol. 2006; 13: 71-9.

[8] Le Ber I, Martinez M, Campion D, Laquerriére A, Bétard C, Bassez G et al. A non-DM1, non-DM2 multisystem myotonic disorder with fronto temporal dementia: phenotype and suggestive mapping of the DM3 locus to chromosome 15q21-24. Brain. 2004; 127: 1979-92.

[9] Cho DH, Tapscott SJ. Myotonic dystrophy: emerging mechanisms for DM1 and DM2. Biochimic Biophysic Acta. 2007; 1772: 195-204.

[10] Brunner HG, Jennekens FGI, Smeets HJM, de Visser M, Wintzen AR. Myotonic dystrophy (Steinert's disease). In: Emery AEH, ed. Diagnostic criteria for neuromuscular disorders. 2º ed. Londres: Royal Society of Medicine Press; 1997. p 27-9.

[11] Kroksmark AK, Ekstrom AB, Bjorck E, Tulinius M. Myotonic dystrophy: muscle involvement in relation to disease type and size of expanded CTG-repeat sequence. Dev Med Child Neurol. 2005; 47: 478-85.

[12] North K. Congenital myopathies. In: Engel AG, Franzini-Armstrong C. Myology. United States of America: McGraw-Hill; 2004. p.1473-533.

[13] Brooke MH. Congenital fiber type disproportion. In: Kakulas BA. Clinical studies in myology. Proc of the 2nd Int. Cong on Muscle Diseases, Perth, Australia, 1971. Part 2. Amsterdam: Excerpta Medica (pub.) 1973. p. 147-59.

[14] Cavanagh NPC, Lake BD, McMeniman P. Congenital fibre type disproportion myopathy. A histological diagnosis with an uncertain clinical outlook. Arch Dis Child. 1979; 54: 735-43.

[15] Clancy RR, Kelts KA, Oehlert JW. Clinical variability in congenital fibre type disproportion. J Neurol Sci.1980; 46: 257-66.

[16] Clarke NF, North KN. Congenital fibre type disproportion – 30 years on. J Neuropathol Exp Neurol. 2003; 62: 977-89.

[17] Sobrido MJ, Fernandez JM, Fontoira E, Pérez-Sousa C, Cabello A, Castro M et al. Autosomal dominant congenital fibre type disproportion: a clinicopathological and imaging study of a large family. Brain. 2005; 128: 1716-27.

[18] Curless RG, Nelson MB. Congenital fiber type disproportion in identical twins. Ann Neurol.1977; 2: 455-9.

[19] Kula RW, Sher JH, Shafiq SA, Hardy-Stashin J. Variability of clinical pathological manifestations in familial fiber type disproportion. Trans Am Neurol Assoc. 1980; 105: 416-8.

[20] Sulaiman AR, Swick HM, Kinder DS. Congenital fibre type disproportion with unusual clinico pathologic manifestations. J Neurol Neurosurg Psychiatry. 1983; 46: 175-82.

[21] Bartholomeus MGT, Gabreels FJM, ter Laak HJ, Van Engelen BGM. Congenital fibre type disproportion a time-locked diagnosis: a clinical and morphological follow-up study. Clin Neurol Neurosurg. 2000; 102: 97-101.

[22] Laing NG, Clarke NF, Dye DE, Liyanage K, Walker KR, Kobayashi Y et al. Actin mutations are one cause of congenital fibre type disproportion. Ann Neurol. 2004; 56: 689-94.

[23] Clarke NF, Kolski H, Dye DE, Lim E, Smith RLL, Patel R et al. Mutation in TPM3 are a common cause of congenital fiber type disproportion. Ann Neurol. 2008; 63: 329-37.

[24] Fowler Jr WM. Management of musculoskeletal complications in neuromuscular diseases: weakness and the role of exercise. Advances in the rehabilitation of neuromuscular diseases. Physic Med Rehabil. 1988; 2: 489-507.

[25] Kurihara T. New classification and treatment for myotonic disorders. Internal Medicine. 2005; 44(10): 1027-32.

[26] Stteg AM, Lankhorst GJ. Screening instruments for disability. Critical Rev Phys Rehabil Med. 1994; 6: 101-2.

[27] Cacho EWA, Melo FRLV, Oliveira R. Avaliação da recuperação motora de pacientes hemiplégicos através do Protocolo de Desempenho Físico de Fugl-Meyer. Rev Neurocienc. 2004; 12(2): 94-102. Errata, 12(4):221.

[28] Bérard C, Payan C, Hodgkinson I, Fermanian J. A motor function measure scale for neuromuscular diseases. Construction and validation study. Neuromuscul Disord. 2005; 15(7): 463-70.

[29] Iwabe C, Miranda-Pfeilsticker BH, Nucci A. Medida da função motora: versão da escala para o português e estudo de confiabilidade. Rev Bras Fisioter. 2008; 12(5): 417-24.

[30] Masuko AH, Carvalho LBC, Machado MAC, Morais JF, Prado LBF, Prado GF. Translation and validation into Brazilian Portuguese of the restless legs syndrome rating scale of the international restless legs syndrome study group. Arq Neuropsiquiatr. 2008; 66(4):832-6.

[31] Miller DK, Malmstrom TK, Andresen EM, Miller JP, Herning MM, Schootman M et al. Development and validation of a short portable sarcopenia measure in the African American Health project. J Gerontol A Biol Sci Med Sci. 2009; 64A(3): 388-94.

[32] Silva MB, Asa SKP, Santa Maria NN, Zanella EM, Fávero FM, Fukujima MM et al. Análise dos instrumentos de avaliação na miopatia. Rev Neurocienc. 2006; 14(2): 29-43.

[33] Forst J, Forst R. Lower limb surgery in Duchenne muscular dystrophy. Neuromuscul Disord. 1999; 9(3): 176-81.

[34] Vondracek P, Bednarik J. Clinical and electrohysiological findings and long-term outcomes in paediatric patients with critical illness polyneuromyopathy. Eur J Paediatr Neurol. 2006; 10(4): 176-81.

[35] Jansa J, Pogacnik T, Gompertz P. An evaluation of the Extended Barthel Index with acute ischemic stroke patients. Neurorehabil Neural Repair. 2004; 18: 37-41.

[36] Tiffreau V, Viet G, Thévenon A. Pain and neuromuscular disease: the results of a survey. Am J Phys Med Rehabil. 2006; 85(9): 756-66.

[37] Nair KP, Vasanth A, Gourie-Devi M, Taly AB, Rao S, Gayathri N et al. Disabilities in children with Duchene muscular dystrophy: a profile. J Rehabil Med. 2001; 33: 147-9.

[38] Martinez JAB, Brunherotti MA, Assis MR, Sobreira CFR. Validação da escala motora funcional EK para a língua portuguesa. Rev Assoc Med Brás. 2006; 52(5): 347-51.

[39] Vandervelde L, Van den Bergh PY, Goemans N, Thonnard JL. ACTIVLIM: a Rasch-built measure of activity limitations in children and adults with neuromuscular disorders. Neuromuscul Disord. 2007; 17(6): 459-69.

[40] Werneck LC, Bonilla E. Dystrophin in the differentiation between Duchenne and Becker muscular dystrophies: an immunihistochemical study compared with clinical stage, serum enzymes and muscle biopsy. Arq Neuropsiquiatr. 1990; 48(4): 454-64.

[41] Werneck LC. Correlation between functional disability, age and serum enzymes in neuromuscular diseases. Arq Neuropsiquiatr. 1995; 53: 60-8.

[42] Thong MK, Bazlin RI, Wong KT. Diagnosis and management of Duchenne muscular dystrophy in a developing country over a 10 year period. Dev Med Child Neurol. 2005; 47(7): 474-7.

[43] Chen JY, Clark MJ. Family function in families of children with Duchenne muscular dystrophy. Fam Community Health. 2007; 30(4): 296-304.

[44] Brunherotti MA, Sobreira C, Rodrigues-Junior AL, de Assis MR, Terra Filho J, Baddini Martinez JA. Correlations of Egen Klassification and Barthel Index scores with pulmonary function parameters in Duchenne muscular dystrophy. Heart Lung. 2007; 36(2): 132-9.

[45] De Cauwer H, Heytens L, Martin JJ. Report of the 89th ENMC international workshop: central core disease. Neuromusc Disord. 2002; 12: 588-95.

[46] Mercuri E, Talim B, Moghadaszadeh B, Petit N, Brockington M, Counsell S et al. Clinical and imaging findings in six cases of congenital muscular dystrophy with rigid spine syndrome linked to chromosome 1p (RSMD1). Neuromusc Disord. 2002b; 12: 631-8.

[47] Nucci A. Miopatia a corpos hialinos. Estudo clinico-laboratorial e de ressonância magnética [Tese - Livre Docência]. Campinas (SP): Universidade Estadual de Campinas; 2006.

[48] Clarke NF, Kidson W, Quijano-Roy S, Estournet B, Ferreiro A, Guicheney P et al. SEPN1: associated with congenital fiber-type disproportion and insulin resistance. Ann Neurol. 2006; 59:546-52.

[49] Mizuno Y, Komiya K. A serial muscle biopsy study in a case of congenital fiber-type disproportion associated with progressive respiratory failure. Brain Dev. 1990; 12(4): 431-6.

[50] Levy JA, Alegro MSC, Lusvarghi ES, Salum PNB, Tsanaclis AMC, Levy A. Desproporção congênita de fibras. Atrofia de fibras tipo 1. Arq Neuropsiquiatr. 1987; 45(2): 153-8.

[51] Jaffe M, Shapira J, Borochowitz Z. Familial congenital fiber type disproportion (CFTD) with an autosomal recessive inheritance. Clin Genet. 1988; 33: 33-7.

[52] Vestergaard H, Klein HH, Hansen T, Muller J, Skovby F, Bjorbaek C et al. Severe insulin-resistant diabetes mellitus in patients with congenital muscle fiber type disproportion myopathy. J Clin Invest. 1995; 95: 1925-32.

[53] Sharma MC, Ralte AM, Atri SK, Gulati S, Kalra V, Sarkar C. Congenital fiber type disproportion: A rare type of congenital myopathy: A report of four cases. Neurol India. 2004; 52(2): 254-6.

[54] Na SJ, Kim WK, Kim TS, Kang SW, Lee EY, Choi YC. Comparison of clinical characteristics between congenital fiber type disproportion myopathy and

congenital myopathy with type fiber predominance. Yonsei Med J. 2006; 47(4): 513-8.

[55] Linssen WHJP, Notermans NC, Van der Graaf Y, Wokke HJ, Van Doorn PA, Howeler CJ et al. Miyoshi - type distal muscular dystrophy. Clinical spectrum in 24 Dutch patients. Brain. 1997; 120: 1989-96.

[56] Mercuri E, Pichiecchio A, Counsell S, Allsop J, Cini C, Jungbluth H et al. A short protocol for muscle MRI in children with muscular dystrophies. Eur J Paediatr Neurol. 2002a; 6: 305-7.

[57] Hogrel JY, Ollivier G, Desnuelli C. Manual and quantitative muscle testing in neuromuscular disorders. How to assess the consistency of strength measurements in clinical trials? Rev Neurol. 2006; 162 (4): 427-36.

[58] Cup EH, Pieterse AJ, Brook Pastoor JM, Munneke M, Van Engelen BG, Hendricks HT et al. Exercise therapy and other types of physical therapy for patients with neuromuscular diseases: a systematic review. Arch Phys Med Rehabil. 2007; 88: 1452-64.

[59] Lindeman E, Leffers P, Reulen J, Spaans F, Drukker J. Quadriceps strength and timed motor performances in myotonic dystrophy Charcot-Marie-Tooth disease, and healthy subjects. Clin Rehabil. 1998; 12: 127-35.

[60] Whittaker RG, Ferenczi E, Hilton Jones D. Myotonic dystrophy: practical issues relating to assessment of strength. J Neurol Neurosurg Psychiatry. 2006: 77: 1282-3.

[61] Lindeman E, Leffers P, Spaans F, Drukker J, Reulen J. Deterioration of motor function in myotonic dystrophy and hereditary motor and sensory neuropathy. Scand J Rehabil Med. 1995a; 27(1): 59-64.

[62] Murakami N, Sakuta R, Takahashi E, Katada Y, Nagai T, Owada M et al. Early onset distal muscular dystrophy with normal dysferlin expression. Brain Dev. 2005; 27: 589-91.

[63] Lamont PJ, Udd B, Mastaglia FL, Visser M, Hedera P, Voit T et al. Laing early onset distal myopathy: slow myosin defect with variable abnormalities on muscle biopsy. J Neurol Neurosurg Psychiatry. 2006; 77: 208-15.

[64] Mathieu J, Boivin H, Richards CL. Quantitative motor assessment in myotonic dystrophy. Can J Neurol Sci. 2003; 30(2): 129-36.

[65] Lindeman E, Drukker J. Specificity of strength training in neuromuscular disorders. J Rehabil Sc. 1994; 7: 13-5.

[66] Lindeman E, Spaans F, Reulen J, Leffers P, Drukker J. Progressive resistance training in neuromuscular patients. Effects on force and surface EMG. J Electromyography Kinesiology. 1999; 9: 379-84.

[67] Hosking JP, Bhat US, Dubowitz V, Edwards RH. Measurements of muscle strength and performance in children with normal and diseased muscle. Arch Dis Child. 1976; 51(12): 957-63.

[68] Milner Brown HS, Miller RG. Muscle strengthening though high resistance weight training in patients with neuromuscular disorders. Arch Phys Med Rehabil. 1988; 69(1): 14-9.

[69] Lue YJ, Chen SS. Strength and functional performance of patients with limb girdle muscular dystrophy. Kaohsuing J Med Sci. 2000; 16(2): 83-90 (abstract).

[70] Kelm J, Ahlhelm F, Regitz T, Pace D, Schmitt E. Controlled dynamic weight training in patients with neuromuscular disorders. Fortschr Neurol Psychiatr. 2001; 69(8): 359-66.

[71] Van der Kooi EL, Lindeman E, Riphagen I. Strength training and aerobic exercise training for muscle disease. Cochrane Database Syst Rev. 2005; 25(1): CD 003907.

[72] Stubgen JP. Limb girdle muscular dystrophy: an interval study of weakness and functional impairment. J Clin Neuromuscul Dis. 2008; 9(3): 333-40.

[73] Shumway-Cook A, Woolacott MH. Reach, grasp and manipulation: changes across the life span. In: Shumway-Cook A, Woolacott MH. Motor control: theory and pratical applications. 2ed. London: Lippincott Williams & Wilkins; 2001. p. 471-96.

[74] McFadyen BJ, Winter DA. An integrated biomechanical analysis of normal stair ascent and descent. J Biomech. 1988; 21: 733-44.

[75] Kotake T, Dohi N, Kajiwara T, Sumi N, Koyama Y, Miura T. An analysis of sit to stand movements. Arch Phys Med Rehabil. 1993; 74: 1095-9.

[76] Lindeman E, Leffers P, Spaans F, Drukker J, Reulen J, Kerckhoffs M et al. Strength training in patients with myotonic dystrophy and hereditary motor and sensory neuropathy: a randomized clinical trial. Arch Phys Med Rehabil. 1995b; 76: 612-20.

[77] Hedberg B, Anvret M, Ansved T. CTG-repeat length in distal and proximal leg muscles of symptomatic and non-symptomatic patients with myotonic dystrophy: relation to muscle strength and degree of histopathological abnormalities. Eur J Neurol. 1999; 6: 341-6.

[78] Kierkegaard M, Tollback A. Reliability and feasibility of the six minute walk test in subjects with myotonic dystrophy. Neuromuscul Disord. 2007; 17: 943-9.

[79] Galassi G, Rowland LP, Hays AP, Hopkins LC, DiMauro S. High serum levels of creatinekinase: asymptomatic prelude to distal myopathy. Muscle Nerve. 1987; 10: 346-50.

[80] Aldelrag AS, Jonsson H, Ansved T. Effects of a hand training programme in five patients with myotonic dystrophy type I. Occup Ther Int. 2005; 12(1): 14-27.

[81] Dawes H, Korpershoek N, Freebody J, Elsworth C, Van Tintelen N, Wade DT et al. A pilot randomized controlled trial of a home based exercise programme aimed at improving endurance and function in adults with neuromuscular disorders. J Neurol Neurosurg Psychiatry. 2006; 77: 959-62.

[82] Ikeda ER, Schenkman ML, Riley PO, Hodge WA. Influence of age on dynamics of rising from a chair. Phys Ther. 1991; 71: 473-81.

[83] VanSant AF. Life span development in functional tasks. Phys Ther. 1990; 70: 788-9.

17

Strength and Functional Measurement for Patients with Muscular Dystrophy

Yen-Mou Lu[1] and Yi-Jing Lue[2,3,4]
[1]Department of Orthopedics, Kaohsiung Medical University Hospital,
[2]Department of Physical Therapy, College of Health Science,
[3]Department of Rehabilitation, Kaohsiung Medical University Hospital,
[4]Department and Graduate Institute of Neurology, School of Medicine, College of Medicine,
[1,2,3,4]Kaohsiung Medical University, Kaohsiung,
Taiwan

1. Introduction

Progressive muscle weakness is the major symptom of patients with muscular dystrophy.

The aims of the chapter are to introduce the strength decrease pattern and functional assessment, and to exam the advantages and disadvantages of these measurements applied to various types of muscular dystrophy. Three parts of the measurement for muscular dystrophy are included: the strength decrease pattern, the common general functional scales, and the disease specific scale.

This chapter places emphasis on patients with more weakness in proximal than distal parts. The most common type of proximal muscular dystrophy is Duchenne muscular dystrophy (DMD). Due to rapid deterioration, DMD can be seen as a severe form of muscular dystrophy. Other types of proximal muscular dystrophies have a slower rate of disease progression compared to DMD, such as Beck muscular dystrophy (BMD), limb girdle muscular dystrophy (LGMD), facioscapulohumeral muscular dystrophy (FSHD) and others.

2. Strength measurement

Muscle strength can be assessed by many methods, such as manual muscle testing (MMT) and using the quantitative methods by instrument. Common instruments include the handheld dynamometer (HHD), and the isokinetic dynamometry or other fixation instruments.

For MMT method, the Medical Research Council (MRC) Scale is the most often used system, with the procedures detecting the magnitude of strength by grading muscle strength from 0 to 5. The MRC scale is an ordinal scale, with grades 0-5 also named as "Zero, Trace, Poor, Fair, Good, and Normal". Grade 0 (Zero) cannot be palpated in muscle contraction. Grade 1 (Trace) has some evidence of slight muscle contraction but the strength is too weak to move the joint. Grade 2 (Poor) strength can move the joint (full range of motion) when gravity is eliminated during the test. The Poor grade is sub-graded as Poor minus (2-), Poor, and Poor plus (2+). The 2- indicates strength able to move the joint but unable to complete the range of motion. The 2+ indicates strength to complete the range of motion and also the ability to resist slight force made by the rater. Grade 3 (Fair) strength can be tested at the antigravity position. Similar to Poor grade, the Fair grade is sub-graded as Fair minus (3-: cannot complete the range of motion), Fair (3: can complete the range of motion), and Fair plus (3+: can against gravity with minimal resistance). Grade 4 (Good) completes the range of motion against gravity with moderate resistance, and Grade 5 (Normal) can resist with strong resistance. We recommend using the MMT method to measure the strength decrease pattern for patients with muscular dystrophy especially in clinical applications. The MMT grading system can clearly provide information as to whether patients can move their body in an antigravity position, and even if the strength is very weak, the strength can be discriminated by grade Poor, Trace or Zero. The weakness strength of patients with muscular dystrophy may be unable to be measured by some instrumentation, as most of these are designed to be measured in an antigravity position and the resistance is added during the measurement. The grading system is also graded (recorded) as different symbol methods. For example, the Kendall system ranked the grade from 0 to 10: it leaves the 0 as Zero, and 10 as Normal, and transforms the strength to a percentage, with a range from 0 to 100 %; the 100% being the grade of "Normal" strength. The percentages of Normal grade strength can be used for calculating the mean strength from many muscles. (Kendall et al., 1993)

For isokinetic dynamometer or other fixation methods in strength measurement, complicated procedures are often not practicable due to the expense and time required to prepare the instruments. Although inconvenient, isokinetic dynamometry has been considered to be the gold standard for assessing dynamic muscle strength and provides much information of various muscle performance characteristics (Mark et al., 2004). The isokinetic strength has been studied in patients with mild or moderate strength impairment (Kilmer et al., 1994; Tiffreau et al., 2007). The patient with DMD with severe progressive muscle weakness highlights the method's limitations for assessment of very weak strength (Bäckman, 1988).

For HHD, it is a convenient, portable and inexpensive device for assessing isometric strength in a clinical setting. The rater handholds the device and presses it against the force that subjects exert with maximal effort. The make test and break test are two methods for HHD. In the make test, the rater resists the patient's maximal isometric contraction, whereas in the break test the rater overcomes the force of the patient produced in eccentric contraction (Bohannon, 1988; Stratford & Balsor, 1994). Both methods have their advantage and disadvantages. To measure the weakness strength of patients with muscular dystrophy, we suggest using the make method. The HHD has been studied in DMD; the strength measured by a force transducer and the data presented in Newtons or kilograms has been seen as real compared to the MMT method where the strength record is in ratio-level parametric data (Scott & Mawson, 2006; Brussock et al., 1992; Stuberg & Metcalf, 1988) However, the main disadvantage of the HHD is the unsure reliability of some muscle strength on the tester when stabilizing the dynamometer (Bohannon, 1999).

3. Strength decrease pattern of various types of muscular dystrophy

3.1 Methods of strength measurement

We previously measured the strength decrease pattern of some common types of muscular dystrophy, such as Duchenne muscular dystrophy (DMD), limb girdle muscular dystrophy

(LGMD) and facioscapulohumeral muscular dystrophy (FSHD) (Lue et al., 1992; Lue & Chen, 2000a; Lue & Chen, 2000b). Patients had been diagnosis by two qualified neurologists and followed up for at least two years. Before the strength measurement, they did not receive medication or a strengthening program for improving muscle strength.

The manual muscle test was used by well trained physical therapists. Thirty-two muscle groups were examined on both sides; the muscle groups included neck and trunk muscles, and upper and lower extremities. The neck and trunk muscles included neck flexors/extensor and the trunk flexors/extensors. In the upper extremities, the shoulder (flexors, extensors, and abductors), elbow (flexors and extensors) and wrist (flexors and extensors) muscle strength were measured. In the lower extremities, the hip (flexors, extensors, and abductors), knee (flexors and extensors) and ankle (dorsi- and plantar-flexors) muscle strength were measured. To calculate the mean strength, we used Kendall's percentage method (Kendall et al., 1993).

3.2 Natural strength decrease pattern of patients with DMD

DMD is a quick deterioration muscular dystrophy, with the strength decrease in a linear pattern positively correlated with age. For every year increment in age, the average strength decreases by about 3.9 percent of normal strength. About half of normal strength will be retained at the age of 12 years. The lower extremities are weaker than the upper extremities. The proximal parts are weaker than distal parts; the weakness of the elbow and wrist extensors is more dominant than that of the flexors. In the lower extremities, hip and knee extensors are weaker than hip and knee flexors. If the strengths of agonist and antagonist muscles of a joint are significantly different, the part of the stronger side becomes shorter and joint contracture easily develops. Therefore, in the upper extremities, elbow and wrist flexion contracture is easily found. Routine active or passive range of motion exercise for patients to maintain the full range of motion is a very important part of any rehabilitation program. Similar to the upper extremities, in the lower extremities, hip flexor contracture is commonly found in early stages of DMD; after the patients are unable to walk, the knee joints may develop severe flexion contracture as the joints are not routinely performing the (normal) range of motion exercises. At the end of life of a patient with DMD, the strength of finger flexors can manage some activities, even though at the age of twenty. Therefore, we recommend using computer games as finger exercises or a leisure activity for patients with DMD, and the keyboard may or may not need modification.

3.3 Natural strength decrease pattern of patients with LGMD

LGMD is also named limb girdle muscular dystrophy syndrome, which is combined with various types of limb girdle muscular dystrophy. Therefore, the strength decrease pattern has greater variation than other types of muscular dystrophy. The speed of muscle strength decrease will become slower than the onset after long disease duration. The strength decrease patterns do not fit well in a linear regression model (R^2 only 0.074), and fit better in an inverse regression model (R^2 equal to 0.154), with the equation as follows: mean muscle strength = 0.61+(0.63/disease duration). No significantly stronger strength in flexor than extensor muscles for extremities are found in patients with LGMD. The limitation of this study needs to be mentioned, as these patients with LGMD may or may not have only one type of LGMD. For more precise study in the future, the gene deficit should be confirmed and including the same type of LGMD for strength study is essential.

3.4 Natural strength decrease pattern of patients with FSHD

Comparing the severity of the strength decrease, the strength decrease of patients with FSHD is the mildest compared to the strength decrease of patients with LGMD or DMD. The shoulder muscle strength is the weakest, followed by elbow muscle strength. The strengths of the trunk area and lower extremities are the best. A special pattern of the strength asymmetry is found in patients with FSHD, as the average right side muscle strength is weaker than the left side. Most of the subjects included in this study were right-handed. The dominant side may increase the use and lead to more prominence of strength decrease, therefore, in clinical applications for patients with FSHMD, too many strengthening programs or overload activity for the upper extremities may not suit such patients. The mechanism for asymmetry of strength found in patients with FSHD still requires further studies to be elucidated.

4. Functional measurements

4.1 The brooke and vignos scales

The common functional scales to rate the grade of disease severity are the Brooke Scale and the Vignos Scale. Both scales were firstly designed for DMD, and nowadays have been used in many neuromuscular diseases. The Brooke scale was designed to assess the upper extremity function. The grades of the Brooke scale range from 1 to 6; 1 means that the subject can elevate their arms full range to the head with the arms straight; while 2 means that the shoulder strength is insufficient to elevate their arms and the subject needs to flex the elbow to elevate the arms; in grades 3 and 4, the subject is unable to elevate the shoulders but can raise hands to the mouth with or without weight respectively; grade 5 refers to the subject being unable to raise hands to the mouth and only some hand movement exists, while grade 6 refers to no useful function of hands (Table 1).

Grade	Description
1	Starting with arms at the sides, the patient can abduct the arms in a full circle until they touch above the head
2	Can raise arms above head only by flexing the elbow (shortening the circumference of the movement) or using accessory muscles
3	Cannot raise hands above head, but can raise an 8-oz glass of water to the mouth
4	Can raise hands to the mouth, but cannot raise an 8-oz glass of water to the mouth
5	Cannot raise hands to the mouth, but can use hands to hold a pen or pick up pennies from the table
6	Cannot raise hands to the mouth and has no useful function of hands

Table 1. Grading system for the Brooke scale.

The Vignos scale was designed to assess the lower extremity function. The grades of the Vignos scale range from 1 to 10; 1 means that the subject can walk and climb stairs without assistance; 2 and 3 means that the strength is insufficient to walk upstairs without assistance as they need to use a rail for climbing stairs (grade 2: in a normal speed; grade 3: slowly);

grades 4 and 5 refer to subjects still having the ability to walk unassisted but unable to climb stairs (grade 4 also can rise from a chair but grade 5 cannot); grades 6 to 8 refer to patients using the long leg brace for walking or standing (grade 6: walk without assistance; grade 7: walk with assistance for balance; grade 8: cannot walk, only for standing); grade 9 refers to the subject being unable to stand, but can sit in a wheelchair; and the final grade 10 refers to the subject being confined to a bed (Table 2).

Grade	Description
1	Walks and climbs stairs without assistance
2	Walks and climbs stair with aid of railing
3	Walks and climbs stairs slowly with aid of railing (over 25 seconds for eight standard steps)
4	Walks unassisted and rises from chair but cannot climb stairs
5	Walks unassisted but cannot rise from chair or climb stairs
6	Walks only with assistance or walks independently with long leg braces
7	Walks in long leg braces but requires assistance for balance
8	Stands in long leg braces but unable to walk even with assistance
9	Is in a wheelchair
10	Is confined to a bed

Table 2. Grading system for the Vignos scale.

4.2 Timed tests

Some studies also record the time needed for some activities as a functional testing for patients with muscular dystrophy. The raters measure the time need for a person to complete the activity. The example of these common activities are climbing some steps of stairs, walking a fixed distance, sitting to standing from a chair, rising from the floor, dressing a cloth and cutting a square.

5. Advantages and disadvantage of the common functional scales of various types of muscular dystrophy

The Brooke and Vignos scales are easy to rate the severity of the patients, but the study found some disadvantages (Lue et al., 2009). We assessed the acceptability of the Brooke and Vignos scales in patients with DMD, BMD, FSHMD, and LGMD from a multi-center study. The patients with DMD were classified as severely progressive group, while the others (BMD, FSHD, and LGMD) were classified as slowly progressive group.

The results showed that the Brooke and Vignos scales were easy to assess, and it took a little time to complete the tests, and the patients did not feel uncomfortable. The Brooke scale is acceptable to grade arm function of the severely progressive group; the DMD, each grade of the Brooke scale is distributed with the acceptable percentage (ranging from 7.1% to 33.3%). However, it is insufficient to discriminate differing levels of severity of the slowly progressive group (BMD, FSHMD, and LGMD). No subject was graded at 4, and only one was graded at 6. The floor effect was large in all types of the slowly progressive group (ranging from 20.0% to 61.9%), especially high in BMD.

In the Vignos scale, using the long leg brace to grade the lower limb function may be a major problem for this scale. Grades 6 to 8 are items using long leg braces for walking or standing; these grades are inapplicable, because some cases did not use long leg braces for walking or standing. The floor effect of the Vignos scale was also large in BMD (23.8%) and in FSHD (50.0%). Among the slowly progressive muscular dystrophies, the function of patients with FSHD was the best; they had better leg function and were less influenced in their daily living activities than other types of slowly progressive muscular dystrophy. Using the two scales in combination with other measures (or instead, to use a complicated instrument for various types of muscular dystrophy) to calculate their function is suggested.

6. The muscular dystrophy functional rating scale

The Muscular Dystrophy Functional Rating Scale (MDFRS) is a disease specific scale designed for various muscular dystrophies. The MDFRS was developed by Lue et al. in 2006. Four domains are included in MDFRS. It was developed in many stages: the preliminary pool of items, the admission of various types of muscular dystrophies and the reliability, validity and responsiveness studies (Lue et al. 2006). The results showed the MDFRS is a reliable and valid disease-specific measure of functional status for patients with muscular dystrophy. The internal consistency was excellent, with the value of the Cronbach' alpha ranging from 0.84 to 0.97. The test-retest reliability and the inter-rater reliability were high (ICC=0.99) for all domains. The MDFRS demonstrated moderate to high correlation with a range of functional rating scales. The confirmatory factor analysis supported a four-dimensional construct. The floor and ceiling effects were small and the responsiveness of various types of muscular dystrophies was well.

The MDFRS combines four domains to rate mobility, basic activities of daily living, arm function and impairment. The number of items of each domain is 9, 6, 7 and 11 respectively (Table 3). The scale offers much important information of muscular dystrophy such as the mobility ability, dependence of daily living, the arm function, and many impairment conditions. The arm function part of the MDFRS effectively conquers the disadvantages of the Brooke scale (Lue et al. 2006; Lue 2010).

Each item of MDFRS is scored on a 4-point scale (1-4), with 1 representing being unable to do the activity and is completely dependent; 2 needing assistance from another person, 3 is independent, without assistance from another person but movement or completion of an activity is slow, and 4 means no problem for the activity and can be done at normal speed. The impairment domain includes the items for measuring contractures and scoliosis, strengths, and respiratory function, and the scoring system was specially designed by the characteristics of the items.

In the mobility domain, the 9 items included measuring the ability of stair climbing, outdoor mobility, indoor mobility, transfers from bed to chair, wheelchair manipulation, standing from sitting, sitting from lying, rolling and changing body position in bed. The items of stair climbing, outdoor and indoor mobility can effectively rate the function of the initial stage of the disease, and the ability of the sitting from lying, rolling and changing body position in bed is needed to examine the condition of the patients with terminal stages of the disease, such as the patients with DMD.

Domains							
Mobility domain		Basic ADL domain		Arm function domain		Impairment domain	
1	Stair climbing	1	Feeding	1	Managing objects over head	1	Severity of upper limb joint contracture
2	Outdoor mobility	2	Combing hair	2	Carrying objects	2	Severity of lower limb joint contractures
3	Indoor mobility	3	Brushing teeth	3	Cleaning table	3	Number of contracted joints in the upper limbs
4	Transfers from bed to chair	4	Dressing upper/lower parts of body	4	Writing	4	Number of contracted joints in the lower limbs
5	Wheelchair manipulation	5	Toileting	5	Turning books	5	Severity of neck contracture
6	Standing from sitting	6	Bathing	6	Picking up small objects	6	Strength of the neck
7	Sitting from lying			7	Managing objects over head	7	Strength of the trunk
8	Rolling					8	Scoliosis
9	Changing body position in bed					9	Orthopnea
						10	Sputum clearance
						11	Ventilator assisted

Table 3. Domains and Items of the Muscular Dystrophy Functional Rating Scale.

In the basic activity daily living domain, the 6 items included measuring the ability of feeding, combing hair, brushing teeth, dressing upper/lower parts of body, toileting and bathing. The bathing activity is the most difficult item, and the feeding and combing hair items are easy activities for patients with muscular dystrophy.

In the arm function domain, the 7 items included measuring the ability of managing objects overhead, carrying objects, clearing a table, writing, turning books, picking up small objects, and manipulating small objects. The items were designed to be more functional as needed for daily routine activities. The ability of managing objects over the head and carrying objects is useful to assess the better upper extremity function for patients with muscular dystrophy.

The part of impairment section of the MDFRS offers simple measurement methods for measuring the condition of the contracture and scoliosis, weakness of the head and trunk muscles to provide head control and sitting balance, and the condition of the pulmonary function. In the impairment domain, the 11 items included measuring the problem of severity of upper and lower limb joint contracture, the number of contracted joints in the upper and lower limbs, the severity of neck contracture, strength of the neck, strength of the trunk, severity of the scoliosis, and three respiratory problems such as orthopnea, sputum clearance ability, and the need to use a ventilator. These impairment items are all important symptoms and signs of the various types of muscular dystrophy, and decreasing the complication of contracture is the most important issue for management of such patients. At the end stage of the disease, vital respiratory care needs to be added, and the 3 items of impairment domain of the MDFRS could offer the general condition of the pulmonary function. Therefore, the assessment from the impairment domain could offer a lot of useful information for clinicians and caregivers to easily know the condition of the patients and provide better care for them at different stages of the disease.

The total scores of each domain sum up the scores of each item, therefore, the range of scores for 4 domains are 9-36 for the mobility domain, 6-24 for the basic activity of daily living domain, 7-28 for the arm domain, and 11-44 for the impairment domain respectively. The scores of each domain can be calculated as a percentage to represent the functional performance of a person compared to normal condition; the equation is as follows: (total scores-number of item) / full total scores and multiple 100. The % of mobility ability = (the sum of score from 9 item -9) / 36 *100; the % of basic activity of daily living ability = (the sum of score from 6 item -6) / 24 *100; the % of arm function ability = (the sum of score from 7 item -7) / 28 *100; and the % of impairment condition = (the sum of score from 11 item -11) / 44 *100.

7. Conclusion

In conclusion, various types of muscular dystrophy present differing speeds of disease progression with decreasing muscular strength in different patterns. Due to some disadvantages of the Brooke and Vignos grading scales applied to patients with muscular dystrophy, clinical application of these scales should be used with caution, especially in patients with slowly progressive muscular dystrophy. We suggest that the applications can be used in combination with MDFRS, which is a multi-domain instrument, a valid and reliable scale, capable of evaluating the various levels of functional status of different types of muscular dystrophy.

8. References

Bäckman, E. (1988). Methods for measurement of muscle function. Methodological aspects, reference values for children, and clinical applications. *Scand J Rehabil Med* Sppl 20:9-95.

Bohannon, R. (1988). Make tests and break tests of elbow flexor muscle strength. *Phys Ther* 68(2): 193–194.

Bohannon, R. (1999). Inter-tester reliability of hand-held dynamometry: a concise summary of published research. *Percept Mot Skills* 88(3): 899-902.

Brussock, C., Haley, S., & Munsat, T. (1992). Measurement of isometric force in children with and without Duchenne's muscular dystrophy. *Phys Ther* 72(2): 105-114.

Kendall, F., McCreary, E., & Provance, P. (1993). Muscles testing and function. 4th ed. Williams & Wilkins, Baltimore.

Kilmer, D., McCrory M., & Wright N. (1994) The effect of a high resistance exercise program in slowly progressive neuromuscular disease. *Arch Phys Med Rehabil* 75 (5): 560-563.

Lue, Y., Jong, Y. & Lin, Y. (1992). The strength and functional performance of patients with Duchenne muscular dystrophy based on natural history. *Kaohsiung J Med Sci* 8(11): 597-604.

Lue, Y., & Chen, S. (2000a). Strength and functional performance of patients with limb-girdle muscular dystrophy. *Kaohsiung J Med Sci* 16(2): 83-90.

Lue, Y., & Chen, S. (2000b). The strength and functional performance of patients with Facioscapulohumeral muscular dystrophy. Kaohsiung J Med Sci 16(5): 248-254.

Lue, Y., Su, C. & Yang, R. (2006). Development and validation of a muscular dystrophy-specific functional rating scale. *Clin Rehab* 20 (9): 804-817.

Lue, Y., Lin, R., & Chen, S. (2009) Measurement of the functional status of patients with different types of muscular dystrophy. *Kaohsiung J Med Sci* 25(6): 325-333.

Lue, Y. (2010). Muscular Dystrophy Functional Rating Scale (MDFRS) In: Registry of Outcome Measures. URL: http://www.researchrom.com/masterlist/view/199. Accessed 2011.7.20.

Mark, B., Martine, A., & Neil, A. (2003). Assessment and interpretation of isokinetic muscle strength during growth and maturation. *Sports Medicine* 33(10): 727-743.

Scott, E., & Mawson, S. (2006). Measurement in Duchenne muscular dystrophy: consideration in the development of a neuromuscular assessment tool. *Dev Med Child Neurol* 48(6): 540-544.

Stratford, P., & Balsor, B. (1994). A comparison of make and break tests using a hand-held dynamometer and the Kin-Com. *J Orthop Sports Phys* 19(1): 28–32.

Stuberg, W., & Metcalf, W. (1988). Reliability of quantitative muscle testing in healthy children and in children with Duchenne muscular dystrophy using a hand-held dynamometer. *Phys Ther* 68(6): 977-982.

Tiffreau, V., Ledoux, I., & Eymard. B. (2007). Isokinetic muscle testing for weak patients suffering from neuromuscular disorders: a reliability study. *Neuromuscul Disord* 17(7):524-531.

Section 4

Therapy

18

Muscle Satellite Cells and Duchenne Muscular Dystrophy

Yuko Miyagoe-Suzuki[1], So-ichiro Fukada[2] and Shin'ichi Takeda[1]
[1]*Department of Molecular Therapy, National Institute of Neuroscience, National Center of Neurology and Psychiatry,*
[2]*Department of Immunology, Graduate School of Pharmaceutical Sciences, Osaka University,*
Japan

1. Introduction

Muscle satellite cells are tissue-specific stem cells in skeletal muscle that play central roles in postnatal muscle growth and regeneration, and therefore are a potential source for cell therapy for Duchenne muscular dystrophy (DMD). However, to date, transplantation of satellite cells-derived myoblasts in human has not been successful. To overcome the limitations of transplantation of myoblasts, we need to better understand the molecular and cellular regulation of satellite cells. In this chapter, we summarize recent advances in satellite cell biology and its role in muscular dystrophies. Then we discuss the roles of the muscle tissue microenvironments in muscle regeneration and muscular dystrophies. Recent results emphasize that mutual interactions among myogenic cells, inflammatory cells, and interstitial mesenchymal cells are important for successful muscle regeneration. The latter two are versatile regulators of muscle regeneration. They promote muscle regeneration in healthy muscle, but when muscle fibers fail to regenerate, they promote fibrosis and fatty degeneration to ensure the continuity of the tissue. In the last part of this chapter, we discuss strategies to generate new muscle stem cells from fibroblasts by transcription factor-mediated reprogramming.

2. Muscle satellite cells

Satellite cells are skeletal muscle-specific stem cells located between the muscle basal lamina and myofibers in a quiescent and undifferentiated state (G0). Satellite cells were first identified by electron microscopy by Mauro in 1961 (Mauro 1961). Ultrastructural data suggests that 2-6% of all nuclei in humans are satellite cells (Schmalbruch & Hellhammer 1976). Satellite cells originate from somites or cranial mesoderm and differentiate into Pax3+Pax7+ muscle progenitor cells, and then take the position of satellite cells (Gros et al 2005; Kassar-Duchossoy et al 2005; Relaix et al 2005). A recent paper, however, demonstrated that all satellite cells (MyoD-negative) originate from MyoD-positive progenitors (Kanisicak et al 2009), suggesting that satellite cells are derived from committed myogenic progenitor cells.

During postnatal development, satellite cells divide to provide new myonuclei to growing muscle fibers (Moss & Leblond 1971), and then enter to an undifferentiated quiescent state in adult skeletal muscle (Schultz et al 1978). In mice, vigorous muscle growth due to satellite cell division is observed until three weeks after birth (White et al 2010). During this period, the number of satellite cells decreases, and then it becomes constant for a long time to maintain skeletal muscle homeostasis.

Skeletal muscle regeneration also depends absolutely on satellite cells. When muscle is injured, satellite cells are activated, proliferate, and differentiate into myofibers, and a minor subset self-renew (**Figure 1**). Their dysfunction is responsible for the loss of muscle mass in muscular dystrophies or during aging. Although many studies indicate that stem cells, which are distinct from satellite cells, contribute to the production of myofibers (Ferrari et al 1998; Fukada et al 2002; Gussoni et al 1999; LaBarge & Blau 2002), there is no doubt that satellite cells are the physiological stem cells for skeletal muscle regeneration.

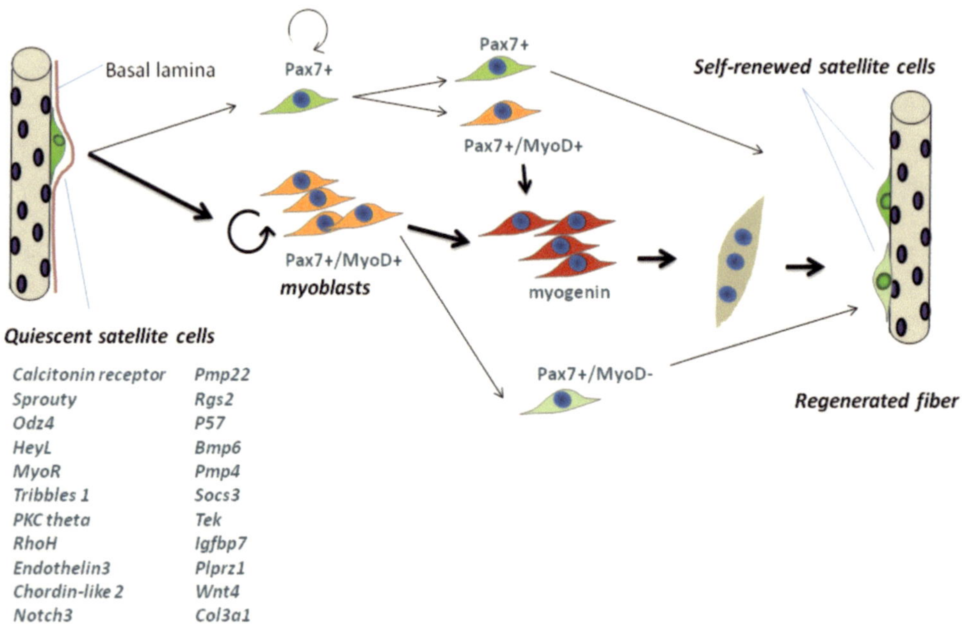

Satellite cells are in a quiescent state in uninjured adult muscle. On injury, satellite cells are activated by mitotic stimuli, vigorously proliferate to reach sufficient cell numbers, and differentiate into myofibers or fuse with pre-existing injured myofibers. A sub-set of cycling satellite cells remains uncommitted by asymmetric division and return to quiescence (Kuang et al 2007). Or a subfraction of MyoD-positive cycling satellite cells withdraw from the cell cycle and returns to the satellite cell niche (Kanisicak et al 2009). Genes up-regulated in quiescent satellite cells are shown as possible regulators of quiescence (Fukada et al 2007).

Fig. 1. Activation, proliferation, differentiation, and self-renewal of satellite cells

2.1 Research tools

Markers: Satellite cells were originally identified by electronic microscopy as mononuclear cells attached to myofibers, but the discovery of M-cadherin expression on satellite cells has made it easier to identify them by light microscopy (Irintchev et al 1994). Pax7 is a marker of satellite cells and is also critical for satellite cell biogenesis, survival and potentially self-renewal (Seale et al 2000). Thanks to an anti-Pax7 monoclonal antibody, which identifies avian, rodent, and human satellite cells (Kawakami et al 1997), Pax7 has become the most widely used marker of satellite cells. Other markers (including c-met, syndecan 3 and 4, SM/C-2.6, integrin-α7, calcitonin receptor, CD34, and CXCR4) have also been established to identify satellite cells by microscopy and flow cytometry (summarized in (Boldrin et al 2010)).

Isolation: Flow cytometric and cell sorting techniques have greatly advanced stem cell studies. Fukada et al. first reported the direct isolation of satellite cells from mouse muscle using their newly developed rat monoclonal antibody, named SM/C-2.6 (Fukada et al 2004). Since then, several groups have reported the purification of satellite cells using CD34, syndecan 4, integrin-α7 or CXCR4 (Boldrin et al 2010; Conboy et al 2010; Fukada et al 2004; Fukada et al 2007; Montarras et al 2005; Sherwood et al 2004; Tanaka et al 2009). A single-fiber culture technique is also widely used for analysis of satellite cells (Rosenblatt et al 1995). In mouse extensor digitorum longus (EDL) muscle, approximately five satellite cells attach to one myofiber, and on isolation of fibers, they are spontaneously activated and migrate from their own myofiber. It is considered that single-fiber culture maintains the satellite cell 'niche' in *in vitro* condition (Collins et al 2005).

Genetic manipulation: Cre-loxP-mediated conditional inactivation of the genes makes it easy to determine the roles of regulatory molecules in a cell of a specific lineage at a specific developmental stage. The Cre-loxP-mediated lineage-tracing system is a powerful method to determine the origins and fates of muscle progenitor cells. These newly established research tools have accelerated research in satellite cell biology. In contrast to the mouse, however, a limited number of markers are available for *in situ* detection of satellite cells in human muscle, and human satellite cells are still isolated by the classical technique.

2.2 Activation, proliferation, differentiation, and self-renewal of satellite cells

Molecular regulators of the activation, proliferation, differentiation, and self-renewal of muscle satellite cells, including paired-box transcription factor Pax7, MyoD families, Six families, epigenetic regulators, or microRNAs, and numerous extracellular components are currently being elucidated (Abou-Khalil et al 2009; Buckingham & Relaix 2007; Chen et al 2010; Crist et al 2009; Dey et al 2011; Dhawan & Rando 2005; Juan et al 2011; Kuang et al 2008; Kuang & Rudnicki 2008; Palacios et al 2010; Yajima et al 2010). Although these molecules are studied mainly on mouse models, similar molecules are believed to regulate human satellite cells.

Self-renewal of satellite cells with stem cell properties is an important process to maintain the stem cell pool throughout life and is one of the main subjects of recent muscle biology research, but it is largely unknown when and how satellite cells self-renew during the regeneration process. Asymmetrical division is proposed to be among the mechanisms by which satellite cells give rise to both stem cells and precursor cells (Conboy & Rando 2002; Conboy et al 2007; Kuang et al 2008; Kuang et al 2007; Shinin et al 2006). It is also possible that some of the activated/proliferating MyoD-positive satellite cells return to the 'niche' of the satellite cells in a stochastic manner. Using $MyoD^{iCre}$ knockin mice and R26R-EYFP or R26R-βgal reporter mice, Kanisicak et al. reported that 99% of satellite cells in limb and body wall muscles originate from MyoD+ progenitors. Their findings suggest that committed MyoD+ myoblasts can return to a dormant state by suppressing MyoD and up-regulating Pax7 (Kanisicak et al 2009). This finding supports the stochastic model and explains well the heterogeneity in myogenic potential within a satellite cell population. Satellite cell activity is impaired in DMD, and how dystrophic environments perturb self-renewal of satellite cells remains to be determined.

Satellite cell behavior is thought to be mainly regulated by the environment. Satellite cells/myoblasts stop dividing just after the size of the regenerated fibers becomes comparable to that of the uninjured muscle and differentiate into myofibers or begin to return to quiescence (Fukada et al 2007; Shea et al 2010). The molecules that signal between the microenvironment and satellite cells are currently being elucidated. Interestingly, Ang1/Tie-2 signaling is such a candidate to regulate self-renewal of satellite cells by controlling the return to quiescence of a subset of them (Abou-Khalil et al 2009).

2.3 Quiescence of satellite cells

Satellite cells are quiescent in uninjured adult muscle. Maintenance of quiescence is important because disruption of cellular quiescence of stem cells leads to a loss of the stem cell pool and impairs tissue repair, but the molecular regulations of satellite cell dormancy are just beginning to be elucidated.

Pax7: Pax7 is highly expressed in quiescent satellite cells and over-expressed Pax7 promote a return to quiescence through repression of MyoD and myogenin (Olguin & Olwin 2004; Olguin et al 2007). Therefore, Pax7 is thought to be central to the maintenance of quiescence. A recent study using a conditional gene inactivation system in mice showed that when Pax7 is inactivated in adult mice, mutant satellite cells can proliferate and reoccupy the sublaminal niche (Lepper et al 2009). Lepper et al. further showed that Pax7 is required in juveniles up to the point when progenitor cells make the transition to quiescence (Lepper et al 2009).

Calcitonin/calcitonin receptor: Fukada et al. performed genome-wide gene expression analysis of quiescent satellite cells freshly isolated from mouse muscle, and reported the molecular signature of quiescent satellite cells (Fukada et al 2007). The authors newly identified genes that are expressed specifically in quiescent satellite cells but down-regulated on activation (including *calcitonin receptor(CTR), Odz4, HeyL/Hesr3, MyoR, tribbles1, PKC theta, Rho H, endothelin 3*)(**Figure 1**), and demonstrated that calcitonin/calcitonin receptor signaling is involved in the maintenance of quiescence of satellite cells (Fukada et al 2007).

Notch: Notch signaling plays a critical role in maintenance of quiescent satellite cells. The *hesr* (*hes-related,* also known as *hey/herp/hrt/gridlock/chf*) families of bHLH transcriptional repressor genes are the primary target of Notch signaling. Fukada at al. demonstrated that genetic ablation of both *Hesr1* and *Hesr3* genes results in a loss of the satellite cell pool and impairs muscle regeneration (Fukada et al., 2011). Intriguingly, satellite cells lacking both *Hesr1* and *Hesr3* expression ectopically express a proliferation marker, MyoD, and a differentiation marker, myogenin.

Sprouty1 (Spry1): Sprouty1 (Spry1) is a candidate molecule involved in the maintenance of satellite cells. In contrast to Pax7 and Hesr1/Hesr3, however, Sprouty1 is not required for maintenance of the satellite cell pool in uninjured muscle, but it is indispensable for the return to quiescence of the self-renewing satellite cells during repair (Abou-Khalil & Brack 2010; Shea et al 2010). Sprouty1 is a negative regulator of receptor tyrosine kinase (RTK) signaling, which suggests that Sprouty1 plays a role in sensing growth factors within the muscle and regulating satellite cell quiescence during muscle regeneration.

Signals from myofibers seem most important to induce cycling satellite cells to return to the quiescent state and maintain them in the niche, because CTR-positive or Sprouty1-positive satellite cells reappear only at a late stage of regeneration (Fukada et al 2007; Shea et al 2010). Interaction between myofibers and satellite cells through cadherins would be required for the maintenance of the quiescent state of satellite cells. Although M-cadherin-null mice did not show any abnormality in skeletal growth and regeneration, the other cadherin families are thought to compensate for the lack of M-cadherin-deficiency (Hollnagel et al 2002).

2.4 Regulation of satellite cells by non-myogenic cells

Mesenchymal cells in skeletal muscle regulate muscle satellite cells. We previously reported a novel side population subset: CD31(-)CD45(-) SP cells (Uezumi et al 2006). They are resident in skeletal muscle and are activated and vigorously proliferate during muscle regeneration. RT-PCR analysis suggested that CD31(-)CD45(-) SP cells are of mesenchymal lineage, and differentiate into adipocytes, osteogenic cells, and muscle cells after specific induction *in vitro* (Uezumi et al 2006). Motohashi et al. further showed by co-transplantation experiments that CD31(-)CD45(-) SP cells promote proliferation and migration of grafted myoblasts (Motohashi et al 2008). They also showed that CD31(-)CD45(-) SP cells produce a variety of cytokines, cytokine receptors, extra-cellular matrix proteins, matrix met al oproteinase families, and other wound healing-related molecules (Motohashi et al 2008). More recently, Joe et al. identified bipotent fibro/adipogenic progenitor cells (FAPs) in muscle. FAPs are CD31(-)CD45(-)α7integrin(-) CD34(-)Sca1(+), and promote differentiation of satellite cells (Joe et al 2010). Although we speculate that CD31(-)CD45(-) SP cells overlap with FAPs, the relationship between them remains to be determined. Interestingly, these studies suggest that mesenchymal progenitor cells themselves are also regulated by the muscle environment.

Macrophages are also versatile regulators of muscle regeneration, exhibiting opposing activities (pro- and anti-inflammatory effects) (Arnold et al 2007; Mann et al 2011; Segawa et al 2008; Tidball & Villalta 2010; Vidal et al 2008; Villalta et al 2009). Possible interaction among macrophages, mesenchymal progenitor cells, and myogenic cells are summarized in **Figure 2.**

3. Satellite cells and Duchenne muscular dystrophy

Duchenne muscular dystrophy is caused by the absence of dystrophin and characterized by progressive muscle weakness and chronic cycles of degeneration and regeneration of skeletal muscle. Satellite cells and their progeny, myoblasts are thought to gradually lose their proliferative and differentiative capacity, and be eventually exhausted in Duchenne muscular dystrophy, due to repeated activation and proliferation and limited self-renewal capacity (Blau et al 1983; Blau et al 1985; Heslop et al 2000). As a result, muscle regeneration

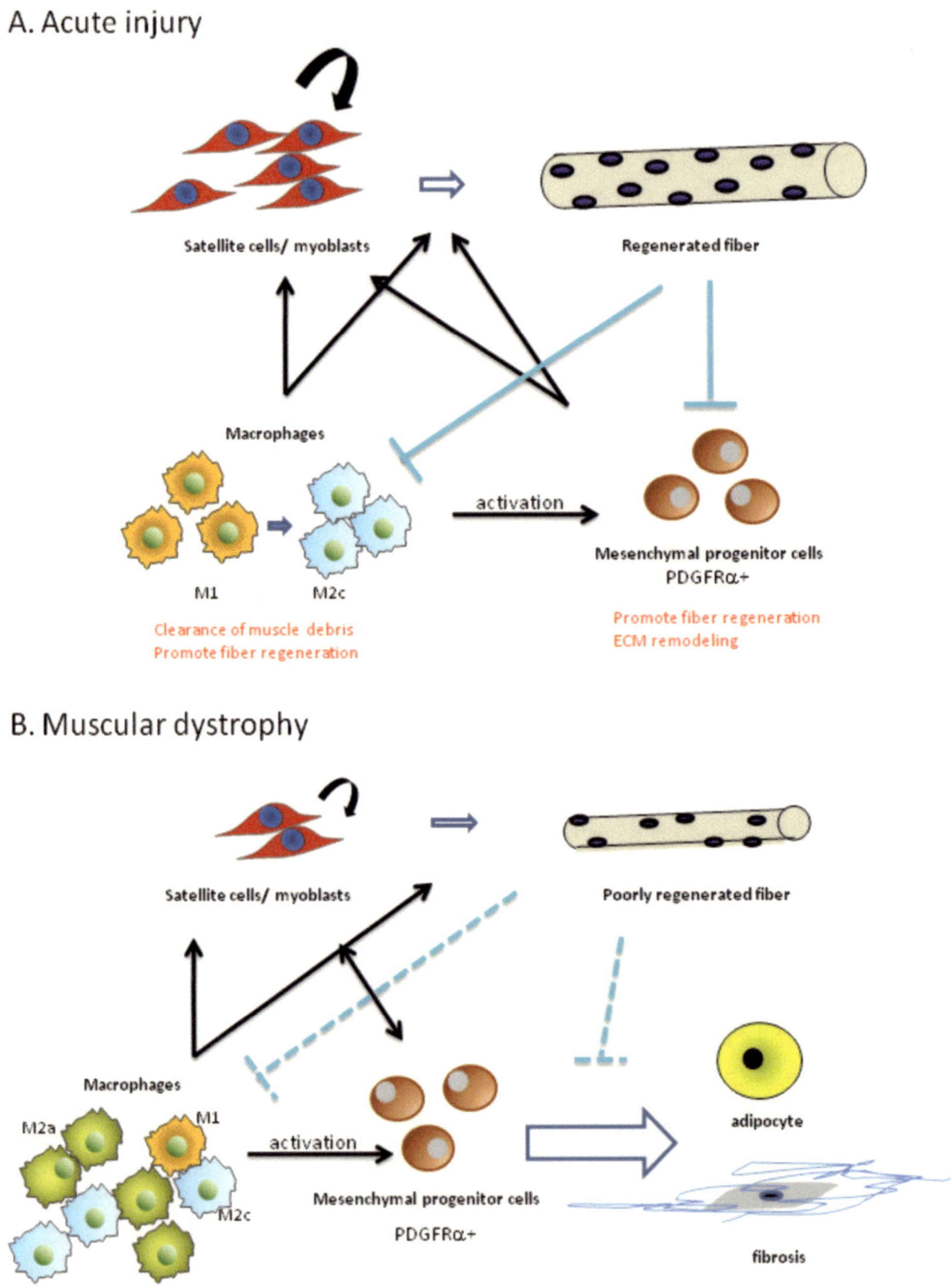

A. In acute muscle injury, resident and infiltrating macrophages first secret pro-inflammatory cytokines, express iNOS, and clear dead fibers by phagocytosis (M1), then release anti-inflammatory cytokines and stimulate myogenesis and fiber growth (M2c: anti-inflammatory macrophages) (Mann et al 2011; Tidball & Villalta 2010). Mesenchymal progenitor cells are rapidly activated, extensively proliferate, and promote proliferation, migration, and differentiation of satellite cells, but almost completely vanish at the completion of myofiber regeneration. M2 macrophages produce pro-fibrotic molecules such as TGF-β and stimulate mesenchymal cells to produce ECM components and ECM-remodeling factors. Successfully regenerated muscle fibers, in turn, seem to calm activated macrophages and mesenchymal cells down.

B. In dystrophic muscle, macrophages continue to release pro-inflammatory cytokines. M2a (alternatively activated) macrophages, which are usually associated with tissue repair, wound-healing and fibrosis, are reported to be abundant in fibrotic muscle of mdx mice, and proposed to be involved in fibrosis development (Vidal et al 2008; Villalta et al 2009). In prolonged inflammation, mesenchymal progenitors differentiate into adipocytes and fibroblastic cells, and promote fatty infiltration and fibrosis. A recent study suggests that regenerated muscle fibers directly inhibit this phenotypic conversion.

Fig. 2. Mutual regulations among macrophages, mesenchymal progenitor cells, and satellite cells in muscle regeneration (model)

is impaired in the advanced state of the disease, and muscle tissue is gradually replaced by adipose and fibrotic tissues. At this stage, gene therapy, exon-skipping therapy, and pharmacological therapy are not effective. Importantly, recent studies show that poor or aberrant muscular regeneration of the diseased muscle cannot be simply ascribed to the exhaustion of satellite cells. Berg et al. recently reported that satellite cells from 10-month-old golden retriever muscular dystrophy dogs, which show severe phenotypes at this age, show proliferation and differentiation potentials equivalent to those of wild-type littermates *in vitro* (Berg et al 2011). The authors suggest that pathological changes in the muscle environment rather than cell-intrinsic defects may be largely implicated in the eventual failure of satellite cell efficacy *in vivo*. For example, prolonged inflammation in dystrophic muscle exposes satellite cells to pro-fibrotic, pro-adipogenic cytokines, and suppresses the myogenic function of satellite cells (reviewed in (Mann et al 2011; Tidball & Villalta 2010). In the next session, we focus on satellite cells in dystrophic conditions, and review the cellular origin of adipogenesis and fibrosis in disease environments. For direct effects of the gene mutations on satellite cells in other muscular dystrophies, please refer to a recent review by Morgan & Zammit (Morgan & Zammit 2010).

3.1 Fibrosis and adipocyte infiltration in DMD muscle

DMD muscle is characterized by chronic inflammation, endomysial fibrosis and adipocyte infiltration (fatty degeneration). It is widely accepted that fibrosis and adipocyte infiltration inhibit not only skeletal muscle function, but also myogenic activities of satellite cells, thereby diminish the amount of target tissue available for therapeutic intervention. Therefore, inhibition of fibrosis and adipogenesis is expected to attenuate DMD progression and increase the success of new cell and gene-based therapies (Mann et al 2011). In fact, many papers show that pharmacological inhibition of fibrosis in *mdx* mice ameliorates the pathology in dystrophin-deficient cardiac and skeletal muscle (Bish et al 2011; Cohn et al 2007; Rafael-Fortney et al 2011; Taniguti et al 2011).

The cellular origin of fatty infiltration has been controversial. Previous studies suggested that satellite cells transdifferentiate into adipocytes and/or fibroblastic cells in pathological conditions. Li et al. reported that TGF-β, a profibrotic cytokine, in skeletal muscle induces the differentiation of C2C12 cells, a myogenic cell line, into fibrotic cells (Li et al 2004). Alexakis et al. also indicated that collagen types I and III were expressed in primary myoblasts derived from mouse satellite cells (Alexakis et al 2007). In contrast, Uezumi et al. (Uezumi et al 2010) and Joe et al.(Joe et al 2010) demonstrated that platelet-derived growth factor receptor alpha (PDGFRα)-positive mesenchymal progenitors or muscle-resident fibro/adipogenic progenitor cells (FAPs) are distinct from satellite cells, and show a strong predisposition towards the generation of adipocytes, and readily differentiate into adipocyte under pathological environments.

Uezumi et al. further provide evidence suggesting that PDGFRα+ mesenchymal progenitors also contribute to fibrosis. The authors demonstrated that PDGFRα+ cells, but not PDGFRα- cells produce fibrosis-related molecules *in vivo* after transplantation, and transforming growth factor (TGF)-βs, known as potent profibrotic cytokines, induce the expression of fibrosis-related genes in PDGFRα+ mesenchymal progenitors, but not in myogenic cells (Uezumi et al 2011). Importantly, imatinib, an inhibitor of several tyrosine kinases including c-abl, c-kit, and PDGFRs, was demonstrated to ameliorate dystrophic phenotypes in *mdx* mice by suppressing the phosphorylation of PDGFRα (Huang et al 2009). In addition, constitutively active PDGFRα-receptor knock-in mice exhibited systemic fibrosis including skeletal muscle tissue (Olson & Soriano 2009). Because PDGFRα is exclusively expressed in mesenchymal progenitors in skeletal muscle, these results strongly suggest that PDGFRα+ mesenchymal progenitors but not satellite cells contribute to connective tissue accumulation in dystrophic muscle.

Mesenchymal progenitor cells never differentiate into adipocytes or produce fibrosis-related molecules in healthy muscle. Why do they preferentially differentiate into collagen-producing fibroblasts or adipocyte in DMD muscle? One plausible explanation is prolonged inflammation due to continuous degeneration/regeneration cycles of muscle and the phenotypic change of macrophages (Mann et al 2011; Tidball & Villalta 2010). Although macrophages promote muscle regeneration (Segawa et al 2008; Tidball & Villalta 2010), macrophages in the advanced stage of mdx are reported to contribute to the development of fibrosis and fatty degeneration by secreting pro-fibrotic and pro-adipogenic cytokines (Mann et al 2011; Tidball & Villalta 2010).

3.2 Limited regenerative potential of human satellite cells

In Duchenne muscular dystrophy, dystrophin deficiency leads to progressive lethal skeletal muscle degeneration. But, dystrophin deficiency does not recapitulate DMD in mice (mdx), which show active regeneration of damaged muscle throughout life, a much milder phenotype than DMD patients, and an almost normal life span.

Sacco et al. demonstrated that mdx mice lacking telomerase activity show shortened telomeres in muscle cells and a severe dystrophic phenotype (Sacco et al 2010). Together with a previous report of a 14-fold greater shortening of telomeres in DMD patients relative to healthy individuals (Decary et al 2000), these studies suggest that a difference in the length of telomeres between humans (5-15 kbs) and mice (>40 kbs) greatly explains the difference in proliferative potential of muscle satellite cells between DMD patients and mdx mice.

On the other hand, Fukada et al. showed that the phenotype of mdx became much more severe when mdx was crossed to with the DBA/2 strain (Fukada et al 2010). The *mdx* mouse (C57BL/10-*Dmd*^{mdx}), first described in 1984, arose in an inbred colony of C57BL/10 mice. Importantly, the proliferation of DBA/2 satellite cells was inferior to that of C57BL/6 (a widely used strain akin to C57BL/10) satellite cells, indicating that the properties of satellite cells and mdx phenotypes greatly depend on the genetic background of the mice.

4. Cell therapy for DMD

In 1989, Partridge et al. demonstrated that transplantation of normal myoblasts restores dystrophin in dystrophin-deficient mdx mice (Partridge et al 1989). In spite of this success, the subsequent myoblast transplantation performed on DMD boys was unsuccessful (Law et al 1992; Mendell et al 1995; Tremblay et al 1993). In this section, we discuss the problems of myoblast-transplantation and other cell sources for cell therapy of DMD.

4.1 Myoblasts transplantation therapy (MTT)

Myoblasts transplantation therapy (MTT) for DMD was tried in the early 90's, but the results were disappointing (Law et al 1992; Mendell et al 1995; Tremblay et al 1993). Although the high-density myoblast transplantation recently performed by Tremblay's team in Canada is promising in some aspects, the effects are still local due to the limited migration and poor survival of grafted cells (Mouly et al 2005; Skuk & Tremblay 2011). In addition, expansion *in vitro* is shown to gradually reduce the regenerative activity of satellite cells (Ikemoto et al 2007; Montarras et al 2005). This is probably because satellite cells have limited proliferative capacities, which are exhausted by expansion in culture. However, currently used culture conditions might simply be inappropriate for the expansion of satellite cells because satellite cells in their niche robustly regenerate injured muscle (Collins et al 2005). Recently, Gilbert et al. pointed out the importance of substrate elasticity in culture (Gilbert et al 2010). When satellite cells were cultured on soft hydrogel substrates that mimic the elasticity of *in vivo* muscle, the cultured cells contributed more extensively to muscle regeneration, indicating that the culture system has much room for improvement. Myoblast transfer therapy is expected to restore muscle function in relatively localized muscle diseases such as oculo-pharyngeal muscular dystrophy (OPMD), by using autologous myoblasts from relatively spared patient muscles (Mouly et al 2005).

4.2 Making satellite cells from non-myogenic cells by reprogramming

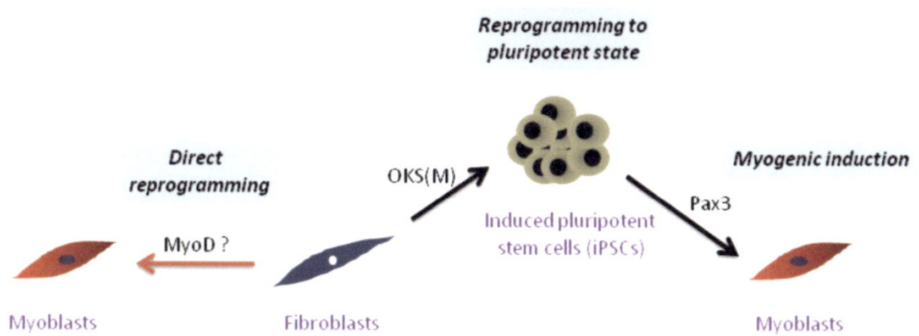

If myogenic cells can be efficiently induced from patient-derived pluripotent stem cells (iPS cells), these cells are candidate sources for cell therapy of muscular dystrophies. On the other hand, direct reprogramming using transcription factors has been reported to successfully convert fibroblasts into clinically relevant cells (neurons, cardiocytes, hepatocytes, chondrocytes, etc). MyoD is a master regulator of myogenesis, but not sufficient to generate myogenic stem cells with high proliferative potential. OKSM: Oct4, Klf4, Sox2 and c-Myc.

Fig. 3. New cell sources for cell therapy of muscular dystrophies

4.3 New cell source for cell therapy of DMD

It is difficult to prepare a large quantity of satellite cells from a donor. In addition, expansion of satellite cells *in vitro* reduces the regenerative activity (Ikemoto et al 2007; Montarras et al 2005). Mesoangioblasts or muscle-derived stem cells (MDSC) are multi-potent stem cells distinct from satellite cells that have been demonstrated to be highly proliferative and able to be delivered to the musculature of the whole body. However, the number of cells, as starting materials, required to restore dystrophin expression in cardiac and respiratory muscle and improve performance of DMD patients remains to be determined in clinical trials. On the other hand, transcription factor-mediated reprogramming of somatic cells into myogenic cells is now being vigorously investigated, and is expected to be a feasible technique in the near future. Two different strategies are proposed to generate myogenic cells from somatic cells **(Figure 3)**. One is to reprogram somatic cells of patients into pluripotent stem cells (iPS cells) using Yamanaka factors, and then induce them to differentiate into transplantable myogenic cells. The other strategy is to directly induce fibroblasts to differentiate into myogenic cells without first passing the cells through a pluripotent state.

4.3.1 Induced pluripotent stem cells (iPS cells)

In 2006, Takahashi and Yamanaka reported that only four factors (Oct4, Klf4, Sox2, and c-Myc, are sufficient to reprogram somatic cells into embryoni stem (ES) cell-like pluripotent stem cells (Takahashi & Yamanaka 2006). The induced cells are called induced pluripotent cells (iPS cells). The next year, the same group and Thompson's group reported the establishment of human iPS cells from skin fibroblasts using slightly different sets of reprogramming factors (Takahashi et al 2007; Yu et al 2007). This technique is groundbreaking, because it enables us to obtain patient-specific iPS cells with pluripotency. Muscular dystrophy patient-specific iPS cells were first reported by Park et al. (Park et al 2008). iPS cells derived from the patients showed human ES-like properties, and therefore may be a promising cell source for cell therapy. If myogenic stem cells can be constantly induced from iPS cells, there will be no limitation in the number of the cells for transplantation. In addition, although a controversial report of immunogenicity appeared recently (Zhao et al 2011), autologous iPS cells are expected to produce tissue-specific stem /progenitor cells that evoke no immune reaction in the host.

4.3.2 Muscle differentiation of ES/iPS cells

The success of iPS cell-based therapy for DMD depends on the efficiency of induction of myogenic progenitor cells from iPS cells. Pax3 and Pax7 have been shown to be a powerful way to derive transplantable myogenic cells from mouse ES cells (Darabi et al 2008; Darabi et al 2011). However, for a clinical trial, integration of viral vectors into the host genome is not desirable. One possibility to avoid the use of viral vectors is to replace Pax3 or Pax7 activity with small bioactive molecules. Purification of myogenic cells from differentiating iPS culture is also important for safe cell transplantation because a culture contains both differentiated and undifferentiated cells. Contamination with undifferentiated cells can cause tumor formation in the host. A research group at Kyoto University described a strategy to sort myogenic cells from differentiating mouse ES cells (Chang et al 2009) or mouse iPS cells (Mizuno et al 2010). The authors cultured embryoid bodies in muscle differentiation medium (10% fetal bovine serum and 5% horse serum in DMEM) for six days and then plated them on Matrigel, and sorted SM/C-2.6-positive cells by FACS before cell transplantation. SM/C-2.6 is a rat monoclonal antibody useful to isolate satellite cells from mouse muscle (Fukada et al 2004). Not all SM/C-2.6-positive cells are myogenic, but the fraction is enriched in myogenic stem cells. Both strategies are promising, but human ES/iPS cells respond to the differentiation signal differently from their mouse equivalents. In addition, human ES/iPS cells differentiate more slowly than their mouse counterparts. In fact, the myogenic differentiation protocol described by Chang et al. for mouse ES/iPS cells was not efficient for human iPS cells (data not shown), and the condition need to be further explored.

4.3.3 Direct reprogramming of fibroblasts by myogenic transcription factors

iPS technology stimulated researchers to seek an appropriate combination of transcriptional factors to reprogram somatic cells into therapeutically relevant cell types *in vitro* and *in vivo* (Hiramatsu et al 2011; Ieda et al 2010; Sekiya & Suzuki 2011; Szabo et al 2010; Vierbuchen et al 2010). However, we already know how to induce myogenic cells from fibroblasts. In 1989, Weintraub and colleagues demonstrated that MyoD is sufficient to convert fibroblasts and numerous other cell types into skeletal muscle (Weintraub et al 1989). This was the first example of transcription factor-based reprogramming of the cell, but this technology has not been successfully applied to regenerative medicine. Recently, Kimura et al. reported that MyoD mediated conversion of fibroblasts *in situ* (Kimura et al 2008). The authors first introduced a tamoxifen-inducible MyoD expression cassette together with a muscle promoter-derived dystrophin expression cassette into mdx-derived fibroblasts, and then transplanted them into mdx muscle. Injection of tamoxifen into the mdx mice resulted in the appearance of dystrophin-positive myofibers in transplanted muscle, but many of them were small and clustered in the interstitial space. Pax3, Pax7 and their co-factors are also candidate transcription factors to reprogram fibroblasts into highly proliferative, systemically transplantable stem cells.

5. Conclusion

Satellite cells are skeletal muscle-specific stem cells involved in muscle growth and regeneration. Their dysfunctions are reported in several pathological conditions. Recent studies emphasize that, in addition to exhaustion of satellite cells, the microenvironment greatly influences satellite cell behaviors. Therefore both satellite cells and their microenvironment are targets of regenerative medicine. Satellite cells are also expected to be a source for cell transplantation therapy, but preparation of viable satellite cells from donors in a large quantity is not realistic. To overcome this limitation, the transcription factor-mediated reprogramming technique is now in the spotlight. MyoD was the first direct reprogramming factor discovered. However, it is not sufficient to generate high-quality myogenic cells from fibroblasts. To overcome this problem, we must fully understand the molecular and cellular regulation of satellite cells. Fortunately, we are now starting to do this.

6. Acknowledgment

We thank all members of Department of Molecular Therapy for valuable discussion.

7. References

Abou-Khalil R, Brack AS. 2010. Muscle stem cells and reversible quiescence: the role of sprouty. *Cell Cycle* 9:2575-80

Abou-Khalil R, Le Grand F, Pallafacchina G, Valable S, Authier FJ, et al. 2009. Autocrine and paracrine angiopoietin 1/Tie-2 signaling promotes muscle satellite cell self-renewal. *Cell Stem Cell* 5:298-309

Alexakis C, Partridge T, Bou-Gharios G. 2007. Implication of the satellite cell in dystrophic muscle fibrosis: a self-perpetuating mechanism of collagen overproduction. *Am J Physiol Cell Physiol* 293:C661-9

Arnold L, Henry A, Poron F, Baba-Amer Y, van Rooijen N, et al. 2007. Inflammatory monocytes recruited after skeletal muscle injury switch into antiinflammatory macrophages to support myogenesis. *J Exp Med* 204:1057-69

Berg Z, Beffa LR, Cook DP, Cornelison DD. 2011. Muscle satellite cells from GRMD dystrophic dogs are not phenotypically distinguishable from wild type satellite cells in ex vivo culture. *Neuromuscul Disord* 21:282-90

Bish LT, Yarchoan M, Sleeper MM, Gazzara JA, Morine KJ, et al. 2011. Chronic losartan administration reduces mortality and preserves cardiac but not skeletal muscle function in dystrophic mice. *PLoS One* 6:e20856

Blau HM, Webster C, Pavlath GK. 1983. Defective myoblasts identified in Duchenne muscular dystrophy. *Proc Natl Acad Sci U S A* 80:4856-60

Blau HM, Webster C, Pavlath GK, Chiu CP. 1985. Evidence for defective myoblasts in Duchenne muscular dystrophy. *Adv Exp Med Biol* 182:85-110

Boldrin L, Muntoni F, Morgan JE. 2010. Are human and mouse satellite cells really the same? *J Histochem Cytochem* 58:941-55

Buckingham M, Relaix F. 2007. The role of Pax genes in the development of tissues and organs: Pax3 and Pax7 regulate muscle progenitor cell functions. *Annu Rev Cell Dev Biol* 23:645-73

Chang H, Yoshimoto M, Umeda K, Iwasa T, Mizuno Y, et al. 2009. Generation of transplantable, functional satellite-like cells from mouse embryonic stem cells. *FASEB J* 23:1907-19

Chen JF, Tao Y, Li J, Deng Z, Yan Z, et al. 2010. microRNA-1 and microRNA-206 regulate skeletal muscle satellite cell proliferation and differentiation by repressing Pax7. *J Cell Biol* 190:867-79

Cohn RD, van Erp C, Habashi JP, Soleimani AA, Klein EC, et al. 2007. Angiotensin II type 1 receptor blockade attenuates TGF-beta-induced failure of muscle regeneration in multiple myopathic states. *Nat Med* 13:204-10

Collins CA, Olsen I, Zammit PS, Heslop L, Petrie A, et al. 2005. Stem cell function, self-renewal, and behavioral heterogeneity of cells from the adult muscle satellite cell niche. *Cell* 122:289-301

Conboy IM, Rando TA. 2002. The regulation of Notch signaling controls satellite cell activation and cell fate determination in postnatal myogenesis. *Dev Cell* 3:397-409

Conboy MJ, Cerletti M, Wagers AJ, Conboy IM. 2010. Immuno-analysis and FACS sorting of adult muscle fiber-associated stem/precursor cells. *Methods Mol Biol* 621:165-73

Conboy MJ, Karasov AO, Rando TA. 2007. High incidence of non-random template strand segregation and asymmetric fate determination in dividing stem cells and their progeny. *PLoS Biol* 5:e102

Crist CG, Montarras D, Pallafacchina G, Rocancourt D, Cumano A, et al. 2009. Muscle stem cell behavior is modified by microRNA-27 regulation of Pax3 expression. *Proc Natl Acad Sci U S A* 106:13383-7

Darabi R, Gehlbach K, Bachoo RM, Kamath S, Osawa M, et al. 2008. Functional skeletal muscle regeneration from differentiating embryonic stem cells. *Nat Med* 14:134-43

Darabi R, Pan W, Bosnakovski D, Baik J, Kyba M, Perlingeiro RC. 2011. Functional Myogenic Engraftment from Mouse iPS Cells. *Stem Cell Rev*

Decary S, Hamida CB, Mouly V, Barbet JP, Hentati F, Butler-Browne GS. 2000. Shorter telomeres in dystrophic muscle consistent with extensive regeneration in young children. *Neuromuscul Disord* 10:113-20

Dey BK, Gagan J, Dutta A. 2011. miR-206 and -486 induce myoblast differentiation by downregulating Pax7. *Mol Cell Biol* 31:203-14

Dhawan J, Rando TA. 2005. Stem cells in postnatal myogenesis: molecular mechanisms of satellite cell quiescence, activation and replenishment. *Trends Cell Biol* 15:666-73

Ferrari G, Cusella-De Angelis G, Coletta M, Paolucci E, Stornaiuolo A, et al. 1998. Muscle regeneration by bone marrow-derived myogenic progenitors. *Science* 279:1528-30

Fukada S, Higuchi S, Segawa M, Koda K, Yamamoto Y, et al. 2004. Purification and cell-surface marker characterization of quiescent satellite cells from murine skeletal muscle by a novel monoclonal antibody. *Exp Cell Res* 296:245-55

Fukada S, Miyagoe-Suzuki Y, Tsukihara H, Yuasa K, Higuchi S, et al. 2002. Muscle regeneration by reconstitution with bone marrow or fetal liver cells from green fluorescent protein-gene transgenic mice. *J Cell Sci* 115:1285-93

Fukada S, Morikawa D, Yamamoto Y, Yoshida T, Sumie N, et al. 2010. Genetic background affects properties of satellite cells and mdx phenotypes. *Am J Pathol* 176:2414-24

Fukada S, Uezumi A, Ikemoto M, Masuda S, Segawa M, et al. 2007. Molecular signature of quiescent satellite cells in adult skeletal muscle. *Stem Cells* 25:2448-59

Fukada S, Yamaguchi M, Kokubo H, Ogawa R, Uezumi A, et al. 2011. Hesr1 and Hesr3 are essential to generate undifferentiated quiescent satellite cells and to maintain satellite cell numbers. *Development*. 138:4609-19.

Gilbert PM, Havenstrite KL, Magnusson KE, Sacco A, Leonardi NA, et al. 2010. Substrate elasticity regulates skeletal muscle stem cell self-renewal in culture. *Science* 329:1078-81

Gros J, Manceau M, Thome V, Marcelle C. 2005. A common somitic origin for embryonic muscle progenitors and satellite cells. *Nature* 435:954-8

Gussoni E, Soneoka Y, Strickland CD, Buzney EA, Khan MK, et al. 1999. Dystrophin expression in the mdx mouse restored by stem cell transplantation. *Nature* 401:390-4

Heslop L, Morgan JE, Partridge TA. 2000. Evidence for a myogenic stem cell that is exhausted in dystrophic muscle. *J Cell Sci* 113 (Pt 12):2299-308

Hiramatsu K, Sasagawa S, Outani H, Nakagawa K, Yoshikawa H, Tsumaki N. 2011. Generation of hyaline cartilaginous tissue from mouse adult dermal fibroblast culture by defined factors. *J Clin Invest* 121:640-57

Hollnagel A, Grund C, Franke WW, Arnold HH. 2002. The cell adhesion molecule M-cadherin is not essential for muscle development and regeneration. *Mol Cell Biol* 22:4760-70

Huang P, Zhao XS, Fields M, Ransohoff RM, Zhou L. 2009. Imatinib attenuates skeletal muscle dystrophy in mdx mice. *Faseb J* 23:2539-48

Ieda M, Fu JD, Delgado-Olguin P, Vedantham V, Hayashi Y, et al. 2010. Direct reprogramming of fibroblasts into functional cardiomyocytes by defined factors. *Cell* 142:375-86

Ikemoto M, Fukada S, Uezumi A, Masuda S, Miyoshi H, et al. 2007. Autologous transplantation of SM/C-2.6(+) satellite cells transduced with micro-dystrophin CS1 cDNA by lentiviral vector into mdx mice. *Mol Ther* 15:2178-85

Irintchev A, Zeschnigk M, Starzinski-Powitz A, Wernig A. 1994. Expression pattern of M-cadherin in normal, denervated, and regenerating mouse muscles. *Dev Dyn* 199:326-37

Joe AW, Yi L, Natarajan A, Le Grand F, So L, et al. 2010. Muscle injury activates resident fibro/adipogenic progenitors that facilitate myogenesis. *Nat Cell Biol* 12:153-63

Juan AH, Derfoul A, Feng X, Ryall JG, Dell'Orso S, et al. 2011. Polycomb EZH2 controls self-renewal and safeguards the transcriptional identity of skeletal muscle stem cells. *Genes Dev* 25:789-94

Kanisicak O, Mendez JJ, Yamamoto S, Yamamoto M, Goldhamer DJ. 2009. Progenitors of skeletal muscle satellite cells express the muscle determination gene, MyoD. *Dev Biol* 332:131-41

Kassar-Duchossoy L, Giacone E, Gayraud-Morel B, Jory A, Gomes D, Tajbakhsh S. 2005. Pax3/Pax7 mark a novel population of primitive myogenic cells during development. *Genes Dev* 19:1426-31

Kawakami A, Kimura-Kawakami M, Nomura T, Fujisawa H. 1997. Distributions of PAX6 and PAX7 proteins suggest their involvement in both early and late phases of chick brain development. *Mech Dev* 66:119-30

Kimura E, Han JJ, Li S, Fall B, Ra J, et al. 2008. Cell-lineage regulated myogenesis for dystrophin replacement: a novel therapeutic approach for treatment of muscular dystrophy. *Hum Mol Genet* 17:2507-17

Kuang S, Gillespie MA, Rudnicki MA. 2008. Niche regulation of muscle satellite cell self-renewal and differentiation. *Cell Stem Cell* 2:22-31

Kuang S, Kuroda K, Le Grand F, Rudnicki MA. 2007. Asymmetric self-renewal and commitment of satellite stem cells in muscle. *Cell* 129:999-1010

Kuang S, Rudnicki MA. 2008. The emerging biology of satellite cells and their therapeutic potential. *Trends Mol Med* 14:82-91

LaBarge MA, Blau HM. 2002. Biological progression from adult bone marrow to mononucleate muscle stem cell to multinucleate muscle fiber in response to injury. *Cell* 111:589-601

Law PK, Goodwin TG, Fang Q, Duggirala V, Larkin C, et al. 1992. Feasibility, safety, and efficacy of myoblast transfer therapy on Duchenne muscular dystrophy boys. *Cell Transplant* 1:235-44

Lepper C, Conway SJ, Fan CM. 2009. Adult satellite cells and embryonic muscle progenitors have distinct genetic requirements. *Nature* 460:627-31

Li Y, Foster W, Deasy BM, Chan Y, Prisk V, et al. 2004. Transforming growth factor-beta1 induces the differentiation of myogenic cells into fibrotic cells in injured skeletal muscle: a key event in muscle fibrogenesis. *Am J Pathol* 164:1007-19

Mann CJ, Perdiguero E, Kharraz Y, Aguilar S, Pessina P, et al. 2011. Aberrant repair and fibrosis development in skeletal muscle. *Skelet Muscle* 1:21

Mauro A. 1961. Satellite cell of skeletal muscle fibers. *J Biophys Biochem Cytol* 9:493-5

Mendell JR, Kissel JT, Amato AA, King W, Signore L, et al. 1995. Myoblast transfer in the treatment of Duchenne's muscular dystrophy. *N Engl J Med* 333:832-8

Mizuno Y, Chang H, Umeda K, Niwa A, Iwasa T, et al. 2010. Generation of skeletal muscle stem/progenitor cells from murine induced pluripotent stem cells. *FASEB J* 24:2245-53

Montarras D, Morgan J, Collins C, Relaix F, Zaffran S, et al. 2005. Direct isolation of satellite cells for skeletal muscle regeneration. *Science* 309:2064-7

Morgan JE, Zammit PS. 2010. Direct effects of the pathogenic mutation on satellite cell function in muscular dystrophy. *Exp Cell Res* 316:3100-8

Moss FP, Leblond CP. 1971. Satellite cells as the source of nuclei in muscles of growing rats. *Anat Rec* 170:421-35

Motohashi N, Uezumi A, Yada E, Fukada S, Fukushima K, et al. 2008. Muscle CD31(-) CD45(-) side population cells promote muscle regeneration by stimulating proliferation and migration of myoblasts. *Am J Pathol* 173:781-91

Mouly V, Aamiri A, Perie S, Mamchaoui K, Barani A, et al. 2005. Myoblast transfer therapy: is there any light at the end of the tunnel? *Acta Myol* 24:128-33

Olguin HC, Olwin BB. 2004. Pax-7 up-regulation inhibits myogenesis and cell cycle progression in satellite cells: a potential mechanism for self-renewal. *Dev Biol* 275:375-88

Olguin HC, Yang Z, Tapscott SJ, Olwin BB. 2007. Reciprocal inhibition between Pax7 and muscle regulatory factors modulates myogenic cell fate determination. *J Cell Biol* 177:769-79

Olson LE, Soriano P. 2009. Increased PDGFRalpha activation disrupts connective tissue development and drives systemic fibrosis. *Dev Cell* 16:303-13

Palacios D, Mozzetta C, Consalvi S, Caretti G, Saccone V, et al. 2010. TNF/p38alpha/polycomb signaling to Pax7 locus in satellite cells links inflammation to the epigenetic control of muscle regeneration. *Cell Stem Cell* 7:455-69

Park IH, Arora N, Huo H, Maherali N, Ahfeldt T, et al. 2008. Disease-specific induced pluripotent stem cells. *Cell* 134:877-86

Partridge TA, Morgan JE, Coulton GR, Hoffman EP, Kunkel LM. 1989. Conversion of mdx myofibres from dystrophin-negative to -positive by injection of normal myoblasts. *Nature* 337:176-9

Rafael-Fortney JA, Chimanji NS, Schill KE, Martin CD, Murray JD, et al. 2011. Early treatment with lisinopril and spironolactone preserves cardiac and skeletal muscle in duchenne muscular dystrophy mice. *Circulation* 124:582-8

Relaix F, Rocancourt D, Mansouri A, Buckingham M. 2005. A Pax3/Pax7-dependent population of skeletal muscle progenitor cells. *Nature* 435:948-53

Rosenblatt JD, Lunt AI, Parry DJ, Partridge TA. 1995. Culturing satellite cells from living single muscle fiber explants. *In Vitro Cell Dev Biol Anim* 31:773-9

Sacco A, Mourkioti F, Tran R, Choi J, Llewellyn M, et al. 2010. Short telomeres and stem cell exhaustion model Duchenne muscular dystrophy in mdx/mTR mice. *Cell* 143:1059-71

Schmalbruch H, Hellhammer U. 1976. The number of satellite cells in normal human muscle. *Anat Rec* 185:279-87

Schultz E, Gibson MC, Champion T. 1978. Satellite cells are mitotically quiescent in mature mouse muscle: an EM and radioautographic study. *J Exp Zool* 206:451-6

Seale P, Sabourin LA, Girgis-Gabardo A, Mansouri A, Gruss P, Rudnicki MA. 2000. Pax7 is required for the specification of myogenic satellite cells. *Cell* 102:777-86

Segawa M, Fukada S, Yamamoto Y, Yahagi H, Kanematsu M, et al. 2008. Suppression of macrophage functions impairs skeletal muscle regeneration with severe fibrosis. *Exp Cell Res* 314:3232-44

Sekiya S, Suzuki A. 2011. Direct conversion of mouse fibroblasts to hepatocyte-like cells by defined factors. *Nature* 475:390-3

Shea KL, Xiang W, LaPorta VS, Licht JD, Keller C, et al. 2010. Sprouty1 regulates reversible quiescence of a self-renewing adult muscle stem cell pool during regeneration. *Cell Stem Cell* 6:117-29

Sherwood RI, Christensen JL, Conboy IM, Conboy MJ, Rando TA, et al. 2004. Isolation of adult mouse myogenic progenitors: functional heterogeneity of cells within and engrafting skeletal muscle. *Cell* 119:543-54

Shinin V, Gayraud-Morel B, Gomes D, Tajbakhsh S. 2006. Asymmetric division and cosegregation of template DNA strands in adult muscle satellite cells. *Nat Cell Biol* 8:677-87

Skuk D, Tremblay JP. 2011. Intramuscular cell transplantation as a potential treatment of myopathies: clinical and preclinical relevant data. *Expert Opin Biol Ther* 11:359-74

Szabo E, Rampalli S, Risueno RM, Schnerch A, Mitchell R, et al. 2010. Direct conversion of human fibroblasts to multilineage blood progenitors. *Nature* 468:521-6

Takahashi K, Tanabe K, Ohnuki M, Narita M, Ichisaka T, et al. 2007. Induction of pluripotent stem cells from adult human fibroblasts by defined factors. *Cell* 131:861-72

Takahashi K, Yamanaka S. 2006. Induction of pluripotent stem cells from mouse embryonic and adult fibroblast cultures by defined factors. *Cell* 126:663-76

Tanaka KK, Hall JK, Troy AA, Cornelison DD, Majka SM, Olwin BB. 2009. Syndecan-4-expressing muscle progenitor cells in the SP engraft as satellite cells during muscle regeneration. *Cell Stem Cell* 4:217-25

Taniguti AP, Pertille A, Matsumura CY, Santo Neto H, Marques MJ. 2011. Prevention of muscle fibrosis and myonecrosis in mdx mice by suramin, a TGF-beta1 blocker. *Muscle Nerve* 43:82-7

Tidball JG, Villalta SA. 2010. Regulatory interactions between muscle and the immune system during muscle regeneration. *Am J Physiol Regul Integr Comp Physiol* 298:R1173-87

Tremblay JP, Malouin F, Roy R, Huard J, Bouchard JP, et al. 1993. Results of a triple blind clinical study of myoblast transplantations without immunosuppressive treatment in young boys with Duchenne muscular dystrophy. *Cell Transplant* 2:99-112

Uezumi A, Fukada S, Yamamoto N, Takeda S, Tsuchida K. 2010. Mesenchymal progenitors distinct from satellite cells contribute to ectopic fat cell formation in skeletal muscle. *Nat Cell Biol* 12:143-52

Uezumi A, Ito T, Morikawa D, Shimizu N, Yoneda T, et al. 2011.Fibrosis and adipogenesis originate from a common mesenchymal progenitor in skeletal muscle. *J Cell Sci.* 124: 3654-64.

Uezumi A, Ojima K, Fukada S, Ikemoto M, Masuda S, et al. 2006. Functional heterogeneity of side population cells in skeletal muscle. *Biochem Biophys Res Commun* 341:864-73

Vidal B, Serrano AL, Tjwa M, Suelves M, Ardite E, et al. 2008. Fibrinogen drives dystrophic muscle fibrosis via a TGFbeta/alternative macrophage activation pathway. *Genes Dev* 22:1747-52

Vierbuchen T, Ostermeier A, Pang ZP, Kokubu Y, Sudhof TC, Wernig M. 2010. Direct conversion of fibroblasts to functional neurons by defined factors. *Nature* 463:1035-41

Villalta SA, Nguyen HX, Deng B, Gotoh T, Tidball JG. 2009. Shifts in macrophage phenotypes and macrophage competition for arginine metabolism affect the severity of muscle pathology in muscular dystrophy. *Hum Mol Genet* 18:482-96

Weintraub H, Tapscott SJ, Davis RL, Thayer MJ, Adam MA, et al. 1989. Activation of muscle-specific genes in pigment, nerve, fat, liver, and fibroblast cell lines by forced expression of MyoD. *Proc Natl Acad Sci U S A* 86:5434-8

White RB, Bierinx AS, Gnocchi VF, Zammit PS. 2010. Dynamics of muscle fibre growth during postnatal mouse development. *BMC Dev Biol* 10:21

Yajima H, Motohashi N, Ono Y, Sato S, Ikeda K, et al. 2010. Six family genes control the proliferation and differentiation of muscle satellite cells. *Exp Cell Res* 316:2932-44

Yu J, Vodyanik MA, Smuga-Otto K, Antosiewicz-Bourget J, Frane JL, et al. 2007. Induced pluripotent stem cell lines derived from human somatic cells. *Science* 318:1917-20

Zhao T, Zhang ZN, Rong Z, Xu Y. 2011. Immunogenicity of induced pluripotent stem cells. *Nature* 474:212-5

19

Exon Skipping and Myoblast Transplantation: Single or Combined Potential Options for Treatment of Duchenne Muscular Dystrophy

T. Iannitti[1,*], D. Lodi[2], V. Sblendorio[3], V. Rottigni[4] and B. Palmieri[4]

[1]Department of Physiology, School of Medicine, University of Kentucky Medical Center, Lexington,
[2]Department of Nephrology, Dialysis and Transplantation, University of Modena and Reggio Emilia Medical School, Modena,
[3]Department of General Surgery and Surgical Specialties, University of Modena and Reggio Emilia Medical School, Surgical Clinic, Modena,
Present address: Unit of Pharmacology, Department of Pharmacobiology, Faculty of Pharmacy, University of Bari,
[4]Department of General Surgery and Surgical Specialties, University of Modena and Reggio Emilia Medical School, Surgical Clinic, Modena,
[1]USA
[2,3,4]Italy

1. Introduction

Edward Meryon, an English doctor, described Duchenne muscular dystrophy (DMD) for the first time, but the symptoms and the histology typical of this condition were firstly described by Duchenne de Boulogne in 1861. The dystrophin gene (dys) was firstly identified by Kunkel and coworkers (Kunkel et al., 1986), while Hoffman and colleagues (Hoffman et al., 1987) identified the gene product dystrophin. This protein is lacking in DMD patients' muscles and, due to its essentiality in membrane stability, its absence induces contraction-related membrane damage and the activation of the inflammatory cascade, leading to muscle failure, necrosis, and fibrosis (Hoffmann and Dressman, 2001; Blake et al., 2002; Palmieri B. and Sblendorio V., 2006). This condition affects primarily human and animal skeletal and cardiac muscle and it is defined as an X-linked recessive disease with the most cases inherited from carrier mothers, and about a third of cases occurring as de novo mutations in the infants. DMD is present at birth, but clinical symptoms are not evident until 3 to 5 years of age (leg weakness, increasing spine kyphosis, and a waddle-like gait) and usually its diagnosis is made on the basis of gait spine abnormalities from 4 to 5 years after birth (Dubowitz et al., 1975; Jennekens et al., 1991). DMD patients display problems in climbing stairs and rising up from the floor; they are unable to run, and in a variable way, most of them lose ambulation by 7 to 12 years (Iannitti et al., 2010). Moreover, other characteristics of this

* Corresponding Author

disease are the progressive loss of respiratory function that can lead to respiratory failure, scoliosis, weight loss, cardiomyopathy, and finally death, as a result of respiratory and cardiac complications (Iannitti et al., 2010). The continuous muscle wasting, that characterizes this pathological condition, puts DMD patients, from 8 to 12 years of age, in wheelchairs with scoliosis developing in 90% of boys who use a wheelchair full-time and die in the late teens or early twenties due to respiratory/cardiac failure after a worsening of symptoms (Emery, 1993). In children with DMD, non-progressive abnormalities of the central nervous system have also been observed. In fact, the mean intelligence quotient of these patients is 82 which is 18 points under the mean value of the healthy population, while 30% of the patients have a quotient under 75 (Bresolin et al., 1994).In particular, verbal intelligence is primarily affected and 80% of DMD patients display atypical electroretinography with the most prominent portion of the normal electroretinogram, the wave b, that is absent (Billard et al., 1992; Sigesmund et al., 1994).

Inflammation, mediated by neutrophils, macrophages and cytokines, also seems to be involved in the damage of dystrophic muscles (Whitehead et al., 2006). Gosselin and colleagues (Gosselin et al., 2004) described the important role played by inflammation showing that a persistent inflammatory response has been observed in dystrophic skeletal muscle leading to an alteration in extracellular environment; it includes an increase in inflammatory cells, such as macrophages and elevated levels of various inflammatory cytokines like tumor necrosis factor alpha (TNF-α) that contributes to muscle degeneration, while pro-fibrotic cytokines, such as transforming growth factor beta (TGF-β), can account for a progressive fibrosis. Experimental studies, using the DMD mdx mouse model, support this fact reporting that the depletion of inflammatory cells, such as neutrophils, cromolyn blockade of mast cell degranulation or pharmacological blockade of TNF, reduces necrosis of dystrophic myofibers (DeSilva et al., 1987).

2. Dystrophin

The human dystrophin gene (13.973 nucleotides), dys, maps at the Xp21.1 locus; it is encoded by a 2.25-Mbp gene with 79 exons and 99.4% of its sequence is composed of introns (the fully processed transcript is only 14 Kbp) (Kunkel et al., 1986). The DMD gene can produce different dystrophin isoforms through alternative promoter usage and splicing of pre-mRNA and the predominant isoform is an approximately 427-kDa cytoskeletal protein that consists of 3685 amino acids constituting 5% of sarcolemmal protein and 0.002% of total striated muscle protein (Hoffman et al., 1987; Koenig et al., 1988).

Four domains constitute the structure of full length dystrophin, i.e. an N-terminal "acting binding" domain, a middle "rod" domain consisting of spectrin-like repeats, a cysteine-rich domain encoded by exons 62 to 70 and a C-terminal domain. The last two domains play a key role in the assembly of the dystroglycan complex and in the sarcolemmal function (Petrof, 2002; Palmieri and Sblendorio, 2006). When a mutation and deletion occur in the dystrophin gene, as observed in DMD patients, the protein cannot be produced leading to its complete absence in muscle fibers. Dystrophin belongs to a group of proteins called dystrophin glycoprotein complex (DGC), which also include cytoskeletal actin, the dystroglycan integral membrane proteins, the syntrophins, dystrobrevins and α-catulin (Brown et al., 1997).Dystrophin links the actin intracellular microfilament network to the extracellular matrix and its absence changes the level and localization of DGC, making the sarcolemma fragile and muscle fibers prone to degeneration during repeated cycles of muscle contraction and relaxation. Actin associates with the N-terminal of dystrophin, in a region displaying two calponin homology domains (Corrado et al., 1994; Norwood et al., 2000; Way et al., 1992), while the other proteins bind to the C-terminal region of dystrophin. The association of b-dystroglycan with dystrophin is mediated by a cysteine-rich region of dystrophin that contains a protein module with two highly conserved tryptophans (WW domain) and 2 EF-handlike motifs (Huang et al., 2000; Jung et al., 1995). Furthermore, b-dystroglycan associates with the extracellular protein a-dystroglycan which, in turn, connects to laminin in the extracellular matrix (ECM) (Henry et al., 1998; Henry et al., 1999; Hohenester et al., 1999).Dystrophin, through its association with actin and dystroglycan, represents a key bridge between the ECM and cytoskeleton, playing an important role in the structural integrity of the muscle cell membrane. The absence or disruption of dystrophin, observed in DMD, also exerts some effects on the central nervous system (CNS) function. In fact the dystrophin role in the positioning of receptors and channels is relevant at the synapse level where the neuromuscular junction exerts an important role on the synapse structure and function (Hall et al., 1993; Sanes et al., 1999). Dystrophin is localized in the deep regions of junctional folds at the post-synaptic face (Bewick et al., 1992; Sealock et al., 1991) and, through its association with its complex of proteins (Fig. 1), dystrophin plays both structural and signalling roles.

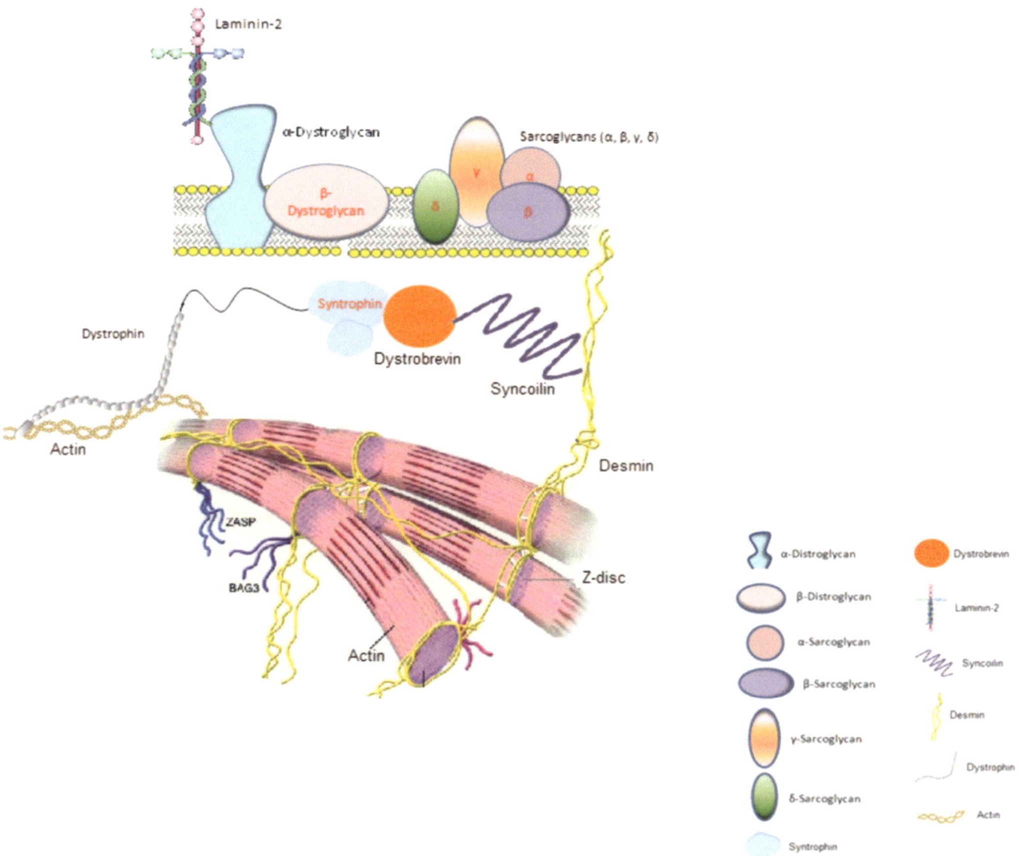

Fig. 1. Complex of proteins associated with dystrophin.

Other clinical aspects of the DMD pathophysiology have been reported. These are cognitive impairment and lower intelligence quotient (IQ) (average = 85) observed in boys with DMD, disordered CNS architecture, abnormalities in dendrites and loss of neurons. Moreover, at the biochemical level, the bioenergetics of the CNS is abnormal, and there is an increase in the concentration of choline-containing compounds, indicative of CNS pathology.

Dystrophin expression is regulated by seven independent promoters, three of which regulate the expression of full-length isoforms, while four intragenic promoters regulate the expression of different short isoforms in various tissues. Two additional isoforms are considered to be full-length and are expressed in the brain. The mutation that affects dystrophin promoter regions and regulates the expression of brain isoforms, may be the cause of neurological symptoms in some patients with DMD. Each of the additional transcripts results in the expression of multiple dystrophin proteins (Dp) that are indicated according to their molecular weight: Dp427 muscle, Dp427 brain, Dp427 purkinje, Dp260, Dp140, Dp116, and Dp71 (Muntoni et al., 2003).These last four variants contain unique first exons and lack the actin binding domain, suggesting that they may have functions that are different from the ones ascribed to full-length dystrophin. Dp260 in the retina and Dp71 in the brain and other tissues restore the integrity of DGC, but only Dp260, the longest of the short isoforms, restores some functional integrity in the dystrophic muscle. These findings suggest that a better bridge between ECM and actin is more necessary for the improvement of dystrophic muscle function than the one provided by the Dp71 variant.

Alternative splicing of exons 71 to 74 and 78 increases the diversity of transcripts; the first splicing regulates interactions with syntrophins. These exons can be spliced singularly or in a different combination, generating a series of in-frame spliced variants.

The elimination of exons 73 and 74 in any of these transcripts generates a functional protein that lacks the syntrophin binding sites (Yang et al., 1995; Newey et al., 2000). The splicing of exons gives a translational frame shift, producing the substitution of the last 13 amino acids of the predominantly hydrophilic C-terminal region with 31 hydrophobic amino acids. This process is regulated in a developmental and tissue- specific way (Tennyson et al., 1996). The hydrophobic splice variant is abundant in the cerebral cortex and retina and it serves to regulate the binding of dystrophin to α-catulin and its associated proteins (Roberts et al., 1998).

3. Searching criteria and aim

We have been searching Pubmed/Medline, using the key words "Duchenne", "Muscular" and "Dystrophy" combined with "Exon", "Skipping", "Immunosuppressant", "Stem", "Cells", "Myoblast" and "Transplantation", in order to collect and analyze all the recent advances in DMD, focusing on clinical trials performed in humans. This chapter highlights the most promising therapeutical approaches to DMD, i.e. exon skipping and myoblast transplantation with some details about the immunosuppressive therapy.

4. Immunosuppressant drugs

Among the scientific community there is a growing interest in the use of immunosuppressant drugs that may potentially give clinical benefits during the DMD course. The interest is due to the host transplant, potential immunosuppressant schedule that should be suitable to increase myoblast or mesangioblast graft survival supporting, in the meantime, the autologous crippled mass function. Among immunosuppressant drugs, corticosteroids slow DMD progression and, in particular, two corticosteroids, i.e. prednisone and deflazacort have been extensively used because of their ability to improve skeletal muscle function. Research has also focused on the use of suppressing drugs acting against TNF level and suppressing calcineurin signals.

The long-term effects of deflazacort treatment has been investigated according to two treatment protocols from Naples (N) and Toronto (T) in boys, aged between 8 and 15 years, who were affected by DMD and had 4 or more years of deflazacort treatment (Biggar et al., 2001).Thirty seven boys were treated with protocol N, using deflazacort at a dose of 0.6 mg/kg per day for the first 20 days of the month and no deflazacort for the remainder of the month.Vitamin D and calcium were administered daily to boys with osteoporosis. Deflazacort treatment started between 4 and 8 years of age. Thirty two were treated with protocol T, using deflazacort at a dose of 0.9 mg/kg per day, plus vitamin D and calcium daily. Treatment started between 6 and 8 years of age. All boys were monitored every 4 to 6 months and the results were compared with age-matched control subjects in the two groups (19 for protocol N and 30 for protocol T). It was observed that: 1) for the boys treated with protocol N, 97% were ambulatory at 9 years (control, 22%), 35% at 12 years (control, 0%) and 25% at 15 years (control, 0%); 2) for the 32 boys treated with protocol T, 100% were ambulatory at 9 years (control, 48%), 83% at 12 years (control, 0%) and 77% at 15 years (control, 0%); 3) in boys aged 13 and older, scoliosis developed in 30% of boys in protocol N, 16% in protocol T, and 90% of control subjects. 30% of boys, who were treated according to protocol T, had asymptomatic cataracts, but they did not require any treatment. Fractures occurred in 19% of boys in protocol N (controls: 16%) and 16% of boys in protocol T (controls: 20%). Summarizing, long term deflazacort treatment has beneficial effects on both protocols, although protocol T seems to be more effective and it is frequently associated with asymptomatic cataracts.

The same group (Biggar et al., 2006) designed a study involving 54 boys (30 treated with deflazacort), aged between 7 and 15 years, affected by DMD, who were reviewed retrospectively. The boys, untreated with deflazacort, stopped walking at 9.8 ± 1.8 years, while 7 out of 30 treated boys stopped walking at 12.3 ± 2.7 years ($P < 0.05$). Among the 23 boys who were still walking, 21 were 10 year older; pulmonary function was significantly greater in 15 year old treated boys (88% ± 18%) than in untreated boys (39% ± 20%) ($P<0.001$). Between 9 and 15 years, the treated boys were shorter and, between 9 and 13 years, the treated boys weighed less. After 13 years, the treated boys maintained their weight, whereas the untreated boys lost weight. Asymptomatic cataracts developed in 10 out of 30 boys who had received deflazacort.

Another clinical study compared the course of 74 boys, aged from 10 to 18 years, and affected by DMD, treated (n = 40) and untreated (n = 34) with deflazacort (Biggar et al., 2006). The treated boys were able to rise from a supine condition to standing, climb stairs, and walk 10 m without aids from 3 to 5 years longer than the untreated boys. After 10 years of age, the treated boys had a significantly better pulmonary function than the untreated boys and, after 15 years of age, 8 out of 17 untreated boys required nocturnal ventilation unlike the 40 treated boys. As for boys older than 15 years of age, 11 out of 17 untreated boys required assistance with feeding unlike the treated boys. Towards 18 years, 30 out of 34 untreated boys had a spinal curve greater than 20° if compared with 4 out of the 40 treated boys. By 18 years of age, 7 out of 34 untreated boys had lost 25% or more of their body weight (treated 0 out of 40) and four of those 7 boys required a gastric feeding tube. By 18 years of age, 20 out of 34 untreated boys had cardiac left ventricular ejection fractions, less than 45% if compared with 4 out of the 40 treated boys and 12 out of 34 died in their second decade (17.6 ± 1.7 years), primarily of cardiorespiratory complications. Two out of 40 boys, treated with deflazacort, died at 13 and 18 years of age from cardiac failure. The treated boys were significantly shorter, did not have excessive weight gain, and 22 out of 40 had asymptomatic cataracts. Long bone fractures occurred in 25% of boys in both the treated and untreated groups. The authors conclude that these long-term observations are the most encouraging. The major benefits of daily deflazacort appear to be the prolonged ambulation, improvement in cardiac and pulmonary functions, delay in the need for spinal instrumentation, and a greater independence for self-feeding. According to the described last two studies, deflazacort has a significant impact on health, quality of life, and healthcare costs for boys with DMD and their families and it is associated with a few side effects.

Houde and coworkers (Houde et al., 2008) collected data over an 8-year period for 79 patients with DMD, 37 of whom were treated with deflazacort. Deflazacort (dose of 0.9 mg/kg adjusted to a maximum of 1 mg/kg according to the side effects) was started when the boys showed a functional decline resulting in ambulating difficulties. The mean length of treatment was 66 months.

The treated boys stopped walking at 11.5 ± 1.9 years, whereas the untreated boys stopped walking at 9.6 ± 1.4 years. The cardiac function, assessed by echocardiography every 6 to 12 months, was better preserved as shown by a normal shortening fraction in treated (30.8% ± 4.5%) versus untreated boys (26.6% ± 5.7%, $P < 0.05$), a higher ejection fraction (52.9% ± 6.3% treated versus 46% ± 10% untreated), and lower frequency of dilated cardiomyopathy (32% treated versus 58% untreated). No change was observed in blood pressure, left ventricle end-diastolic diameter, or cardiac mass. Scoliosis was much less severe in treated (14° ± 22.5°) than in untreated boys (46° ± 224°) and no spinal surgery was necessary in treated boys. Limb fractures occurred in 24% of treated and in 26% of untreated boys, whereas vertebral fractures occurred in the treated group only (7 out of 37 compared with zero in the untreated group). In both groups, weight excess was observed at 8 years of age, and its frequency tripled between the ages of 8 and12 years. More patients had weight excess in the treated group (13 out of 21 [62%]) than in the untreated group (6 out of 11 [55%]), at 12 years of age. Cataracts developed in 49% of treated patients and, in almost all of these patients, they developed after at least 5 year treatment. This study underlines that deflazacort use in DMD prolongs walking for at least 2 years, slows the decline of vital capacity, and postpones the need for mechanical ventilation. The quality of life seems to improve in terms of prolonged independence in transfers and rolling over in bed, as well as sitting comfortably without having to resort to surgery.

A study determined and compared the long-term effects of prednisone and deflazacort on 49 boys, aged between 12 and 15 years, with DMD over a 7-year follow up period (Balaban et al., 2005). Eighteen boys were treated with prednisone, 12 with deflazacort, and 19 had no drug treatment. Analyzing their lower and upper limb motor functions, pulmonary function, prevalence of surgery for scoliosis and side effects, they reached these results: the boys in the steroid groups were significantly more functional and performed better on all tests than the untreated boys ($P < 0.05$); there was no significant difference between deflazacort- and prednisone-treated groups ($P > 0.05$); the number of boys having scoliosis surgery among the treated groups was significantly less than the one of untreated boys ($P<0.05$); the control group's capacity had decreased and was significantly less than the one of both the prednisone and deflazacort treated boys; both deflazacort and prednisone had beneficial effects on the pulmonary function and scoliosis; cataracts, hypertension, behavioural changes, excessive weight gain, and vertebral fracture were noted as serious side effects. The results of this long-term study are very encouraging and both prednisone and deflazacort seem to have a significant beneficial effect on slowing the disease progress. Their use in DMD may prolong ambulation and upper limb function with similar potency. Both steroids are also able to improve pulmonary function, more than delay the need for spinal interventions, with similar therapeutic profiles.

A study was performed in 17 patients affected by DMD, aged between 17 and 22 years, treated with deflazacort (0.9 mg/kg/day) and compared with DMD patients who did not receive any treatment, in order to evaluate the involvement of cardiac and sternocleidomastoid muscles by means of magnetic resonance imaging (MRI) measurement of T2 relaxation time and the left ventricular systolic function (Mavrogeni et al., 2009). This study showed that DMD patients, treated with deflazacort, present a better cardiac and skeletal profile compared to DMD patients without medication ($p<0.001$).

Dubowitz and colleagues (Dubowitz et al., 2002) reported a 5-year follow up of two 4-year-old boys, with classic DMD with an out-of-frame deletion in the Duchenne gene and absence of dystrophin in their muscle, who had a quite remarkable response to an intermittent, low dosage regime of prednisolone (0.75 mg/kg per day for 10 days each month or alternating 10 days on and 10 days off). In the first case, there was a complete remission of all clinical signs of dystrophy, sustained, almost fully, up to the present time; in the second case, the initial response was almost as marked, sustained for almost 5 years before showing a fairly rapid decline over the ensuing year that resulted in loss of independent ambulation at the age of 10. Both boys remained around the 50th percentile as for height and weight and showed no evidence of demineralization of bone on consecutive dual x-ray absorptiometry scanning of the spine nor any signs of chronic prednisolone toxicity. Although this study involved a limited number of patients, it showed that there might be an optimal window for treatment in the early stages of the disease and further larger-scale controlled studies should be targeted more selectively at this stage of the disease. This report also showed that a regime of low-dosage, intermittent prednisolone, with cycles of 10 day treatment, either per month or alternating with 10 days off treatment, is well tolerated in children affected by DMD.

Markham and colleagues (Markham et al., 2005) studied the effect of steroids in the cardiac function of patients with DMD. They evaluated the left ventricular systolic function and cardiac geometry of those subjects through a transthoracic echocardiogram; 111 patients, aged 21 years or younger, affected by DMD, were selected. They were divided into two groups: untreated (never exposed or treated for less than 6 months) and steroid-treated (steroids were administered longer than 6 months); the subjects did not differ in age, height, weight, body mass index, systolic and diastolic blood pressure, or left ventricular mass. Among the treated patients, 29 received prednisone and 19 received deflazacort. This study showed that treatment, either with prednisone or deflazacort, appears to have an impact on the decline in cardiac function seen with DMD. The shortening fraction was significantly lower in the untreated group than in the steroid-treated one. The authors concluded that deflazacort and prednisone were equally effective in preserving the cardiac function. This study shows that the progressive decline in cardiac muscle function can be altered by steroid treatment. In particular steroid treatment brings a clinical improvement in respiratory and cardiac function in DMD patients, during and beyond their treatment period. Moreover, it has the potential to prolong their survival.

A randomized controlled trial of prednisone and azathioprine, involving 99 boys aged between 5 and 15 years and affected by DMD, was conducted with the aim to assess the longer-term effects of prednisone and to determine whether azathioprine, alone or in combination with prednisone, is able to improve strength (Griggs et al., 1993). The patients were divided into 3 groups: placebo; 0.3 mg/kg prednisone per day; 0.75 mg/kg prednisone per day. After 6 months, 2 to 2.5 mg/kg azathioprine per day was added to the first two groups and placebo added to the third group. The study showed that the beneficial effect of prednisone (0.75mg/kg per day) is maintained for at least 18 months and it is associated with a 36% increase in muscle mass. Weight gain, growth retardation, and other side effects were associated with prednisone and azathioprine did not have any beneficial effect. The authors conclude that prednisone beneficial effect is not the result of immunosuppression.

Kirschner et al. (Kirschner et al., 2008) conducted a randomized, multicenter, double-blind placebo-controlled trial. One hundred and fifty three patients were randomized to receive either placebo or 4 mg/kg ciclosporin A (CsA). After 3 months, both groups received additional treatment with intermittent prednisone (0.75 mg/kg, 10 days on/10 days off) for 12 months more. In each group, 73 patients were available for intention to treat analysis. Baseline characteristics were comparable in both groups. There was no significant difference between the two groups concerning primary (manual muscle strength according to the Medical Research Council) and secondary (myometry, loss of ambulation, side effects) outcome measures. Peak CsA values were measured blindly and ranged from 12 to 658 ng/mL (mean, 210 ng/mL) in the verum group. According to this study CsA does not improve muscle strength as a monotherapy and the efficacy of intermittent prednisone in DMD. Calcineurin inhibitors induced chronic nephrotoxicity as reported in a previous study (Naesens et al., 2009).

Sharma and coworkers (Sharma et al., 1993) tested CsA in 15 patients affected by DMD and observed an increase in the muscular force generation, measuring the titanic force and maximum voluntary contraction (MVC) of both anterior tibial muscles. Normally the titanic force and MVC declined during 4 months in patients with DMD. During 8 week CsA treatment (5 mg/kg per day), the titanic force significantly increased (25.8% 6 6.6%) and MVC (13.6% 6 4.0%) occurred in two weeks' time. The CsA side effects, gastrointestinal and flu-like symptoms were transient and self-limiting. Straathof and colleagues (Straathof et al., 2009) retrospectively analyzed 35 DMD patients' data, who were treated with 0.75 mg/kg prednisone per day intermittently, 10 days on/10 days off. Prednisone was started during the ambulant phase at the age 3.5 up to 9.7 years. The median period of treatment was 27 months. The authors reported the following results: the median age at which ambulation was lost was 10.8 years; 9 patients (26%) had excessive weight gain; 8 boys (21%) had a bone fracture that happened when four of those 8 children lost the ability to walk. Treatment was stopped in 2 obese patients, 2 hyperactive boys, and 1 patient after a fracture. Based on the previously described data, the authors conclude that prednisone, 10 days on/10 days off, has relatively few side effects and extends the ambulant phase for 1 year if compared to historical controls.

5. Exon skipping

DMD is caused by mutations in the dystrophin gene (Aartsma-Rus et al., 2006; Muntoni, 2003), leading to disruption of the open reading frame (Fig. 2a). Monaco et al. (Monaco et al., 1988) found that frame shift mutations in the DMD gene will lead to a truncated and non-functional dystrophin. Patients with such mutations present less severe Becker muscular dystrophy. This reading frame rule holds true for ~91% of DMD cases (Aartsma-Rus et al., 2006) and has inspired the development of the exon skipping strategy which employs antisense oligonucleotides (AON). These small synthetic RNA molecules are complimentary to exonic or splice site sequences, thereby, upon hybridization, they are able to modulate exon inclusion by the splicing machinery (Manzur et al., 2009; Trollet et al., 2009; van Ommen et al., 2008). Although the functionality of the resulting protein may vary, this treatment could delay or even stop disease progression and improve function in the remaining muscle (Melis et al., 1998; Helderman-van den Enden et al., 2010). The antisense oligonucleotides are chemically modified to resist nucleases and promote RNA binding and are designed to have high sequence specificity. A lot of studies have provided the proof of principle of the therapeutic feasibility of the AON to reframe dystrophin transcripts and restore dystrophin synthesis, both in vitro (Aartsma-Rus et al., 2002, 2003, 2004) and in vivo using the mdx and DMD mice (Mann et al., 2002; Bremmer-Bout et al., 2004; Heemskerk et al., 2009). In studies in the mdx mouse model, oligonucleotides with chemical properties, similar to the ones of 2′-O-methyl-phosphorothioate (2′OMePS) RNA, were taken up in dystrophin-deficient muscle up to 10 times as much as in healthy muscle tissue, most likely owing to increased permeability of the muscle myofiber membrane. In addition, 4 to 8 weeks′ subcutaneous delivery of the oligonucleotides resulted in a steady increase in oligonucleotides levels, exon skipping and dystrophin levels (Heemskerk et al., 2010).

Exon skipping provides a mutation-specific, and so potentially personalized, therapeutic approach for patients with DMD (Fig. 2b). Since mutations cluster around exons 45-55 of DMD, the skipping of one specific exon may be therapeutic for patients with a variety of mutations. The skipping of exon 51 affects the largest subgroup of patients (approximately 13%), including the ones with deletions of exons 45 to 50, 48 to 50, or 52 (Aartsma-Rus et al., 2009). Subsequent clinical trials have shown that two different AON chemistries, either 2′OMePS (van Deutekom et al., 2007) or phosphorodiamidate morpholino oligomer (PMO) (Kinali et al., 2009), targeting DMD exon 51, can restore local dystrophin synthesis in DMD patients with no or minimum side effects. However, some relevant points of pathophysiologic DMD cascade, such as severe muscle wasting, fibrosis and deficient muscle regeneration, may reduce the efficacy of the DMD exon skipping therapy. In addition, as DMD patients suffer from muscle degeneration from their early life, myoblasts undergo extensive division in an attempt to regenerate, eventually leading to exhaustion of the muscle regenerative potential (Yoshida et al., 1998; Hawke et al., 2001; Blau et al., 1985). To overcome these problems, there have been several additional therapies in which myostatin inhibition has received considerable interest (Kemaladewi et al., 2011).

Here we report the three clinical trials based on the exon skipping approach which have been performed to date and we describe the trials that are still ongoing. A study, consisting in the injection of 0.8 mg of PRO051 into the tibialis anterior muscle, was performed by van Deutekom and colleagues (van Deutekom et al., 2007). PRO051 is a 2'OMePS antisense oligoribonucleotide complementary to a 20-nucleotide sequence within exon 51. Four patients with DMD were included in this study and they all had deletions that were correctable by exon-51skipping and had no evidence of dystrophin in the previously made diagnostic muscle biopsy. For every patient mutational status and positive exon-skipping response to PRO051 in vitro were confirmed, and T1-weighted MRI was used to determine the condition of the tibialis anterior muscle. The intramuscular injection of PRO051 induced exon-51 skipping, corrected the reading frame, and thus introduced dystrophin in the muscle in all four patients affected by DMD. PRO051 restored dystrophin to levels between 3-12% or 17- 35%, basing on quantification relative to total protein or myofiber content. The poorest results that were obtained in a patient, who had the most advanced disease, led the authors to underline the importance of using patients at a relatively young age, since in them relatively little muscle tissue has been replaced by fibrotic and adipose tissue. Among the adverse effects, mild local pain at the injection site was reported by a patient. Mild-to-moderate pain, after the muscle biopsy, was also reported. Blistering under the bandages used for wound closure was reported by two patients. In the period of time elapsing between injection and biopsy, flu-like symptoms were observed in two patients and a mild diarrhea in a patient.

A dose escalation intramuscular trial was performed in 7 patients (2 patients received 0·09 mg and 5 patients received 0·9 mg of AVI-4658) who received injections in one extensor digitorum brevis (EDB) muscle, while the contralateral EDB muscle was injected with 900 μL normal saline (Kinali et al., 2009). The 7 patients had deletions in the open reading frame of DMD that are responsive to exon 51 and were selected on the basis of the preservation of EDB muscle, as assessed by MRI, and the response of cultured fibroblasts from a skin biopsy to AVI-4658. Muscles were biopsied between 3 and 4 weeks after injection. No adverse events, related to AVI-4658, were reported in this study and they showed an increased dystrophin expression in all treated EDB muscles. Immunostaining of EDB-treated muscle for dystrophin was performed. In the areas of the immunostained sections that were close to the needle track through which AVI-4658 was given, 44–79% of myofibres had increased expression of dystrophin. In randomly chosen sections of treated EDB muscles, the mean intensity of dystrophin staining ranged from 22% to 32% of the mean intensity of dystrophin in healthy control muscles (mean 26·4%), and the mean intensity was 17% (range 11–21%) greater than the intensity in the contralateral saline-treated muscle. In the dystrophin-positive fibres, the intensity of dystrophin staining was up to 42% of that in healthy muscle. Western blot analysis detected increased expression of dystrophin in the AVI-4658-treated muscle of all patients who received the high dose, and the immunoblot detected expression of dystrophin of the expected molecular weight in all patients. This study has led to a dose-ranging systemic study of AVI-4658 in ambulant patients affected by DMD (ClinicalTrials.gov, number NCT00844597).

A phase 1-2a study has been conducted to assess the safety, pharmacokinetics and molecular and clinical effects of systemically administered PRO051 (Goemans et al., 2011). PRO051 was administered subcutaneously for 15 weeks in 12 patients, with each of four possible doses (0.5, 2.0, 4.0, and 6.0 mg per kilogram of body weight) given to 3 patients. Irritation at the administration site and, during the extension phase, mild and variable proteinuria and increased urinary α(1)-microglobulin levels were reported. The mean terminal half-life of PRO051 in the circulation was 29 days. PRO05, at the dose of 2.0 mg per kilogram or higher, induced specific exon-51 skipping. In 10 patients new dystrophin expression was observed between approximately 60% and 100% of muscle fibers, as observed in post-treatment biopsy. New dystrophin expression increased dose-dependently up to 15.6% of the expression in healthy muscle. After the 12 week extension phase, a modest improvement was observed in the 6 minute walk test (Netherlands National Trial Register number, NTR1241).

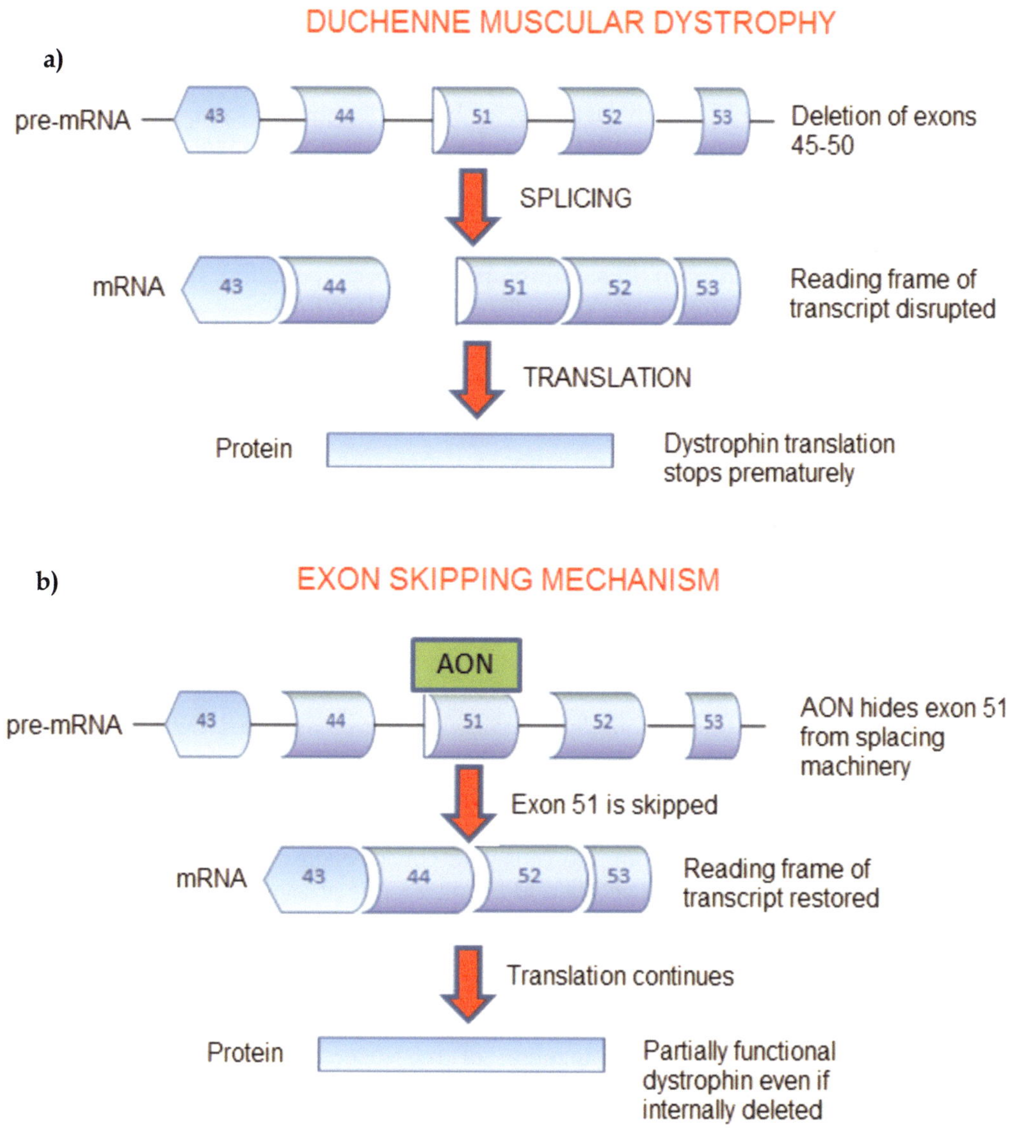

Fig. 2. a) Duchenne muscular dystrophy is caused by mutations in the dystrophin gene, leading to disruption of the open reading frame; b) Exon skipping mechanism in Duchenne muscular dystrophy.

6. Ongoing clinical trials

Several clinical trials, involving DMD patients, and based on the exon skipping approach are ongoing. A phase 1 trial is testing a drug (GSK2402968) that has been designed to skip exon 51 of the dystrophin gene, assessing the safety and tolerability of the drug in boys/adolescents who are unable to walk. The absorption and processing of the drug in their bodies will be also studied. This trial is expected to end in September 2011. A Phase 1/2 trial is investigating whether the experimental drug PRO044 is safe and effective as a therapy for people with DMD with a mutation in a specific region of the dystrophin gene, i.e. exon 44. The expecting end date of the trial is December 2011. Another phase 2 trial is investigating GSK2402968 (two different doses), a drug that has been designed to skip exon 51 of the dystrophin gene. The aim of the study is to determine if an intermittent treatment with GSK2402968 will lead to a better long-term safety profile, while maintaining its effectiveness. This trial is expected to end in September 2012. A phase 3 trial is undergoing testing a drug (GSK2402968) that has been designed to skip exon 51 of the dystrophin gene. It will assess the effect of GSK2402968 on the muscle function of boys with DMD and will monitor the safety of the drug. It is expected to end in December 2012 (The information contained in this paragraph has been collected from the website http://www.musculardystrophy.org/research/clinical_trials/0/duchenne+muscular+dystrophy accessed on 18/05/2011).

7. Cell-based therapy

The cell-based therapy, or cell transplantation, involves different procedures with injected cell pool to correct some functional tissue or organ impairment. Depending on the pathology to be treated, the protocol of cell graft is specific. In genetic disorders, cells are genetically corrected with ex vivo procedure and grafted. In degenerative disorders, cells are amplified and injected. In cancer or infectious pathologies, the cells are selected on the base of immunoreacting or immunomodulating properties, amplified and injected in patients. The cells can derive from other species (xenotransplantation), other subjects (heterologous) or the receiver (autologous). Using cells deriving from other organism, xenotransplantation and heterologous transplantation are associated with the immunosuppressive therapy which reduces host immune-reaction against graft. It is important to decide which cell type to transplant. Based on remaining differentiate ability and plasticity, it is possible to choose the stem cell origin (embryonic, foetal or adult), progenitor cells or terminally committed cells, and collect them from the tissue of interest. Based on remaining differentiated ability and plasticity, it is possible to choose the stem cell origin (embryonic, foetal or adult), progenitor cells or terminally committed cells, from a selected specific tissue and followed by a process and purification before graft. They are frequently amplified and specifically stimulated to increase and improve grafted pool. In autologous transplantation treating genetic disorder, the cells are genetically handled to revert mutation. Depending on localization of the disorder, the cells are locally or systemically injected. The strategies of the cell-based therapy, adopted for DMD, are two: ex vivo genetic correction in autologous cells, followed by graft or heterologous injection of cells. It allows to evaluate rapidly the improvement or disadvantages of the therapy, avoiding severe complications due to impairment in vital muscles. Heterologous transplantation allows to inject low-handled healthy cells with the certainty of avoiding dys mutations. Unfortunately, the immunosuppressive therapy is necessary to protect graft from host immune system.

8. Cell types

In these last few years, stem cells have received a lot of attention for their potential use in cell-based therapies for various human diseases including DMD (Lodi et al., 2011; Farini et al., 2009). For several years, after they were discovered, the satellite cells were considered as the only cells responsible for the growth and maintenance of the skeletal muscle (Le Grand and Rudnicki, 2007a; Le Grand and Rudnicki, 2007b). With the improvements of cell-isolation technology, a number of markers were described to identify a lot of muscular and nonmuscular subpopulations able to actively participate in myogenesis. Recent works have described the partial identification and characterization of multilineage stem cells derived in culture from numerous adult tissues. In the skeletal muscle itself, rather than satellite cells, alternative adult multi-lineage progenitor cell populations showed to have a myogenic potential: muscle-derived stem cells (MDSCs) (Sarig et al., 2006), muscle side-population (mSP) cells (Wognum et al., 2003) and muscle-derived CD133+ progenitors (Peault et al., 2007). Several works have described how nonmuscular resident stem cells could participate in myogenesis: the bone marrow-derived mesenchymal stem cells (BMMSCs) can differentiate into mesodermal cells, including myoblasts (Pittenger et al., 1999; Prockop, 1997) and adult tissue host cells can also contribute to endodermal and ectodermal cell lineages (Krause et al., 2001; Mezey et al., 2000). A subpopulation of CD133+ cells that play an important role in myogenic development, has been isolated from blood (Torrente et al., 2004). Furthermore, other stem cells have been identified in the dorsal aorta of avian and mammalian species, the so-called mesoangioblasts (Cossu and Bianco, 2003), while the pericytes were found in the basement membrane of the vessels (Dellavalle et al., 2007).

9. Satellite cells

Satellite cells derive from a progenitor population paired box protein 3 and 7 (Pax3 and Pax7, muscle and neural crest development markers) +/+ localized in the central portion of the dermomyotome, the dorso-lateral part of the somite. During the fetal development, the resident progenitor population generates cells in satellite position around myofibers, which are marked by the expression of Pax7, while the limb muscle satellite cells arise from hypaxial cells expressing Pax3. (Le Grand and Rudnicki, 2007b). The satellite cells are located beneath the basal lamina of mature skeletal muscle fibres, and they are ideally positioned to repair degenerating muscle fibres. These quiescent cells are activated to proliferate upon muscle injury or when heavily used during activities such as weight lifting or running. This proliferation step is necessary to generate sufficient numbers of myoblasts for muscle differentiation and myotube formation. In humans, these mononuclear cells are most plentiful at birth (estimated at 32% of sublaminar nuclei). Their frequency declines postnatally, stabilizing between 1% and 5% of skeletal muscle nuclei in the adult muscle. In humans, the proportion of satellite cells in skeletal muscles also decreases with age, and it could explain the decreased efficiency of muscle regeneration in older subjects. Satellite cells from aged muscle also display reduced proliferative and fusion capacity, as well as a tendency to store fat, thus deteriorating their regeneration potential. Satellite cells present an extended proliferative potential and can repopulate extensively the host's muscle with an efficiency unknown in any other experimental situation (Cooper et al., 2006).

10. Multipotent muscle-derived stem cells

Recent studies have demonstrated the existence of a population of multipotent muscle-derived stem cells (MMDSCs), distinct from satellite cells, with high myogenic potential in vitro, even after being appropriately stimulated to differentiate into other lineages, such as haematopoietic. MMDSCs reside in skeletal muscle sharing the ability to self-renew and differentiate into other mesodermal cell types (Farini et al., 2009). MDSCs were isolated on the base of their adhesion ability. The cells, obtained by enzymatic digestion of muscle tissue, are seeded on a culture dish and, after 1 hour, the medium and non-adherent cells are transferred to another dish (preplating). Then, analogous preplates are repeated at 24 hour intervals until preplate 6 (pp6) is completed. The cells, which rapidly attach to the surface, are mainly fibroblasts (pp1), cells which adhere within 24-48 hours. They are predominantly satellite cells (pp2 - pp4) and the population, which settle at the most slowest speed on a flask, consists of multipotential stem cells (pp-6). The phenotype of fraction pp6 is described as stem cell antigen-1 (sca-1), CD34+ (marker of hematopoietic and satellite cells), CD45-, c-kit- (markers of hematopoietic cells) with the expression of desmin (marker of myogenic cells) on a different level. MDSCs, cultured in vitro, differentiate spontaneously into myotubes but, when appropriately stimulated, these cells can also give rise either to osteoblasts , chondroblasts , hematopoietic cells or endothelial cells. MDSCs firmly adhere to endothelium in mdx muscles microcirculation and then participate in muscle regeneration, following an intramuscular injection. Interestingly, they have also been found in muscles, after intravenous administration, and their number was higher in muscles, previously injured, than in the control ones. The expression of desmin gradually decreases with subsequent preplates and in pp6 population only about 10-20% of cells are positive for this protein. However, pp6 cells, cultured in standard conditions, spontaneously enter the myogenic pathway that is associated with an increased desmin expression. It has also been demonstrated that the majority of MDSCs is positive as for desmin. The studies, regarding cell viability after transplantation, have shown that more MDSCs survive following intramuscular administration, if compared to more differentiated cells (myoblasts). After the injection of the same number of either MDSCs or early preplate (EP) cells, the contribution to muscle regeneration, 30 and 90 days later, has been even 10 times higher in MDSC group. Marked differences have probably been associated with the distinct immunogenicity between MDSCs and EP cells. The evaluation of major histocompatibility complex (MHC-1) expression in cell membranes of both cell types has revealed that MHC-1 is present in 63% of EP cells, whereas only in 0.5% of MDSCs. However, MDSCs are a much less numerous cell population if compared to "typical" satellite cells which dominate in EP group. Only one clone of MDSCs can be obtained from 10^5 of cells originally isolated from muscle tissue (Lee-Pullen and Grounds, 2005). MMDSCs could also be distinguished by flow cytometry. After staining with Hoechst 33324, it was possible to characterize a cell population, called skeletal muscle side population (SMSP) or simply side population (SP), which is able to extrude dye via ATP-binding cassette G2 (ABCG2) multi-drug resistant pump. SP expresses several surface markers associated with haematopoietic stem cells (HSCs) including CD45, c-kit, Sca-1 and CD34, but no satellite cell markers such as M-cadherin, Pax7 or desmin. SP cells can give rise to all hematopoetic lines, both in vitro and in vivo. The question of myogenic potential is more complex. The SP cells, harvested in vitro, do not differentiate spontaneously into myocytes. However, cell-mediated inductive interactions trigger myogenic potential of SP cells. These cells contain two distinct fractions with myogenic potential, such as CD45+ and CD45-, both exhibiting the potential to constitute myogenic cells after a co-culture with primary myoblasts. In particular, CD45+ SP are able to integrate into regenerating muscle fibres after an intramuscular injection, while the sub-fraction CD45- SP has the potential to give rise to adipocytes and osteocyte. Regardless of hematopoietic and myogenic potential, SP also displays endothelial trait (CD31+). Moreover, it has been shown that SP expresses angiopoietin 2 and the Tie2 receptor, which is bound and activated by angiopoietins. It means, that most of the SP cells share partially signalling pathways with endothelial/hematopoietic precursor cell populations. SP cells demonstrate that lack of Pax7 gene in experimental animals does not influence the number of muscle SP cells. Furthermore, Pax7-/- SP cells can differentiate into myotubes when co-cultured with myoblasts. It indicates that Pax7 gene is not required for myogenic specification of SP cells. Finally, forced expression of MyoD induces myogenic differentiation of Pax7-/- SP cells, but not pax7-/- myoblasts. All these data suggest that SMSP and satellite cells are distinct populations and probably have different origin (Burdzinska et al., 2008).

11. Blood- and muscle-derived CD133+ progenitors

CD133+ cells are considered to be haematopoietic and endothelial stem cells of bone marrow origin that could give rise to both endothelial cells and myoblasts. Circulating human CD133+ cells demonstrate stemness properties and the ability to restore dystrophin expression and eventually regenerate the satellite cell pool in dystrophic scid/mdx mouse after intra-muscular and intra-arterial delivery. Skeletal muscle CD133+ stem cell have the potential to differentiate towards both muscle and endothelium lineages. Dystrophic human CD133+ are able to express an exon-skipped version of human dystrophin, after transduction with a lentivirus, carrying a construct designed to skip exon 51; therefore their ability to participate in muscle regeneration has been examined after transplantation into scid/mdx mice. The comparison of two distinct CD133+ cell populations, one from blood and one from skeletal muscle, show that the muscle-derived CD133+ stem cells have the potential to differentiate towards both muscle and endothelium lineages. Skipped blood and muscle-derived Δ49–50 stem cells, fused in vivo with regenerative fibres, express a functional human dystrophin and restructure the dystrophin-associated protein complex, as shown by plasmalemmal re-expression of a and b-sarcoglycan proteins. Moreover, being sometimes located beneath the basal lamina, and distributed along freshly isolated fibres, it is interesting to assess whether muscle-derived CD133+ stem cells are able to differentiate into satellite cells. Genetically engineered DMD muscle-derived CD133+ cells show a better muscle regeneration in terms of spreading and number of positive fibres in comparison with the results obtained from blood-derived stem cells. DMD muscle-derived CD133+ cells are more efficient than their blood counterpart in the improvement of morphology and restoration of the normal skeletal muscle function in dystrophic murine muscles. Human CD133+ cells, isolated from muscle or blood, are able to promote muscular- and endothelial-differentiation after intra-arterial and intra-muscular delivery. These cells can be injected safely in DMD patients, not only without side effects, but also promoting an increase in the number of capillaries per muscle fibres. Moreover, DMD CD133+ cells can be genetically modified to re-express a functional dystrophy. Unfortunately, several things need to be ameliorated, such as the potential to enhance proliferation of blood-derived CD133+ cells in culture and storage for repeated treatments, the relative efficiency of blood-derived cells, compared with muscle-derived cells to contribute to muscle nuclei, the strategy to deliver myogenic cells chronically to the various sites of sporadic regeneration that occur in muscular dystrophies (Farini et al., 2009; Peault et al., 2007).

12. Mesenchymal stem cells

Mesenchymal stem cells (MSCs) are conventionally defined as adherent, non-hematopoietic cells expressing markers such as CD90, CD105, and CD73, and being negative for CD14, CD34, and CD45. While originally identified in the bone marrow, MSCs have been extracted from numerous tissues including adipose tissue, heart, Wharton's jelly, dental pulp, peripheral blood, cord blood menstrual blood, and, more recently, Fallopian tube. One of the major properties of MSCs is the ability to differentiate into various tissues. The traditional differentiation properties of MSCs are their ability to become adipocytes, chondrocytes, and osteocytes in vitro, after treatment with induction agents. Non-orthodox differentiation into other tissues, for example, cells resembling neurons, muscles, hepatocytes and pancreatic islets, has also been reported. There is some evidence that MSCs may differentiate selectively into tissues that have been injured. The ease of obtaining bone marrow sample and myogenic potential of MSCs makes this population an attractive candidate for cellular transplantation in cases of diseases associated with muscle dysfunction. However, there are still a lot of controversies around the level of myogenic potential of mesenchymal cells. Numerous studies were focused on the methodology of induction of MSC differentiation into muscle cells. Contrasting results were obtained treating MSCs with DNA methyltransferase inhibitor, such as 5-azacitidine, or galectin-1 as the factor initializing myogenesis of MSCs (Chan et al., 2006; Liu et al., 2003). Regarding BMMSC myogenic potential, interesting results were achieved culturing the cells by a mixture of cytokines and growth factors (fibroblast growth factor beta (βFGF), forskolin, plateled derived growth factor (PDGF), neuregulin and subsequently transfected with gene encoding Notch 1 intracellular domain (NICD). Following this procedure, cells differentiated into muscle cells with the efficacy of 89% (Dezawa et al., 2005). An alternative approach to induce myogenesis in MSCs, is the exposure of these cells to myogenic environment. MSCs, co-cultured with cardiomycytes or satellite cells, differentiated into either cardiac cells or myotubes respectively (Fukuhara et al., 2003; Lee et al., 2005). However, the differentiation rate in these conditions was highly limited. The fate of MSCs, injected into either skeletal or cardiac muscle, was also analyzed (Shi et al., 2004). It has been demonstrated that undifferentiated MSCs can undergo myogenesis after an intramuscular administration but, similarly to the in vitro studies, the proportion of differentiated cells was barely detectable, only 0,44% of transplanted MSCs fused in myotubes. Gene-corrected DMD MSCs restored dystrophin expression in co-cultured dystrophic myoblasts through spontaneous cell fusion (Goncalves et al., 2006a). Furthermore, a study where dystrophic MSCs transfected by recombinant adenovirus, which contains human microdystrophin cDNA, were injected into mdx mouse, showed that expression of dystrophin was detected in dystrophic tissue (Xiong et al., 2007). A study has also compared MSCs transplantation with and without prior differentiation. Cells were injected around the myocardial infarcted area of a rabbit model. The improvement in left ventricular function, vascular density and reduction of infarcted area did not differ significantly between the two groups. The perspective to transplant undifferentiated mesenchymal stem cells seems to be promising because it does not require time-consuming and expensive extracorporeal manipulations in cells (Ichim et al., 2010).

13. Mesoangioblasts

Mesoangioblasts are multipotent progenitors of mesodermal tissues, physically associated with the embryonic dorsal aorta in avian and mammalian species. Mesoangioblasts are able to differentiate into various mesodermal phenotypes. Mesoangioblast-like cells have been isolated from vessels of post-natal tissues. Post-natal cells generally express pericytes rather than endothelial cell markers, but they are otherwise similar to their embryonic counterparts in terms of proliferation and differentiation potency. When wild-type or dystrophic, genetically corrected mesoangioblasts are delivered intra-arterially to dystrophic muscle of α-sarcoglycan- null mice (a model for limb girdle muscular dystrophy), they induce a dramatic functional amelioration of the dystrophic phenotype. This is due to the widespread distribution of the donor's cells through the capillary network and to an intrinsic defect of proliferation in the resident satellite cells, a situation that creates a selective advantage for the injected donor cells. To proceed with clinical experimentation, it has been considered to be crucial that the delivery and muscle homing of mesoangioblasts may be optimized to characterize human cells in depth and the protocol needs to be tested in a large animal model. Recently, it has been reported that the enhancing delivery of mesoangioblasts leads to the complete reconstitution of downstream skeletal muscles in α-sarcoglycan-null dystrophic mice. Mesoangioblasts, exposed in vitro to either stromal cell derived factor-1 or TNF-α, have showed enhanced transmigration in vitro and migration into dystrophic muscle in vivo. Transient expression of α-4 integrins or l-selectin have also produced a several-fold increase in migration, both in vitro and in vivo. Mesoangioblasts, transduced with a lentiviral vector expressing human microdystrophin and injected scid/mdx mice and immunosuppressed dystrophic golden retriever muscular dystrophy (GRMD) dogs, have showed a modified mesoangioblasts-induced dystrophin positivity in myofibres. In particular, the results of these injections have been promising in the dystrophic dogs with improvements in their muscle function and mobility together with an increased dystrophin expression. In order to ameliorate the efficiency of the muscle repair by mesoangioblasts, cell migration to skeletal muscle has been improved and unspecific trapping in the capillary filters of the body, such as liver and lung, has been reduced (Farini et al., 2009).

14. Bone marrow stem cells

In the last decade, it has been discovered the contribution of various nonmyogenic cells in the regeneration of skeletal muscle, such as bone marrow-derived cells (BMDCs) and the circulating haematopoietic cells. With the advent of more sensitive markers, it has been demonstrated that BMDCs can enter the sites of muscle regeneration and also contribute to the formation of new muscle fibres. Furthermore, similar cells, resident in skeletal muscle, appeared to reconstitute the bone marrow and, via this route, enter again and contribute to the regeneration of skeletal muscle. In this sense, it has been demonstrated that the intravenous injection of either normal HSCs or a novel population of MDSCs into irradiated mdx mice resulted in the reconstitution of the haematopoietic compartment of the transplanted recipients, the incorporation of donor-derived nuclei into muscle, and the partial restoration of dystrophin expression in the affected muscle. Similarly, after the transplantation into immunodeficient mice, BMDCs migrated into areas of induced muscle degeneration, underwent myogenic differentiation, and participated in the regeneration of the damaged fibres. Following the transplantation in irradiated mice ablated of endogenous satellite cells, the transplanted BMDCs were able to occupate the niche of those satellite cells. Furthermore, BMDC satellite cells participated in the regeneration of multinucleated muscle fibres at high frequency, becoming heritably myogenic. As these results were obtained using the whole bone marrow as transplant source, and since it is known to contain haematopoietic and non-haematopoietic progenitors, it is possible to speculate that the bone marrow could contain such progenitors for muscle and blood. On the other hand, a common progenitor with haematopoietic potential could generate myogenic cells due to either physiological stimuli and fusion with a myogenic cell (Farini et al., 2009).

15. Pericytes

Pericytes wrap around the vascular tube and interdigitate with the endothelial cells in the basement membrane of the vessels, playing a fundamental role in the maintenance of microcirculation functionality. Pericytes can be mobilized from the adult bone marrow under ischemic conditions, and utilized for their contractile capabilities and their multiple cytoplasmic processes. It has been demonstrated that pericytes have a high capacity of myogenic differentiation because they give rise to a high number of muscular fibres, when injected into scid/mdx mice. It has been proposed that the pericyte could be released from its position on a vascular tube in the case of a focal injury, functioning as an immunomodulatory and trophic mesenchymal stem cell. The activity of the pericyte ensures that the field of damage remains limited and that tissue-intrinsic progenitors replace the expired cells. As provided by this evidence, these stem cells could represent a good candidate for the muscle therapy because they could be isolated from a muscle biopsy and therefore easily accessible. They can be cultured in vitro without loss of stem-cell properties and are able to regenerate skeletal muscle after muscular and arterial injection. Nevertheless, it would be important to determine whether transplanted pericytes can fully reconstitute the satellite cell niche as a real functional stem cell. More information are needed about the role of pericytes, in both normal and dystrophic skeletal muscle, in order to avoid that the injection of these cells into human dystrophic muscle environment could elicit pericyte-derived tumours.

16. Adipocytes

Adipocytes share the same mesodermal origin with skeletal muscle. An inverse relationship, between skeletal muscle mass and adipose tissue mass, is apparent in murine models of skeletal muscle dystrophic pathology such as mdx where the relative level of fat tissue, within the diseased muscle, has increased. Moreover, in the myostatin-/- mouse, where the skeletal muscle mass has hugely increased, the fat tissue mass is reduced substantially. Moreover, cell culture studies have demonstrated that myogenic cell lines, when made to overexpress adipogenic transcription factors peroxisome proliferator-activated receptor gamma (PPARγ) and CCAAT/enhancer-binding protein alpha (C/EBPα) lose their myogenic marker expression and differentiate into adipocytes, suggesting that the adult myoblasts are capable of being reprogrammed to become adipocytes. Furthermore, the satellite cell population has been shown to be capable of conversion into the adipocyte lineage, given the correct cues. A more recent work has provided good evidence that the adipocyte lineage can also undergo conversion into myoblasts. An adipocyte-specific stem cell population that expressed high levels of CD13, CD44, CD73 and CD90 and was negative for CD34, CD45, CD56 and CD184, suggesting mesenchymal stem cell-like characteristics, was recently isolated and has shown to display myogenic markers and fuse with maturing myofibres when co-cultured with myoblast cell lines. Furthermore, it has been demonstrated that cells, isolated from the stromal vascular fraction of adipose tissue, which have been shown to differentiate in vitro into adipogenic, chondrogenic, osteogenic and myogenic cells, can spontaneously form myotubes when cultured under standard conditions in vitro. Furthermore, these cells are able to fuse into myotubes following in vitro expansion and following injection into ischaemic murine hind limbs. They also form new myofibres and are capable of restoring dystrophin expression in mdx mice, thus displaying a therapeutic potential. More recently, a more specific CD45- side population of adipocyte progenitor cells, purified from the stromal vascular fraction, has been shown to form myofibres in vivo. An array analysis of murine brown fat precursor cell populations has recently shown that certain myogenic transcription factors, including myogenin, Myf5 and MyoD, are expressed at levels comparable with C2C12 cells within these progenitors. These data are in keeping with the previous lineage-tracing studies that showed a dermomyotomal origin for brown, but not white, fat precursor cells. Moreover, brown fat lineage cells also express the known myogenic microRNAs miR-1 miR-133a and miR-206, suggesting that brown adipocytes share a common ancestor with myogenic cells. Subsequently, it has been demonstrated that the transcription factor PRD1-BF1-RIZ1 homologous domain containing 16 (PRDM16), is sufficient and necessary to drive the conversion of white adipocytes into brown adipocytes, through an up-regulation of uncoupling protein and PPARγ coactivator-1alpha (PGC1-α) expression. It shows to be a key regulator in the formation of the brown fat lineage. PRDM16 drives the brown fat lineage by forming a transcriptional complex with C-terminal binding protein 1 or 2, whereby it acts to repress white fat-specific genes or complexing with PGC1-α, and PPARγ Coactivator 1-beta (PGC1-β) according to which it enhances expression of brown fat genes. Recently, it has been elegantly shown that brown fat cells arise from a Myf5+ common precursor that was previously only thought to form skeletal muscle cells. Furthermore, PRDM16 overexpression causes brown fat cells to undergo a lineage switch, forming skeletal myoblasts through the activation of PPAR-γ, whereas PRDM16- /- brown fat has elevated myogenic gene transcription and reduced uncoupling ability. Subsequently, it has been shown that human skeletal muscle contains a population of brown fat precursor cells that up-regulates uncoupling protein 1 following PPAR-γ agonist treatment. Finally, human adipose tissue-derived mesenchymal stem cells have been shown to differentiate into myofibres spontaneously as well as induce dystrophin expression following co-culture with human DMD myoblasts in vitro through a cell fusion. These data show that adipogenic stem cells may be used for therapeutic applications (Otto et al., 2009).

17. Clinical trials

Myoblast transplantation is a possible treatment for DMD. Promising results in vivo nude/mdx mouse transplantation was obtained and in the 90's a series of clinical trials on DMD patients was conducted. Huard et al. (Huard, et al. 1991; Huard, et al. 1992) transplanted myoblasts from an immunocompatible donor into the limb muscles of 4 DMD patients in the advanced stages of the disease. A different degree of dystrophin was detected by immunostaining in the patients, but this change slowly decayed over time and it was not associated to a strength improvement. Although no immunosuppressive treatment was used, no patient showed any clinical sign of rejection. The effects of myoblast transplantations, without an immunosuppressive treatment on muscle strength and the formation of dystrophin-positive fibers, were studied in five young boys with DMD, using a triple blind design. No increase in the static contraction was detected. The expression of dystrophin in myoblast-injected fibers was generally low and it decreased to control level in 6 months. These results strongly suggest that myoblast transplantations, as well as gene therapy for DMD, cannot be done without immunosuppression (Tremblay et al., 1993). Karpati et al. (Karpati et al., 1993) used cyclophosphamide as an immunosuppressive agent to improve the myoblast transfer; however, subsequent experiments demonstrated that this antitumour drug killed the transplanted myoblasts, as well as any other rapidly proliferating cells. Normal dystrophin was detected, by reverse-transcriptase polymerase chain reaction, in DMD patients after myoblast transplantation, but it was not associated to an increase in the percentage of dystrophin-positive fibers (Gussoni et al., 1992). Immunosuppression of DMD boys by cyclosporine, during myoblast transplantation, improved force generation, but it was not effective in replacing clinically significant amounts of dystrophin in DMD muscle (Miller et al., 1997). Mendell et al. (Mendell et al., 1995) injected myoblast, once a month for six months, in 12 DMD patients, but this treatment failed to improve strength. Law et al. (Law et al., 1992) demonstrated the feasibility and safety of myoblast transplantation, but with a poor clinical improvement. At the end of the 90's, a careful overview of the previous initial trials brought several research teams to identify three problems responsible for the limited results observed: (1) 3 days after the graft, at least 75% of the transplanted myoblasts died (Fan et al., 1996; Guerette et al., 1997; Huard et al., 1994); (2) myoblasts were not able to migrate more than 200 μm away from the intramuscular injection trajectory (Skuk et al., 1999); (3) if immunosuppression was not adequate, the myoblasts were rapidly rejected in less than 2 weeks (Guerette et al., 1994) or were induced to activate apoptosis, such as cyclophosphamide usage (Hardiman et al., 1993; Hong et al., 2002). There are now some solutions to overcome these problems. The rapid death of a large percentage of myoblasts can be compensated by the transplantation of a high number of cells. Indeed the transplantation of 30 million cells per mm^3 has given very good results in monkeys (Skuk et al., 1999). In monkeys, the low migration distance of myoblasts was avoided by a high number of adjacent intramuscular injections, i.e. 100 injections per cm^2 of muscle surface. High density of intramuscular injections of myoblast in 11 DMD patients were also well tolerated. One patient received a total of 4,000 intramuscular injections without any complication. No infection or other complication, related to the procedure, was registered (Skuk et al., 2007). An interesting improvement in myoblast migration injected in muscle was obtained by the modulation of MyoD expression (El Fahime et al., 2000; Smythe and Grounds, 2001). Similarly, it has been observed the restoration of 26–30% dystrophin expression in muscle fibers in the environment of the irradiated muscle, suggesting an improvement in myoblast migration induced by factors released with the irradiated muscle (Cousins et al., 2004; Skuk et al., 2006; Skuk et al., 2007; Skuk et al., 2004). The immunosuppression problem was tackled introducing new drugs. FK506 (Tacrolimus or Prograf®; Astellas Pharma, Deerfield, IL, USA) allowed to obtain very good transplantation results, not only in mice, but also in monkeys (Kinoshita et al., 1996; Kinoshita et al., 1994). Unfortunately, FK506 may induce adverse effects in patients (nephrotoxicity, diabetes, increased risk of cancer) if used on an ongoing, long-term basis (Palmieri et al., 2010). Many therapeutic protocols were developed to induce specific immunological tolerance towards the donor's myoblasts and through the creation of mixed chimerism and central tolerance (Camirand et al., 2004; Stephan et al., 2006). Another support to immunosuppression therapy was the transplantation of genetically modified autologous myoblasts (Floyd et al., 1998; Goncalves et al., 2006b; Quenneville et al., 2007), or avoidance of gradual senescence of differentiated cells, autologous pluripotent stem cells (Di Rocco et al., 2006). Other researchers refocus their efforts to optimise the therapy searching cell populations thought to be more primitive and less immunologic than myoblasts. They include MDSCs (Sarig et al., 2006), mSP cells (Wognum et al., 2003) and muscle-derived CD133+ progenitors (Farini et al., 2009). In a double-blind phase I clinical trial, Torrente et al. (Torrente et al., 2007) transplanted autologous CD133+ cells, extracted from muscle biopsies by intramuscular injection, into eight boys with DMD and sampled after 7 months. The cells were not genetically corrected, their fate was not monitored, and the boys were not immunosuppressed, because the experiment was designed only to test the safety of the implanted cells (grown in culture for only 48 hours). No adverse effects were observed. Afterwards, thanks to these observations, the cell therapy was combined with a genetic approach: ex vivo introduction of corrective genes into dystrophic CD133+ myogenic cells and their subsequent autologous transplantation. The use of exon-skipping for the expression of human dystrophin, within the DMD CD133+ cells, allows the use of the patient's own stem cells, thus minimizing the risk of immunological graft rejection (Riviere et al., 2006). The exon-skipping therapeutic approach is applicable to gene defects up to 70% of DMD patients, and avoids the problems associated with the delivery of the prohibitively large full length dystrophin gene or a (less functional) truncated mini-gene. Blood- and muscle-derived DMD CD133+ cells were isolated and characterized for their ability to express an exon-skipped version of human dystrophin, after infection with a lentivirus carrying a construct designed to skip exon 5 (Denti et al., 2006; Goyenvalle et al., 2004). The skipped blood and muscle-derived Δ49–50 stem cells were able to fuse in vivo with regenerative fibres and expressed, not only a functional human dystrophin, but also the dystrophin-associated proteins a and b-sarcoglycans. However, intramuscular transplantations lead only to local and focused regeneration, whereas DMD pathology affects the whole body musculature and its effective treatment requires some methods to distribute the injected cells to the dispersed sites. In future clinical trials, we speculate that these stem cells, purified from DMD patients, could be ex vivo engineered and reinjected in the initial donor intra-arterially. The intra-arterial injections of the patients'own infected stem cells allow the distribution of the cells to the whole body musculature so that it could be possible to take care of severely affected patients that have a reduced body mass. One of the most important problem to solve, for a future clinical application, is the amelioration in safety procedures of the gene modifications. Ichim et al. (Ichim et al., 2010) reported the case study of a 22 year-old male diagnosed with DMD, treated with a combination of endometrial regenerative cells (ERC) and CD34+ umbilical cord blood. Three months later, the patient received another course of therapy including placental matrix derived mesenchymal stem cells. The improvement in muscular strength, clinical respiratory function and general level of activity are maintained to date. No adverse events have been associated with the stem cell infusion. The innovation introduced by this trial was the usage of "adjuvant" cellular population which provides a more suitable environment for muscle regeneration. The local intramuscular MSCs are able to add chemotactic/ trophic support for the intravenously administered CD34. It has been reported that mesoangioblasts, which reside within the CD34 population, as well as cord blood CD34 cells, have had positive activity on DMD in animal models, although they appear to be short-lived (Jazedje et al., 2009; Nunes et al., 2007; Otto et al., 2009). Mesoangioblasts have been the main contributors to de novo myogenesis and were selectively attracted into the dystrophic tissue. It is known that CD34 cells express very late antigen-4 (VLA-4), which is the ligand for Vascular Cell Adhesion Molecule 1 (VCAM-1), whose expression is elevated in dystrophic muscles (Gavina et al., 2006). Furthermore, CD34 chemokines such as Macrophage inflammatory protein-1 alpha (MIP-1α) and Regulated upon activation normal T-cell expressed and secreted (RANTES) expression have been found in dystrophic muscle (Demoule et al., 2005).

18. Conclusions

According to this review, the attempts to treat DMD with different genetic and cellular approaches open new perspectives in the muscular function restoration, although it is very difficult to predict, at the moment, what strategy would be more successful. From a lifelong perspective, it is reasonable to conceive an integrated schedule of treatment protocols, subdivided by decades of age.On this basis, cell transplantation is supposed to be the final answer to replace the irreversibly impaired muscle mass with healthy myocytes. It is therefore important to choose the best age for the transplant and the best timing schedule is probably before the crash of the muscular framework that will be replaced with fibrous and adipose tissue. Alternatively , in the very early period of life, when the disease is not phenotipically expressed yet, and it is just a genetic biochemical trait, the timing could be perfect for either exon skipping or cell transplant approaches that could be more easily integrated in the muscular structure. Furthermore, in the homologous cell transplantation, a longstanding immunosuppressive phase, which is strongly adversed by the ethical committees, is at the moment mandatory in order to achieve an adequate survival of nonidentical transplanted cells. These cells should be reasonably replaced with a series of transplant sessions in the follow up, as long as their vital cycle will decline to apoptosis. Probably, in the next future,even histocompatible cadaver sources might be helpful in the long run.

As to the cell administration route, the transplant procedure, addressed by Cossu and coworkers (Sampaolesi et al., 2003; Díaz-Manera et al., 2010), through intra-arterial regional perfusion, has to be validated and compared with the more cumbersome repeated intramuscular injections for which automatically injecting devices, a proper anesthesia and, probably, laparoscopic-thoracoscopic schedule will be required, especially for the deep muscles, like diaphragm and heart. In the procedure described by Cossu (Sampaolesi et al., 2006), according to the results obtained in dog models of DMD, the mesangioblasts can easily trespass the endothelial barrier and reach the muscular areas to be restored by new healthy myocytes. On the other hand, in the direct intramuscular injections, the operator chooses the topography of injections, and, on the basis of mathematical and geometrical models, and with the hopeful aid of robotization, a systematic and well arranged replacement of several millions of myocytes can be achieved, during each session, on a very accurately, individually tailored protocol. The exon-skipping approach is very appealing due to the progress observed in the clinical trials, but it is very hard to conceive that this genetic correction of the dystrophin gene will be enough effective to support the muscular strength in the developing child, guaranteeing long lasting surrogate effect if introduced in a lifelong administration schedule. In this scenario, the oral route is certainly preferred to the subcutaneous one, and toxicological studies in mice let us suppose that the compounds are safe, but clinical trials in humans require further commitments, especially regarding the clinical monitoring of the follow up to determine possible side effects.

In conclusion, we think that, at the moment, due to brand new strong technological weapons, we could achieve a normal life span and quality of life for DMD kids and their families. At the same time, we need the collaboration of the centers working on DMD to design new clinical trials in order to reach the best effective therapeutic protocol as soon as possible. In the "Global Village", based on the World Wide Web, it is possible to plan panels of evidence-based medicine clinical studies by a single international World Wide Web based committee, eventually organized by the World Health Organization. This committee will be a powerful instrument to meet the urgent demand of the generation of kids with DMD who claim to achieve the goal of a fully autonomous life.

19. Statement of authorship

The authors hereby certify that all work contained in this review is original work of Tommaso Iannitti, Daniele Lodi, Valeriana Sblendorio, Valentina Rottigni and Beniamino Palmieri. All the information, taken from other articles, including tables and pictures, have been referenced in the "Bibliography" section. The authors claim full responsibility for the contents of the article.

20. Conflict of interest statement

The authors certify that there is no conflict of interest with any financial organization regarding the material discussed in the manuscript.

21. Acknowledgments

The authors contributed equally to this work. This review was not supported by grants.

22. Abbreviations

2'OMePS: 2'-O-methyl-phosphorothioate
ABCG2: ATP Binding Cassette G2
AON: Antisense Oligonucleotide
BMDC: Bone Marrow Derived Cell
BMMSC: Bone Marrow Mesenchymal Stem Cell
βFGF: Fibroblast Growth Factor beta
C/EBPα: CCAAT/Enhancer Binding Protein alpha
CNS: Central Nervous System
CsA: Ciclosporin A
DGC: Dystrophin Glycoprotein Complex
DMD: Duchenne Muscular Dystrophy
Dp: Dystrophin proteins
Dys: Dystrophin

ECM: Extracellular matrix
EDB: Extensor Digitorum Brevis
EP: Early Preplate
ERC: Endometrial Regenerative Cell
GRMD: Golden Retriever Muscular Dystrophy
HSC: Haematopoietic Stem Cell
IQ: Intelligence Quotient
MDSC: Muscle Derived Stem Cell
MHC: Major Histocompatibility Complex
MIP-1α: Macrophage Inflammatory Protein-1 alpha
MMDSC: Multipotent Muscle Derived Stem Cell
MRI: Magnetic Resonance Imaging
MSC: Mesenchymal Stem Cell
mSP: muscle Side Population
MVC: Maximum Voluntary Contraction
N: Naples
NICD: Notch1 Intracellular Domain
NTR: Netherlands National Trial Register
PDGF: Plateled Derived Growth Factor
PGC1-α: PPARγ Coactivator 1-alpha
PGC1-β: PPARγ Coactivator 1-beta
PMO: Phosphorodiamidate Morpholino Oligomer
PPARγ: Peroxisome Proliferator Activated Receptor gamma
pp6: preplate 6
RANTES: Regulated upon Activation, Normal T-cell Expressed and Secreted
SMSP: skeletal muscle side population
SP: Side Population
T: Toronto
TGF-β: Transforming Growth Factor beta
TNF-α: Tumor Necrosis Factor-alpha
VCAM-1: Vascular Cell Adhesion Molecule 1
VLA-4: Very Late Antigen-4

23. References

Aartsma-Rus A, Bremmer-Bout M, Janson AA, den Dunnen JT, van Ommen GJ, van Deutekom JC. Targeted exon skipping as a potential gene correction therapy for Duchenne muscular dystrophy. Neuromuscul Disord 2002;12 Suppl 1:S71-77.

Aartsma-Rus A, Janson AA, Kaman WE, Bremmer-Bout M, den Dunnen JT, Baas F, van Ommen GJ, van Deutekom JC. Therapeutic antisense-induced exon skipping in cultured muscle cells from six different DMD patients. Hum Mol Genet 2003;12:907-14.

Aartsma-Rus A, Janson AA, Kaman WE, Bremmer-Bout M, den Dunnen JT, van Ommen GJ, van Deutekom JC. Antisense-induced multiexon skipping for Duchenne muscular dystrophy makes more sense. Am J hum Genet 2004;74:83-92.

Aartsma-Rus A, Kaman WE, Weij R, den Dunnen JT, van Ommen GJ, van Deutekom JC. Exploring the frontiers of therapeutic exon skipping for Duchenne muscular dystrophy by double targeting within one or multiple exons. Mol Ther 2006;14: 401 - 07.

Aartsma-Rus A, van Deutekom JC, Fokkema IF, van Ommen GJ, den Dunnen JT. Entries in the Leiden Duchenne muscular dystrophy database: an overwiew of mutation typesand paradoxical cases that confirm the reading-frame rule. Muscle Nerve 2006;34:135-144.

Aartsma-Rus A, van Vliet L, Hirschi m, et al. Guidelines for antisense oligo-nucleotide design and insight into splice-modulating mechanisms. Mol Ther 2009,17:548-53.

Balaban B, Matthews DJ, Clayton GH, et al. Corticosteroid treatment and functional improvement in Duchenne muscular dystrophy: long-term effect. Am J Phys Med Rehabil. 2005;84:843–850.

Bewick GS, Nicholson LV, Young C, et al. Diffferent distributions of dystrophin and related proteins at nerve-muscle junctions. Neuroreport. 1992;3;857–860.

Biggar WD, Gingras M, Fehlings DL, et al. Deflazacort treatment of Duchenne muscular dystrophy. J Pediatr. 2001;138:45–50.

Biggar WD, Harris VA, Eliasoph L, et al. Long-term benefits of deflazacort treatment for boys with Duchenne muscular dystrophy in their second decade. Neuromuscul Disord. 2006;16:249–255.

Billard C, Gillet P, Signoret JL, et al. Cognitive function in Duchenne muscular dystrophy and spinal muscular atrophy. Neuromuscul Disord. 1992;2:371–378.

Blake DJ, Weir A, Newey SE, Davies KE. Function and genetics of dystrophin and dystrophin-related proteins in muscle. Physiol Rev. 2002;82:291–329

Blau HM, Webster C, Pavlath GK, Chiu CP. Evidence for defective myoblasts in Duchenne muscular dystrophy. Adv Exp Med Biol 1985;182:85-110.

Bremmer-Bout M, Aartsma-Rus A, de Meijer EK, Kaman WE, Janson AA, Vossen RH, van Ommen GJ, den Dunnen JT, van Deutekom JC. Targeted exon skipping in transgenic hDMD mice: a model for direct preclinical screening of human-specific antisense oligonucleotides. Mol Ther 2004;10:232-40.

Bresolin N, Castelli E, Comi GP, et al. Cognitive impairment in Duchenne muscular dystrophy. Neuromuscul Disord. 1994;4:359–369.

Brown Jr RH. Dystrophin associated proteins and the muscular dystrophy. Annu Rev Med. 1997;48:457–466.

Burdzinska A, Gala K Paczek L. Myogenic stem cells. Folia Histochem Cytobiol. 2008;46(4):401-12.

Camirand G, Rousseau J, Ducharme ME, Rothstein DM, Tremblay JP. Novel Duchenne muscular dystrophy treatment through myoblast transplantation tolerance with anti-CD45RB, anti-CD154 and mixed chimerism. Am J Transplant. 2004;4(8):1255-65.

Chan J, O'Donoghue K, Gavina M et. al. Galectin-1 induces skeletal muscle differentiation in human fetal mesenchymal stem cells and increases muscle regeneration. Stem Cells. 2006;24:1879-1891.

Cooper RN, Butler-Browne GS, Mouly V. Human muscle stem cells. Curr Opin Pharmacol. 2006;6(3):295-300.

Corrado K, Mills PL, Chamberlain JS. Deletion analysis of the dystrophin-actin binding domain. FEBS Lett. 1994;344:255–260.

Cossu G, Bianco P. Mesoangioblasts vascular progenitors for extravascular mesodermal tissues. Curr Opin Genet Dev. 2003;13(5):537-42.

Cousins JC, Woodward KJ, Gross JG, Partridge TA, Morgan JE. Regeneration of skeletal muscle from transplanted immortalised myoblasts is oligoclonal. J Cell Sci. 2004;117(Pt 15):3259-69.

Dellavalle A, Sampaolesi M, Tonlorenzi R, Tagliafico E, Sacchetti B, Perani L, Innocenzi A, Galvez BG, Messina G, Morosetti R, Li S, Belicchi M, Peretti G, Chamberlain JS, Wright WE, Torrente Y, Ferrari S, Bianco P, Cossu G. Pericytes of human skeletal muscle are myogenic precursors distinct from satellite cells. Nat Cell Biol. 2007;9(3):255-67

Demoule A, Divangahi M, Danialou G, Gvozdic D, Larkin G, Bao W, Petrof BJ. Expression and regulation of CC class chemokines in the dystrophic (mdx) diaphragm. Am J Respir Cell Mol Biol. 2005;33(2):178-85.

Denti MA, Rosa A, D'Antona G, Sthandier O, De Angelis FG, Nicoletti C, Allocca M, Pansarasa O, Parente V, Musarò A, Auricchio A, Bottinelli R, Bozzoni I. Chimeric adeno-associated virus/antisense U1 small nuclear RNA effectively rescues dystrophin synthesis and muscle function by local treatment of mdx mice. Hum Gene Ther. 2006;17(5):565-74

DeSilva S, Drachman DB, Mellits D, et al. Prednisone treatment in Duchenne muscular dystrophy: Long term benefit. Arch Neurol. 1987;44:818–822.

Dezawa M, Ishikawa H, Itokazu Y et. al. Bone marrow stromal cells generate muscle cells and repair muscle degeneration. Science. 2005;309:314-317.

Di Rocco G, Iachininoto MG, Tritarelli A, Straino S, Zacheo A, Germani A, Crea F, Capogrossi MC. Myogenic potential of adipose-tissue-derived cells. J Cell Sci. 2006;119(Pt 14):2945-52.

Díaz-Manera J, Touvier T, Dellavalle A, Tonlorenzi R, Tedesco FS, Messina G, Meregalli M, Navarro C, Perani L, Bonfanti C, Illa I, Torrente Y, Cossu G. Partial dysferlin reconstitution by adult murine mesoangioblasts is sufficient for full functional recovery in a murine model of dysferlinopathy. Cell Death Dis. 2010 Aug 5;1:e61.

Dubowitz V, Kinali M, Main M, et al. Remission of clinical signs in early Duchenne muscular dystrophy on intermittent low-dosage prednisolone therapy. Eur J Paediatr Neurol. 2002;6:153–159.

Dubowitz V. Neuromuscular disorders in childhood. Old dogmas, new concepts. Arch Dis Child. 1975;50:335–346.

El Fahime E, Torrente Y, Caron NJ, Bresolin MD, Tremblay JP. In vivo migration of transplanted myoblasts requires matrix metalloproteinase activity. Exp Cell Res. 2000;258(2):279-87.

Emery AE. Duchenne Muscular Dystrophy, 2nd edition. Cary, NC: Oxford University Press, 1993.

Fan Y, Maley M, Beilharz M, Grounds M. Rapid death of injected myoblasts in myoblast transfer therapy. Muscle Nerve. 1996;19(7):853-60.

Farini A, Razini P, Erratico S, Torrente Y, Meregalli M. Cell based therapy for Duchenne muscular dystrophy. J Cell Physiol. 2009;221(3):526-34.

Fukuhara S, Tomita S, Yamashiro S et. al. Direct cell-cell interaction of cardiomyocytes is key for bone marrow stromal cells to go into cardiac lineage in vitro. J Thorac Cardiovasc Surg. 2003;125:1470-14

Floyd SS Jr, Clemens PR, Ontell MR, Kochanek S, Day CS, Yang J, Hauschka SD, Balkir L, Morgan J, Moreland MS, Feero GW, Epperly M, Huard J. Ex vivo gene transfer using adenovirus-mediated full-length dystrophin delivery to dystrophic muscles. Gene Ther. 1998;5(1):19-30.

Gavina M, Belicchi M, Rossi B, Ottoboni L, Colombo F, Meregalli M, Battistelli M, Forzenigo L, Biondetti P, Pisati F, Parolini D, Farini A, Issekutz AC, Bresolin N, Rustichelli F, Constantin G, Torrente Y. VCAM-1 expression on dystrophic muscle vessels has a critical role in the recruitment of human blood-derived CD133+ stem cells after intra-arterial transplantation. Blood. 2006;108(8):2857-66.

Goemans NM, Tulinius M, van den Akker JT, Burm BE, Ekhart PF, Heuvelmans N, Holling T, Janson AA, Platenburg GJ, Sipkens JA, Sitsen JM, Aartsma-Rus A, van Ommen GJ, Buyse G, Darin N, Verschuuren JJ, Campion GV, de Kimpe SJ, van Deutekom JC. Systemic administration of PRO051 in Duchenne's muscular dystrophy. N Engl J Med. 2011 Apr 21;364(16):1513-22. Epub 2011 Mar 23.

Goncalves MA, de Vries AA, Holkers M, van de Watering MJ, van der Velde I, van Nierop GP, Valerio D, Knaän-Shanzer S. Human mesenchymal stem cells ectopically expressing full-length dystrophin can complement Duchenne muscular dystrophy myotubes by cell fusion. Hum Mol Genet. 2006a;15(2):213-21.

Gonçalves MA, Holkers M, Cudré-Mauroux C, van Nierop GP, Knaän-Shanzer S, van der Velde I, Valerio D, de Vries AA. Transduction of myogenic cells by retargeted dual high-capacity hybrid viral vectors: robust dystrophin synthesis in duchenne muscular dystrophy muscle cells. Mol Ther. 2006b;13(5):976-86.

Gosselin LE, McCormick KM. Targeting the immune system to improve ventilator function in muscular dystrophy. Med Sci Sports Exerc. 2004;36:44–51.

Goyenvalle A, Vulin A, Fougerousse F, Leturcq F, Kaplan JC, Garcia L, Danos O. Rescue of dystrophic muscle through U7 snRNA-mediated exon skipping. Science. 2004;306(5702):1796-9.

Griggs RC, Griggs RC, Moxley RT 3rd, et al. Duchenne dystrophy: randomized, controlled trial of prednisone (18 months) and azathioprine (12 months). Neurology. 1993;43:520-527.

Guérette B, Asselin I, Skuk D, Entman M, Tremblay JP. Control of inflammatory damage by anti-LFA-1: increase success of myoblast transplantation. Cell Transplant. 1997;6(2):101-7.

Guérette B, Asselin I, Vilquin JT, Roy R, Tremblay JP. Lymphocyte infiltration following allo- and xenomyoblast transplantation in mice. Transplant Proc. 1994;26(6):3461-2.

Gussoni, E, Pavlath GK, Lanctot AM, Sharma KR, Miller RG, Steinman L, Blau HM. Normal dystrophin transcripts detected in Duchenne muscular dystrophy patients after myoblast transplantation. Nature. 1992;356(6368):435-8.

Hall ZW, Sanes JR. Synaptic structure and development: The neuromuscular junction. Cell. 1993;72 (Suppl):99–121.

Hardiman OR, Sklar M, Brown RH Jr. Direct effects of cyclosporin A and cyclophosphamide on differentiation of normal human myoblasts in culture. Neurology. 1993;43(7):1432-4.

Hawke TJ, Garry DJ. Myogenic satellite cells: physiology to molecular biology. J Appl Physiol 2001;91:534-51.

Heemskerk H, de Winter C, van Kuik P, et al. Preclinical PK and PD studies on 2′-O-methyl-phosphorothioate RNA antisense oligonucleotides in the mdx mouse model. Mol Ther 2010;18:1210-7.

Heemskerk H, de Winter Cl, de Kimpe SJ, van Kuik-Romeijn P, Heuvelmans N, Platenburg GJ, van Ommen GJ, van Deutekom JC, Aartsma-Rus A. in vivo comparison of 2′-O-methyl phosphorothioate and mopholino antisense oligonucleotides for Duchenne muscular dystrophy exon skipping. J Gene Med 2009;11:257-66.

Helderman-van den Enden AT, Straathof CS, Aartsma-Rus A, et al. Becker muscular dystrophy patients with deletions around exon 51: a promising outlook for xon skipping therapy in Duchenne patients. Neuromuscul Disord 2010;20:251-4.

Henry MD, Campbell KP. A role for dystroglican in basement membrane assembly. Cell. 1998;95:859–870.

Henry MD, Campbell KP. Dystroglican inside and out. Curr Opin Cell Biol. 1999;11:602–607.

Hoffman EP, Brown Jr RH, Kunkel LM. Dystrophin: The protein product of the Duchenne muscular dystrophy locus. Cell. 1987;51:919–928.

Hoffman EP, Dressman D. Molecular pathophysiology and targeted therapeutics for muscular dystrophy. Trends Pharmacol Sci 2001;22: 465–70

Hohenester E, Tisi D, Talts JF, et al. The crystal structure of a laminin G-like module reveals the molecular basis of alpha-destroglycan binding to laminins, perlecan, and agrin. Mol Cell. 1999;4:783–792.

Hong, F, Lee J, Song JW, Lee SJ, Ahn H, Cho JJ, Ha J, Kim SS. Cyclosporin A blocks muscle differentiation by inducing oxidative stress and inhibiting the peptidyl-prolyl-cis-trans isomerase activity of cyclophilin A: cyclophilin A protects myoblasts from cyclosporin A-induced cytotoxicity. Faseb J. 2002;16(12):1633-5.

Houde S, Filiatrault M, Fournier A, et al. Deflazacort use in Duchenne muscular dystrophy: an 8-year follow-up. Pediatr Neurol. 2008;38:200–206.

Huang X, Poy F, Zhang E, et al. Structure of a WW domain containing fragment of dystrophin in complex with beta-dystroglican. Nat Struct Biol. 2000;7:634–638.

Huard J, Acsadi G, Jani A, Massie B, Karpati G. Gene transfer into skeletal muscles by isogenic myoblasts. Hum Gene Ther. 1994;5(8):949-58.

Huard J, Bouchard JP, Roy R, Labrecque C, Dansereau G, Lemieux B, Tremblay JP. Myoblast transplantation produced dystrophin-positive muscle fibres in a 16-year-old patient with Duchenne muscular dystrophy. Clin Sci (Lond). 1991;81(2):287-8.

Huard J, Bouchard JP, Roy R, Malouin F, Dansereau G, Labrecque C, Albert N, Richards CL, Lemieux B, Tremblay JP. Human myoblast transplantation: preliminary results of 4 cases. Muscle Nerve. 1992;15(5):550-60.

Iannitti T, Capone S, Feder D, Palmieri B. Clinical use of immunosuppressants in duchenne muscular dystrophy. J Clin Neuromuscul Dis. 2010;12(1):1-21.

Ichim TE, Alexandrescu DT, Solano F, Lara F, Campion Rde N, Paris E, Woods EJ, Murphy MP, Dasanu CA, Patel AN, Marleau AM, Leal A, Riordan NH. Mesenchymal stem cells as anti-inflammatories: implications for treatment of Duchenne muscular dystrophy. Cell Immunol. 2010;260(2):75-82.

Jazedje T, Secco M, Vieira NM, Zucconi E, Gollop TR, Vainzof M, Zatz M. Stem cells from umbilical cord blood do have myogenic potential, with and without differentiation induction in vitro. J Transl Med. 2009;14; 7:6.

Jennekens FG, ten Kate LP, de Visser M et al. Diagnostic criteria for Duchenne and Becker muscular dystrophy and myotonic dystrophy. Neuromuscul Disord. 1991;1:389–391.

Jung D, Yang B, Meyer J, et al. Identification and characterizion of the dystrophin anchoring site on betadystroglican. J Biol Chem. 1995;270:27305–27310.

Karpati, G, Ajdukovic D, Arnold D, Gledhill RB, Guttmann R, Holland P, Koch PA, Shoubridge E, Spence D, Vanasse M. Myoblast transfer in Duchenne muscular dystrophy. Ann Neurol. 1993;34(1):8-17.

Kemaladewi DU, Hoogaars WM, van Heiningen SH, Terlouw S, de Gorter DJ, den Dunnen JT, van Ommen GJ, Aartsma-Rus A, Ten Dijke P, 't Hoen PA. Dual exon skipping in myostatin and dystrophin for Duchenne muscular dystrophy. BMC Med Genomics. 2011;4:36.

Kinali M, Arechavala-Gomeza V, Feng L, Cirak S, Hunt D, Adkin C, Guglieri M, Ashton E, Abbs S, Nihoyannopoulos P, Garralda ME, Rutherford M, McCulley C, Popplewell L, Graham IR, Dickson G, Wood MJ, Wells DJ, Wilton SD, Kole R, Straub V, Bushby K, Sewry C, Morgan JE, Muntoni F. Local restoration of dystrophin expression with the morpholino oligomer AVI-4658 in Duchenne muscular dystrophy: a single-blind, placebo-controlled, dose-escalation, proof-of-concept study. Lancet Neurol. 2009 Oct;8(10):918-28. Epub 2009 Aug 25. Erratum in: Lancet Neurol. 2009 Dec;8(12):1083.

Kinoshita I, Roy R, Dugré FJ, Gravel C, Roy B, Goulet M, Asselin I, Tremblay JP. Myoblast transplantation in monkeys: control of immune response by FK506. J Neuropathol Exp Neurol. 1996;55(6):687-97.

Kinoshita I, Vilquin JT, Guérette B, Asselin I, Roy R, Tremblay JP. Very efficient myoblast allotransplantation in mice under FK506 immunosuppression. Muscle Nerve. 1994;17(12):1407-15.

Kirschner J, Schessl J, Ihorst G, et al; Muskeldystrophie Netzwerk MD-NET. Treatment of Duchenne muscular dystrophy with cyclosporin A—a randomized, double-blind, placebo controlled trial. Neuropediatrics. 2008;44:39.

Koenig M, Monaco AP, Kunkel LM. The complete sequence of dystrophin predicts a rod-shaped cytoskeletal protein. Cell. 1988;53:219–226.

Krause DS, Theise ND, Collector MI, Henegariu O, Hwang S, Gardner R, Neutzel S, Sharkis SJ. Multi-organ, multi-lineage engraftment by a single bone marrow-derived stem cell. Cell. 2001;105(3):369-77.

Kunkel LM. Analysis of deletions in DNA from patients with Becker and Duchenne muscular dystrophy. Nature. 1986;622:73–77.

Law PK, Goodwin TG, Fang Q, Duggirala V, Larkin C, Florendo JA, Kirby DS, Deering MB, Li HJ, Chen M. Feasibility, safety, and efficacy of myoblast transfer therapy on Duchenne muscular dystrophy boys. Cell Transplant. 1992;1(2-3):235-44.

Le Grand F, Rudnicki M. Satellite and stem cells in muscle growth and repair. Development. 2007a;134(22):3953-7.

Le Grand F, Rudnicki M. Skeletal muscle satellite cells and adult myogenesis. Curr Opin Cell Biol. 2007b;19(6):628-33.

Lee-Pullen TF, Grounds MD. Muscle-derived stem cells: implications for effective myoblast transfer therapy. IUBMB Life. 2005;57(11):731-6.

Lee JH, Kosinski PA, Kemp DM. Contribution of human bone marrow stem cells to individual skeletal myotubes followed by myogenic gene activation. Exp Cell Res. 2005;307:174-182.

Liu Y, Song J, Liu W, Wan Y, Chen X, Hu C. Growth and differentiation of rat bone marrow stromal cells: does 5-azacytidine trigger their cardiomyogenic differentiation? Cardiovasc Res. 2003;58:460-468.

Lodi D, Iannitti T, Palmieri B. Stem cells in clinical practice: applications and warnings. J Exp Clin Cancer Res. 2011;30:9.

Mann CJ, Honeyman K, McClorey G, Fletcher S, Wilton SD. Improved antisense oligonucleotide induced exon skipping in the mdx mouse model of muscular dystrophy. J Gene Med 2002;4:644-54.

Manzur AY, Muntoni F. Diagnosis and new treatments in muscular dystrophies. J Neurol Neurosurg Psychiatry 2009;80:706-14.

Markham LW, Spicer RL, Khoury PR, et al. Steroid therapy and cardiac function in Duchenne muscular dystrophy. Pediatr Cardiol. 2005;26:768–771.

Mavrogeni S, Papavasiliou A, Douskou M, Kolovou G, Papadopoulou E, Cokkinos DV. Effect of deflazacort on cardiac and sternocleidomastoid muscles in Duchenne musculardystrophy: a magnetic resonance imaging study. Eur J Paediatr Neurol. 2009 Jan;13(1):34-40. Epub 2008 Apr 11.

Melis MA, Cau M, Muntoni F, et al. Elevation of serum creatine kinase as the only manifestation of an intragenic dletion of the dystrophin gene in three unrelated families. Eur J Paediatr neurol 1998; 2:255-61.

Mendell JR, Kissel JT, Amato AA, King W, Signore L, Prior TW, Sahenk Z, Benson S, McAndrew PE, Rice R. Myoblast transfer in the treatment of Duchenne's muscular dystrophy. N Engl J Med. 1995;333(13):832-8

Mezey E, Chandross KJ, Harta G, Maki RA, McKercher SR. Turning blood into brain: cells bearing neuronal antigens generated in vivo from bone marrow. Science. 2000;290(5497):1779-82.

Miller RG, Sharma KR, Pavlath GK, Gussoni E, Mynhier M, Lanctot AM, Greco CM, Steinman L, Blau HM. Myoblast implantation in Duchenne muscular dystrophy: the San Francisco study. Muscle Nerve. 1997;20(4):469-78.

Monaco AP, Bertelson CJ, Liechti-gallati S, Moser H, Kunkel LM. An explanation for the phenotypic differences between patients bearing partial deletions of the DMD locus. Genomics 1988;2:90-95.

Muntoni F, Torelli S, Ferlini A. Dystrophin and mutations: one gene, several proteins, multiple phenotypes. Lancet Neurol. 2003;2:731–740.

Naesens M, Kuypers DR, Sarwal M. Calcineurin inhibitor nephrotoxicity. Clin J Am Soc Nephrol. 2009;4:481–508.

Nassiri SM, Khaki Z, Soleimani M, Ahmadi SH, Jahanzad I, Rabbani S, Sahebjam M, Ardalan FA, Fathollahi MS. The similar effect of transplantation of marrow-derived mesenchymal stem cells with or without prior differentiation induction in experimental myocardial infarction. J Biomed Sci. 2007 Nov;14(6):745-55. Epub 2007 Jul 1.

Newey SE, Benson MA, Pointing CP, et al. Alternative splicing of dystrobrevin regulates the stoichiometry of syntrophin binding to the dystrophin protein complex. Curr Biol. 2000;10:1295–1298.

Norwood FL, Sutherland-Smith AJ, Keep NH, et al. The structure of the N-terminal actin-binding domain of human dystrophin and how mutations in this domain maybe cause Duchenne or Becker muscular dystrophy. Structure Fold Des. 2000;8:481–491.

Nunes VA, Cavaçana N, Canovas M, Strauss BE, Zatz M. Stem cells from umbilical cord blood differentiate into myotubes and express dystrophin in vitro only after exposure to in vivo muscle environment. Biol Cell. 2007;99(4):185-96.

Otto A, Collins-Hooper H, Patel K. The origin, molecular regulation and therapeutic potential of myogenic stem cell populations. J Anat. 2009;215(5):477-97.

Palmieri B, Sblendorio V. Duchenne Muscular Dystrophy: An Update, Part I. Journal of Clinical Neromuscular Disease 8 (2) 2006.

Palmieri B, Tremblay JP, Daniele L. Past, present and future of myoblast transplantation in the treatment of Duchenne muscular dystrophy. Pediatr Transplant. 2010;14(7):813-9.

Peault B, Rudnicki M, Torrente Y, Cossu G, Tremblay JP, Partridge T, Gussoni E, Kunkel LM, Huard J. Stem and progenitor cells in skeletal muscle development, maintenance, and therapy. Mol Ther. 2007;15(5):867-77.

Petrof BJ. Molecular pathophysiology of myofiber injury in deficiencies of the dystrophin-glycoprotein complex. Am. J. Phys. Med. Rehabil. 2002;81, S162-S174.

Pittenger MF, Mackay AM, Beck SC, Jaiswal RK, Douglas R, Mosca JD, Moorman MA, Simonetti DW, Craig S, Marshak DR. Multilineage potential of adult human mesenchymal stem cells. Science. 1999;284(5411):143-7.

Prockop DJ. Marrow stromal cells as stem cells for nonhematopoietic tissues. Science. 1997;276(5309):71-4.

Quenneville SP, Chapdelaine P, Skuk D, Paradis M, Goulet M, Rousseau J, Xiao X, Garcia L, Tremblay JP. Autologous transplantation of muscle precursor cells modified with a lentivirus for muscular dystrophy: human cells and primate models. Mol Ther. 2007;15(2):431-8.

Rivière C, Danos O, Douar AM. Long-term expression and repeated administration of AAV type 1, 2 and 5 vectors in skeletal muscle of immunocompetent adult mice. Gene Ther. 2006;13(17):1300-8

Roberts RG, Bobrow M. Dystrophins in vertebrates and invertebrates. Hum Mol Genet. 1998;7:589–595.

Sampaolesi M, Blot S, D'Antona G, Granger N, Tonlorenzi R, Innocenzi A, Mognol P, Thibaud JL, Galvez BG, Barthélémy I, Perani L, Mantero S, Guttinger M, Pansarasa O, Rinaldi C, Cusella De Angelis MG, Torrente Y, Bordignon C, Bottinelli R, Cossu G. Mesoangioblast stem cells ameliorate muscle function in dystrophic dogs. Nature. 2006 Nov 30;444(7119):574-9. Epub 2006 Nov 15.

Sampaolesi M, Torrente Y, Innocenzi A, Tonlorenzi R, D'Antona G, Pellegrino MA, Barresi R, Bresolin N, De Angelis MG, Campbell KP, Bottinelli R, Cossu G. Cell therapy of alpha-sarcoglycan null dystrophic mice through intra-arterial delivery of mesoangioblasts. Science. 2003 Jul 25;301(5632):487-92. Epub 2003 Jul 10.

Sanes JR, Lichtam JW. Development of the vertebrate neuromuscular junction. Ann Rev Neurosci. 1999;22:389–442.

Sarig, R, Baruchi Z, Fuchs O, Nudel U, Yaffe D. Regeneration and transdifferentiation potential of muscle-derived stem cells propagated as myospheres. Stem Cells. 2006;24(7):1769-78.

Sealock R, Butler MH, Kramarcy NR, et al. Localization of dystrophin relative to acetylcholine receptor domains in electric tissue and adult and cultured skeletal muscle. J Cell Biol. 1991;113:1133–1144.

Sharma KR, Mynhier MA, Miller RG. Cyclosporine increases muscular force generation in Duchenne muscular dystrophy. Neurology. 1993;43:527–532.

Shi D., Reinecke H, Murry CE, Torok-Storb B. Myogenic fusion of human bone marrow stromal cells, but not hematopoiecti cells. Blood. 2004;104:290-294.

Sigesmund DA, Weleber RG, Pillers DA, et al. Characterization of the ocular phenotype of Duchenne and Becker muscular dystrophy. Ophthalmology. 1994;101:856–865.

Skuk D, Goulet M, Roy B, Chapdelaine P, Bouchard JP, Roy R, Dugré FJ, Sylvain M, Lachance JG, Deschênes L, Senay H, Tremblay JP. Dystrophin expression in muscles of duchenne muscular dystrophy patients after high-density injections of normal myogenic cells. J Neuropathol Exp Neurol. 2006;65(4):371-86.

Skuk D, Goulet M, Roy B, Piette V, Côté CH, Chapdelaine P, Hogrel JY, Paradis M, Bouchard JP, Sylvain M, Lachance JG, Tremblay JP. First test of a "high-density injection" protocol for myogenic cell transplantation throughout large volumes of muscles in a Duchenne muscular dystrophy patient: eighteen months follow-up. Neuromuscul Disord. 2007;17(1):38-46.

Skuk D, Roy B, Goulet M, Chapdelaine P, Bouchard JP, Roy R, Dugré FJ, Lachance JG, Deschênes L, Hélène S, Sylvain M, Tremblay JP Dystrophin expression in myofibers of Duchenne muscular dystrophy patients following intramuscular injections of normal myogenic cells. Mol Ther. 2004;9(3):475-82.

Skuk D, Roy B, Goulet M, Tremblay JP. Successful myoblast transplantation in primates depends on appropriate cell delivery and induction of regeneration in the host muscle. Exp Neurol. 1999;155(1):22-30.

Smythe GM, Grounds MD. Absence of MyoD increases donor myoblast migration into host muscle. Exp Cell Res. 2001;267(2):267-74.

Stephan L, Pichavant C, Bouchentouf M, Mills P, Camirand G, Tagmouti S, Rothstein D, Tremblay JP. Induction of tolerance across fully mismatched barriers by a nonmyeloablative treatment excluding antibodies or irradiation use. Cell Transplant. 2006;15(8-9):835-46.

Straathof CS, Overweg-Plandsoen WC, van den Burg GJ, van der Kooi AJ, Verschuuren JJ, de Groot IJ. Prednisone 10 days on/10 days off in patients with Duchenne muscular dystrophy. J Neurol. 2009 May;256(5):768-73. Epub 2009 Mar 22.

Tennyson CN, Dally GY, Ray PN, et al. Expression of the dystrophin isoform Dp71 in differentiating human fetal myogenic cultures. Hum Mol Genet. 1996;5:1559–1566.

Torrente Y, Belicchi M, Marchesi C, Dantona G, Cogiamanian F, Pisati F, Gavina M, Giordano R, Tonlorenzi R, Fagiolari G, Lamperti C, Porretti L, Lopa R, Sampaolesi M, Vicentini L, Grimoldi N, Tiberio F, Songa V, Baratta P, Prelle A, Forzenigo L, Guglieri M, Pansarasa O, Rinaldi C, Mouly V, Butler-Browne GS, Comi GP, Biondetti P, Moggio M, Gaini SM, Stocchetti N, Priori A, D'Angelo MG, Turconi A, Bottinelli R, Cossu G, Rebulla P, Bresolin N. Autologous transplantation of muscle-derived CD133+ stem cells in Duchenne muscle patients. Cell Transplant. 2007;16(6):563-77.

Torrente Y, Belicchi M, Sampaolesi M, Pisati F, Meregalli M, D'Antona G, Tonlorenzi R, Porretti L, Gavina M, Mamchaoui K, Pellegrino MA, Furling D, Mouly V, Butler-Browne GS, Bottinelli R, Cossu G, Bresolin N. Human circulating AC133(+) stem cells restore dystrophin expression and ameliorate function in dystrophic skeletal muscle. J Clin Invest. 2004;114(2):182-95.

Tremblay JP, Malouin F, Roy R, Huard J, Bouchard JP, Satoh A, Richards CL. Results of a triple blind clinical study of myoblast transplantations without immunosuppressive treatment in young boys with Duchenne muscular dystrophy. Cell Transplant. 1993;2(2):99-112.

Trollet C, Athanasopoulos T, Popplewell L, Malerba A, Dickson G. Gene therapy for muscular dystrophy: current progress and future prospects. Expert Opinion on Biologicla Therapy 2009; 9:849-66.

van Deutekom JC, Janson AA, Ginjaar IB, Frankhuizen WS, Aartsma-Rus A, Bremmer-Bout M, den Dunnen JT, Koop K, van der Kooi AJ, Goemans NM, de Kimpe SJ, Ekhart PF, Venneker EH, Platenburg GJ, Verschuuren JJ, van Ommen GJ. Local dystrophin restoration with antisense oligonucleotide PRO051. N Engl J Med. 2007 Dec 27;357(26):2677-86.

van Ommen GJ, van Deutekom J, Aartsma-Rus A. The therapeutic potential of antisense-mediated exon skiping. Curr Opin Mol Ther 2008,10:140-9.

Way M, Pope B, Cross RA, et al. Expression of the N-terminal domain of dystrophin in E. Coli and demonstration of binding of F-actin. FEBS Lett. 1992;301:243–245.

Whitehead NP, Yeung EW, Allen DG. Muscle damage in mdx (dystrophic) mice: role of calcium and reactive oxygen species. Clin Exp Pharmacol Physiol. 2006;33:657–662.

Wognum AW, Eaves AC, Thomas TE. Identification and isolation of hematopoietic stem cells. Arch Med Res. 2003;34(6):461-75.

Xiong, F, Zhang C, Xiao SB, Li MS, Wang SH, Yu MJ, Shang YC. Construction of recombinant adenovirus including microdystrophin and expression in the mesenchymal cells of mdx mice. Sheng Wu Gong Cheng Xue Bao. 2007;23(1):27-32.

Yang B, Jung D, Rafael JA, et al. Identification of alpha-syntrophin binding to syntrophin triplet, dystrophin, and utrophin. J Biol Chem. 1995;270:4975–4978.

Yoshida N, Yoshida S, Koishi K, Masuda K, Nabeshima Y. Cell heterogeneity upon myogenic differentiation: down-regulation of MyoD and Myf-5 generates 'reverse cells'. J Cell Sci 1998;111:769-79.

20

Duchenne Muscular Dystrophy: Therapeutic Approaches to Restore Dystrophin

Pietro Spitali and Annemieke Aartsma-Rus
Leiden University Medical Center, The Netherlands

1. Introduction

Duchenne muscular dystrophy (DMD) is a progressive neuromuscular disorder. The first symptoms involve the lower limbs and appear between the third and fifth year. Due to weakness of the knee and hip extensors, patients rise from a sitting position using the Gower's maneuver. Muscle weakness progresses to the shoulder girdle-, upper arm and trunk-muscles and patients loose ambulation before the age of 12 (Emery, 1993). Histological changes involve variation in fiber size with atrophic and hypertrophic fibers, degeneration and regeneration of the muscle fibers, infiltration of inflammatory cells and fibrosis. The fiber necrosis results in leakage of the enzyme creatine kinase (CK), resulting in very high serum CK levels in DMD patients (20,000 to 50,000 U/L compared to 80 to 250 U/L in unaffected individuals). These levels decline as patients get older and the overall muscle mass decreases progressively. The pathology is caused by mutations in the *DMD* gene, which was known to be on the X chromosome long before the responsible gene was cloned due to an X-linked recessive inheritance pattern. The protein product of the gene is a 427 KDa protein called dystrophin. In the early 80s several groups were collaborating on the regional cloning of the gene responsible for DMD (Burghes et al., 1987; Monaco et al., 1985) which happened to co-localize with the locus for Becker muscular dystrophy (BMD) (Kingston et al., 1984). This is a milder disease, where patients are diagnosed in adolescence or adulthood, remain ambulant longer and survival is generally only slightly decreased (Emery, 2002). After a couple of years Monaco and colleagues confirmed that deletions in the identified locus caused DMD (Monaco et al., 1985) and BMD (Hoffman et al., 1988). In the following years, the coding sequence of the gene was identified, which turned out to occupy a huge genomic region. The complete cDNA and protein product of the *DMD* gene were published in 1987 (Hoffman et al., 1987; Koenig et al., 1987). The cloning of the genomic and coding sequence of the *DMD* gene allowed the development of tools for the molecular diagnosis of DMD. Deletions of one or more exons were found to be most common (65% of patients) and mainly localized in two hotspot regions in the gene (exons 2-20 and 45-53). This led Chamberlain and colleagues to develop a multiplex PCR able to detect the most frequent mutations (Chamberlain et al., 1988). This technique has been used for years, but recently multiple ligation-dependent probe amplification (MLPA) has been developed that allows an exact characterization of exons involved in deletions and duplications (Janssen et al., 2005; Schwartz & Duno, 2004). For small mutations a more labour-intensive method of PCR analysis of each exon, followed by direct sequencing is required (Spitali et al., 2009). The study of mutations and clinical features in DMD and BMD patients led to a deeper understanding of the disease, the gene and disease causing mutations. This made it possible to correlate genotype and phenotype and explain the discrepancy that mutations in one gene could lead to a severe DMD and a milder BMD phenotype. In 1989 two groups postulated that frame disrupting mutations were responsible for DMD while BMD was caused by frame maintaining mutations (Koenig et al., 1989; Monaco, 1989). This has been crucial for the development of certain potential therapies such as exon skipping and microdystrophins.

2. Dystrophin and the associated glycoprotein complex (DGC)

Dystrophin consists of 3685 amino acids and is a 427 kDa protein (Koenig et al., 1988). Dystrophin is composed of 4 domains, the first 240 N-terminal aminoacids define the actin-binding domain, which contains two actin-binding sites (Jarrett & Foster, 1995; Koenig & Kunkel, 1990). This domain is followed by a central rod shaped domain, consisting of 24 spectrin-like repeat units interrupted by 4 proline-rich hinge regions (Koenig & Kunkel, 1990). It has been demonstrated that an extra actin binding domain is present between repeats 11 and 17 (Rybakova et al., 1996) and that repeat 16 and 17 contain an nNOS binding site (Lai et al., 2009). The cysteine-rich domain encompasses aminoacids 3080 to 3360 and includes 15 cysteines, two EF hand motifs and a ZZ domain (Koenig et al., 1988) and binds to β-dystroglycan. Finally the C-terminal domain consists of the last 325 amino acids involved in protein-protein interactions. Dystrophin is part of the dystrophin-associated glycoprotein complex (DGC) (Figure 1). The cysteine-rich and C-terminal domains of dystrophin bind to several parts of the DGC, which can be divided into the dystroglycan complex, the sarcoglycan-sarcospan complex and the cytoplasmatic, dystrophin containing complex (Blake et al., 2002; Yoshida et al., 1994). In skeletal muscle the dystroglycan complex consists of α-dystroglycan and β-dystroglycan, which are both heavily glycosylated (Ibraghimov-Beskrovnaya et al., 1992). Dystrophin binds to β-dystroglycan, a transmembrane protein that binds to the extra-cellular α-dystroglycan; α-dystroglycan on its part binds to the extracellular matrix component laminin-2 (Hohenester et al., 1999; Rentschler et al., 1999; Suzuki et al., 1994). The sarcoglycan-sarcospan complex includes α-, β-, γ- and δ-sarcoglycan and sarcospan (Blake et al., 2002). The cytoplasmatic part of the DGC includes dystrophin itself, syntrophin and α-dystrobrevin, which binds to both dystrophin and syntrophin (Ahn et al., 1996). Alpha-syntrophin also binds to dystrophin and, additionally, it recruits the enzyme nNOS to the sarcolemma (Ahn & Kunkel, 1995; Brenman et al., 1995; Yoshida et al., 1995), although it has been recently demonstrated that the recruitment of nNOS by dystrophin repeats 16 and 17 is more important (Lai et al., 2009). Dystrophin also binds to and influences microtubules organization in the cytoplasm (Prins et al., 2009). In BMD patients, internally deleted dystrophins maintaining the N-terminal and C-terminal domains are able to bind to the DGC complex at the sarcolemma (Matsumura et al., 1994; Matsumura et al., 1993; Mirabella et al., 1998), while in DMD patients the absence of dystrophin results in the complete loss or decrease of other DGC proteins, and in the loss of nNOS at the sarcolemma (Brenman et al., 1995; Ervasti et al., 1990; Ohlendieck & Campbell, 1991). The function of the DGC is still largely unknown. However, since the complex forms a mechanical link between the cytoskeleton and the extracellular matrix, it is assumed that the DGC has a function in maintaining sarcolemma stability during contraction (Matsumura & Campbell, 1994).

3. Pathology

Dystrophin loss leads to a high susceptibility of muscle fibers to injury after repeated eccentric contractions. This results in a chronic inflammation state, which provokes damage and necrosis. Muscle tissue is lost and replaced by fibrosis after exhausted cycles of damage and repair. Recent data suggest that stretched contractions activate reactive oxygen species (ROS) production, which causes opening of stretch-activated channels (SACs) and Ca2+ entry via src kinase activation induced by caveolin-3 (Allen et al., 2010). Oxidative stress may amplify the process inducing activation of the inflammatory transcription factor NF-κB, and thus functional impairment of force-generating capacity (Lawler, 2011).

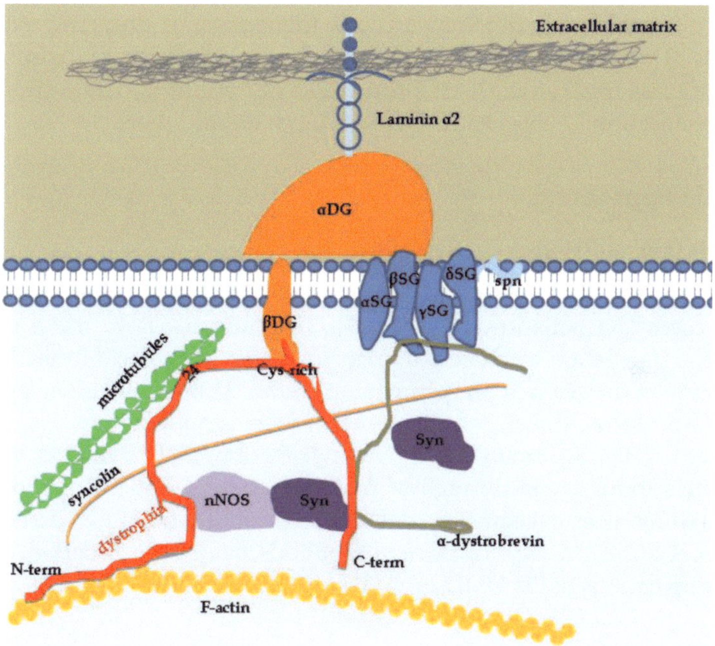

Fig. 1. Schematic representation of the dystrophin associated glycoprotein complex (DGC). αDG: α-dystroglycan; βDG: β-dystroglycan; αSG: α-sarcoglycan; βSG: β-sarcoglycan; γSG: γ-sarcoglycan; δSG: δ-sarcoglycan; spn: sarcospan; N-term: dystrophin aminoterminal domain; Cys-rich: dystrophin cystein rich domain; C-term: dystrophin carboxyterminal domain; nNOS: neuronal nitric oxide synthase; Syn: syntrophin.

4. Current treatment

There is currently no therapy for DMD. Nevertheless the lifespan and quality of life of DMD patients has significantly improved during the last 2 decades due to improved health care, especially assisted ventilation (Eagle et al., 2002). The mean age of death in the 1960s was 14.4 years, whereas for those ventilated since 1990 it was 25.3 years. The chances of survival to 25 years have increased from 0% in the 1960s to 4% in the 1970s and 12% in the 1980s, and that the impact of nocturnal ventilation has further improved this chance to 53% for those ventilated since 1990. Another crucial step has been the use of corticosteroids (mainly prednisone (Moxley, III & Pandya, 2011) and deflazacort (Biggar et al., 2001)), which reduce the inflammatory response in patients' muscle and the accompanied damage and fibrosis, thus longer maintaining muscle quality. The benefit of corticosteroids has been clearly demonstrated for DMD patients in a double-blind randomized controlled trial in more than 100 boys (Mendell et al., 1989). Corticosteroids treatment extends the ambulation of patients for about 2 years and reduces scoliosis (King et al., 2007). The prolonged use of corticosteroids has however known side effects, which include weight gain, hypertension, bone demineralization, vertebral compression fractures and sometimes behavior disorders. Guidelines for DMD patients' management have been published in order to harmonize the standards of clinical practice (Bushby et al., 2010a; Bushby et al., 2010b).

There are numerous therapeutic approaches under development for DMD. Some aim at addressing specific issues of pathology such as Idebenone, or green tea extract to reduce oxidative stress (Dorchies et al., 2009; Nagy & Nagy, 1990), or myostatin inhibition to increase muscle mass (Bish et al., 2011; Dumonceaux et al., 2010), while others directly aim at dystrophin restoration. In this chapter we will focus on the latter.

5. Therapeutic approaches

5.1 Stop codon read-through

This approach has been developed to address nonsense mutations, which are responsible for 14% of DMD cases (Aartsma-Rus et al., 2009). The rationale is to use a compound that interacts with the translation machinery to incorporate an amino acid instead of terminating protein translation at the site of a premature stop codon. This will result in a protein that is - aside from a one amino acid change at the location of the stop mutation - completely normal (Aurino & Nigro, 2006; Kaufman, 1999; Linde & Kerem, 2008; Malik et al., 2010a). This approach can also induce read-through of real stop codons, but this is thought to be less efficient due to differences in sequence context and location of real vs. aberrant stop codons (Manuvakhova et al., 2000). So far, three compounds have been reported induce efficient read-through stop codons in the DMD mRNA.

5.1.1 Gentamicin

Gentamicin is an aminoglycoside antibiotic binding to the 40S ribosomal subunit when this recognizes a stop codon (Palmer et al., 1979; Singh et al., 1979; Yoshizawa et al., 1998). This causes the insertion of an amino acid at the stop codon position. It has first been shown that it can act on each type of stop codon without any preference in vitro (Howard et al., 2004). Gentamicin (and negamycin) can induce the read-through stop codon in the mdx mouse (Arakawa et al., 2003; Barton-Davis et al., 1999), the most used mouse model for DMD which carries a nonsense mutation in exon 23 (Danko et al., 1992). However, in another report gentamicin was unable to restore dystrophin expression in the same mouse model (Dunant et al., 2003). It was later revealed that there are a number of gentamicin isomers, which all have different read-through efficiencies, and that different gentamicin batches consist of different mixes of these isomers, which can explain these controversial results (Aartsma-Rus et al., 2010; Yoshizawa et al., 1998). Three different clinical trials have been undertaken in

DMD patients using gentamicin (Malik et al., 2010b; Politano et al., 2003; Wagner et al., 2001). In the last one Malik and colleagues used the most active gentamicin isomer and treated the patients for 6 months. For 3 out of 12 patients the number of dystrophin positive fibers increased as assessed by immune histochemical analysis, while the effect was less clear by western blot analysis, as dystrophin was already visible before treatment, possibly due to spontaneous read-through or exon skipping (see below). Since chronic gentamicin use, is known to result in reversible kidney toxicity and irreversible ototoxicity, long term treatment with gentamicin - which would be required for DMD patients - is not realistic.

5.1.2 Ataluren

Ataluren, also called PTC124, was identified via in vitro screening in a luciferase assay. It is more selective for premature stop codons than regular ones, and it can be taken orally unlike gentamicin, which is administered intravenously. Studies in the mdx mouse showed that dystrophin expression could be restored after subcutaneous ataluren treatment (Welch et al., 2007). The compound was first tested in healthy volunteers where it was well tolerated (Hirawat et al., 2007). Then different doses were tested in DMD patients and an increase in dystrophin was reported for 18/38 patients (http://www.drugs.com/clinical_trials/ptc-therapeutics-announces-additional-results-phase-2-study-ptc124-duchenne-muscular-dystrophy-2308.html). In a subsequent placebo-controlled phase IIb trial 174 DMD and BMD patients were treated with two doses or placebo for 48 weeks, and then all were treated with the high dose in an open label extension study (Finkel, 2010). Treatment was well tolerated, but the primary outcome - set at 30 meter increase compared to placebo treated patients in the six minute walk test (6MWT) - was not reached, and the extension study was put on hold. From the data released (http://ptct.client.shareholder.com/releasedetail.cfm?ReleaseID=518941) it could be inferred that the low dose worked better than the high dose. It has been postulated that ataluren efficiency works through a bell shaped curve, which could explain this finding. Dystrophin analysis is pending, and different analyses of subgroups of patients is currently ongoing, as well as studies to identify the most optimal dose. Recently (May 2011) Genzyme and PTC Therapeutics announced that they are planning a follow-up clinical study for DMD patients who previously participated in the clinical trials in the UK, Europe, Israel and Australia, starting December 2011. This will provide access to ataluren to patients who have been involved in earlier clinical trials, as the trial in the USA had already been reinititated.

It has been recently published that the results obtained with the in vitro luciferase screening used to identify ataluren may have been biased, as atluren derivatives can stabilize the luciferase enzyme, giving rise to a false positive (Auld et al., 2010; Auld et al., 2009). However, it has been shown that ataluren has at least some read-through potential (Du et al., 2008; Welch et al., 2007), though it is uncertain whether the levels of dystrophin restoration will be sufficient to restore muscle function.

5.1.3 RTC13

RTC13 is a new compound for stop codon read through. Promising preliminary data were presented at the 14th annual meeting of the American Society of Gene and Cell Therapy (http://www.cureduchenne.org/site/PageServer?pagename=research_index). In the mdx mouse model RTC13 was able to restore dystrophin expression as assessed by western blot and immune-fluorescent analyses. Muscle fiber uptake was improved compared to the previous tested compounds. After 6 weeks of treatment mice showed improvement in muscle strength that was dependent on dystrophin recovery. Serum CK levels dropped and no toxicity was detected. Research to assess if RTC13 oral treatment is feasible is ongoing.

5.1.4 Nonsense mediated decay

A modifying factor which can play a role in the stop codon-read through is nonsense-mediated decay (NMD). This mechanism breaks down mRNAs that carry premature stop codons, thus resulting in less target mRNAs for stop codon read through compounds. It is known that NMD efficiency varies among individuals, for different stop codons, location within the mRNA, and sequence context. In a study of cystic fibrosis patient-derived cell cultures carrying premature stop mutations in their *CFTR* gene, it was shown that NMD was more active in patients who did not respond to gentamicin treatment than in patients who did respond to gentamicin patients (Linde et al., 2007). When NMD was blocked in non-responders' cells, they became more responsive to gentamicin treatment (Linde et al., 2007). It is anticipated that NMD influences other stop codon read through approaches.

5.2 Exon skipping

The idea of the exon skipping approach is based on the observation that the milder BMD phenotype is due to mutations in which the mRNA reading frame is maintained, while the more severe DMD phenotype is caused by frame disrupting mutations. The rationale is to restore the open reading frame. Most (~65%) of the DMD causing mutations are deletions (Aartsma-Rus et al., 2009). Scientists have tried to reframe these mutations by inducing the skipping of additional exons adjacent to the out of frame deletions during pre-mRNA splicing (Figure 2). The reframed mRNA will then allow translation into a smaller, partially functional, BMD-like dystrophin protein. Several groups have worked on this approach using antisense oligonucleotides (AONs) or snRNAs to induce the specific exon skipping in patients' cells in vitro and in several animal models.

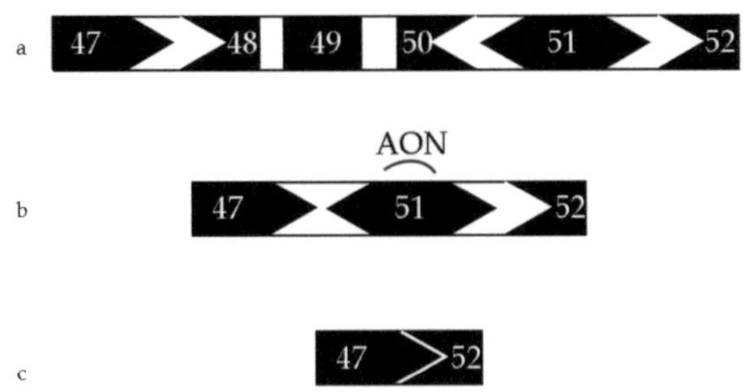

Fig. 2. a. Schematic representation of the DMD genomic region encompassing exons 47 to 52. b. Deletion of exons 48 to 50 leads to an out-of-frame mRNA which can be corrected into an in-frame deletion with the use of antisense oligonucleotides (c).

There are two AON chemistries used in clinical trials for DMD: 2-O-Methyl-Phosphorothioates (2OMePS) and phosphorodiamidate morpholino oligomers (PMOs).

5.2.1 2OMePS studies

2OMePS have a methyl group at the 2'-O position of the ribose, which increases the AON affinity for RNA and avoids RNase H activation of RNA:RNA hybrids (Dominski & Kole, 1993; Sproat et al., 1989). The PS modification is required to further increase the AON nuclease resistance, enhance cellular uptake and increase the serum half-life in vivo.

Proof of principle for the exon skipping approach and dystrophin restoration has been achieved in DMD derived cells and in murine cells (Aartsma-Rus et al., 2003; Errington et al., 2003; Mann et al., 2002; Van Deutekom et al., 2001). To test the feasibility of the approach in vivo the mdx mouse model was mainly used. The premature stop codon in exon 23 leads to a complete absence of dystrophin, and a mild dystrophic phenotype in mice, probably due to a better regenerative capacity. Mouse dystrophin exon 23 is an in frame exon, so it is possible to skip this exon, inducing an exon 22-exon 24 junction which preserves the reading frame. Intramuscular injection of AONs targeting the exon 23 donor splice site resulted in exon 23 skipping and dystrophin synthesis (Lu et al., 2003; Mann et al., 2002). This was accompanied by rescued sarcoglycan expression at the sarcolemma, improved titanic force, while no antibodies against the newly synthesized dystrophin were found in the serum. Gene expression profiling to evaluate AON efficacy and safety was tested in preclinical experiments. AONs were delivered using different carriers (PEI - F127 - Optison) to enhance muscle fibers uptake, or with recombinant adeno-associated virus (rAAV) expressing antisense sequences incorporated in a U7 snRNP gene. Exon skipping induced a shift towards wild type expression levels, which became statistically significant when high exon skipping levels were induced ('t Hoen et al., 2006). Since AON-PEI complexes worsened the muscle inflammation, while F127 and Optison did not enhance AON efficacy in vivo, following experiments were performed using naked AONs. These studies all tested local intramuscular injection, while whole body treatment is required for DMD. It is known that 2OMePS AONs have a favorable serum half-life, as the PS backbones binds to serum proteins with low affinity, which prevents renal filtration and excretion in urine. Normally, 2OMePS AONs are primarily taken up by liver and kidney and the uptake in muscle is poor. However, due to the dystrophic pathology of skeletal muscle in DMD patients, AON uptake is up to 10-fold higher, resulting in sufficient AON levels for exon skipping and dystrophin restoration in skeletal muscles in mdx mice after systemic AON administration (Heemskerk et al., 2009; Lu et al., 2005). In a comparison of intravenous, subcutaneous and intraperitoneal delivery, subcutaneous and intraperitoneal delivery showed the most preferable pharmacokinetic and pharmacodynamic profiles (lower uptake by liver and kidney), while slightly higher exon skipping levels were achieved by intravenous injections (Heemskerk et al., 2010). Based on these results and the relative easy and low invasiveness of subcutenaous injection, this delivery route was selected for systemic clinical trials.

5.2.1.1 Clinical trials with 2OMePS

Since the exon skipping is a mutation specific approach clinical experimentation started with the largest patient cohort that would potentially benefit of skipping a single exon, i.e. exon 51 (13% of all DMD patients (Aartsma-Rus et al., 2009)). Deep phenotypic screening of two BMD patients carrying deletions that could result from exon 51 skipping, showed that these dystrophins can be largely functional (Helderman-van den Enden AT et al., 2010). A first clinical trial was coordinated by Prosensa/GSK in collaboration with the Leiden

University Medical Center, using an AON targeting exon 51 (PRO051, currently called GSK2402968). This trial involved 4 patients who were each injected intramuscularly with 0.8 mg GSK2402968 in their tibialis anterior muscle. This induced specific exon 51 skipping and dystrophin recovery in 64-97% of muscle fibers at levels of 17-35% and 3-12% when quantified by immune-histochemical and western blot analysis, respectively) (Van Deutekom et al., 2007). After these encouraging results, the same AON was used in a subsequent Phase I/IIb clinical trial in which patients were subcutaneously injected and divided into 4 cohorts of 3 patients each based on the dose used (0.5 – 2 - 4 - 6 mg/kg). The AON was well tolerated, and patients showed a dose dependent dystrophin recovery in 60-100% of fibers (Goemans et al., 2011). Dystrophin amounts were quantified via fluorescent signal intensities in immune-histochemical analysis (4 to 11% dystrophin recovery) and via western blot analysis (2 to 20% dystrophin recovery). All patients were included in an open label extension study where they received weekly, subcutaneous treatments of the highest dose (6 mg/kg). The 6-minutes walk test was used as a functional outcome parameter and for most of the patients an improvement in walking distance was found after 3 months (Goemans et al., 2011). This trial did not have a placebo group, so these results, while promising, have to be interpreted with caution. A phase III double blind clinical trial in 180 DMD patients is ongoing to determine whether long term treatment with 6 mg/kg/week GSK2402968 is safe and effective ((http://clinicaltrials.gov/ct2/show/NCT01254019?term=duchenne&rank=4). Furthermore, a trial comparing weekly and biweekly dosing at 6 mg/kg is ongoing (http://clinicaltrials.gov/ct2/show/NCT01153932?term=duchenne&rank=11). Finally, a phase I double-blind, escalating dose, randomized, placebo-controlled study assessing pharmacokinetics, safety, and tolerability in non-ambulant DMD patients is ongoing (http://clinicaltrials.gov/ct2/show/NCT01128855?term=GSK2402968&rank=3) in which patients will receive different dosages (3 – 6 - 9 -12 mg/kg).

5.2.2 PMOs

PMOs contain a morpholino moiety instead of the ribose sugar and phosphoroamidate intersubunit linkages instead of phosphodiester bonds (Kurreck, 2003). PMOs have an affinity for RNA that is comparable to DNA oligos, are nuclease resistant and non-toxic (Summerton, 1999). Their backbone is uncharged, which makes them difficult to transfect in vitro, and as they do not bind serum proteins, their serum half-life is limited as they are filtered out by the kidneys. PMOs have been shown to induce exon skipping and dystrophin restoration in the mdx mouse after intramuscular (Gebski et al., 2003) and systemic injections (Alter et al., 2006; Malerba et al., 2011a; Wu et al., 2010). Upon direct comparison with 2OMePS they were shown to be more effective in inducing exon 23 skipping in the mdx mouse (Heemskerk et al., 2009). However, in all studies exon skipping and dystrophin restoration was only observed in skeletal muscle and not in heart, or only at very low levels unless heroic doses (up to 3 g/kg!) or microbubbles to improve uptake in heart were used (Alter et al., 2009; Wu et al., 2010). It has become clear that repeated low dose injections are more effective than single high dosage injections (Malerba et al., 2011b; Malerba et al., 2009), probably because of the fast PMOs clearance from the body by the kidneys (Heemskerk et al., 2010). Survival studies show that high doses of PMOs could correct the pathology and were well tolerated (Wu et al., 2011b). PMOs have also been used to restore dystrophin expression in the canine model of Duchenne, the golden retriever muscular dystrophy model (GRMD). GRMD dogs carry a splice site mutation in intron 6 leading exon 7 skipping. The skipping of exons 6 and 8 produces an in-frame exon-exon junction. Three dogs have been treated with an equimolar mixture of 3 morpholinos (2 targeting exon 6 and 1 targeting exon 8 in a cumulative dose of 120-200 mg/kg). PMOs were injected 5 to 11 times at weekly or biweekly intervals and tissue examination was performed 2 weeks after the last injection. Dystrophin restoration was achieved showing that exon skipping represents a possible choice also for complex mutations for which more than one exon needs to be skipped (Yokota et al., 2009).

5.2.2.1 Clinical trials with PMOs

Before starting clinical studies optimization of PMOs targeting exon 51 was done in cells and in the hDMD mouse (Arechavala-Gomeza et al., 2007). Clinical studies in DMD patients using PMOs targeting exon 51 (AVI-4658) were performed in the UK by the MDEX consortium in collaboration with AVI Biopharma. Local intramuscular injection in the extensor digitorum longus (EDL) muscle induced exon skipping and dystrophin restoration. After baseline correction for the controlateral, saline injected muscle, 44 to 79% of dystrophin positive fibers were observed (Kinali et al., 2009) at 22-32% of wild type levels (controlateral muscle showed dystrophin levels between 4 and 14%). This led to a Phase I/IIb clinical trial in which 19 patients received 12 weekly intravenous doses of PMO. Patients were divided in cohorts based on six different doses (0.5 - 1 - 2 - 4 - 10 - 20 mg/kg). PMOs were not toxic and well tolerated. The 2 high dosage cohorts showed an increase in the fluorescent intensity per fiber and dystrophin was restored in 7/19 patients. Three patients responded very well showing up to 55% of dystrophin positive fibers with an increase above 10% in mean fluorescence intensity per fiber (Cirak et al., 2011). Based on the varying response it was concluded that dosing was not yet optimal. In a subsequent study recently initiated, weekly intravenous doses of 30 mg/kg and 50 mg/kg for 24 weeks are tested (http://clinicaltrials.gov/ct2/show/NCT01396239?term=AVI-4658&rank=1).

It is difficult to compare results for the experiments performed with the PMOs and 2OMePS, as they were performed by different groups and different analyses were used to quantify dystrophin. In a direct comparison using equal molar amounts of PMO and 2OMePS in the mdx mouse, PMOs targeting exon 23 showed higher exon skipping percentages and higher dystrophin rescue. However, experiments performed in the hDMD mouse model, carrying a copy of the complete human *DMD* gene, there was no clear difference between 2OMePS and PMO AONs targeting exon 44, 45, 46 and 51 upon intramuscular injection (Heemskerk et al., 2009). Differences in the systemic trials for GSK2402968 and AVI-4658 are probably also due to the different pharmacokinetic and pharmacodynamic properties of the AONs. PMOs are extremely stable, but due to their uncharged nature they are filtered out by the kidney and their serum half-life is ~1 hour, so the time for tissue uptake is limited. The 2OMePS AONs by contrast bind serum proteins due to the PS backbone. This prevents renal clearance and increases their serum half-life to weeks. This may underlie the different staining patterns observed between PMO trials (patchy) and 2OMePS trials (more homogeneous).

5.2.3 AON chemistry development

While results in clinical trials are encouraging, ways to improve delivery to muscle tissues, allowing lower AON dosages would be preferred. Many approaches have been tested. Cell penetrating peptides (Jearawiriyapaisarn et al., 2008; Jearawiriyapaisarn et al., 2010; Wu et al., 2008; Yin et al., 2008), muscle targeting peptides connected to cell penetrating peptides (Yin et al., 2009) and guanidine analogs (Hu et al., 2010; Wu et al., 2009) showed the most promising results in the mdx mouse and in the hDMD mouse model (Wu et al., 2011a). Notably, pPMOs (containing arginine-rich peptides covalently bound to the morpholino AONs) have shown great potential in the mdx mouse, inducing high levels of exon skipping in skeletal muscles and heart and high levels of dystrophin rescue. Promising results using pPMOs have also been achieved in the severe mdx-utrophin$^{-/-}$ mouse model, which is defective for dystrophin and its homologue utrophin gene. Normally these mice do not survive beyond 3 months, but survival was increased to over a year after pPMO treatment (Goyenvalle et al., 2010). Unfortunately, preliminary tests in non-human primates showed mild tubular degeneration in the kidney after 4 weekly injections of 9 mg/kg of pPMOs (Moulton & Moulton, 2010). Additional peptide conjugates will hopefully be less toxic (Yin et al., 2011).

5.2.4 Antisense snRNP mediated exon skipping

Due to AON turnover and clearance, life-long treatment would be required. An alternative approach uses viral vectors expressing antisense sequences incorporated in a small nuclear ribonucleoprotein (snRNP). Adeno-associated viral vectors (AAVs) have been used to deliver the modified snRNPs as they have the best capacity to infect the muscle tissue. Different serotypes have been investigated and two molecular strategies which make use of modified U7 and U1 snRNAs have been developed. These snRNAs ensure an efficiently nuclear localization of the antisense construct, specific exon skipping and sustained dystrophin rescue in the mdx mouse model (Denti et al., 2006a; Denti et al., 2006b; Goyenvalle et al., 2004). Optimization for human exons using splicing enhancers has been also performed (Goyenvalle et al., 2009). Preclinical studies show the long-term benefit of the approach for up to 1 year (Denti et al., 2008). However the clinical translation of this approach is complicated by immune response to the viral vector (see section 5.4). Thus immune-suppression will be required, especially for patients for which multiple injections to treat muscles or muscle groups will be required.

5.3 Gene editing

Gene editing is a process in which the endogenous mutated gene is modified to produce a functional dystrophin, either by correcting the DMD causing mutation or by introducing a second mutation which will rescue the effect of the first mutation. This approach has been developed using chimeric RNA-DNA oligonucleotides (RDOs or "chimeraplasts") which anneal to genomic DNA, inducing homologous recombination between the endogenous gene and the RDO, or activating the mismatch repair system. Proof of principle was demonstrated in the mdx mouse muscle (Rando et al., 2000), in muscle precursor cells in vitro and in vivo (Bertoni & Rando, 2002). It has been demonstrated that correction is more efficient when the RDOs target the coding strand (the non transcribed strand) (Bertoni et al., 2005). Unfortunately, the gene conversion efficiency is as yet too low for clinical application and systemic delivery of RDOs in larger animals needs to be optimized further.

Recently another group has pioneered the use of meganucleases to correct the effect of the genetic mutation. The rationale is to correct the reading frame by introducing a microdeletion or micro-insertion into the *DMD* gene. This is done by specific double strand breaks at the end of an exon which precedes a deletion or at the beginning of an exon following a deletion. Meganucleases can be engineered to specifically cut at a certain genomic position causing non-homologous end joining (NHEJ) or homologous recombination when a donor corrected sequence is present. During this process often small deletions or insertions occur, which can restore the reading frame. Proof of principle for this approach has been recently demonstrated in vitro and after local delivery in vivo, albeit at low levels (Chapdelaine et al., 2010). The challenge of this approach will be the delivery of the meganucleases and the limited recognition of target sequences of meganucleases. The recently developed TALE nuclease system (Miller et al., 2011) allows targeting of almost all human sequences, and may provide a better alternative.

5.4 Gene therapy

Gene therapy approaches focus on providing an exogenous functional copy of the mutated gene. Gene therapy approaches are divided into 2 groups based on the type of delivery method used (viral or non-viral vector mediated). Muscle is a difficult target tissue for viral delivery (see below). Furthermore, the huge size of the *DMD* gene and its 11 Kb long full length cDNA sequence (FLDYS) has been one of the bottlenecks in developing this strategy, until smaller dystrophin versions were developed to make them fit into viral vector capsids. These smaller dystrophin coding sequences, called mini-dystrophins (mDYS) and micro-dystrophins (µDys), were designed based on the observations that BMD patients with minor dystrophic phenotype can carry very large deletions (England et al., 1990).

5.4.1 Viral vector based gene therapy

5.4.1.1 Lentiviral vectors

Lentiviral vectors have been used to treat mdx mice locally restoring dystrophin expression at different efficiencies (Kobinger et al., 2003; Li et al., 2005). Kimura and colleagues showed that a lentivirus encoding µDys intramuscularly injected into 2 weeks old mdx^{4cv} mice could restore dystrophin in up to 400-1200 fibers in the tibialis anterior muscle. Mice were sacrificed at 4 different time points (4 weeks - 4 months - 1 year - 2 years) and results were comparable over time. The virus was capable of infecting satellite cells ensuring long-term treatment efficacy (Kimura et al., 2010). However, this may also pose a safety risk, since the transgene expression is ensured by the integration of the viral genome into the host genome. This process can cause neoplastic mutations due to the integration of the viral genome which mainly occurs close to promoter sequences (Maruggi et al., 2009). Systemic delivery of lentiviral vectors to muscle tissue is very challenging, as muscle is post-mitotic and fibers bundles are surrounded by layers of connective tissue that filter out most viruses (>30 nm).

5.4.1.2 Adeno-associated viral vectors

Due to their small size (20 nm) adeno-associated viral vectors (AAVs) are able to efficiently infect muscles. They have been more broadly used for gene therapy for muscle diseases. They do not integrate into the host genome, making them safer than lentiviruses. At least five of the many serotypes known, show a high tropism for muscle tissues (serotypes 1, 2, 6, 8 and 9). Due to the low vector capacity mDYS and µDys have been used and efficiently delivered to skeletal muscle (Gregorevic et al., 2004) and heart. Very promising studies performed in the mdx mouse showed high dystrophin recovery with AAV1 (Wang et al., 2008) and AAV2 (Wang et al., 2000), while studies in the dog model with AAV2, AAV6 (Wang et al., 2007) and AAV8 (Ohshima et al., 2009) raised the issue of cytotoxic immune response against the viral capsid proteins. AAV8 has also been tested in non human primates to delivery human μDys and levels up to 80% were obtained. Unfortunately these levels dropped to 40%when antibodies against the viral vector were present before the injection (Rodino-Klapac et al., 2010).

A clinical study has been also carried out in 6 DMD patients (aged 5-11 years) who received an intramuscular injection into the biceps muscle of a recombinant AAV (rAAV) vector carrying a μDYS gene (Mendell et al., 2010). This μDYS encoded the amino-terminal actin binding domain (ABD), 5 rod repeat domains (R1, R2, R22, R23, and R24), 3 hinge domains (H1, H3 and H4), and the cysteine-rich (CR) domain of the human *DMD* gene. The human cytomegalovirus (CMV) immediate early promoter regulated transgene expression. Vector genomes were packaged in AAV2.5, a serotype 2 capsid variant that contains five AAV1 amino acids (one insertion and four substitutions) in the AAV2 VP1 background. AAV2.5 offers improved muscle transduction properties of AAV1 with minimal recognition by serum neutralizing antibodies. Dystrophin recovery was only very limited (a few fibers for 2 patients). Mendell and colleagues further showed the presence of T-cells recognizing dystrophin epitopes in the circulation of some of the patients. For one patient the recognized epitopes were present in the μDys and deleted in the patient *DMD* gene, so this perhaps was not unexpected. Interestingly, for 2 patients T-cells able to recognize dystrophin expressed in revertant fibers were identified before and after treatment. However, the continuous presence of revertant fibers suggests that the immunity against dystrophin in the blood, did not lead to an auto-immune response in the muscle tissue.

5.5 Cell therapy

Another approach to restore dystrophin expression is based on the use of stem cells with myogenic potential, which can help repair the muscle damage and also delivery a healthy (when donor cells are used) or corrected (when autologous cells are used) *DMD* gene.

Initial efforts focused on the transplantation of adult myoblasts able to fuse with resident damaged muscle fibers creating hybrid muscle fibers (Brussee et al., 1999; Gussoni et al., 1997). However, this approach turned out to be hindered by poor cell survival, inability of the cells to extravagate into the muscle from the circulation, and limited migration of the injected cells within the host muscle (Qu et al., 1998). Results of clinical studies were discouraging (Tremblay et al., 1993). To compensate for the poor migration within muscle, a multiple injection technique has been used (up to 250 injections per square cm) (Skuk et al., 2006), but this is only feasible for small superficial muscles.

Many adult stem cells have been tested for their ability to fuse with muscle fibers in the host dystrophic muscles in murine and canine models. Cells have been grown in vitro and then transplanted in vivo with different efficiencies. Characterization of these cells has been based on their adhesion properties in vitro or on their membrane markers. Muscle side-populations cells, bone-marrow-derived stem cells, muscle-derived stem cells, mesangioblasts, blood and muscle derived CD133+ stem cells and pericytes have been identified (Asakura & Rudnicki, 2002; Benchaouir et al., 2007; Dezawa et al., 2005; Doherty et al., 1998; Gavina et al., 2006; Palumbo et al., 2004; Qu-Petersen et al., 2002). Among all, satellite cells, mesangioblasts and pericytes have shown the most promising characteristics.

Satellite cells are small progenitor cells that lie between the basement membrane and the sarcolemma of the muscle fibers. They are normally in a quiescent state but they can be activated to form new muscle fibers or to fuse with damaged ones upon muscle fiber injury. They are characterized by the expression of *pax3* and *pax7* and they have been shown to restore dystrophin expression after transplantation in dystrophic dog muscle (Montarras et al., 2005). Satellite cells have a great myogenic potential that is unfortunately lost when they are expanded in vitro. Encouraging results obtained in a mouse model led to a phase I clinical trial in DMD patients. Donor satellite cells were isolated from muscle biopsies from first-degree relatives of the affected children and were grown in culture (Daston et al., 1996; Seale et al., 2004). Dystrophin production in muscle fibers was very low (~1%) and no functional or clinical improvement in the children was observed (Peault et al., 2007).

Mesangioblasts express early but not late epithelial markers, they can transmigrate from blood vessels in tissues and they can differentiate in to muscle (Meregalli et al., 2010).

Autologous corrected and donor mesangioblasts have shown to recover dystrophin expression in dystrophic dogs, although some dogs died due to pneumonia which may be caused by accumulation of these cells in the lungs (Sampaolesi et al., 2006). At the moment mesangioblasts are tested in a clinical safety trial in DMD patients.

Pericytes share various markers with mesangioblasts, they can be isolated from skeletal muscle (Dellavalle et al., 2007) and also from non-muscular tissues (Crisan et al., 2008). Dellavalle and coworkers demonstrated that pericytes have high myogenic capacity when injected into SCID/mdx mice. It still needs to be determined whether transplanted pericytes can fully reconstitute the satellite cell niche as real functional stem cells (Morgan & Muntoni, 2007) and whether systemic delivery can be performed.

The main hurdles facing stem cell treatment for DMD are the abundance of muscle (up to 40% of the bodyweight in men), which, combined with the poor efficiency of delivery of cells to muscle tissue (generally (much) below 10%), creates the need for the transplantation of huge numbers of cells in order to generate clinical benefit.

Finally the use of donor stem cells would need constant immune suppression to avoid a specific immune response against the newly formed myofibers. This issue can be solved using autologous stem cells modified ex vivo. However, this process reduces the myogenic properties of cells using current culturing methods, and may impact the behavior of the cells once they are re-injected in the patients.

6. Conclusion

In the last 20-25 years we have seen how basic science findings have been translated into clinical research. Many therapeutic approaches have been developed in vitro, in preclinical animal models and some of them have advanced to the clinical stage. Among all therapeutic approaches the exon skipping is at the moment the most promising for clinical application in the near future.

7. References

't Hoen, P. A., van der Wees, C. G., Aartsma-Rus, A., Turk, R., Goyenvalle, A., Danos, O., Garcia, L., van Ommen, G. J., den Dunnen, J. T., & Van Deutekom, J. C. (April 2006). Gene expression profiling to monitor therapeutic and adverse effects of antisense therapies for Duchenne muscular dystrophy. *Pharmacogenomics.*, Vol.7,No.3, (April 2006), pp. 281-297, ISSN

Aartsma-Rus, A., den Dunnen, J. T., & van Ommen, G. J. (December 2010). New insights in gene-derived therapy: the example of Duchenne muscular dystrophy. *Ann.N.Y.Acad.Sci.*, Vol.1214,No.December 2010), pp. 199-212, ISSN

Aartsma-Rus, A., Fokkema, I., Verschuuren, J., Ginjaar, I., van, D. J., van Ommen, G. J., & den Dunnen, J. T. (March 2009). Theoretic applicability of antisense-mediated exon skipping for Duchenne muscular dystrophy mutations. *Hum.Mutat.*, Vol.30,No.3, (March 2009), pp. 293-299, ISSN

Aartsma-Rus, A., Janson, A. A., Kaman, W. E., Bremmer-Bout, M., den Dunnen, J. T., Baas, F., van Ommen, G. J., & Van Deutekom, J. C. (April 2003). Therapeutic antisense-induced exon skipping in cultured muscle cells from six different DMD patients. *Hum.Mol.Genet.*, Vol.12,No.8, (April 2003), pp. 907-914, ISSN

Ahn, A. H., Freener, C. A., Gussoni, E., Yoshida, M., Ozawa, E., & Kunkel, L. M. (February 1996). The three human syntrophin genes are expressed in diverse tissues, have distinct chromosomal locations, and each bind to dystrophin and its relatives. *J.Biol.Chem.*, Vol.271,No.5, (February 1996), pp. 2724-2730, ISSN

Ahn, A. H. and Kunkel, L. M. (February 1995). Syntrophin binds to an alternatively spliced exon of dystrophin. *J.Cell Biol.*, Vol.128,No.3, (February 1995), pp. 363-371, ISSN

Allen, D. G., Gervasio, O. L., Yeung, E. W., & Whitehead, N. P. (February 2010). Calcium and the damage pathways in muscular dystrophy. *Can.J.Physiol Pharmacol.*, Vol.88,No.2, (February 2010), pp. 83-91, ISSN

Alter, J., Lou, F., Rabinowitz, A., Yin, H., Rosenfeld, J., Wilton, S. D., Partridge, T. A., & Lu, Q. L. (February 2006). Systemic delivery of morpholino oligonucleotide restores dystrophin expression bodywide and improves dystrophic pathology. *Nat.Med.*, Vol.12,No.2, (February 2006), pp. 175-177, ISSN

Alter, J., Sennoga, C. A., Lopes, D. M., Eckersley, R. J., & Wells, D. J. (June 2009). Microbubble stability is a major determinant of the efficiency of ultrasound and microbubble mediated in vivo gene transfer. *Ultrasound Med.Biol.*, Vol.35,No.6, (June 2009), pp. 976-984, ISSN

Arakawa, M., Shiozuka, M., Nakayama, Y., Hara, T., Hamada, M., Kondo, S., Ikeda, D., Takahashi, Y., Sawa, R., Nonomura, Y., Sheykholeslami, K., Kondo, K., Kaga, K., Kitamura, T., Suzuki-Miyagoe, Y., Takeda, S., & Matsuda, R. (November 2003). Negamycin restores dystrophin expression in skeletal and cardiac muscles of mdx mice. *J.Biochem.*, Vol.134,No.5, (November 2003), pp. 751-758, ISSN

Arechavala-Gomeza, V., Graham, I. R., Popplewell, L. J., Adams, A. M., Aartsma-Rus, A., Kinali, M., Morgan, J. E., Van Deutekom, J. C., Wilton, S. D., Dickson, G., & Muntoni, F. (September 2007). Comparative analysis of antisense oligonucleotide sequences for targeted skipping of exon 51 during dystrophin pre-mRNA splicing in human muscle. *Hum.Gene Ther.*, Vol.18,No.9, (September 2007), pp. 798-810, ISSN

Asakura, A. and Rudnicki, M. A. (November 2002). Side population cells from diverse adult tissues are capable of in vitro hematopoietic differentiation. *Exp.Hematol.*, Vol.30,No.11, (November 2002), pp. 1339-1345, ISSN

Auld, D. S., Lovell, S., Thorne, N., Lea, W. A., Maloney, D. J., Shen, M., Rai, G., Battaile, K. P., Thomas, C. J., Simeonov, A., Hanzlik, R. P., & Inglese, J. (March 2010). Molecular basis for the high-affinity binding and stabilization of firefly luciferase by PTC124. *Proc.Natl.Acad.Sci.U.S.A*, Vol.107,No.11, (March 2010), pp. 4878-4883, ISSN

Auld, D. S., Thorne, N., Maguire, W. F., & Inglese, J. (March 2009). Mechanism of PTC124 activity in cell-based luciferase assays of nonsense codon suppression. *Proc.Natl.Acad.Sci.U.S.A*, Vol.106,No.9, (March 2009), pp. 3585-3590, ISSN

Aurino, S. and Nigro, V. (June 2006). Readthrough strategies for stop codons in Duchenne muscular dystrophy. *Acta Myol.*, Vol.25,No.1, (June 2006), pp. 5-12, ISSN

Barton-Davis, E. R., Cordier, L., Shoturma, D. I., Leland, S. E., & Sweeney, H. L. (August 1999). Aminoglycoside antibiotics restore dystrophin function to skeletal muscles of mdx mice. *J.Clin.Invest*, Vol.104,No.4, (August 1999), pp. 375-381, ISSN

Benchaouir, R., Meregalli, M., Farini, A., D'Antona, G., Belicchi, M., Goyenvalle, A., Battistelli, M., Bresolin, N., Bottinelli, R., Garcia, L., & Torrente, Y. (December 2007). Restoration of human dystrophin following transplantation of exon-skipping-engineered DMD patient stem cells into dystrophic mice. *Cell Stem Cell*, Vol.1,No.6, (December 2007), pp. 646-657, ISSN

Bertoni, C., Morris, G. E., & Rando, T. A. (January 2005). Strand bias in oligonucleotide-mediated dystrophin gene editing. *Hum.Mol.Genet.*, Vol.14,No.2, (January 2005), pp. 221-233, ISSN

Bertoni, C. and Rando, T. A. (April 2002). Dystrophin gene repair in mdx muscle precursor cells in vitro and in vivo mediated by RNA-DNA chimeric oligonucleotides. *Hum.Gene Ther.*, Vol.13,No.6, (April 2002), pp. 707-718, ISSN

Biggar, W. D., Gingras, M., Fehlings, D. L., Harris, V. A., & Steele, C. A. (January 2001). Deflazacort treatment of Duchenne muscular dystrophy. *J.Pediatr.*, Vol.138,No.1, (January 2001), pp. 45-50, ISSN

Bish, L. T., Sleeper, M. M., Forbes, S. C., Morine, K., Reynolds, C., Singletary, G. E., Trafny, D., Pham, J., Bogan, J., Kornegay, J. N., Vandenborne, K., Walter, G. A., & Sweeney, H. L. (July 2011). Long-term systemic myostatin inhibition via liver-targeted gene transfer in Golden Retriever Muscular Dystrophy. *Hum.Gene Ther.*, Vol.July 2011), pp.

Blake, D. J., Weir, A., Newey, S. E., & Davies, K. E. (April 2002). Function and genetics of dystrophin and dystrophin-related proteins in muscle. *Physiol Rev.*, Vol.82,No.2, (April 2002), pp. 291-329, ISSN

Brenman, J. E., Chao, D. S., Xia, H., Aldape, K., & Bredt, D. S. (September 1995). Nitric oxide synthase complexed with dystrophin and absent from skeletal muscle sarcolemma in Duchenne muscular dystrophy. *Cell*, Vol.82,No.5, (September 1995), pp. 743-752, ISSN

Brussee, V., Tardif, F., Roy, B., Goulet, M., Sebille, A., & Tremblay, J. P. (June 1999). Successful myoblast transplantation in fibrotic muscles: no increased impairment by the connective tissue. *Transplantation,* Vol.67,No.12, (June 1999), pp. 1618-1622, ISSN

Burghes, A. H., Logan, C., Hu, X., Belfall, B., Worton, R. G., & Ray, P. N. (July 1987). A cDNA clone from the Duchenne/Becker muscular dystrophy gene. *Nature,* Vol.328,No.6129, (July 1987), pp. 434-437, ISSN

Bushby, K., Finkel, R., Birnkrant, D. J., Case, L. E., Clemens, P. R., Cripe, L., Kaul, A., Kinnett, K., McDonald, C., Pandya, S., Poysky, J., Shapiro, F., Tomezsko, J., & Constantin, C. (January 2010a). Diagnosis and management of Duchenne muscular dystrophy, part 1: diagnosis, and pharmacological and psychosocial management. *Lancet Neurol.,* Vol.9,No.1, (January 2010a), pp. 77-93, ISSN

Bushby, K., Finkel, R., Birnkrant, D. J., Case, L. E., Clemens, P. R., Cripe, L., Kaul, A., Kinnett, K., McDonald, C., Pandya, S., Poysky, J., Shapiro, F., Tomezsko, J., & Constantin, C. (February 2010b). Diagnosis and management of Duchenne muscular dystrophy, part 2: implementation of multidisciplinary care. *Lancet Neurol.,* Vol.9,No.2, (February 2010b), pp. 177-189, ISSN

Chamberlain, J. S., Gibbs, R. A., Ranier, J. E., Nguyen, P. N., & Caskey, C. T. (December 1988). Deletion screening of the Duchenne muscular dystrophy locus via multiplex DNA amplification. *Nucleic Acids Res.,* Vol.16,No.23, (December 1988), pp. 11141-11156, ISSN

Chapdelaine, P., Pichavant, C., Rousseau, J., Paques, F., & Tremblay, J. P. (July 2010). Meganucleases can restore the reading frame of a mutated dystrophin. *Gene Ther.,* Vol.17,No.7, (July 2010), pp. 846-858, ISSN

Cirak, S., Arechavala-Gomeza, V., Guglieri, M., Feng, L., Torelli, S., Anthony, K., Abbs, S., Garralda, M. E., Bourke, J., Wells, D. J., Dickson, G., Wood, M. J., Wilton, S. D., Straub, V., Kole, R., Shrewsbury, S. B., Sewry, C., Morgan, J. E., Bushby, K., & Muntoni, F. (August 2011). Exon skipping and dystrophin restoration in patients with Duchenne muscular dystrophy after systemic phosphorodiamidate morpholino oligomer treatment: an open-label, phase 2, dose-escalation study. *Lancet,* Vol.378,No.9791, (August 2011), pp. 595-605, ISSN

Crisan, M., Yap, S., Casteilla, L., Chen, C. W., Corselli, M., Park, T. S., Andriolo, G., Sun, B., Zheng, B., Zhang, L., Norotte, C., Teng, P. N., Traas, J., Schugar, R., Deasy, B. M., Badylak, S., Buhring, H. J., Giacobino, J. P., Lazzari, L., Huard, J., & Peault, B. (September 2008). A perivascular origin for mesenchymal stem cells in multiple human organs. *Cell Stem Cell,* Vol.3,No.3, (September 2008), pp. 301-313, ISSN

Danko, I., Chapman, V., & Wolff, J. A. (July 1992). The frequency of revertants in mdx mouse genetic models for Duchenne muscular dystrophy. *Pediatr.Res.,* Vol.32,No.1, (July 1992), pp. 128-131, ISSN

Daston, G., Lamar, E., Olivier, M., & Goulding, M. (March 1996). Pax-3 is necessary for migration but not differentiation of limb muscle precursors in the mouse. *Development,* Vol.122,No.3, (March 1996), pp. 1017-1027, ISSN

Dellavalle, A., Sampaolesi, M., Tonlorenzi, R., Tagliafico, E., Sacchetti, B., Perani, L., Innocenzi, A., Galvez, B. G., Messina, G., Morosetti, R., Li, S., Belicchi, M., Peretti,

G., Chamberlain, J. S., Wright, W. E., Torrente, Y., Ferrari, S., Bianco, P., & Cossu, G. (March 2007). Pericytes of human skeletal muscle are myogenic precursors distinct from satellite cells. *Nat.Cell Biol.*, Vol.9,No.3, (March 2007), pp. 255-267, ISSN

Denti, M. A., Incitti, T., Sthandier, O., Nicoletti, C., De Angelis, F. G., Rizzuto, E., Auricchio, A., Musaro, A., & Bozzoni, I. (June 2008). Long-term benefit of adeno-associated virus/antisense-mediated exon skipping in dystrophic mice. *Hum.Gene Ther.*, Vol.19,No.6, (June 2008), pp. 601-608, ISSN

Denti, M. A., Rosa, A., D'Antona, G., Sthandier, O., De Angelis, F. G., Nicoletti, C., Allocca, M., Pansarasa, O., Parente, V., Musaro, A., Auricchio, A., Bottinelli, R., & Bozzoni, I. (March 2006a). Body-wide gene therapy of Duchenne muscular dystrophy in the mdx mouse model. *Proc.Natl.Acad.Sci.U.S.A*, Vol.103,No.10, (March 2006a), pp. 3758-3763, ISSN

Denti, M. A., Rosa, A., D'Antona, G., Sthandier, O., De Angelis, F. G., Nicoletti, C., Allocca, M., Pansarasa, O., Parente, V., Musaro, A., Auricchio, A., Bottinelli, R., & Bozzoni, I. (May 2006b). Chimeric adeno-associated virus/antisense U1 small nuclear RNA effectively rescues dystrophin synthesis and muscle function by local treatment of mdx mice. *Hum.Gene Ther.*, Vol.17,No.5, (May 2006b), pp. 565-574, ISSN

Dezawa, M., Ishikawa, H., Itokazu, Y., Yoshihara, T., Hoshino, M., Takeda, S., Ide, C., & Nabeshima, Y. (July 2005). Bone marrow stromal cells generate muscle cells and repair muscle degeneration. *Science*, Vol.309,No.5732, (July 2005), pp. 314-317, ISSN

Doherty, M. J., Ashton, B. A., Walsh, S., Beresford, J. N., Grant, M. E., & Canfield, A. E. (May 1998). Vascular pericytes express osteogenic potential in vitro and in vivo. *J.Bone Miner.Res.*, Vol.13,No.5, (May 1998), pp. 828-838, ISSN

Dominski, Z. and Kole, R. (September 1993). Restoration of correct splicing in thalassemic pre-mRNA by antisense oligonucleotides. *Proc.Natl.Acad.Sci.U.S.A*, Vol.90,No.18, (September 1993), pp. 8673-8677, ISSN

Dorchies, O. M., Wagner, S., Buetler, T. M., & Ruegg, U. T. (May 2009). Protection of dystrophic muscle cells with polyphenols from green tea correlates with improved glutathione balance and increased expression of 67LR, a receptor for (-)-epigallocatechin gallate. *Biofactors*, Vol.35,No.3, (May 2009), pp. 279-294, ISSN

Du, M., Liu, X., Welch, E. M., Hirawat, S., Peltz, S. W., & Bedwell, D. M. (February 2008). PTC124 is an orally bioavailable compound that promotes suppression of the human CFTR-G542X nonsense allele in a CF mouse model. *Proc.Natl.Acad.Sci.U.S.A*, Vol.105,No.6, (February 2008), pp. 2064-2069, ISSN

Dumonceaux, J., Marie, S., Beley, C., Trollet, C., Vignaud, A., Ferry, A., Butler-Browne, G., & Garcia, L. (May 2010). Combination of myostatin pathway interference and dystrophin rescue enhances tetanic and specific force in dystrophic mdx mice. *Mol.Ther.*, Vol.18,No.5, (May 2010), pp. 881-887, ISSN

Dunant, P., Walter, M. C., Karpati, G., & Lochmuller, H. (May 2003). Gentamicin fails to increase dystrophin expression in dystrophin-deficient muscle. *Muscle Nerve*, Vol.27,No.5, (May 2003), pp. 624-627, ISSN

Eagle, M., Baudouin, S. V., Chandler, C., Giddings, D. R., Bullock, R., & Bushby, K. (December 2002). Survival in Duchenne muscular dystrophy: improvements in life expectancy since 1967 and the impact of home nocturnal ventilation. *Neuromuscul.Disord.*, Vol.12,No.10, (December 2002), pp. 926-929, ISSN

Emery, A. E. (July 1993). Duchenne muscular dystrophy--Meryon's disease. *Neuromuscul.Disord.*, Vol.3,No.4, (July 1993), pp. 263-266, ISSN

Emery, A. E. (February 2002). The muscular dystrophies. *Lancet*, Vol.359,No.9307, (February 2002), pp. 687-695, ISSN

England, S. B., Nicholson, L. V., Johnson, M. A., Forrest, S. M., Love, D. R., Zubrzycka-Gaarn, E. E., Bulman, D. E., Harris, J. B., & Davies, K. E. (January 1990). Very mild muscular dystrophy associated with the deletion of 46% of dystrophin. *Nature*, Vol.343,No.6254, (January 1990), pp. 180-182, ISSN

Errington, S. J., Mann, C. J., Fletcher, S., & Wilton, S. D. (June 2003). Target selection for antisense oligonucleotide induced exon skipping in the dystrophin gene. *J.Gene Med.*, Vol.5,No.6, (June 2003), pp. 518-527, ISSN

Ervasti, J. M., Ohlendieck, K., Kahl, S. D., Gaver, M. G., & Campbell, K. P. (May 1990). Deficiency of a glycoprotein component of the dystrophin complex in dystrophic muscle. *Nature*, Vol.345,No.6273, (May 1990), pp. 315-319, ISSN

Finkel, R. S. (September 2010). Read-through strategies for suppression of nonsense mutations in Duchenne/ Becker muscular dystrophy: aminoglycosides and ataluren (PTC124). *J.Child Neurol.*, Vol.25,No.9, (September 2010), pp. 1158-1164, ISSN

Gavina, M., Belicchi, M., Rossi, B., Ottoboni, L., Colombo, F., Meregalli, M., Battistelli, M., Forzenigo, L., Biondetti, P., Pisati, F., Parolini, D., Farini, A., Issekutz, A. C., Bresolin, N., Rustichelli, F., Constantin, G., & Torrente, Y. (October 2006). VCAM-1 expression on dystrophic muscle vessels has a critical role in the recruitment of human blood-derived CD133+ stem cells after intra-arterial transplantation. *Blood*, Vol.108,No.8, (October 2006), pp. 2857-2866, ISSN

Gebski, B. L., Mann, C. J., Fletcher, S., & Wilton, S. D. (August 2003). Morpholino antisense oligonucleotide induced dystrophin exon 23 skipping in mdx mouse muscle. *Hum.Mol.Genet.*, Vol.12,No.15, (August 2003), pp. 1801-1811, ISSN

Goemans, N. M., Tulinius, M., van den Akker, J. T., Burm, B. E., Ekhart, P. F., Heuvelmans, N., Holling, T., Janson, A. A., Platenburg, G. J., Sipkens, J. A., Sitsen, J. M., Aartsma-Rus, A., van Ommen, G. J., Buyse, G., Darin, N., Verschuuren, J. J., Campion, G. V., de Kimpe, S. J., & Van Deutekom, J. C. (April 2011). Systemic administration of PRO051 in Duchenne's muscular dystrophy. *N.Engl.J.Med.*, Vol.364,No.16, (April 2011), pp. 1513-1522, ISSN

Goyenvalle, A., Babbs, A., Powell, D., Kole, R., Fletcher, S., Wilton, S. D., & Davies, K. E. (January 2010). Prevention of dystrophic pathology in severely affected dystrophin/utrophin-deficient mice by morpholino-oligomer-mediated exon-skipping. *Mol.Ther.*, Vol.18,No.1, (January 2010), pp. 198-205, ISSN

Goyenvalle, A., Babbs, A., van Ommen, G. J., Garcia, L., & Davies, K. E. (July 2009). Enhanced exon-skipping induced by U7 snRNA carrying a splicing silencer sequence: Promising tool for DMD therapy. *Mol.Ther.*, Vol.17,No.7, (July 2009), pp. 1234-1240, ISSN

Goyenvalle, A., Vulin, A., Fougerousse, F., Leturcq, F., Kaplan, J. C., Garcia, L., & Danos, O. (December 2004). Rescue of dystrophic muscle through U7 snRNA-mediated exon skipping. *Science*, Vol.306,No.5702, (December 2004), pp. 1796-1799, ISSN

Gregorevic, P., Blankinship, M. J., Allen, J. M., Crawford, R. W., Meuse, L., Miller, D. G., Russell, D. W., & Chamberlain, J. S. (August 2004). Systemic delivery of genes to striated muscles using adeno-associated viral vectors. *Nat.Med.*, Vol.10,No.8, (August 2004), pp. 828-834, ISSN

Gussoni, E., Blau, H. M., & Kunkel, L. M. (September 1997). The fate of individual myoblasts after transplantation into muscles of DMD patients. *Nat.Med.*, Vol.3,No.9, (September 1997), pp. 970-977, ISSN

Heemskerk, H., de, W. C., van, K. P., Heuvelmans, N., Sabatelli, P., Rimessi, P., Braghetta, P., van Ommen, G. J., de, K. S., Ferlini, A., Aartsma-Rus, A., & Van Deutekom, J. C. (June 2010). Preclinical PK and PD studies on 2'-O-methyl-phosphorothioate RNA antisense oligonucleotides in the mdx mouse model. *Mol.Ther.*, Vol.18,No.6, (June 2010), pp. 1210-1217, ISSN

Heemskerk, H. A., de Winter, C. L., de Kimpe, S. J., van Kuik-Romeijn, P., Heuvelmans, N., Platenburg, G. J., van Ommen, G. J., Van Deutekom, J. C., & Aartsma-Rus, A. (March 2009). In vivo comparison of 2'-O-methyl phosphorothioate and morpholino antisense oligonucleotides for Duchenne muscular dystrophy exon skipping. *J.Gene Med.*, Vol.11,No.3, (March 2009), pp. 257-266, ISSN

Helderman-van den Enden AT, Straathof, C. S., Aartsma-Rus, A., den Dunnen, J. T., Verbist, B. M., Bakker, E., Verschuuren, J. J., & Ginjaar, H. B. (April 2010). Becker muscular dystrophy patients with deletions around exon 51; a promising outlook for exon skipping therapy in Duchenne patients. *Neuromuscul.Disord.*, Vol.20,No.4, (April 2010), pp. 251-254, ISSN

Hirawat, S., Welch, E. M., Elfring, G. L., Northcutt, V. J., Paushkin, S., Hwang, S., Leonard, E. M., Almstead, N. G., Ju, W., Peltz, S. W., & Miller, L. L. (April 2007). Safety, tolerability, and pharmacokinetics of PTC124, a nonaminoglycoside nonsense mutation suppressor, following single- and multiple-dose administration to healthy male and female adult volunteers. *J.Clin.Pharmacol.*, Vol.47,No.4, (April 2007), pp. 430-444, ISSN

Hoffman, E. P., Brown, R. H., Jr., & Kunkel, L. M. (December 1987). Dystrophin: the protein product of the Duchenne muscular dystrophy locus. *Cell*, Vol.51,No.6, (December 1987), pp. 919-928, ISSN

Hoffman, E. P., Fischbeck, K. H., Brown, R. H., Johnson, M., Medori, R., Loike, J. D., Harris, J. B., Waterston, R., Brooke, M., Specht, L., & . (May 1988). Characterization of dystrophin in muscle-biopsy specimens from patients with Duchenne's or Becker's muscular dystrophy. *N.Engl.J.Med.*, Vol.318,No.21, (May 1988), pp. 1363-1368, ISSN

Hohenester, E., Tisi, D., Talts, J. F., & Timpl, R. (November 1999). The crystal structure of a laminin G-like module reveals the molecular basis of alpha-dystroglycan binding to laminins, perlecan, and agrin. *Mol.Cell*, Vol.4,No.5, (November 1999), pp. 783-792, ISSN

Howard, M. T., Anderson, C. B., Fass, U., Khatri, S., Gesteland, R. F., Atkins, J. F., & Flanigan, K. M. (March 2004). Readthrough of dystrophin stop codon mutations induced by aminoglycosides. *Ann.Neurol.*, Vol.55,No.3, (March 2004), pp. 422-426, ISSN

Hu, Y., Wu, B., Zillmer, A., Lu, P., Benrashid, E., Wang, M., Doran, T., Shaban, M., Wu, X., & Lu, Q. L. (April 2010). Guanine analogues enhance antisense oligonucleotide-induced exon skipping in dystrophin gene in vitro and in vivo. *Mol.Ther.*, Vol.18,No.4, (April 2010), pp. 812-818, ISSN

Ibraghimov-Beskrovnaya, O., Ervasti, J. M., Leveille, C. J., Slaughter, C. A., Sernett, S. W., & Campbell, K. P. (February 1992). Primary structure of dystrophin-associated glycoproteins linking dystrophin to the extracellular matrix. *Nature*, Vol.355,No.6362, (February 1992), pp. 696-702, ISSN

Janssen, B., Hartmann, C., Scholz, V., Jauch, A., & Zschocke, J. (February 2005). MLPA analysis for the detection of deletions, duplications and complex rearrangements in the dystrophin gene: potential and pitfalls. *Neurogenetics.*, Vol.6,No.1, (February 2005), pp. 29-35, ISSN

Jarrett, H. W. and Foster, J. L. (March 1995). Alternate binding of actin and calmodulin to multiple sites on dystrophin. *J.Biol.Chem.*, Vol.270,No.10, (March 1995), pp. 5578-5586, ISSN

Jearawiriyapaisarn, N., Moulton, H. M., Buckley, B., Roberts, J., Sazani, P., Fucharoen, S., Iversen, P. L., & Kole, R. (September 2008). Sustained dystrophin expression induced by peptide-conjugated morpholino oligomers in the muscles of mdx mice. *Mol.Ther.*, Vol.16,No.9, (September 2008), pp. 1624-1629, ISSN

Jearawiriyapaisarn, N., Moulton, H. M., Sazani, P., Kole, R., & Willis, M. S. (February 2010). Long-term improvement in mdx cardiomyopathy after therapy with peptide-conjugated morpholino oligomers. *Cardiovasc.Res.*, Vol.85,No.3, (February 2010), pp. 444-453, ISSN

Kaufman, R. J. (August 1999). Correction of genetic disease by making sense from nonsense. *J.Clin.Invest*, Vol.104,No.4, (August 1999), pp. 367-368, ISSN

Kimura, E., Li, S., Gregorevic, P., Fall, B. M., & Chamberlain, J. S. (January 2010). Dystrophin delivery to muscles of mdx mice using lentiviral vectors leads to myogenic progenitor targeting and stable gene expression. *Mol.Ther.*, Vol.18,No.1, (January 2010), pp. 206-213, ISSN

Kinali, M., Arechavala-Gomeza, V., Feng, L., Cirak, S., Hunt, D., Adkin, C., Guglieri, M., Ashton, E., Abbs, S., Nihoyannopoulos, P., Garralda, M. E., Rutherford, M., McCulley, C., Popplewell, L., Graham, I. R., Dickson, G., Wood, M. J., Wells, D. J., Wilton, S. D., Kole, R., Straub, V., Bushby, K., Sewry, C., Morgan, J. E., & Muntoni, F. (October 2009). Local restoration of dystrophin expression with the morpholino oligomer AVI-4658 in Duchenne muscular dystrophy: a single-blind, placebo-controlled, dose-escalation, proof-of-concept study. *Lancet Neurol.*, Vol.8,No.10, (October 2009), pp. 918-928, ISSN

King, W. M., Ruttencutter, R., Nagaraja, H. N., Matkovic, V., Landoll, J., Hoyle, C., Mendell, J. R., & Kissel, J. T. (May 2007). Orthopedic outcomes of long-term daily corticosteroid treatment in Duchenne muscular dystrophy. *Neurology*, Vol.68,No.19, (May 2007), pp. 1607-1613, ISSN

Kingston, H. M., Sarfarazi, M., Thomas, N. S., & Harper, P. S. (1984). Localisation of the Becker muscular dystrophy gene on the short arm of the X chromosome by linkage to cloned DNA sequences. *Hum.Genet.*, Vol.67,No.1, (1984), pp. 6-17, ISSN

Kobinger, G. P., Louboutin, J. P., Barton, E. R., Sweeney, H. L., & Wilson, J. M. (October 2003). Correction of the dystrophic phenotype by in vivo targeting of muscle progenitor cells. *Hum.Gene Ther.*, Vol.14,No.15, (October 2003), pp. 1441-1449, ISSN

Koenig, M., Beggs, A. H., Moyer, M., Scherpf, S., Heindrich, K., Bettecken, T., Meng, G., Muller, C. R., Lindlof, M., Kaariainen, H., & . (October 1989). The molecular basis for Duchenne versus Becker muscular dystrophy: correlation of severity with type of deletion. *Am.J.Hum.Genet.*, Vol.45,No.4, (October 1989), pp. 498-506, ISSN

Koenig, M., Hoffman, E. P., Bertelson, C. J., Monaco, A. P., Feener, C., & Kunkel, L. M. (July 1987). Complete cloning of the Duchenne muscular dystrophy (DMD) cDNA and preliminary genomic organization of the DMD gene in normal and affected individuals. *Cell*, Vol.50,No.3, (July 1987), pp. 509-517, ISSN

Koenig, M. and Kunkel, L. M. (March 1990). Detailed analysis of the repeat domain of dystrophin reveals four potential hinge segments that may confer flexibility. *J.Biol.Chem.*, Vol.265,No.8, (March 1990), pp. 4560-4566, ISSN

Koenig, M., Monaco, A. P., & Kunkel, L. M. (April 1988). The complete sequence of dystrophin predicts a rod-shaped cytoskeletal protein. *Cell*, Vol.53,No.2, (April 1988), pp. 219-228, ISSN

Kurreck, J. (April 2003). Antisense technologies. Improvement through novel chemical modifications. *Eur.J.Biochem.*, Vol.270,No.8, (April 2003), pp. 1628-1644, ISSN

Lai, Y., Thomas, G. D., Yue, Y., Yang, H. T., Li, D., Long, C., Judge, L., Bostick, B., Chamberlain, J. S., Terjung, R. L., & Duan, D. (March 2009). Dystrophins carrying spectrin-like repeats 16 and 17 anchor nNOS to the sarcolemma and enhance exercise performance in a mouse model of muscular dystrophy. *J.Clin.Invest*, Vol.119,No.3, (March 2009), pp. 624-635, ISSN

Lawler, J. M. (May 2011). Exacerbation of pathology by oxidative stress in respiratory and locomotor muscles with Duchenne muscular dystrophy. *J.Physiol*, Vol.589,No.Pt 9, (May 2011), pp. 2161-2170, ISSN

Li, S., Kimura, E., Fall, B. M., Reyes, M., Angello, J. C., Welikson, R., Hauschka, S. D., & Chamberlain, J. S. (July 2005). Stable transduction of myogenic cells with lentiviral vectors expressing a minidystrophin. *Gene Ther.*, Vol.12,No.14, (July 2005), pp. 1099-1108, ISSN

Linde, L., Boelz, S., Nissim-Rafinia, M., Oren, Y. S., Wilschanski, M., Yaacov, Y., Virgilis, D., Neu-Yilik, G., Kulozik, A. E., Kerem, E., & Kerem, B. (March 2007). Nonsense-mediated mRNA decay affects nonsense transcript levels and governs response of cystic fibrosis patients to gentamicin. *J.Clin.Invest*, Vol.117,No.3, (March 2007), pp. 683-692, ISSN

Linde, L. and Kerem, B. (November 2008). Introducing sense into nonsense in treatments of human genetic diseases. *Trends Genet.*, Vol.24,No.11, (November 2008), pp. 552-563, ISSN

Lu, Q. L., Mann, C. J., Lou, F., Bou-Gharios, G., Morris, G. E., Xue, S. A., Fletcher, S., Partridge, T. A., & Wilton, S. D. (August 2003). Functional amounts of dystrophin produced by skipping the mutated exon in the mdx dystrophic mouse. *Nat.Med.*, Vol.9,No.8, (August 2003), pp. 1009-1014, ISSN

Lu, Q. L., Rabinowitz, A., Chen, Y. C., Yokota, T., Yin, H., Alter, J., Jadoon, A., Bou-Gharios, G., & Partridge, T. (January 2005). Systemic delivery of antisense oligoribonucleotide restores dystrophin expression in body-wide skeletal muscles. *Proc.Natl.Acad.Sci.U.S.A*, Vol.102,No.1, (January 2005), pp. 198-203, ISSN

Malerba, A., Boldrin, L., & Dickson, G. (August 2011a). Long-term systemic administration of unconjugated morpholino oligomers for therapeutic expression of dystrophin by exon skipping in skeletal muscle: implications for cardiac muscle integrity. *Nucleic Acid Ther.*, Vol.21,No.4, (August 2011a), pp. 293-298, ISSN

Malerba, A., Sharp, P. S., Graham, I. R., Arechavala-Gomeza, V., Foster, K., Muntoni, F., Wells, D. J., & Dickson, G. (February 2011b). Chronic systemic therapy with low-dose morpholino oligomers ameliorates the pathology and normalizes locomotor behavior in mdx mice. *Mol.Ther.*, Vol.19,No.2, (February 2011b), pp. 345-354, ISSN

Malerba, A., Thorogood, F. C., Dickson, G., & Graham, I. R. (September 2009). Dosing regimen has a significant impact on the efficiency of morpholino oligomer-induced exon skipping in mdx mice. *Hum.Gene Ther.*, Vol.20,No.9, (September 2009), pp. 955-965, ISSN

Malik, V., Rodino-Klapac, L. R., Viollet, L., & Mendell, J. R. (November 2010a). Aminoglycoside-induced mutation suppression (stop codon readthrough) as a therapeutic strategy for Duchenne muscular dystrophy. *Ther.Adv.Neurol.Disord.*, Vol.3,No.6, (November 2010a), pp. 379-389, ISSN

Malik, V., Rodino-Klapac, L. R., Viollet, L., Wall, C., King, W., Al-Dahhak, R., Lewis, S., Shilling, C. J., Kota, J., Serrano-Munuera, C., Hayes, J., Mahan, J. D., Campbell, K. J., Banwell, B., Dasouki, M., Watts, V., Sivakumar, K., Bien-Willner, R., Flanigan, K. M., Sahenk, Z., Barohn, R. J., Walker, C. M., & Mendell, J. R. (June 2010b). Gentamicin-induced readthrough of stop codons in Duchenne muscular dystrophy. *Ann.Neurol.*, Vol.67,No.6, (June 2010b), pp. 771-780, ISSN

Mann, C. J., Honeyman, K., McClorey, G., Fletcher, S., & Wilton, S. D. (November 2002). Improved antisense oligonucleotide induced exon skipping in the mdx mouse model of muscular dystrophy. *J.Gene Med.*, Vol.4,No.6, (November 2002), pp. 644-654, ISSN

Manuvakhova, M., Keeling, K., & Bedwell, D. M. (July 2000). Aminoglycoside antibiotics mediate context-dependent suppression of termination codons in a mammalian translation system. *RNA.*, Vol.6,No.7, (July 2000), pp. 1044-1055, ISSN

Maruggi, G., Porcellini, S., Facchini, G., Perna, S. K., Cattoglio, C., Sartori, D., Ambrosi, A., Schambach, A., Baum, C., Bonini, C., Bovolenta, C., Mavilio, F., & Recchia, A. (May 2009). Transcriptional enhancers induce insertional gene deregulation independently from the vector type and design. *Mol.Ther.*, Vol.17,No.5, (May 2009), pp. 851-856, ISSN

Matsumura, K., Burghes, A. H., Mora, M., Tome, F. M., Morandi, L., Cornello, F., Leturcq, F., Jeanpierre, M., Kaplan, J. C., Reinert, P., & . (January 1994). Immunohistochemical analysis of dystrophin-associated proteins in Becker/Duchenne muscular dystrophy with huge in-frame deletions in the NH2-terminal and rod domains of dystrophin. *J.Clin.Invest*, Vol.93,No.1, (January 1994), pp. 99-105, ISSN

Matsumura, K. and Campbell, K. P. (January 1994). Dystrophin-glycoprotein complex: its role in the molecular pathogenesis of muscular dystrophies. *Muscle Nerve*, Vol.17,No.1, (January 1994), pp. 2-15, ISSN

Matsumura, K., Nonaka, I., Tome, F. M., Arahata, K., Collin, H., Leturcq, F., Recan, D., Kaplan, J. C., Fardeau, M., & Campbell, K. P. (August 1993). Mild deficiency of dystrophin-associated proteins in Becker muscular dystrophy patients having in-frame deletions in the rod domain of dystrophin. *Am.J.Hum.Genet.*, Vol.53,No.2, (August 1993), pp. 409-416, ISSN

Mendell, J. R., Campbell, K., Rodino-Klapac, L., Sahenk, Z., Shilling, C., Lewis, S., Bowles, D., Gray, S., Li, C., Galloway, G., Malik, V., Coley, B., Clark, K. R., Li, J., Xiao, X., Samulski, J., McPhee, S. W., Samulski, R. J., & Walker, C. M. (October 2010). Dystrophin immunity in Duchenne's muscular dystrophy. *N.Engl.J.Med.*, Vol.363,No.15, (October 2010), pp. 1429-1437, ISSN

Mendell, J. R., Moxley, R. T., Griggs, R. C., Brooke, M. H., Fenichel, G. M., Miller, J. P., King, W., Signore, L., Pandya, S., Florence, J., & . (June 1989). Randomized, double-blind six-month trial of prednisone in Duchenne's muscular dystrophy. *N.Engl.J.Med.*, Vol.320,No.24, (June 1989), pp. 1592-1597, ISSN

Meregalli, M., Farini, A., Parolini, D., Maciotta, S., & Torrente, Y. (August 2010). Stem cell therapies to treat muscular dystrophy: progress to date. *BioDrugs.*, Vol.24,No.4, (August 2010), pp. 237-247, ISSN

Miller, J. C., Tan, S., Qiao, G., Barlow, K. A., Wang, J., Xia, D. F., Meng, X., Paschon, D. E., Leung, E., Hinkley, S. J., Dulay, G. P., Hua, K. L., Ankoudinova, I., Cost, G. J., Urnov, F. D., Zhang, H. S., Holmes, M. C., Zhang, L., Gregory, P. D., & Rebar, E. J. (February 2011). A TALE nuclease architecture for efficient genome editing. *Nat.Biotechnol.*, Vol.29,No.2, (February 2011), pp. 143-148, ISSN

Mirabella, M., Galluzzi, G., Manfredi, G., Bertini, E., Ricci, E., De, L. R., Tonali, P., & Servidei, S. (August 1998). Giant dystrophin deletion associated with congenital cataract and mild muscular dystrophy. *Neurology*, Vol.51,No.2, (August 1998), pp. 592-595, ISSN

Monaco, A. P. (October 1989). Dystrophin, the protein product of the Duchenne/Becker muscular dystrophy gene. *Trends Biochem.Sci.*, Vol.14,No.10, (October 1989), pp. 412-415, ISSN

Monaco, A. P., Bertelson, C. J., Middlesworth, W., Colletti, C. A., Aldridge, J., Fischbeck, K. H., Bartlett, R., Pericak-Vance, M. A., Roses, A. D., & Kunkel, L. M. (August 1985). Detection of deletions spanning the Duchenne muscular dystrophy locus using a tightly linked DNA segment. *Nature*, Vol.316,No.6031, (August 1985), pp. 842-845, ISSN

Montarras, D., Morgan, J., Collins, C., Relaix, F., Zaffran, S., Cumano, A., Partridge, T., & Buckingham, M. (September 2005). Direct isolation of satellite cells for skeletal muscle regeneration. *Science*, Vol.309,No.5743, (September 2005), pp. 2064-2067, ISSN

Morgan, J. and Muntoni, F. (March 2007). Mural cells paint a new picture of muscle stem cells. *Nat.Cell Biol.*, Vol.9,No.3, (March 2007), pp. 249-251, ISSN

Moulton, H. M. and Moulton, J. D. (December 2010). Morpholinos and their peptide conjugates: therapeutic promise and challenge for Duchenne muscular dystrophy. *Biochim.Biophys.Acta*, Vol.1798,No.12, (December 2010), pp. 2296-2303, ISSN

Moxley, R. T., III and Pandya, S. (August 2011). Weekend high-dosage prednisone: A new option for treatment of Duchenne muscular dystrophy. *Neurology*, Vol.77,No.5, (August 2011), pp. 416-417, ISSN

Nagy, K. and Nagy, I. (November 1990). The effects of idebenone on the superoxide dismutase, catalase and glutathione peroxidase activities in liver and brain homogenates, as well as in brain synaptosomal and mitochondrial fractions. *Arch.Gerontol.Geriatr.*, Vol.11,No.3, (November 1990), pp. 285-291, ISSN

Ohlendieck, K. and Campbell, K. P. (December 1991). Dystrophin-associated proteins are greatly reduced in skeletal muscle from mdx mice. *J.Cell Biol.*, Vol.115,No.6, (December 1991), pp. 1685-1694, ISSN

Ohshima, S., Shin, J. H., Yuasa, K., Nishiyama, A., Kira, J., Okada, T., & Takeda, S. (January 2009). Transduction efficiency and immune response associated with the administration of AAV8 vector into dog skeletal muscle. *Mol.Ther.*, Vol.17,No.1, (January 2009), pp. 73-80, ISSN

Palmer, E., Wilhelm, J. M., & Sherman, F. (January 1979). Phenotypic suppression of nonsense mutants in yeast by aminoglycoside antibiotics. *Nature*, Vol.277,No.5692, (January 1979), pp. 148-150, ISSN

Palumbo, R., Sampaolesi, M., De, M. F., Tonlorenzi, R., Colombetti, S., Mondino, A., Cossu, G., & Bianchi, M. E. (February 2004). Extracellular HMGB1, a signal of tissue damage, induces mesoangioblast migration and proliferation. *J.Cell Biol.*, Vol.164,No.3, (February 2004), pp. 441-449, ISSN

Peault, B., Rudnicki, M., Torrente, Y., Cossu, G., Tremblay, J. P., Partridge, T., Gussoni, E., Kunkel, L. M., & Huard, J. (May 2007). Stem and progenitor cells in skeletal muscle development, maintenance, and therapy. *Mol.Ther.*, Vol.15,No.5, (May 2007), pp. 867-877, ISSN

Politano, L., Nigro, G., Nigro, V., Piluso, G., Papparella, S., Paciello, O., & Comi, L. I. (May 2003). Gentamicin administration in Duchenne patients with premature stop codon. Preliminary results. *Acta Myol.*, Vol.22,No.1, (May 2003), pp. 15-21, ISSN

Prins, K. W., Humston, J. L., Mehta, A., Tate, V., Ralston, E., & Ervasti, J. M. (August 2009). Dystrophin is a microtubule-associated protein. *J.Cell Biol.*, Vol.186,No.3, (August 2009), pp. 363-369, ISSN

Qu, Z., Balkir, L., Van Deutekom, J. C., Robbins, P. D., Pruchnic, R., & Huard, J. (September 1998). Development of approaches to improve cell survival in myoblast transfer therapy. *J.Cell Biol.*, Vol.142,No.5, (September 1998), pp. 1257-1267, ISSN

Qu-Petersen, Z., Deasy, B., Jankowski, R., Ikezawa, M., Cummins, J., Pruchnic, R., Mytinger, J., Cao, B., Gates, C., Wernig, A., & Huard, J. (May 2002). Identification of a novel population of muscle stem cells in mice: potential for muscle regeneration. *J.Cell Biol.*, Vol.157,No.5, (May 2002), pp. 851-864, ISSN

Rando, T. A., Disatnik, M. H., & Zhou, L. Z. (May 2000). Rescue of dystrophin expression in mdx mouse muscle by RNA/DNA oligonucleotides. *Proc.Natl.Acad.Sci.U.S.A*, Vol.97,No.10, (May 2000), pp. 5363-5368, ISSN

Rentschler, S., Linn, H., Deininger, K., Bedford, M. T., Espanel, X., & Sudol, M. (April 1999). The WW domain of dystrophin requires EF-hands region to interact with beta-dystroglycan. *Biol.Chem.*, Vol.380,No.4, (April 1999), pp. 431-442, ISSN

Rodino-Klapac, L. R., Montgomery, C. L., Bremer, W. G., Shontz, K. M., Malik, V., Davis, N., Sprinkle, S., Campbell, K. J., Sahenk, Z., Clark, K. R., Walker, C. M., Mendell, J. R., & Chicoine, L. G. (January 2010). Persistent expression of FLAG-tagged micro dystrophin in nonhuman primates following intramuscular and vascular delivery. *Mol.Ther.*, Vol.18,No.1, (January 2010), pp. 109-117, ISSN

Rybakova, I. N., Amann, K. J., & Ervasti, J. M. (November 1996). A new model for the interaction of dystrophin with F-actin. *J.Cell Biol.*, Vol.135,No.3, (November 1996), pp. 661-672, ISSN

Sampaolesi, M., Blot, S., D'Antona, G., Granger, N., Tonlorenzi, R., Innocenzi, A., Mognol, P., Thibaud, J. L., Galvez, B. G., Barthelemy, I., Perani, L., Mantero, S., Guttinger, M., Pansarasa, O., Rinaldi, C., Cusella De Angelis, M. G., Torrente, Y., Bordignon, C., Bottinelli, R., & Cossu, G. (November 2006). Mesoangioblast stem cells ameliorate muscle function in dystrophic dogs. *Nature*, Vol.444,No.7119, (November 2006), pp. 574-579, ISSN

Schwartz, M. and Duno, M. (2004). Improved molecular diagnosis of dystrophin gene mutations using the multiplex ligation-dependent probe amplification method. *Genet.Test.*, Vol.8,No.4, (2004), pp. 361-367, ISSN

Seale, P., Ishibashi, J., Scime, A., & Rudnicki, M. A. (May 2004). Pax7 is necessary and sufficient for the myogenic specification of CD45+:Sca1+ stem cells from injured muscle. *PLoS.Biol.*, Vol.2,No.5, (May 2004), pp. E130-

Singh, A., Ursic, D., & Davies, J. (January 1979). Phenotypic suppression and misreading Saccharomyces cerevisiae. *Nature*, Vol.277,No.5692, (January 1979), pp. 146-148, ISSN

Skuk, D., Goulet, M., Roy, B., Chapdelaine, P., Bouchard, J. P., Roy, R., Dugre, F. J., Sylvain, M., Lachance, J. G., Deschenes, L., Senay, H., & Tremblay, J. P. (April 2006). Dystrophin expression in muscles of duchenne muscular dystrophy patients after high-density injections of normal myogenic cells. *J.Neuropathol.Exp.Neurol.*, Vol.65,No.4, (April 2006), pp. 371-386, ISSN

Spitali, P., Rimessi, P., Fabris, M., Perrone, D., Falzarano, S., Bovolenta, M., Trabanelli, C., Mari, L., Bassi, E., Tuffery, S., Gualandi, F., Maraldi, N. M., Sabatelli-Giraud, P., Medici, A., Merlini, L., & Ferlini, A. (November 2009). Exon skipping-mediated dystrophin reading frame restoration for small mutations. *Hum.Mutat.*, Vol.30,No.11, (November 2009), pp. 1527-1534, ISSN

Sproat, B. S., Lamond, A. I., Beijer, B., Neuner, P., & Ryder, U. (May 1989). Highly efficient chemical synthesis of 2'-O-methyloligoribonucleotides and tetrabiotinylated derivatives; novel probes that are resistant to degradation by RNA or DNA specific nucleases. *Nucleic Acids Res.*, Vol.17,No.9, (May 1989), pp. 3373-3386, ISSN

Summerton, J. (December 1999). Morpholino antisense oligomers: the case for an RNase H-independent structural type. *Biochim.Biophys.Acta*, Vol.1489,No.1, (December 1999), pp. 141-158, ISSN

Suzuki, A., Yoshida, M., Hayashi, K., Mizuno, Y., Hagiwara, Y., & Ozawa, E. (March 1994). Molecular organization at the glycoprotein-complex-binding site of dystrophin. Three dystrophin-associated proteins bind directly to the carboxy-terminal portion of dystrophin. *Eur.J.Biochem.*, Vol.220,No.2, (March 1994), pp. 283-292, ISSN

Tremblay, J. P., Malouin, F., Roy, R., Huard, J., Bouchard, J. P., Satoh, A., & Richards, C. L. (March 1993). Results of a triple blind clinical study of myoblast transplantations without immunosuppressive treatment in young boys with Duchenne muscular dystrophy. *Cell Transplant.*, Vol.2,No.2, (March 1993), pp. 99-112, ISSN

Van Deutekom, J. C., Bremmer-Bout, M., Janson, A. A., Ginjaar, I. B., Baas, F., den Dunnen, J. T., & van Ommen, G. J. (July 2001). Antisense-induced exon skipping restores dystrophin expression in DMD patient derived muscle cells. *Hum.Mol.Genet.*, Vol.10,No.15, (July 2001), pp. 1547-1554, ISSN

Van Deutekom, J. C., Janson, A. A., Ginjaar, I. B., Frankhuizen, W. S., Aartsma-Rus, A., Bremmer-Bout, M., den Dunnen, J. T., Koop, K., van der Kooi, A. J., Goemans, N. M., de Kimpe, S. J., Ekhart, P. F., Venneker, E. H., Platenburg, G. J., Verschuuren, J. J., & van Ommen, G. J. (December 2007). Local dystrophin restoration with antisense oligonucleotide PRO051. *N.Engl.J.Med.*, Vol.357,No.26, (December 2007), pp. 2677-2686, ISSN

Wagner, K. R., Hamed, S., Hadley, D. W., Gropman, A. L., Burstein, A. H., Escolar, D. M., Hoffman, E. P., & Fischbeck, K. H. (June 2001). Gentamicin treatment of Duchenne and Becker muscular dystrophy due to nonsense mutations. *Ann.Neurol.*, Vol.49,No.6, (June 2001), pp. 706-711, ISSN

Wang, B., Li, J., Qiao, C., Chen, C., Hu, P., Zhu, X., Zhou, L., Bogan, J., Kornegay, J., & Xiao, X. (August 2008). A canine minidystrophin is functional and therapeutic in mdx mice. *Gene Ther.*, Vol.15,No.15, (August 2008), pp. 1099-1106, ISSN

Wang, B., Li, J., & Xiao, X. (December 2000). Adeno-associated virus vector carrying human minidystrophin genes effectively ameliorates muscular dystrophy in mdx mouse model. *Proc.Natl.Acad.Sci.U.S.A*, Vol.97,No.25, (December 2000), pp. 13714-13719, ISSN

Wang, Z., Kuhr, C. S., Allen, J. M., Blankinship, M., Gregorevic, P., Chamberlain, J. S., Tapscott, S. J., & Storb, R. (June 2007). Sustained AAV-mediated dystrophin expression in a canine model of Duchenne muscular dystrophy with a brief course of immunosuppression. *Mol.Ther.*, Vol.15,No.6, (June 2007), pp. 1160-1166, ISSN

Welch, E. M., Barton, E. R., Zhuo, J., Tomizawa, Y., Friesen, W. J., Trifillis, P., Paushkin, S., Patel, M., Trotta, C. R., Hwang, S., Wilde, R. G., Karp, G., Takasugi, J., Chen, G., Jones, S., Ren, H., Moon, Y. C., Corson, D., Turpoff, A. A., Campbell, J. A., Conn, M. M., Khan, A., Almstead, N. G., Hedrick, J., Mollin, A., Risher, N., Weetall, M., Yeh, S., Branstrom, A. A., Colacino, J. M., Babiak, J., Ju, W. D., Hirawat, S., Northcutt, V. J., Miller, L. L., Spatrick, P., He, F., Kawana, M., Feng, H., Jacobson, A., Peltz, S. W., & Sweeney, H. L. (May 2007). PTC124 targets genetic disorders caused by nonsense mutations. *Nature*, Vol.447,No.7140, (May 2007), pp. 87-91, ISSN

Wu, B., Benrashid, E., Lu, P., Cloer, C., Zillmer, A., Shaban, M., & Lu, Q. L. (2011a). Targeted skipping of human dystrophin exons in transgenic mouse model systemically for antisense drug development. *PLoS.One.*, Vol.6,No.5, (2011a), pp. e19906-

Wu, B., Li, Y., Morcos, P. A., Doran, T. J., Lu, P., & Lu, Q. L. (May 2009). Octa-guanidine morpholino restores dystrophin expression in cardiac and skeletal muscles and ameliorates pathology in dystrophic mdx mice. *Mol.Ther.*, Vol.17,No.5, (May 2009), pp. 864-871, ISSN

Wu, B., Lu, P., Benrashid, E., Malik, S., Ashar, J., Doran, T. J., & Lu, Q. L. (January 2010). Dose-dependent restoration of dystrophin expression in cardiac muscle of dystrophic mice by systemically delivered morpholino. *Gene Ther.*, Vol.17,No.1, (January 2010), pp. 132-140, ISSN

Wu, B., Moulton, H. M., Iversen, P. L., Jiang, J., Li, J., Li, J., Spurney, C. F., Sali, A., Guerron, A. D., Nagaraju, K., Doran, T., Lu, P., Xiao, X., & Lu, Q. L. (September 2008). Effective rescue of dystrophin improves cardiac function in dystrophin-deficient mice by a modified morpholino oligomer. *Proc.Natl.Acad.Sci.U.S.A*, Vol.105,No.39, (September 2008), pp. 14814-14819, ISSN

Wu, B., Xiao, B., Cloer, C., Shaban, M., Sali, A., Lu, P., Li, J., Nagaraju, K., Xiao, X., & Lu, Q. L. (March 2011b). One-year treatment of morpholino antisense oligomer improves skeletal and cardiac muscle functions in dystrophic mdx mice. *Mol.Ther.*, Vol.19,No.3, (March 2011b), pp. 576-583, ISSN

Yin, H., Moulton, H. M., Betts, C., Seow, Y., Boutilier, J., Iverson, P. L., & Wood, M. J. (November 2009). A fusion peptide directs enhanced systemic dystrophin exon skipping and functional restoration in dystrophin-deficient mdx mice. *Hum.Mol.Genet.*, Vol.18,No.22, (November 2009), pp. 4405-4414, ISSN

Yin, H., Moulton, H. M., Seow, Y., Boyd, C., Boutilier, J., Iverson, P., & Wood, M. J. (December 2008). Cell-penetrating peptide-conjugated antisense oligonucleotides restore systemic muscle and cardiac dystrophin expression and function. *Hum.Mol.Genet.*, Vol.17,No.24, (December 2008), pp. 3909-3918, ISSN

Yin, H., Saleh, A. F., Betts, C., Camelliti, P., Seow, Y., Ashraf, S., Arzumanov, A., Hammond, S., Merritt, T., Gait, M. J., & Wood, M. J. (July 2011). Pip5 transduction peptides direct high efficiency oligonucleotide-mediated dystrophin exon skipping in heart and phenotypic correction in mdx mice. *Mol.Ther.*, Vol.19,No.7, (July 2011), pp. 1295-1303, ISSN

Yokota, T., Lu, Q. L., Partridge, T., Kobayashi, M., Nakamura, A., Takeda, S., & Hoffman, E. (June 2009). Efficacy of systemic morpholino exon-skipping in Duchenne dystrophy dogs. *Ann.Neurol.*, Vol.65,No.6, (June 2009), pp. 667-676, ISSN

Yoshida, M., Suzuki, A., Yamamoto, H., Noguchi, S., Mizuno, Y., & Ozawa, E. (June 1994). Dissociation of the complex of dystrophin and its associated proteins into several unique groups by n-octyl beta-D-glucoside. *Eur.J.Biochem.*, Vol.222,No.3, (June 1994), pp. 1055-1061, ISSN

Yoshida, M., Yamamoto, H., Noguchi, S., Mizuno, Y., Hagiwara, Y., & Ozawa, E. (July 1995). Dystrophin-associated protein A0 is a homologue of the Torpedo 87K protein. *FEBS Lett.*, Vol.367,No.3, (July 1995), pp. 311-314, ISSN

Yoshizawa, S., Fourmy, D., & Puglisi, J. D. (November 1998). Structural origins of gentamicin antibiotic action. *EMBO J.*, Vol.17,No.22, (November 1998), pp. 6437-6448, ISSN

21

Stem Cell Based Therapy for Muscular Dystrophies: Cell Types and Environmental Factors Influencing Their Efficacy

Jennifer Morgan[1] and Hala Alameddine[2]
[1]*The Dubowitz Neuromuscular Centre, UCL Institute of Child Health, London,*
[2] *UMRS 974, UMR7215, Institut de Myologie, Paris*
[1]*UK*
[2]*France*

1. Introduction

Muscular dystrophies are inherited disorders in which muscle fibers are unusually susceptible to damage, leading to progressive loss of muscle structure and function. Some types of muscular dystrophy affect heart muscles, other involuntary muscles and other organs. The most common form of muscular dystrophy, Duchenne Muscular Dystrophy (DMD), is due to genetic deficiency of the protein dystrophin (Monaco et al., 1985). This protein is one of several partners that interact to link intracellular cytoskeleton to extracellular matrix (ECM) hence consolidating the scaffold necessary for maintaining structural integrity of skeletal muscle fibers. Dystrophin deficiency destabilizes muscle fibers, which become less resistant to contractions leading to muscle fiber necrosis and subsequent regeneration.

Skeletal muscle repair, maintenance and regeneration are mediated by muscle-specific stem cells: the satellite cells (Mauro, 1961), located underneath basal lamina of muscle fibers. In DMD muscles, fat and connective tissue often replace muscle fibers in the late stages of muscular dystrophy, indicating that muscle regeneration does not keep up with fiber loss. Defective muscle regeneration could be due to exhaustion of proliferative capacity of satellite cells (Blau et al., 1983; Webster & Blau, 1990) or to environmental factors that are not conducive to their function. The healing process usually includes sequential and overlapping events of muscle fiber degeneration, inflammatory reaction, regeneration and remodeling of ECM components that require tightly regulated orchestration of the interactive cross-talk that conditions the outcome of the regenerative process. Uncontrolled wound-healing, in response to chronic injury and inflammation, results in tissue fibrosis and scarring which impacts on the efficiency of muscle regeneration, hence contributing to the degradation of muscle function.

At present, we still have no cure for any form of muscular dystrophy, but medications and therapy can slow the course of the disease to allow people with muscular dystrophy to remain mobile for as long as possible. Nevertheless, experimental therapeutic strategies have been initiated in light of basic and technical advances of skeletal muscle biology and pathophysiology. The description of the muscle regeneration process and the identification of the cells responsible for myofiber regeneration led to stem cell therapy being considered as a potential strategy to alleviate muscle deficiency in DMD patients. Alternatively, the identification of gene defects and the sophistication of molecular biology technologies have opened perspectives for gene therapy, either by providing the deficient gene, or by restoring gene function. Other strategies combining both approaches have been considered and imply the correction of patients' own stem cells before grafting them into the diseased muscles. These promising strategies have been challenged in animal models of muscular dystrophies and although they achieved a certain success, they also identified a number of limitations. Moreover, the failure of myogenic cell grafting to improve muscle function and to restore dystrophin expression in clinical trials of DMD patients, underscored the need to improve the efficiency of cell therapy. Cell environment, which comprises ECM and extracellular matrix deposited factors such as growth factors, cytokines and chemokines, regulate diverse cellular functions. These molecules are metabolized by Matrix MetalloProteinases (MMPs) that play a central role as regulators of tissue microenvironment. In normal situations, precise spatiotemporal repertoires of MMPs balanced by inhibitors, among which are the four Tissue Inhibitors of MatrixmetalloProteinases (TIMPs), regulate extracellular signaling networks and maintain tissue homeostasis. On the contrary, increased MMPs expression or activity has been demonstrated in various disease situations including, practically every known inflammatory disease (Manicone & McGuire, 2008). Such disruption of the dynamic equilibrium between MMPs and TIMPs may affect diverse cellular functions including cell proliferation, migration, adhesion and apoptosis (Holmbeck et al., 2005; Hulboy et al., 1997; Vu & Werb, 2000). In DMD, for example, inflammation and fibrosis are major hurdles in the path of therapeutic strategies (Wells et al., 2002) and their resolution is expected to positively impact on the efficiency of any form of therapy, but more specifically, on the efficiency of cell therapy. Indeed, myogenic stem cells have limited migratory capacity, which is further aggravated by excessive proliferation of connective tissue. Therefore, improving the efficiency of cell therapy could be achieved either by myogenic cells better able to digest accumulated ECM components or, alternatively, by other types of stem cells that can be recruited from a resident or circulating pool and are capable of migrating through one or several tissue barriers to home into skeletal muscles. In this chapter, we consider the use of stem cell therapy to treat muscular dystrophies. By going through the different cell types that have been used, we will try to define the best cell type to use, how to handle and expand these cells before transplantation and the best route of delivery. Moreover, the possibility of using genetically-modified autologous stem cells for transplantation will be presented. This would only be possible if the stem cell had not been deleteriously affected by the dystrophic environment. Finally, we will consider the host environment as a modulator of cell behaviour and the dual role MMPs play in the control of this environment and their impact on transplanted cells migration, differentiation and self-renewal.

2. Potential therapies for duchenne muscular dystrophy

Muscular dystrophies are a heterogeneous group of inherited neuromuscular disorders, including X-linked recessive as in DMD, autosomal recessive as in limb-girdle muscular dystophy type 2, or autosomal dominant as in facioscapulohumeral muscular dystophy, myotonic dystrophy, and limb-girdle muscular dystophy type 1 (Emery, 2002). In the last two decades, different types of dystrophies have been genetically characterized. The most frequent and most severe form, DMD, is a progressive, incurable X-linked recessive disorder that affects 1 in 3500 newborn boys and leads to death in the second or third decade of life (Bushby et al., 2010). DMD patients lack the protein dystrophin while in-frame mutations of the same gene led to expression of a partially functional protein, resulting in the milder Becker muscular dystrophies (BMD). As a result of the absence of dystrophin, muscle fibers of DMD patients undergo necrosis followed by regeneration which, in the long run, fails to keep up with the recurrent cycles of degeneration-regeneration and muscle fibers are lost and replaced by fibro-fatty tissue. Interruption of these cycles can be achieved by dystrophin restoration to the muscle fiber membrane (Meng et al., 2011a). Several strategies can now be used to restore dystrophin to the muscle fibers of affected patients. They include virally-mediated gene therapy, read-through of stop codons, up-regulation of compensatory genes, or skipping of mutated dystrophin exons to give rise to a shorter, but still functional dystrophin protein. However, all of these have possible drawbacks (reviewed (Goyenvalle & Davies, 2011; Guglieri & Bushby, 2010; Hoffman et al., 2011; Sugita & Takeda, 2010)). Either gene therapy, or application of antisense oligonucleotides to skip mutated dystrophin exons, requires that the patient has sufficient muscle fibers remaining for treatment. In addition, exon skipping is mutation-dependent and not all patients have mutations amenable to this approach.

3. Stem cell therapy for the treatment of DMD

The concept of a cell-based therapy to alleviate loss of muscle structure and function in muscular dystrophy originated with the observation of the intrinsic ability of myogenic stem cells to fuse either with each other to form multinucleated myofibers, or with necrotic muscle fibers to form mosaic fibers. In theory, functional correction could be achieved in DMD by the generation of either hybrid muscle fibers where the donor nuclei provide the missing gene product and/or the regeneration of normal myofibers from the fusion of normal donor cells to replace lost muscle fibers. Cell therapy was the first biologically based approach applied for the treatment of DMD and required the use of animal models to explore the beneficial effects of this therapy. The ability of cultured myogenic cells to regenerate new muscle fibers, that reconstitute the same architectural organization of the original muscle and induce functional recovery, has been validated using an experimental model of irreversible injury to adult rodent muscle associating auto-transplantation of skeletal muscle to X-irradiation (Alameddine et al., 1989; Alameddine et al., 1991; Alameddine et al., 1994).

3.1 Stem cells

Stem cells are defined as cells that can both self-renew and give rise to more differentiated cell type, whereas precursor cells do not have the ability to self-renew. Both cell types present a great advantage for the treatment of muscular dystrophies as they could repair segmental necrosis and also give rise to regenerated muscle fibers to replace those that are lost as a consequence of the dystrophy. They could therefore be effective at later stages of the dystrophy, when muscle fibers have already been lost. Donor cells derived from a normal individual will automatically express dystrophin when they differentiate into a muscle fiber, but the quantity and distribution of dystrophin within the fiber will depend on the number of donor myonuclei and the size of segments of the fiber to which they contribute. However, the recipient and donor will need to be HLA-matched, so that stem cells from one normal donor could not be used to treat all patients.

Although many different stem or precursor cells have been shown to contribute to muscle regeneration in animal models, many of these give rise to only limited amount of muscle, for example haematopoietic stem cells (Ferrari et al., 1998) and mesenchymal stem cells (Chan et al., 2006; Meng et al., 2010). Satellite cells are the archetypal skeletal muscle stem cell, but they are by definition quiescent cells underneath the basal lamina of muscle fibers and it would be impossible to obtain enough of them for therapeutic application. However, the progeny of satellite cells, muscle precursor cells or myoblasts, could be prepared in sufficient quantity for transplantation. In this review, therefore, we will focus on cells that can be expanded in culture and that have been shown to contribute to muscle regeneration-myoblasts, cells derived from blood-vessel associated pericytes (termed mesoangioblasts) and skeletal muscle-derived AC133+ cells. There are several recent reviews on stem cells to treat muscular dystrophies, which cover most of the cell types that have been studied (Meng et al., 2011a; Negroni et al., 2011; Palmieri et al., 2010; Skuk & Tremblay, 2011; Tedesco et al., 2010).

3.2 Models and markers

To investigate the potential contribution of a particular cell type to muscle regeneration, the standard experiment is to graft the cells into an animal model of DMD and measure their contribution to skeletal muscle fibers, which may be quantified by either counting the number of dystrophin-positive fibers, or measuring the amount of dystrophin on western blot. Several animal models of DMD exist but the most widely-used is the dystrophin-deficient *mdx* mouse (Bulfield et al., 1984) used in 1,940 pubmed publications, as of 21 July 2011. Other models of DMD include the golden retriever muscular dystrophy (GRMD also known as Canine X-linked Muscular Dystrophy CXMD) dog and zebrafish (reviewed (Banks & Chamberlain, 2008; Collins & Morgan, 2003)). Mouse and dog models have been used to investigate different potential therapies for DMD, including precursor/stem cell transplantation (Nakamura & Takeda, 2011). However, when grafting cells from one donor to another, the host must either be immunodeficient or immunosuppressed. Therefore, *mdx* mice with different types of immunodeficiency have been used as hosts in cell transplantation experiments, including *mdx* nu/nu (Boldrin et al., 2009; Collins et al., 2005; Partridge et al., 1989), SCID *mdx* (Benchaouir et al., 2007; Dellavalle et al., 2007; Torrente et al., 2004), $Rag^{-/-}$ *mdx* (Gerard et al., 2011), or *mdx* mice immunosuppressed with FK506 (Kinoshita et al., 1994b), but to what extent these different hosts are comparable, being on different genetic backgrounds and having different mechanisms and degrees of immunodeficiency, has not been ascertained (reviewed (Meng et al., 2011b)). Immunodeficient mice are more convenient to work with than mice that have to be immunosuppressed and seem to permit greater donor-myoblast-derived muscle regeneration (Partridge et al., 1989). However, it is important to consider the effect of the immunological system on donor-derived muscle regeneration, as DMD patients will not be immunodeficient. Non-dystrophic mice or monkeys, whose muscles have been injured to mimic the degeneration and regeneration that occurs in dystrophic muscles, have also been used as recipients to test cell transplantation (Cooper et al., 2001; Morgan et al., 2002; Sacco et al., 2008; Skuk et al., 1999), as have mice that model different types of dystrophy, e.g. sarcoglycan (Sampaolesi et al., 2003) and dysferlin-deficient mice (Diaz-Manera et al., 2010).

A major consideration when using both dystrophic and non-dystrophic animal models to test stem cells is that the host muscle usually has to be injured in some way to enhance donor cell engraftment. This is surprising, as the muscle fiber degeneration and regeneration that is already occurring in dystrophic muscle would be thought to be sufficient to promote donor stem cells to contribute to muscle regeneration. However, muscle fiber necrosis is often focal and only cells located nearby contribute to regeneration (Yokota et al., 2006). Therefore, if the transplanted stem cell is located a distance away, it may not either receive the correct signals, or be able to migrate to the damaged fibers. As many of these injury regimes are very severe, for example, cryoinjury (Brimah et al., 2004; Irintchev et al., 1997; Negroni et al., 2009) or use of snake venoms (Lefaucheur & Sebille, 1995; Silva-Barbosa et al., 2005) to induce degeneration and regeneration in host muscles, they could not be used in patients. Even in dystrophin-deficient *mdx* nu/nu host mice, satellite cells contribute little, if any, to muscle regeneration (Boldrin et al., 2009; Collins et al., 2005) although myoblasts contribute to muscle regeneration to a greater extent (Morgan et al., 2002; Partridge et al., 1989). This poor contribution of donor cells to muscle regeneration is likely to be due to the fact that *mdx* mouse muscles, in contrast to those of DMD patients, regenerate very well. We therefore blocked muscle regeneration in *mdx* muscles by applying local high doses of radiation, to obtain a model more similar to DMD, in which the muscle degenerates and atrophies but does not regenerate (Morgan et al., 1990; Pagel & Partridge, 1999; Wakeford et al., 1991). If host muscle is irradiated with 18 Gy before donor cell grafting, satellite cell and myoblast contribution to muscle regeneration is significantly augmented (Boldrin et al., 2009; Collins et al., 2005; Morgan et al., 2002). This may be due to prevention of competition from local host stem or satellite cells, as irradiated *mdx* muscles do not regenerate (Pagel & Partridge, 1999; Wakeford et al., 1991) unless a severe injury, e.g. injection of snake venom notexin, is imposed on them, which evokes rare radiation-resistant stem cells to regenerate (Gross & Morgan, 1999; Heslop et al., 2000). Other models that could be used to test whether a wholly or partially emptied satellite cell niche is necessary for efficient donor muscle stem cell engraftment include Pax7 knockout mice (Seale et al., 2000) that lack satellite cells, or the *mdx* mouse that also lacks telomerase (mTR) activity and therefore shows a reduction in the regenerative capacity of myogenic stem cells (Sacco et al., 2010).

Another important consideration is the marker(s) to be used to assess the contribution of donor cells to regenerated muscle fibers and/or satellite cells (reviewed (Meng et al., 2011a)). As the aim is to produce dystrophin in host muscle fibers, it is sensible to quantify dystrophin restoration in the host muscles (Partridge et al., 1989). Because "revertant" fibers that spontaneously express dystrophin are present in animal models of DMD (Hoffman et al., 1990) and in DMD patients (Arechavala-Gomeza et al., 2010) and because clusters of revertant fibers increase in number with time (Hoffman et al., 1990; Yokota et al., 2006), revertant fibers must be controlled for, particularly if dystrophin is being used alone as a marker of donor-derived muscle fibers and especially in time course studies. If grafting human cells into mouse, a human-specific dystrophin antibody (e.g. Novocastra Dys3 (Brimah et al., 2004)) may be used, that will not identify mouse revertant fibers. Because of the existence of revertant fibers, many groups use a second marker of either muscle fibers or cells of donor origin, e.g. by using donor cells from genetically-modified mice, e.g. myosin 3f nLacZ-E, that is expressed in myonuclei of donor origin, Myf5 nLacZ/$^{+}$ that is expressed in satellite cells of donor origin (Collins et al., 2005), or ubiquitously (Morgan et al., 2002) or muscle-specifically (Kinoshita et al., 1994a) expressed β-gal or GFP. Donor cells may alternatively be marked in culture with constructs expressing a marker protein (Blaveri et al., 1999; Cousins et al., 2004; Diaz-Manera et al., 2010; Morgan et al., 2002). However, caution should be used in interpreting results, as GFP is notoriously difficult to use in skeletal muscle (Jackson et al., 2004), some markers spread further along a mosaic muscle fiber than others (Blaveri et al., 1999) and others are switched off in vivo (Boldrin et al.,2009).

3.3 Contribution of locally-delivered donor stem cells to muscle regeneration.

A large body of evidence can be found in the literature to illustrate the contribution of myoblasts to skeletal muscle regeneration, although the number of donor-derived muscle fibers is limited (Figure 1). However, the host muscle environment that permits regeneration from myoblasts of mouse and human origin appears to be different, although a comparative experiment to establish this point has not been performed: human myoblasts form more muscle within host muscles that have been cryoinjured prior to grafting (Brimah et al., 2004), whereas mouse myoblasts form significantly more muscle in irradiated host muscles (Boldrin and Morgan, manuscript in preparation).

Different muscle injury models used for intra-muscular grafting of putative muscle stem cells may also give rise to discrepancies between groups. Some groups have grafted cells into muscles of non-dystrophic mice that had been cryo-injured immediately prior to grafting (Brimah et al., 2004; Cooper et al., 2001; Ehrhardt et al., 2007), but others grafted cells into muscles of *mdx* SCID mice that had been injected 48 hours previously with cardiotoxin, (Dellavalle et al., 2007) or into cryo–injured muscles of immunodeficient Rag2$^{-/-}$ gamma chain-non-dystrophic mice (Pisani et al., 2010). Vauchez et al. grafted into muscles of non-dystrophic SCID mice, injuring the muscles prior to grafting by a combination of irradiation and notexin (Vauchez et al., 2009); Zheng et al. grafted cells into muscles of SCID mice that had been injured by cardiotoxin one day previously (Zheng et al., 2007). How these different injury regimes mimic the dystrophic muscle environment and to what extent the local environment, genetic background and immunological status of the host mouse affect muscle stem cell behavior are important to determine, for the identification of robust methodologies which could reliably be used for therapeutic trials in muscular dystrophies.

Interestingly, although they contributed to much muscle regeneration after intra-arterial injection, pericytes only gave rise to very small numbers of muscle fibers after intra-muscular transplantation: CD56^{+}/ALP^{-} cells (satellite-cell derived myoblasts) gave rise to more muscle than CD56^{+}/ALP^{+} cells (pericytes), but CD56^{-}/ALP^{-} cells, taken to be fibroblasts, made very few donor muscle fibers (Dellavalle et al., 2007). Meng et al. also found that both CD56^{+} and CD56^{-} skeletal muscle-derived cells contributed to muscle regeneration, CD56^{+} cells making significantly more muscle than either CD56^{-}, or non-fractionated cells after intra-muscular transplantation. CD56^{+} cells contributed predominantly to nuclei inside the basal lamina of muscle fibers, i.e. within muscle fibers and/or satellite cells. But CD56^{-} or non-sorted cells contributed to significantly more nuclei outside the basal lamina, confirming that there were more non-myogenic cells within CD56^{-} cell population (Meng et al., 2011b). Zheng et al showed that human skeletal muscle-derived CD56^{+} cells that also expressed CD34 and CD144 (myoendothelial cells) contributed to more muscle regeneration than did CD56^{+}/CD34^{-}/CD144^{-} cells (myoblasts) (Zheng et al., 2007) in contrast to the findings of Meng suggesting that pericytes, rather than endothelial cells, are the major CD56^{-} contributor to muscle regeneration (Meng et al., 2011b)

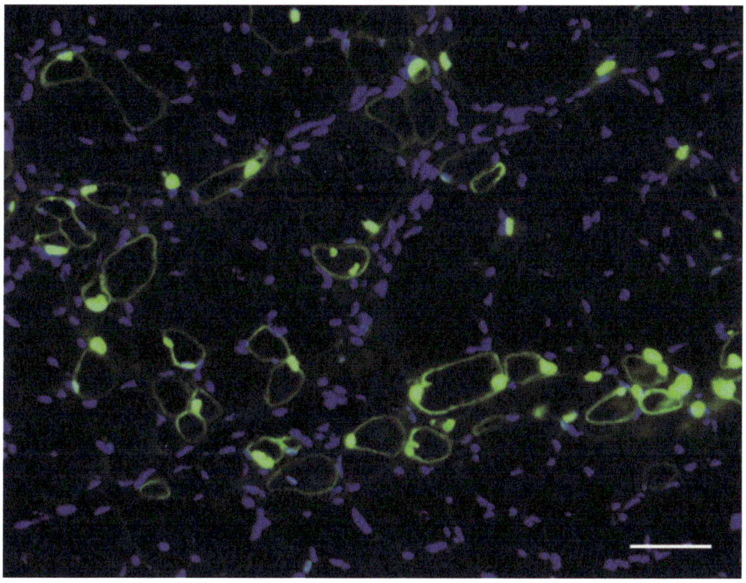

Fig. 1. 7 μm transverse cryosection of *mdx* nu/nu host *tibialis anterior* muscle, that had been cryoinjured and grafted with 5 x 10^5 human skeletal muscle-derived stem cells 4 weeks previously. Stained with antibodies to human spectrin and human specific lamin a/c, that recognise muscle fibers and nuclei of human origin respectively. Counterstained with DAPI. Bar= 50 μm. (Courtesy of Dr Jinhong Meng).

3.4 Contribution of systemically-delivered donor stem cells to muscle regeneration

The contribution of blood vessel-derived cells (both from skeletal muscle and embryonic dorsal aorta) to skeletal muscle regeneration *in vivo* after their systemic delivery has been demonstrated in several publications (Dellavalle et al., 2007; Sampaolesi et al., 2003; Sampaolesi et al., 2006)(reviewed (Sancricca et al., 2010)), however these promising findings could not be replicated by others (Meng et al., 2011b). For long-term efficacy, it would be useful to know whether a grafted pericyte self-renews to give more functional pericytes and if so, what contribution these have to further muscle regeneration. Another stem cell that is promising for systemic delivery to skeletal muscle is the AC133+ cell, derived from either blood (Torrente et al., 2004), or skeletal muscle (Benchaouir et al., 2007).

3.5 Death and proliferation of grafted cells

Donor myoblasts die on intra-muscular grafting (Beauchamp et al., 1999; Skuk et al., 2002; Smythe et al., 2000) possibly as a result of one or a combination of various factors: cell dissociation, trophic factor withdrawal, oxidative stress, excito-toxicity, hypoxia and, possibly, anoikis (reviewed (Gerard et al., 2011; Skuk & Tremblay, 2011)) and much effort has been expended to prevent this death (reviewed (Skuk & Tremblay, 2011)). Recent experiments have indicated that the number and density of cells transplanted into one site intra-muscularly may also be critical factors influencing their survival and proliferation (Pellegrini & Beilharz, 2011) and that more cells may not give rise to more muscle fibers of donor origin (Pellegrini & Beilharz, 2011; Praud et al., 2003; Rando & Blau, 1994), possibly because cells in the centre of dense pellets undergo more apoptosis. But another theory is that the cells that die are irrelevant, as those that survive proliferate extensively under appropriate environmental conditions, to reconstitute the host muscle (Beauchamp et al., 1999). It is however unclear whether other types of muscle stem cell undergo death after transplantation, or if they proliferate within the grafted muscles.

3.6 Signals inducing muscle stem cells to contribute to muscle regeneration

Intra-arterial injection of mesoangioblasts has shown that only a very small percentage reach downstream skeletal muscles, most being trapped in the filter organs. To enable cells to exit blood vessels, the vessels must express the appropriate adhesion molecules for that cell type. Molecules that have been shown to be important for mesangioblast extravasation into skeletal muscle include HMGB1, SDF-1 and TNF-α (Palumbo et al., 2004). Expression of the adhesion molecules L-selectin and alpha 4 integrin on mesoangioblasts improved their migration into skeletal muscle (Galvez et al., 2006). Pre-treatment with nitric oxide was shown to augment the positive effects of TNF-α, TGF-β and VEGF on mesangioblast migration (Sciorati et al., 2006).

Once the donor stem cells have entered the muscles, they must migrate to sites of injury, proliferate to give a pool of muscle precursor cells and then differentiate to form muscle fibers, either by fusing with each other or by repairing necrotic segments of dystrophic fibers. This will require them to respond to a new series of signals, which might be more appropriate for satellite cells than for stem cells.

In order to have long term benefit, the donor stem cells muscle repopulate a stem cell niche within the muscle and must retain the properties of a functional muscle stem cell within this niche. It is not clear if pericytes within their niche contribute to muscle regeneration, so the best niche to occupy would be the satellite cell niche. However, efficient repopulation of any niche, for example, the satellite cell niche, would only be possible if it were emptied as a consequence of the dystrophy and if the niche environment remains permissive for donor-derived stem cell function. As satellite cell of donor origin are most commonly found on fibers containing myonuclei of donor origin, they may not be called upon to regenerate, as the fiber on which they are situated will already have been strengthened by the new dystrophin and may not undergo further necrosis, at least at the sites where dystrophin is expressed. A means of activating these cells and drawing them towards more distant areas of injury is therefore required to enable them to respond to future muscle fiber necrosis elsewhere within the muscle.

3.7 Autologous cell transplantation

An attractive proposition for treating muscular dystrophies is to use genetically-corrected autologous stem cells. The use of autologous stem cells should circumvent the need for immunosuppression, although tissue culture components or expression of novel protein isotypes *in vivo* may evoke an immunological reaction. But, if the stem cells are skeletal-muscle derived, their function may be impaired by either the primary genetic defect, or secondary environmental consequences of the primary defect.

In some muscular dystrophies, the gene responsible is not expressed in satellite cells (reviewed (Morgan & Zammit, 2010)); for example, dystrophin is not expressed in satellite cells (or other types of muscle stem cell), so satellite cells in DMD muscles would therefore be expected to have normal function. However, the satellite cells may have undergone many divisions in their previous attempts to repair the dystrophic fibers and could therefore be close to senescence (Decary et al., 1996; Decary et al., 1997; Webster & Blau, 1990). They would consequently be of little use for autologous therapy, as they would undergo insufficient divisions *in vitro* to be genetically modified and then to proliferate following transplantation. But although human myoblasts are exhausted in DMD (Decary et al., 1996; Decary et al., 1997; Webster & Blau, 1990), *mdx* satellite cells do not appear to suffer the same consequence of dystrophin deficiency (Bockhold et al., 1998). Recent evidence has indicated that *mdx* satellite cells are highly functional following transplantation into irradiated *mdx* nu/nu muscles (Boldrin and Morgan, unpublished observations). So although satellite cells may not be lost in DMD (reviewed (Boldrin et al., 2010)), their function is compromised, which may be due to telomere shortening leading to reduced proliferative capacity, or a change in the timing or extent of differentiation. However, caution must be taken when comparing *mdx* and DMD cells, as there are differences in telomere biology between mice and humans: inbred mouse strains have extremely long telomeres (20–150 kilobases) compared with humans (up to 15 kilobases) (Bekaert et al., 2005) and telomerase activity is lower in human compared to mouse cells (reviewed (Mather et al., 2011)).

It is unclear whether skeletal muscle-resident cells other than satellite cells contribute to muscle regeneration in muscular dystrophies, or even to maintenance and repair of normal muscle. If they had not actively contributed to the cycles of degeneration and regeneration that occur in DMD, they would be capable of many more divisions than the satellite-cell derived myoblasts and therefore be a more attractive candidate for autologous therapy. However, if they do not contribute to muscle regeneration in DMD, why do they not do so? And why would they be effective after transplantation, if they are not functional *in situ*? Possibly they are not recruited to muscle fiber maintenance and regeneration when they are in their natural niche *in vivo*, but do so after they encounter the site of muscle damage after either intra-muscular or systemic injection.

An ideal autologous stem cell would be derived non-invasively, e.g. from the peripheral blood, or a skin biopsy. However, to date there is only one report of blood-derived stem cells that make reasonable amounts of muscle after their systemic delivery (Torrente et al., 2004).

3.7.1 Genetic modification of autologous cells.

Genetic correction of autologous stem cells has been successfully used as a therapeutic option in other conditions and encouraging preclinical results have also been recently obtained in animal models of DMD (Meregalli et al., 2008). However key questions that need to be resolved before this approach could be used in DMD include the optimal vector configuration and the safety profile of the gene delivery methodology. Lentiviral vectors efficiently infect quiescent cells, including stem cells (S. Li et al., 2005) and give long-term, heritable, gene expression because they integrate into the host genome. Drawbacks with lentiviral vectors include possible gene silencing, or mutagenesis (Wilson & Cichutek, 2009), due to the site at which the virus inserts into the host genome. Although lentiviruses integrate preferentially into active transcription sites (Ciuffi, 2008) the development of third generation lentiviruses with advanced SIN design (Bokhoven et al. 2009), physiological promoters and cell-specific envelope proteins (Rahim et al., 2009) and enhancer-less regulatory elements, e.g. the ubiquitously acting chromatin opening element (UCOE) (Montini et al., 2006; Zhang et al., 2007) should circumvent these problems.

A lentiviral vector has been used to insert a 6.8 kb dystrophin mini gene (S. Li et al., 2005), to give rise to a shorter dystrophin protein in regenerated muscle fibers. While these engineered mini-dystrophins appear to retain most of the functional properties of full-length dystrophin, they nevertheless miss important domains, such as the nitric oxide synthase anchoring domain (Lai et al., 2009). Considering the cloning capacity of lentiviral vectors (up to 10kb (M. Kumar et al., 2001)), it should be possible to further optimise a vector so that it accommodates most of the functionally relevant coding region of dystrophin. An optimal dystrophin construct in a lentiviral vector could be used to treat patients with different mutations, in contrast to the U7 constructs, which, although they can be placed in a lentiviral vector and induce dystrophin expression in stem cells *in vitro* and following their transplantation *in vivo* (Quenneville et al., 2007), are mutation-specific.

4. Matrix Metalloproteinases: modulators of microenvironment and cell function in skeletal muscles

The Matrix Metalloproteinases (MMPs) are a large group of zinc-dependent extracellular endopeptidase proteinases within the Metzincin superfamily of protease that also includes a disintegrin and metalloproteinases (ADAM) and ADAM with thrombospondin motifs (ADAMTS). MMPs family comprises 23 members in humans that share common modular domains and form 5 main sub-groups based on their structure and substrate: collagenases, gelatinases, matrilysins, stromelysins and membrane-type (Figure 2). With the exception of membrane bound MMPs, the other members of the group are secreted in the extracellular space where they are present in latent forms and become activated by other proteases or in response to signaling events. Their activity is regulated at the transcriptional and post-transcriptional levels as well as by their physiological inhibitors, Tissue Inhibitors of Matrix Metalloproteinases (TIMPs). Collectively, they are able to degrade all components of the ECM. Initially confined to the degradation of ECM, their function has progressively evolved and they are now regarded as major regulators of tissue environment and cell functions (Murphy, 2010; Rodriguez et al., 2010). They modulate cell proliferation, adhesion, migration and signaling (Fanjul-Fernandez et al., 2010).

4.1 Matrix Metalloproteinases in remodeling muscles

The adult skeletal muscle is a very stable tissue yet it is endowed with a high capacity to adapt to modification of functional demands, trauma or disease. In normal situations, the dynamic equilibrium between MMPs and TIMPs maintains homeostasis of ECM that provides a dynamic support and stores a number of growth factors that are liberated during ECM remodeling. In response to remodeling situations, dysregulation of this balance occurs in favor of MMPs, to allow necessary hydrolysis of ECM which results in the liberation of neo-epitopes from basement membrane components, as well as various growth factors and signaling molecules that modulate cell response to environmental modifications. Such imbalance may be temporary and the equilibrium is restored upon the disappearance of remodeling stimuli.

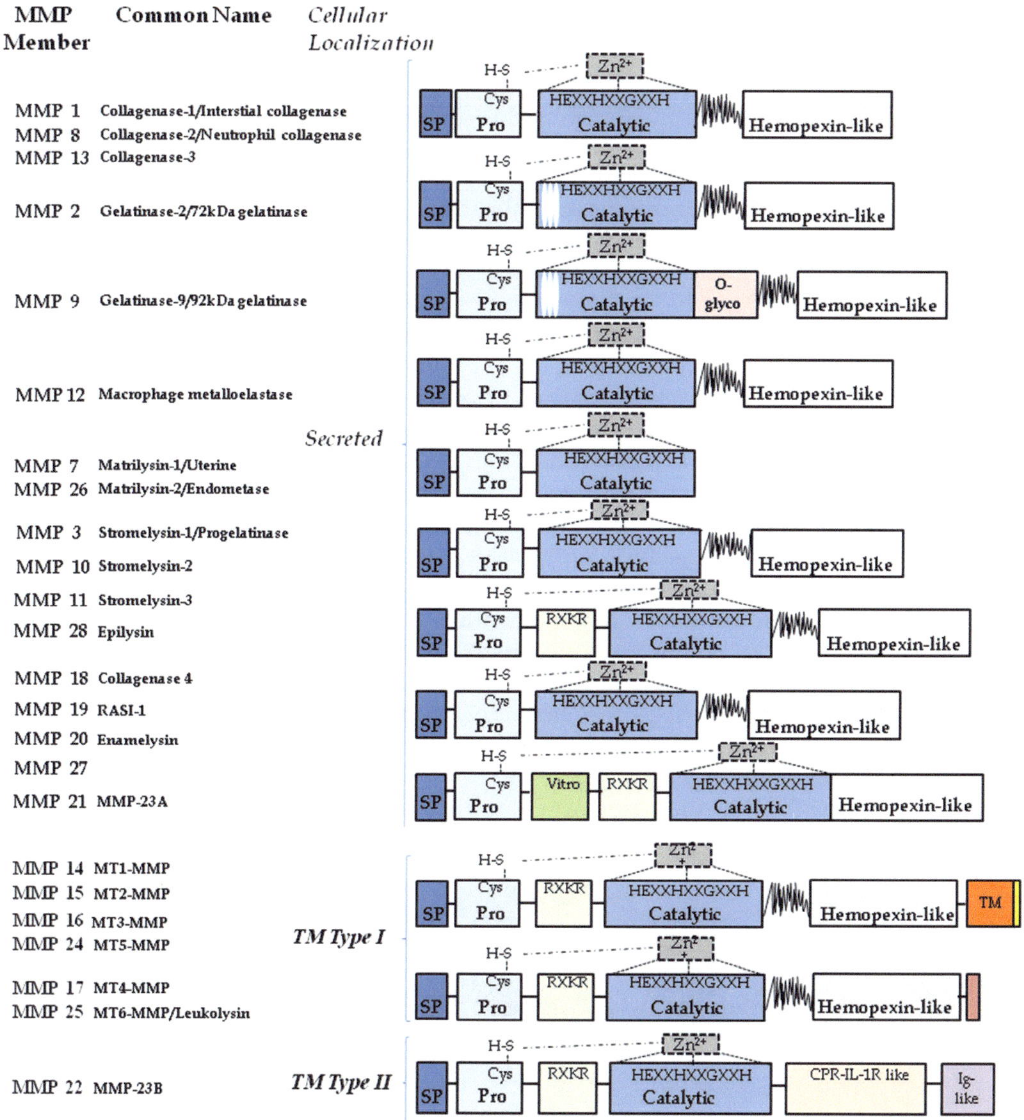

Fig. 2. Structural domains and nomenclature of the matrix metalloproteinases, A: Schematic representation of modular domains composing MMPs which are translated as inactive zymogens with an amino terminal signal peptide (SP), a pro-domain which folds over the zinc ion, in the catalytic site, to maintain latency (Pro), a catalytic domain that carries zinc at the active site, a hemopexin that confers the specificity to and interaction with the substrates or inhibitors (TIMPs) and presents the substrate to the catalytic site via a highly flexible hinge domain. Membrane-type (MT-) MMPs are anchored to the membrane either with a hydrophobic domain and a short cytoplasmic tail (Type I transmembrane protein) or with a glycosyl-phosphatidyl-inositol (GPI) domain. Gelatinases A and B also contain three collagen-binding fibronectin type II repeats within the catalytic domain and MMP-9 has an additional Serine-Threonine and proline rich O-Glycosylated domain. Some MMP have a furin-like motif

between the pro- and catalytic domains that allow their activation before they are secreted or localize to the membrane. MMP- 22 has a cysteine/proline rich, interleukin-1R domain and an Immunoglobulin-like domain. Compiled from (Bourboulia & Stetler-Stevenson, 2010; Fanjul-Fernandez et al., 2010; Rosenberg, 2009; Sternlicht & Werb, 2001).

In skeletal muscles, normal muscle development, limb immobilisation, electrical stimulation and muscle injury are all remodeling situations characterized by MMPs/TIMPs dysregulation. However, the nature of MMPs that is upregulated and the time frame of this upregulation depend, a great deal, on the model used. Immobilization or unloading, that result in muscle fiber atrophy, induce upregulation of both MMP-2 and MMP-9 and downregulation of TIMPs (Berthon et al., 2007; Giannelli et al., 2005; Reznick et al., 2003; Stevenson et al., 2003; Wittwer et al., 2002) (Berthon et al., 2007; Giannelli et al., 2005; Reznick et al., 2003; Stevenson et al., 2003; Wittwer et al., 2002) but only MMP-2 is active (Liu et al., 2010). Whereas a single bout of degeneration-regeneration, induced by experimental injury to the muscle, also results in upregulation of these two proteases but the time frame and intensity differ according to the type/extent of injury (Ferre et al., 2007; Frisdal et al., 2000; Kherif et al., 1999). In a cardiotoxin injury model that induced massive myofiber necrosis, gelatinase activity progressively increased and peaked at day 7, when muscle fiber formation was the most active. It then returned to normal at later stages. This increase was due to simultaneous and consecutive steps of gelatinases regulation- both expression and activation. Within hours after tissue injury, MMP-9 was induced in the tissue that expressed only MMP-2 in the normal situation. It correlated with inflammatory cells infiltration of necrotic muscle fibers that exhibit high gelatinase intracellularly, in contrast to pericellular localization of gelatinase in normal muscles (Figure 3). Simultaneously, MMP-2 expression and activation decreased within the first 24 hours and was followed by a progressive reconstitution of these forms afterwards. MMP-9 transcripts localized to

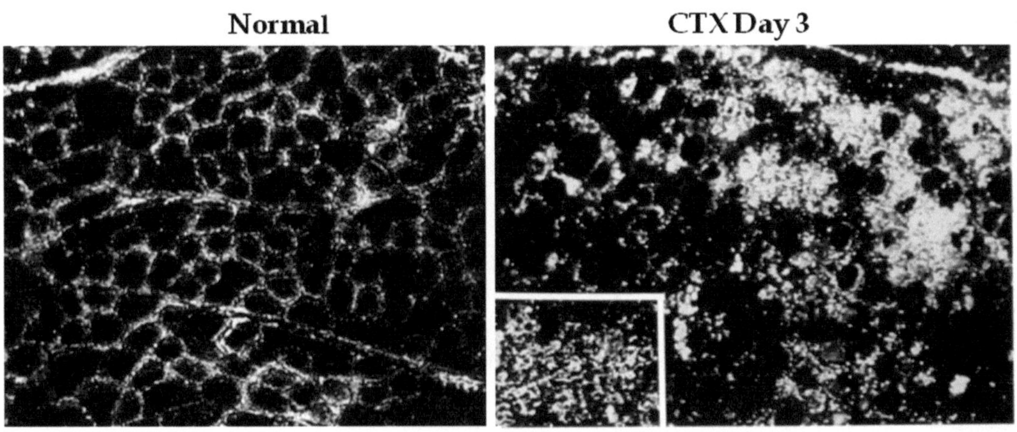

Fig. 3. *In situ* zymography of normal and cardiotoxin injured muscle 3 days after injury. In normal muscles, gelatinase activity (shown in white) localized to the endomysium and mononucleated cells present at the vicinity of muscle fibers. In injured muscles, gelatinase activity localizes to inflammatory cells. At early time points when necrotic muscle fibers are invaded by inflammatory cells, gelatinase activity is detected within degenerating muscle fibers that are invaded by inflammatory cells. Original magnification, X40 (Alameddine, Unpublished results).

inflammatory cells and mononucleated cells at satellite cell position (Kherif et al., 1999). The possibility that myogenic cells upregulate MMP-9 has been confirmed recently. When exposed to debris of damaged myotubes, the myogenic cells upregulated MMP-9, monocyte chemoattractant protein (MCP)-1 and other factors necessary for angiogenesis, tissue regeneration, and phagocyte recruitment (Dehne et al., 2011). Latent MT1-MMP (63kDA), which contributes with TIMP-2 to MMP-2 activation, is processed to its active (50kDa) form that retained its ability to process MMP-2 and was preceded by TIMP-2 decrease (Barnes et al., 2009). MMP-3 and TIMP-1 transcripts were also shown to be upregulated within the first 24 hours following cold injury. TIMP-1 started to decrease 72 hours post injury and early increase was followed by a decrease of active MMP-3 (Urso et al., 2010).

4.2 Matrix Metalloproteinases in dystrophic muscles

In dystrophic *mdx* and CXMD muscles, MMP-2 and MMP-9 are found in muscle extracts whereas only MMP-2 is found in normal muscles (Fukushima et al., 2007; Kherif et al., 1999). MMP-9 is upregulated in both muscles and serum of *mdx* mice (H. Li et al., 2009) throughout their lifespan (Alameddine et al., unpublished results). MT1-MMP, TIMP-1 and TIMP-2 are also upregulated in CXMD muscles and gelatinase activity localized to necrotic fibers and endomysium, demonstrated by *in situ* zymography (Fukushima et al., 2007). Differences in MMP expression and activity patterns detected in different adult *mdx* muscles - gastrocnemius, soleus and diaphragm- led Bani (Bani et al., 2008) to hypothesize that the microenvironment of distinct skeletal muscles may influence a particular kinetic pattern of MMP activity, which ultimately favors persistent inflammation and myofiber regeneration at different stages of the myopathy in *mdx* mice. Gene array analysis revealed profound modification of mRNA levels of several MMPs and other associated proteins in gastrocnemius and *tibialis anterior* muscles of *mdx* mice. MMP-3, -8, -9,-10,-12, -14 and -15 Adamts2 and Timp-1 mRNA levels are increased, MMP-11 as well as Adamts1, Adamts5, Adamts8 and Timp-2 and Timp-3 were downregulated (A. Kumar et al., 2010).

In DMD muscles, TIMP-1, TIMP-2 and MMP-2 transcripts are upregulated and MMP-2 activity is increased (von Moers et al., 2005). TIMP-1 levels, usually increased in the serum and plasma of patients with fibrotic diseases, are elevated in serum, plasma, and muscle extracts of muscular dystrophy patients and animal models. It correlated with TGFβ1 levels in DMD and in congenital muscular dystrophy (CMD) patients but not with Becker muscular dystrophy patients (Sun et al., 2010). In muscle tissue from dystrophin deficient and LAMA2-mutated muscular dystrophy patients, pro-fibrotic TGF-β1 is increased partly through a positive autocrine feedback loop and is released from decorin that is degraded by MMP-2. DMD fibroblasts have been shown to produce more soluble collagen, biglycan, decorin, TGF-β1 and MMP-7 and less MMP-1 than normal fibroblasts. TGF-β1 is known to modulate the ability of cells to synthesize various ECM components and was shown to modify the protein pattern produced by DMD fibroblasts upon their transformation to myofibroblasts. It increased MMP-7 thought to contribute to fibrosis (Fadic et al., 2006; Simona Zanotti et al., 2010; S. Zanotti et al., 2007).

In Emery-Dreifuss muscular dystrophy, screening of MMP-2, MMP-9 and MT1-MMP levels in the serum showed an increase of MMP-2 levels in both the autosomal and X- linked forms, suggesting it may serve as biomarker for the detection of cardiac involvement in patients with no subjective cardiac symptoms (Niebroj-Dobosz et al., 2009).

4.3 MMPs and inflammation in the development of fibrosis

End-stage DMD muscles are characterized by an almost complete disappearance of muscle fibers and their replacement by fibro-fatty tissue. Although DMD is not a fibrotic disease *per se*, their muscle biopsies are generally characterized by excessive production, deposition, and contraction of extracellular matrix. This accumulation results from factors, produced in diseased muscles, that influence the normal balance between production and/or hydrolysis of ECM components. Clearly, structural and functional changes of tissue microenvironment in dystrophic muscles are not equivalent to those that accompany normal muscle development. The permanent induction of wound-healing response with its inflammatory component may be essential contributors to the development of fibrosis in dystrophic muscles. Acute or chronic inflammation includes exudation of plasma proteins, recruitment of leukocytes and activation of cell and plasma derived inflammatory mediators as well as increased expression of MMPs (Manicone & McGuire, 2008). When inflammation is continuous or excessive, it is thought to contribute to tissue injury, organ dysfunction or chronic disease states. Inversely, decrease of MMP activity has been incriminated in the development of fibrotic conditions. Decreased MMP activity may result from dysregulation of the balance between MMPs and TIMPs. Upregulation of MMPs or downregulation of TIMPs activity could be applied for resolution of tissue fibrosis (reviewed (Hemmann et al., 2007)).

Experimental evidence shows that inflammatory cells such as macrophages, eosinophiles and T lymphocytes, the major infiltrating cell types, contribute to increased fibrosis (J. Morrison et al., 2000). Inflammatory cells produce cytokines/chemokines that regulate MMPs expression. In their turn, MMPs modulate the activities of cytokines and their receptors at the cell surface. The list of validated ECM components, growth factors (receptors and binding proteins) and cytokines/chemokines substrates is compiled in table 1.

Studies using gene microarrays have demonstrated that dystrophic muscles are characterized by an inflammatory "molecular signature", in which CC chemokines are prominent (Y. W. Chen et al., 2000; Y. W. Chen et al., 2005; Porter et al., 2003; Porter et al., 2002). Similarly, CC chemokines are greatly upregulated in normal skeletal muscles after experimental injury (Hirata et al., 2003). CC chemokine receptors (CCRs 1, 2, 3, 5) and ligands (macrophage inflammatory protein-1α, RANTES) are expressed at higher levels in dystrophic than in wild-type muscles across age groups (6, 12, and 24 wk). Moreover, chemokine ligand expression and muscle inflammation are significantly higher in dystrophic diaphragms than in limb muscles of the same animals. *In vitro*, CCR1 is constitutively expressed by myotubes formed from primary myoblasts derived from diaphragm muscles. Stimulation of myotubes by proinflammatory cytokines (tumor necrosis factor-α, interleukin-1α, interferon-γ) found within the *in vivo* dystrophic muscle environment, upregulates CCR1 in *mdx* and wild-type myoblast cultures, and also increases expression of its ligand RANTES to a significantly greater degree (Demoule et al., 2005).

In damaged muscles, various cytokines and growth factors are also released during necrosis and regeneration of muscle fibers. The most widely documented pro-fibrotic agent that is over-expressed in dystrophic muscles is TGF-β. It is upregulated in dystrophic muscles, after invasion of the damaged muscle by inflammatory cells (Y. W. Chen et al., 2005; Zhou et al., 2006) that were shown to express TGF-β mRNA although these cells may not be the sole contributors to its production (Bernasconi et al., 1999; Gosselin et al., 2004).

Enzyme	Enzymes ECM substrates	Growth factors & Cytokines/Chemokines
Secreted-type MMP		
Collagenases		
Interstitial collagenase MMP-1	Aggrecan; Collagens I,- III, VII, VIII, X, XI; Entactin; Fn; Gelatins; Ln; Link protein; Tenascin; Vn; Perlecan;	CTGF; IL1-β; IGFBPs; MCP-1, MCP-2, MCP-3, MCP-4; TNF-α
Neutrophil collagenase MMP-8	Aggrecan; Collagens I- III; Gelatins; link protein	LIX/CXCL5
Collagenase-3 MMP-13	Aggrecan; Collagens I-III,VI, IX, X, XIV; Fibrillin; Fn; Gelatins; Osteonectin; Ln; Perlecan	CTGF; MCP-3/CCL7, TGF-β; SDF-1/CXCL12
Collagenase-4 MMP-18	Collagen I	
Gelatinases		
Gelatinase A MMP-2	Aggrecan; Collagens I, III-V, VII, X- XI; Decorin; Elastin; Entactin; Fibrillin; Fn; Fibulins; Gelatins; Ln; Link protein; Osteonectin; Tenascin;	CTGF; FGFR1; CX_3CL1; IL1-β; IGFBPs; MCP-3/CCL7; TGF-β; TNF-α; SDF-1/CXCL12
Gelatinase B MMP-9	Aggrecan; Collagens III, IV-V, XI; Decorin; Elastin; Entactin; Fibrillin; Gelatins; Ln; Link protein; Osteonectin; N-telopeptide of collagen I; Vn	MCP-3; CCL11; CCL17; Fractalkine; GRO-alpha; IGFBP-3; IL1-β; IL-2Rα; IL-8/CXCL8; Kit-L; LIF; TGF-β; TNF-α; SDF-1/CXCL12; VEGF
Stromelysins		
Stromelysin-1 MMP-3	Aggrecan; Collagens III-V, VII, IX- XI; Decorin; Elastin; Entactin; Fibrillin; Fn; Gelatins;Ln; link protein; Osteonectin; Perlecan; Tenascin; Vn;	CTGF; HB-EGF; IL1-β; IGFBPs; MCP-1, MCP-2, MCP-3, MCP-4; IL-1β; TGF-β1; TNF-α; SDF-1/CXCL12;
Stromelysin-2 MMP-10	Aggrecan; Collagens III-V; Elastin; Fn; Gelatin; Link protein	
Matrilysins		
Matrilysin-1 (MMP-7)	Aggrecan; Collagens I, IV; Decorin; Elastin; Entactin; Fn; Fibulins; Gelatins; Ln; Link protein; Osteonectin; Osteopontin; Tenascin; Vn; Syndecan-1,	CTGF; Fas-L; HB-EGF; IGFBP-3; TNF-α; RANKL
Matrilysin-2 MMP-26	Collagen IV; Fn; Fibrinogen; Gelatin; Vn	

Furin-activated MMP		
Stromelysin-3 MMP-11	Aggrecan; Fn; Gelatins; Ln;	IGFBP-1
Epilysin MMP-28	Unknown	
Other secreted-type MMP		
Metalloelastase MMP-12	Aggrecan; Collagen I, IV; Elastin; Entactin; Fibrillin; Fn; Gelatin; Ln; Osteonectin; Vn;	TNF-α
RASI-1 (MMP-19)	Aggrecan; Collagen I, IV; COMP; Fn; Gelatin; Ln; Tenascin;	IGFBP-3
Enamelysin (MMP-20)	Aggrecan; Amelogenin; COMP; Gelatin;	Unknown
MMP-21	Unknown	Unknown
MMP-27	Unknown	Unknown
Membrane-anchored MMP		
Type I transmembrane-type MMP		
MT1-MMP MMP-14	Aggrecan; Collagens I-III, VI; Entactin; Fibrillin; Fn; Gelatins; Ln; Osteonectin; Vn;	CTGF; IL-8; MCP-3/CCL7; TNF-α
MT2-MMP MMP-15	Aggrecan; Entactin	
MT3-MMP MMP-16	Collagen III; Fn; Gelatins	
MT5-MMP MMP-24	PG	
GPI-linked MMP		
MT4-MMP MMP-17	Gelatin;	
MT6-MMP MMP-25	collagen IV; Fibrin; Fn; Gelatin; Ln	
Type II transmembrane-type MMP MMP-23	Gelatins	

CCL11, CC chemokine ligand 11; CCL17, CC chemokine ligand 17, COMP, cartilage oligomeric matrix protein; CTGF, connective tissue growth factor; Fas-L, Fas ligand; FGF, Fibroblast Growth Factor;, FGFR1, Fibroblast growth factor receptor 1; Fn, fibronectin; HB-EGF, heparin-binding epidermal growth factor like growth factor; IGFBP, insulin-like growth factor binding proteins; IL1-β, interleukin-1β; IL-2Rα, Interleukin 2 receptor; IL-8, interleukin 8; Kit-L, kit ligand; Ln, laminin; LIF, Leukimia inhibitory factor; LIX-CXL, lipopolysaccharide induced CXC chemokine, MCP-, monocyte chemotactic protein-; PCPE, Procollagen C protein enhancer; PG, proteoglycan; Pro, proteinase type; SDF-1/CXCL12, Stromal cell derived factor, TNF-α, tumor necrosis factor-α; TGF-β, transforming growth factor β; RASI-1, rheumatoid arthritis synovium inflamed-1; RANKL, receptor activator for nuclear factor κ B ligand.

Table 1. Validated MMPs substrates that include ECM and non-ECM proteins. Of the long list of non-ECM substrates, only growth factors, receptors and cytokines/chemokines have been extracted because of the role they play in the modification of tissue environment and the modulation of cell functions (Manicone & McGuire, 2008; C. J. Morrison et al., 2009; Shiomi et al., 2010; Sternlicht & Werb, 2001).

TGF-β is thought to play a prominent role in the pathogenesis of muscle fibrosis. Its short-term neutralization by decorin administration resulted in a 40% decline in type I collagen mRNA expression in *mdx* mice. *In vitro,* it stimulates collagen synthesis and inhibits collagen degradation in fibroblasts (Grande et al., 1997; Ignotz & Massague, 1986; Sharma & Ziyadeh, 1994)}. Myoblast stimulation by TGF-β1 induced autocrine production of TGF-β1, downregulation of myogenic proteins, production of fibrosis-related proteins and phenotypic transformation of myogenic cells to fibrobroblast/myofibroblast cell types *in vitro* (Yong Li et al., 2004). TGF-β treatment of myogenic cells also upregulated Connective Tissue Growth Factor (CTGF) (Maeda et al., 2005) incriminated in various fibrotic diseases. CTGF is overexpressed in dystrophic muscles and is thought to contribute, with TGF-β, to the development of fibrosis (Sun et al., 2008). Interestingly, both factors are validated MMPs substrates and could be modulated through MMPs action.

Tumor necrosis factor-(TNF-α), also upregulated in muscular dystrophy (Porreca et al., 1999) may exert direct adverse effects on skeletal muscle function and regeneration potential. Blockade of TNF-α by inhibitory antibodies reduced necrosis and contractile dysfunction in response to eccentric exercise (Piers et al., 2011; Radley et al., 2008). *In vitro* TNF-α has been shown to stimulate collagen synthesis in fibroblasts (Lurton et al., 1999) hence contributing directly to muscle fibrosis. *In vivo,* short-term pharmacological blockade of TNF-α in *mdx* mice significantly reduced the level of both TGF-β1 and type I collagen mRNA (Gosselin et al., 2004). Whether TNF-α mediates muscle fibrosis directly or indirectly (by upregulating the expression of TGF-β1) remains an open question. However, TNF-α induces MMP-9 upregulation in myogenic cells (Torrente et al., 2003).

Concomitance between inflammation and upregulation of MMPs in mouse models or human diseases with inflammatory conditions, led several groups to propose MMPs as potential therapeutic targets in pathological conditions with aberrant MMP expression and activity (reviewed (Clutterbuck et al., 2009)). Inhibition of MMPs has been recently investigated in *mdx* mice. MMP-9 inhibition either by the administration of nuclear factor-kappa B inhibitory peptide, gene deletion or by L-arginine treatment was reported to reduce muscle injury, inflammation, fibrosis and decrease pro-inflammatory cytokine release (Hnia et al., 2008; A. Kumar et al., 2010; H. Li et al., 2009). However, whether this inhibition is acting directly on the development of fibrosis or through prevention of muscle fibers necrosis and tissue scarring remains an open question.

Extreme precaution has to be taken into consideration regarding MMPs inhibition in muscular dystrophy particularly as animal models of MMP gain- or loss- of function and clinical trials of MMP inhibition in cancer patients have unraveled the dual role an individual MMP could exert, depending on tissue type or stage of the disease (protective/detrimental) (reviewed (Fanjul-Fernandez et al., 2010). In skeletal muscles, the beneficial effect of certain MMPs has been documented, underscoring the necessity for better knowledge of the role MMPs are playing in muscle diseases (Alameddine manuscript in preparation). Indeed, Mmp-2 gene ablation has been shown to impair the growth of muscle fibers by downregulating VEGF and nNOS (Miyazaki et al., 2011). Moreover, proteinases upregulation, during satellite cells activation, is essential for dismantling the satellite cells niche (Pallafacchina et al., 2010) and MMP-1 has been shown to reduce muscle fibrosis (Kaar et al., 2008).

4.4 MMPs favor cell migration

Myogenic cells have been reported to express various MMPs -MMP-1, -2, -3, -7, -9, -10, -14 and -16, either constitutively or after treatment with growth factors, cytokines or phorbol esters (Balcerzak et al., 2001; Caron et al., 1999; El Fahime et al., 2000; Guérin & Holland, 1995; Kherif et al., 1999; Lewis et al., 2000; Lluri & Jaworski, 2005; Nishimura et al., 2008; Ohtake et al., 2006). Cytokines and growth factors differentially modulate MMPs expression in myogenic cells. Treatment of adult mouse myoblasts by soluble serum fibronectin, PDGF-BB, TGF-β or IGF-1 had no effect on the expression of MMP-9 expression, whereas TNF-α and b-FGF reproducibly induced the expression of MMP-9 expression 30- and 10-folds. Other MMPs, such as MMP-1 and MMP-2, were not significantly affected by any of these growth factors (Allen et al., 2003; Torrente et al., 2003).

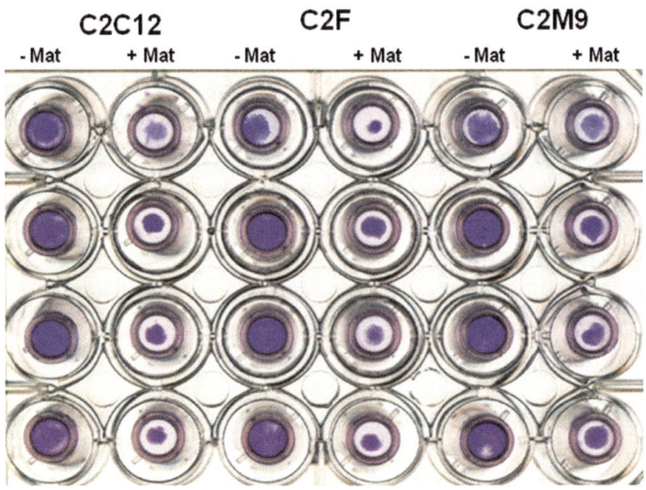

	C2C12	C2F	C2M9
MMP9	178	37	446
MMP2	1786	2635	1538
Total	1964	2672	1964

Fig. 4. Invasion assay establishing the correlation between migratory capacity of myogenic cells and MMP-9 expression levels. Three different cell types, C2C12 and 2 variant clones, expressing different levels of MMP-2 and MMP-9, that were quantified in the same zymography gels with Image J, were assayed in a two chamber migration assay with (+Mat) or without (-Mat) growth factor reduced Matrigel as substrate. The invasive capacity is measured by the ratio between cells that migrated through Matrigel and those diffused through the porous membrane. MMP-2, MMP-9 and total gelatinase values are expressed in arbitrary units. Invasive capacity of C2M9 was > to C2C12>C2F cells.

The role MMPs/TIMPs play in myogenic cells migration and potentially in cell fusion has been confirmed by overexpression and inhibition studies. Myoblasts overexpressing MMP-7 had a higher propensity to form myotubes than parental controls and generated more fibers when transplanted into a single site (Caron et al., 1999). MMP-1 enhanced C2C12 myoblast migration in a wound healing assay *in vitro* by increasing the expression of migration related marker proteins such as N-cadherin, β-catenin, latent MMP-2 and TIMP-1 (Wang et al., 2009). C2C12 cells stably transfected with MMP-2 and MMP-14 cDNA significantly increased the number of myonuclei without affecting the number of myotubes formed (Echizenya et al.,

2005). MT1-MMP has been proposed as a major MMP checkpoint regulator of myotube formation, as shMT1-MMP partly inhibited muscle cell fusion at a specific stage (Ohtake et al., 2006). MMP-9 and TIMP-1 have also been suspected to play a role in myogenesis *in vitro*. MMP-9 expression in human myogenic cells favored their migration on fibronectin and its inhibition by a blocking antibody decreased two dimensional cell migration (Lewis et al., 2000). Cells overexpressing MMP-9 have also better three dimensional migratory capacities (Figure 4). They exhibit higher migration when seeded on top of a Matrigel gel that better mimics ECM and their migration is inhibited in the presence of a specific MMP-9 inhibitor (Morgan et al., 2010). Of relevance to this review is that these cells have also higher engraftment capacities. Upon transplantation in a single site in irradiated and non-irradiated muscles of *mdx* nu/nu mice, they formed more dystrophin positive muscle fibers over larger areas, indicating they migrated better in a dystrophic environment (Morgan et al., 2010).

5. Conclusion

Although promising, there are several challenges to be overcome before stem or precursor cells could be used to treat muscular dystrophies. Apart from reliably and reproducibly identifying and purifying the cells of interest, their characteristics have to be maintained on expansion in culture: attempts at re-creating the niche *in vitro* may facilitate the retention of stem cell characteristics (Cosgrove et al., 2009; Gilbert et al., 2010). Encouraging results from one laboratory should be independently confirmed, before any particular stem cell is considered for therapeutic application.

Systemic delivery would involve turning a cell into a leukocyte to cross the blood vessel endothelium (Springer, 1994) and then switching on survival, migration, proliferative and myogenic regulatory factors once the cells are within the muscle. Even if it does not prove possible to treat muscles body-wide, transplanting stem cells locally into a small, vital, muscle, e.g. in the finger, may prove more practicable and although not life-saving, would improve the quality of life of DMD patients.

But for successful local as well as systemic delivery of stem cells to skeletal muscle, the inhospitable muscle environment remains a major hurdle. Studies on the factors and signaling pathways that hinder donor cell survival, proliferation and migration within both normal and dystrophic muscle and how these may be modified to augment the regenerative capacity of transplanted cells, remain vital for the successful use of stem cells in neuromuscular diseases. More importantly, elucidation of the role MMPs in general and individual MMPs in particular, play in the modulation of the dystrophic microenvironment and stem cell response to this environment warrants further study. In light of our present knowledge, it is tempting to propose that MMPs are temporally upregulated to permit migration and fusion of stem cells, then down-regulated, after donor-derived muscle has been formed, to reduce inflammation and fibrosis and thus improve muscle function. However, it is not clear whether the presence of either stem cells of normal origin, or muscle fibers expressing dystrophin, are sufficient to prevent the uncontrolled wound healing response that occurs in dystrophic muscles.

6. Acknowledgments

J.E.M is funded by a Wellcome Trust University award, the Muscular Dystrophy Campaign, the Duchenne Parent Project (Netherlands), the International Collaborative Effort for

Duchenne muscular dystrophy, and the Medical Research Council. H.S.A is funded by Association Institut de Myologie/Association Française contre les Myopathies and by INSERM (France).

7. References

Alameddine, H.S.; Dehaupas, M. & Fardeau, M. (1989). Regeneration of skeletal muscle fibers from autologous satellite cells multiplied in vitro. An experimental model for testing cultured cell myogenicity. *Muscle Nerve,* Vol.12, No.7, (Jul), pp. 544-55, ISSN 0148-639X

Alameddine, H.S.; Hantaï D.; Dehaupas, M.; & Fardeau, M. (1991). Role of persisting basement membrane in the reorganization of myofibres originating from myogenic cell grafts in the rat. *Neuromuscular Disorders,* Vol.1, No.2, pp. 143-52, ISSN 0960-8966

Alameddine, H.S.; Louboutin,J.P.; Dehaupas, M.; Sebille,A. & Fardeau, M. (1994). Functional recovery induced by satellite cell grafts in irreversibly injured muscles. *Cell Transplantation,* Vol.3, No.1, (Jan-Feb), pp. 3-14, ISSN 0963-6897

Allen, D.L.; Teitelbaum, D.H. & Kurachi, K. (2003). Growth factor stimulation of matrix metalloproteinase expression and myoblast migration and invasion in vitro. *American Journal of Physiology - Cell Physiology,* Vol.284, No.4, (Apr 1), pp. C805-C815,

Arechavala-Gomeza, V.; Kinali, M.; Feng, L.; Guglieri, M.; Edge, G.; Main, M.; Hunt, D.; Lehovsky, J.; Straub, V.; Bushby, K.; Sewry, C.A.; Morgan, J.E. & Muntoni, F. (2010). Revertant fibres and dystrophin traces in Duchenne muscular dystrophy: implication for clinical trials. *Neuromuscular Disorders,* Vol.20, No.5, (May), pp. 295-301, ISSN 1873-2364

Balcerzak, D.; Querengesser, L.; Dixon, W.T. & Baracos, V.E. (2001). Coordinated expression of matrix-degrading proteinases and their activators and inhibitors in bovine skeletal muscle. *Journal Animal Sciences,* Vol.79, No.1, (Jan 1), pp. 94-107,

Bani, C.; Lagrota-Candido, J.; Pinheiro, D.F.; Leite, P.E.; Salimena, M.C.; Henriques-Pons, A. & Quirico-Santos, T. (2008). Pattern of metalloprotease activity and myofiber regeneration in skeletal muscles of mdx mice. *Muscle Nerve,* Vol.37, No.5, (May), pp. 583-92, ISSN 0148-639X

Banks, G.B. & Chamberlain, J.S. (2008). The value of mammalian models for Duchenne muscular dystrophy in developing therapeutic strategies. *Current Topics in Developmental Biology,* Vol.84, pp. 431-53,

Barnes, B.R.; Szelenyi,E.R.; Warren, G.L. & Urso, M.L. (2009). Alterations in mRNA and protein levels of metalloproteinases-2, -9, and -14 and tissue inhibitor of metalloproteinase-2 responses to traumatic skeletal muscle injury. *American Journal of Physiology – Cell Physiology,* Vol.297, No.6, (Dec), pp. C1501-8, ISSN 1522-1563

Beauchamp, J.R.; Morgan, J.E.; Pagel, C.N. & Partridge, T.A. (1999). Dynamics of myoblast transplantation reveal a discrete minority of precursors with stem cell-like properties as the myogenic source. *The Journal of Cell Biology,* Vol.144, No.6, (Mar 22), pp. 1113-22,

Bekaert, S.; De Meyer, T. & Van Oostveldt, P. (2005). Telomere attrition as ageing biomarker. *Anticancer Research,* Vol.25, No.4, (Jul-Aug), pp. 3011-21, ISSN 0250-7005

Benchaouir, R.; Meregalli, M.; Farini ,A.; D'Antona, G.; Belicchi, M.; Goyenvalle, A.; Battistelli, M.; Bresolin, N.; Bottinelli, R.; Garcia, L. & Torrente, Y. (2007). Restoration of human dystrophin following transplantation of exon-skipping-engineered DMD patient stem cells into dystrophic mice. *Cell Stem Cell*, Vol.1, No.6, (Dec 13), pp. 646-57,

Bernasconi, P.; Di Blasi, C.; Mora, M.; Morandi, L.; Galbiati, S.; Confalonieri, P.; Cornelio, F.& Mantegazza, R. (1999). Transforming growth factor-[beta]1 and fibrosis in congenital muscular dystrophies. *Neuromuscular Disorders*, Vol.9, No.1, (Jan 1), pp. 28-33,

Berthon, P.; Duguez, S.; Favier, F.B.; Amirouche, A.; Feasson, L.; Vico, L.; Denis, C. & Freyssenet, D. (2007). Regulation of ubiquitin-proteasome system, caspase enzyme activities, and extracellular proteinases in rat soleus muscle in response to unloading. *Pflügers Archives*, Vol.454, No.4, (Jul), pp. 625-33, ISSN 0031-6768

Blau, H.M.; Webster, C. & Pavlath, G.K. (1983). Defective myoblasts identified in Duchenne muscular dystrophy. *Proceedings of the National Academy of Science USA*, Vol.80, No.15, (Aug), pp. 4856-60, ISSN 0027-8424

Blaveri, K.; Heslop, L.; Yu, D.S.; Rosenblatt, J.D.; Gross, J.G.; Partridge, T.A. & Morgan, J.E. (1999). Patterns of repair of dystrophic mouse muscle: studies on isolated fibers. *Developmental Dynamics*, Vol.216, No.3, pp. 244-56., ISSN

Bockhold, K.J.; Rosenblatt J.D. & Partridge, T.A. (1998). Aging normal and dystrophic mouse muscle: analysis of myogenicity in cultures of living single fibers. *Muscle Nerve*, Vol.21, No.2, (Feb), pp. 173-83,

Bokhoven, M.; Stephen, S.L.; Knight, S.; Gevers, E.F.; Robinson, I.C.; Takeuchi, Y. & Collins, M.K. (2009). Insertional gene activation by lentiviral and gammaretroviral vectors. *Journal of Virology*, Vol.83, No.1, (Jan), pp. 283-94,

Boldrin, L.; Muntoni, F. & Morgan, J.E. (2010). Are human and mouse satellite cells really the same? *Journal of Histochemistry & Cytochemistry*, Vol.58, No.11, (Nov), pp. 941-55, ISSN 1551-5044

Boldrin, L.; Zammit, P.S.; Muntoni, F. & Morgan, J.E. (2009). Mature adult dystrophic mouse muscle environment does not impede efficient engrafted satellite cell regeneration and self-renewal. *Stem Cells*, Vol.27, No.10, pp. 2478-2487, ISSN 1549-4918

Bourboulia, D. & Stetler-Stevenson, W.G. (2010). Matrix metalloproteinases (MMPs) and tissue inhibitors of metalloproteinases (TIMPs): Positive and negative regulators in tumor cell adhesion. *Seminars in Cancer Biology*, Vol.15, No.11, (Nov), pp. 1109-24,

Brimah, K.; Ehrhardt, J.; Mouly, V.; Butler-Browne, G.S.; Partridge, T.A. & Morgan, J.E. (2004). Human muscle precursor cell regeneration in the mouse host is enhanced by growth factors. *Human Gene Therapy*, Vol.15, No.11, (Nov), pp. 1109-24,

Bulfield, G.; Siller, W.G.; Wight, P.A. & Moore, K.J. (1984). X chromosome-linked muscular dystrophy (mdx) in the mouse. *Proceedings of the National Academy of Science USA*,Vol.81, No.4, (Feb), pp. 1189-92,

Bushby, K.; Finkel, R.; Birnkrant, D.J.; Case, L.E.; Clemens, P.R.; Cripe, L.; Kaul, A.; Kinnett, K.; McDonald, C.; Pandya, S.; Poysky, J.; Shapiro, F.; Tomezsko, J. & Constantin, C. (2010). Diagnosis and management of Duchenne muscular dystrophy, part 1: diagnosis, and pharmacological and psychosocial management. *Lancet Neurology*, Vol.9, No.1, (Jan), pp. 77-93, ISSN 1474-4465

Caron, N.J.; Asselin, I.; Morel, G. & Tremblay, J.P. (1999). Increased myogenic potential and fusion of matrilysin-expressing myoblasts transplanted in mice. *Cell Transplantation,* Vol.8, No.5, (Sep-Oct), pp. 465-76, ISSN 0963-6897

Chan, J.; O'Donoghue, K.; Gavina, M.; Torrente, Y.; Kennea, N.; Mehmet, H.; Stewart, H.; Watt ,D.J.; Morgan, J.E. & Fisk, N.M. (2006). Galectin-1 induces skeletal muscle differentiation in human fetal mesenchymal stem cells and increases muscle regeneration. *Stem Cells,* Vol.24, No.8, (Aug), pp. 1879-91,

Chen, Y.W.; Zhao, P.; Borup, R. & Hoffman, E. (2000). Expression profiling in the muscular dystrophies: identification of novel aspects of molecular pathophysiology. *The Journal of Cell Biology,* Vol.151, pp. 1321–36,

Chen, Y.W.; Nagaraju, K.; Bakay, M.; McIntyre, O.; Rawat, R.; Shi, R. & Hoffman, E.P. (2005). Early onset of inflammation and later involvement of TGF{beta} in Duchenne muscular dystrophy. *Neurology,* Vol.65, No.6, (Sep 27), pp. 826-834,

Ciuffi, A. (2008). Mechanisms governing lentivirus integration site selection. *Current Gene Therapy,* Vol.8, No.6, (Dec), pp. 419-29,

Clutterbuck, A.L.; Asplin, K.E.; Harris, P.; Allaway, D. & Mobasheri, A. (2009). Targeting matrix metalloproteinases in inflammatory conditions. *Current Drug Targets,* Vol.10, No.12, (Dec), pp. 1245-54, ISSN 1873-5592

Collins, C.A. & Morgan, J.E. (2003). Duchenne's muscular dystrophy: animal models used to investigate pathogenesis and develop therapeutic strategies. *International Journal of Experimental Pathology,* Vol.84, No.4, (Aug), pp. 165-72,

Collins, C.A.; Olsen, I.; Zammit, P.S.; Heslop, L.; Petrie, A.; Partridge T.A. & Morgan,. J.E. (2005). Stem cell function, self-renewal, and behavioral heterogeneity of cells from the adult muscle satellite cell niche. *Cell,* Vol.122, No.2, pp. 289-301,

Cooper, R.N.; Irintchev, A.; Di Santo, J.P.; Zweyer, M.; Morgan, J.E.; Partridge, T.A.; Butler-Browne, G.S.; Mouly, V. & Wernig, A. (2001). A new immunodeficient mouse model for human myoblast transplantation. *Human Gene Therapy,* Vol.12, No.7, (May 1), pp. 823-31,

Cosgrove, B.D.; Sacco, A.; Gilbert, P.M. & Blau, H.M. (2009). A home away from home: challenges and opportunities in engineering in vitro muscle satellite cell niches. *Differentiation,* Vol.78, No.2-3, (Sep-Oct), pp. 185-94, ISSN 1432-0436

Cousins, J.C.; Woodward, K.J.; Gross, J.G.; Partridge, T.A. & Morgan, J.E. (2004). Regeneration of skeletal muscle from transplanted immortalised myoblasts is oligoclonal. *Journal of Cell Science,* Vol.117, No.15, (Jul 1), pp. 3259-3269,

Decary, S.; Mouly, V. & Butler-Browne, G.S. (1996). Telomere length as a tool to monitor satellite cell amplification for cell-mediated gene therapy. *Human Gene Therapy,* Vol.7, No.11, (Jul 10), pp. 1347-50,

Decary, S.; Mouly, V.; Hamida, C.B.; Sautet, A.; Barbet, J.P. & Butler-Browne, G.S. (1997). Replicative potential and telomere length in human skeletal muscle: implications for satellite cell-mediated gene therapy. *Human Gene Therapy,* Vol.8, No.12, (Aug 10), pp. 1429-38,

Dehne, N.; Kerkweg, U.; Flohe, S.B.; Brune, B. & Fandrey, J. (2011). Activation of HIF-1 in skeletal muscle cells after exposure to damaged muscle cell debris. *Shock,* Vol. 35, No.6, (Jun), pp. 632-8., ISSN 1073-2322

Dellavalle, A.; Sampaolesi, M.; Tonlorenzi, R.; Tagliafico, E.; Sacchetti, B.; Perani, L.; Innocenzi, A.; Galvez, B.G.; Messina, G.; Morosetti, R.; Li, S.; Belicchi, M.; Peretti,

G.; Chamberlain, J.S.; Wright, W.E.; Torrente, Y.; Ferrari, S.; Bianco P. & Cossu, G. (2007). Pericytes of human skeletal muscle are myogenic precursors distinct from satellite cells. *Nature Cell Biology*, Vol.9, No.3, (Mar), pp. 255-67,

Demoule, A.; Divangahi, M.; Danialou, G.; Gvozdic, D.; Larkin, G.; Bao; W.& Petrof, B.J. (2005). Expression and regulation of CC class chemokines in the dystrophic (mdx) diaphragm. *American Journal of Respiratory Cell and Molecular Biology*, Vol.33, No.2, (Aug), pp. 178-185,

Diaz-Manera, J.; Touvier, T.; Dellavalle, A.; Tonlorenzi, R.; Tedesco, F.S.; Messina, G.; Meregalli, M.; Navarro, C.; Perani, L.; Bonfanti, C.; Illa, I.; Torrente, Y.& Cossu, G. (2010). Partial dysferlin reconstitution by adult murine mesoangioblasts is sufficient for full functional recovery in a murine model of dysferlinopathy. *Cell death & disease*, Vol.1, pp. e61, ISSN 2041-4889

Echizenya, M.; Kondo, S.; Takahashi, R.; Oh, J.; Kawashima, S.; Kitayama, H.; Takahashi, C. & Noda, M. (2005). The membrane-anchored MMP-regulator RECK is a target of myogenic regulatory factors. *Oncogene*, Vol.24, No.38, pp. 5850-5857,

Ehrhardt, J.; Brimah, K.; Adkin, C.; Partridge, T. & Morgan, J. (2007). Human muscle precursor cells give rise to functional satellite cells in vivo. *Neuromuscular Disorders*, Vol.17, No.8, (Aug), pp. 631-8,

El Fahime, E.; Torrente, Y.; Caron, N.J.; Bresolin, M.D. & Tremblay, J.P. (2000). In vivo migration of transplanted myoblasts requires Matrix Metalloproteinase activity. *Experimental Cell Research*, Vol.258, No.2, (Aug), pp. 279-287,

Emery, A.E. (2002). The muscular dystrophies. *Lancet*, Vol.359, No.9307, (Feb 23), pp. 687-95, ISSN 0140-6736

Fadic, R.; Mezzano, V.; Alvarez, K.; Cabrera, D.; Holmgren, J. & Brandan, E. (2006). Increase in decorin and biglycan in Duchenne Muscular Dystrophy: role of fibroblasts as cell source of these proteoglycans in the disease. *Journal of Cellular and molecular medicine*, Vol.10, No.3, (Jul-Sep), pp. 758-69, ISSN 1582-1838

Fanjul-Fernandez, M.; Folgueras, A.R.; Cabrera, S. & Lopez-Otin, C. (2010). Matrix metalloproteinases: evolution, gene regulation and functional analysis in mouse models. *Biochimica Biophysica Acta*,Vol.1803, No.1, (Jan), pp. 3-19, ISSN 0006-3002

Ferrari, G.; Cusella-De Angelis, G.; Coletta, M.; Paolucci, E.; Stornaiuolo, A.; Cossu, G. & Mavilio, F. (1998). Muscle regeneration by bone marrow-derived myogenic progenitors. *Science*, Vol.279, No.5356, (Mar 6), pp. 1528-30,

Ferre, P.J.; Liaubet, L.; Concordet, D.; SanCristobal, M.; Uro-Coste, E.; Tosser-Klopp, G.; Bonnet, A.; Toutain, P.L.; Hatey, F. & Lefebvre, H.P. (2007). Longitudinal analysis of gene expression in porcine skeletal muscle after post-injection local injury. *Pharmaceutical Research*, Vol.24, No.8, (Aug), pp. 1480-9, ISSN 0724-8741

Frisdal, E.; Teiger, E.; Lefaucheur, J.P.; Adnot, S.; Planus, E.; Lafuma, C.& D'Ortho, M. P.. (2000). Increased expression of gelatinases and alteration of basement membrane in rat soleus muscle following femoral artery ligation. *Neuropathology and Applied Neurobiology*, Vol.26, No.1, (Feb), pp. 11-21, ISSN 0305-1846

Fukushima, K.; Nakamura, A.; Ueda, H.; Yuasa, K.; Yoshida, K.; Takeda, S. & Ikeda, S. (2007). Activation and localization of matrix metalloproteinase-2 and -9 in the skeletal muscle of the muscular dystrophy dog (CXMDJ). *BMC Musculoskeletal Disorders*, Vol.8, pp. 54, ISSN 1471-2474

Galvez, B.G.; Sampaolesi, M.; Brunelli, S.; Covarello, D.; Gavina, M.; Rossi, B.; Constantin, G.; Torrente, Y. & Cossu, G. (2006). Complete repair of dystrophic skeletal muscle by mesoangioblasts with enhanced migration ability. *The Journal of Cell Biology,* Vol.174, No.2, (Jul 17), pp. 231-43,

Gerard, C.; Forest, M.A.; Beauregard, G.; Skuk, D. & Tremblay, J.P.. (2011). Fibrin gel improves the survival of transplanted myoblasts. *Cell Transplantation,* Vol.20, No.5, (Apr 29), pp. ISSN 1555-3892

Giannelli, G.; De Marzo, A.; Marinosci, F. & Antonaci, S. (2005). Matrix metalloproteinase imbalance in muscle disuse atrophy. *Histology & Histopathology,* Vol.20, No.1, (Jan), pp. 99-106, ISSN 0213-3911

Gilbert, P.M.; Havenstrite, K.L.; Magnusson, K.E.; Sacco, A.; Leonardi, N.A.; Kraft, P.; Nguyen, N.K.; Thrun, S.; Lutolf, M.P. & Blau, H.M. (2010). Substrate elasticity regulates skeletal muscle stem cell self-renewal in culture. *Science,* Vol.329, No.5995, (Aug 27), pp. 1078-81, ISSN 1095-9203

Gosselin, L.E.; Williams, J.E.; Deering, M.; Brazeau, D.; Koury, S. & Martinez, D.A. (2004). Localization and early time course of TGF-β1 mRNA expression in dystrophic muscle. *Muscle Nerve,* Vol.30, No.5, pp. 645-653, ISSN 1097-4598

Goyenvalle, A. & Davies, K.E. (2011). Challenges to oligonucleotides-based therapeutics for Duchenne muscular dystrophy. *Skeletal muscle,* Vol.1, No.1, pp. 8, ISSN 2044-5040

Grande, J.P.; Melder, D.C. & Zinsmeister, A.R. (1997). Modulation of collagen gene expression by cytokines: stimulatory effect of transforming growth factor-beta1, with divergent effects of epidermal growth factor and tumor necrosis factor-alpha on collagen type I and collagen type IV. *Journal of Laboratory and Clinical Medicine,* Vol.130, pp. 476–486.,

Gross, J.G. & Morgan, J.E. (1999). Muscle precursor cells injected into irradiated mdx mouse muscle persist after serial injury. *Muscle Nerve,* Vol.22, No.2, pp. 174-85.,

Guérin, C.W. & Holland, P.C. (1995). Synthesis and secretion of matrix-degrading metalloproteases by human skeletal muscle satellite cells. *Developmental Dynamics,* Vol.202, No.1, (Jan), pp. 91-99,

Guglieri, M. & Bushby, K. (2010). Molecular treatments in Duchenne muscular dystrophy. *Current Opinion in Pharmacology,* Vol.10, No.3, (Jun), pp. 331-7, ISSN 1471-4973

Hemmann, S.; Graf, J.; Roderfeld, M. & Roeb, E. (2007). Expression of MMPs and TIMPs in liver fibrosis - a systematic review with special emphasis on anti-fibrotic strategies. *Journal of Hepatology,* Vol.46, No.5, pp. 955-975,

Heslop, L.; Morgan, J.E. & Partridge, T.A. (2000). Evidence for a myogenic stem cell that is exhausted in dystrophic muscle. *Journal of Cell Science,* Vol.113 (Pt 12), (Jun), pp. 2299-308,

Hirata, A.; Masuda, S.; Tamura, T.; Kai, K.; Ojima, K.; Fukase, A.; Motoyoshi, K.; Kamakura, K.; Miyagoe-Suzuki, Y. & Takeda, S. (2003). Expression profiling of cytokines and related genes in regenerating skeletal muscle after cardiotoxin injection: a role for osteopontin. *American Journal of Pathology,* Vol.163, pp. 203–15,

Hnia, K.; Gayraud, J.; Hugon, G.; Ramonatxo, M.; De La Porte, S.; Matecki, S.& Mornet, D. (2008). L-arginine decreases inflammation and modulates the nuclear factor-kappaB/matrix metalloproteinase cascade in mdx muscle fibers. *American Journal of Pathology,* Vol.172, No.6, (Jun), pp. 1509-19, ISSN 1525-2191

Hoffman, E.P.; Morgan, J.E.; Watkins, S.C. & Partridge, T.A. (1990). Somatic reversion/suppression of the mouse mdx phenotype in vivo. *Journal of the Neurological Sciences*, Vol.99, No.1, (Oct), pp. 9-25,

Hoffman, E.P.; Bronson, A.; Levin, A.A.; Takeda, S.; Yokota, T.;. Baudy, A.R & Connor, E.M. (2011). Restoring dystrophin expression in duchenne muscular dystrophy muscle progress in exon skipping and stop codon read through. *American Journal of Pathology*, Vol.179, No.1, (Jul), pp. 12-22, ISSN 1525-2191

Holmbeck, K.; Bianco, P.; Pidoux, I.; Inoue, S.; Billinghurst, R.C.; Wu, W.; Chrysovergis, K.; Yamada, S.; Birkedal-Hansen, H.& Poole, A.R. (2005). The metalloproteinase MT1-MMP is required for normal development and maintenance of osteocyte processes in bone. *Journal of Cell Science*, Vol.118, No.Pt 1, (Jan 1), pp. 147-56, ISSN 0021-9533

Hulboy, D.L.; Rudolph, L.A. & Matrisian, L.M. (1997). Matrix metalloproteinases as mediators of reproductive function. *Molecular Human Reproduction*, Vol.3, No.1, (Jan), pp. 27-45, ISSN 1360-9947

Ignotz, R.A. & Massague, J. (1986). Transforming growth factor-beta stimulates the expression of fibronectin and collagen and their incorporation into the extracellular matrix. *Journal of Biological Chemistry*, Vol.261, pp. 4337–4345.,

Irintchev, A.; Langer, M.; Zweyer, M.; Theisen R. & Wernig, A. (1997). Functional improvement of damaged adult mouse muscle by implantation of primary myoblasts. *Journal of Physiology*, Vol.500 (Pt 3), (May 1), pp. 775-85,

Jackson, K.A.; Snyder, D.S. & Goodell, M.A. (2004). Skeletal muscle fiber-specific green autofluorescence: potential for stem cell engraftment artifacts. *Stem Cells*, Vol.22, No.2, pp. 180-7, ISSN 1066-5099

Kaar, J.L.; Li, Y.; Blair, H.C.; Asche, G.; Koepsel, R.R.; Huard, J. & Russell, A.J. (2008). Matrix metalloproteinase-1 treatment of muscle fibrosis. *Acta Biomaterialia*, Vol.4, No.5, (Sep), pp. 1411-20, ISSN 1742-7061

Kherif, S.; Lafuma, C.; Dehaupas, M.; Lachkar, S.; Fournier, J.G.; Verdiere-Sahuque, M.; Fardeau, M. & Alameddine, H.S. (1999). Expression of matrix metalloproteinases 2 and 9 in regenerating skeletal muscle: a study in experimentally injured and mdx muscles. *Developmental Biology*, Vol.205, No.1, (Jan 1), pp. 158-70, ISSN 0012-1606

Kinoshita, I.; Huard J. & Tremblay, J.P. (1994a). Utilization of myoblasts from transgenic mice to evaluate the efficacy of myoblast transplantation. *Muscle Nerve*, Vol.17, No.9, (Sep), pp. 975-80, ISSN 0148-639X

Kinoshita, I.; Vilquin, J.T.; Guerette, B.; Asselin, I.; Roy, R.; Lille S. & Tremblay, J.P. (1994b). Immunosuppression with FK 506 insures good success of myoblast transplantation in mdx mice. *Transplantation Proceedings*, Vol.26, No.6, (Dec), pp. 3518, ISSN 0041-1345

Kumar, A.; Bhatnagar, S. & Kumar, A. (2010). Matrix metalloproteinase inhibitor batimastat alleviates pathology and improves skeletal muscle function in dystrophin-deficient mdx mice. *American Journal of Pathology*, Vol.177, No.1, (Jul), pp. 248-60, ISSN 1525-2191

Kumar, M.; Keller, B.; Makalou, N. & Sutton, R.E. (2001). Systematic determination of the packaging limit of lentiviral vectors. *Human Gene Therapy*, Vol.12, No.15, (Oct 10), pp. 1893-905,

Lai, Y.; Thomas, G.D.; Yue, Y.; Yang, H.T.; Li, D.; Long, C.; Judge, L.; Bostick, B.; Chamberlain, J.S.; Terjung, R.L. & Duan, D. (2009). Dystrophins carrying spectrin-like repeats 16 and 17 anchor nNOS to the sarcolemma and enhance exercise performance in a mouse model of muscular dystrophy. *The Journal of Clinical Investigation,* Vol.119, No.3, (Mar), pp. 624-35,

Lefaucheur, J.P. & Sebille, A. (1995). Basic fibroblast growth factor promotes in vivo muscle regeneration in murine muscular dystrophy. *Neuroscience Letters,* Vol.202, No.1-2, (Dec 29), pp. 121-4,

Lewis, M.P.; Tippett, H.L.; Sinanan, A.C.; Morgan, M.J. & Hunt, N.P. (2000). Gelatinase-B (matrix metalloproteinase-9; MMP-9) secretion is involved in the migratory phase of human and murine muscle cell cultures. *Journal of Muscle Research and Cell Motility,* Vol.21, No.3, pp. 223-233,

Li, H.; Mittal, A.; Makonchuk, D.Y.; Bhatnagar, S. & Kumar, A. (2009). Matrix metalloproteinase-9 inhibition ameliorates pathogenesis and improves skeletal muscle regeneration in muscular dystrophy. *Human Molecular Genetics,* Vol.18, No.14, (Jul 15), pp. 2584-98, ISSN 1460-2083

Li, S.; Kimura, E.; Fall, B.M.; Reyes, M.; Angello, J.C.; Welikson, R.; Hauschka, S.D. & Chamberlain, J.S. (2005). Stable transduction of myogenic cells with lentiviral vectors expressing a minidystrophin. *Gene Therapy ,* Vol.12, No.14, (Jul), pp. 1099-108,

Li, Y.; Foster, W.; Deasy, B.M.; Chan, Y.; Prisk, V.; Tang ,Y.; Cummins, J. & Huard, J. (2004). Transforming Growth Factor-{beta}1 induces the differentiation of myogenic cells into fibrotic cells in injured skeletal muscle: A key event in muscle fibrogenesis. *American Journal of Pathology,* Vol.164, No.3, (March 1, 2004), pp. 1007-1019,

Liu, X.; Lee, D.J.; Skittone, L.K.; Natsuhara, K. & Kim, H.T. (2010). Role of gelatinases in disuse-induced skeletal muscle atrophy. *Muscle Nerve,* Vol.41, No.2, (Feb), pp. 174-8, ISSN 1097-4598

Lluri, G. & Jaworski, D.M. (2005). Regulation of TIMP-2, MT1-MMP, and MMP-2 expression during C2C12 differentiation. *Muscle Nerve,* Vol.32, No.4, (Oct), pp. 492-9, ISSN 0148-639X

Lurton, J.; Soto, H.; Narayanan, A. & Raghu, G. (1999). Regulation of human lung fibroblast C1q-receptors by transforming growth factor-beta and tumor necrosis factor-alpha. *Experimental Lung Research,* Vol.25, pp. 151–164,

Maeda, N.; Kanda, F.; Okuda, S.; Ishihara, H. & Chihara, K. (2005). Transforming growth factor-beta enhances connective tissue growth factor expression in L6 rat skeletal myotubes. *Neuromuscular Disorders,* Vol.15, No.11, (Nov), pp. 790-3,

Manicone, A.M. & McGuire, J.K. (2008). Matrix metalloproteinases as modulators of inflammation. *Seminars of Cell and Developmental Biology,* Vol.19, No.1, (Feb), pp. 34-41, ISSN 1084-9521

Mather, K.A.; Jorm, A.F.; Parslow, R.A. & Christensen, H. (2011). Is telomere length a biomarker of aging? A review. *The Journals of Gerontology. Series A, Biological sciences and medical sciences,* Vol.66, No.2, (Feb), pp. 202-13, ISSN 1758-535X

Mauro, A. (1961). Satellite cell of skeletal muscle fibers. *Journal of Biophysical and Biochemical Cytology,* Vol.9, (Feb), pp. 493-5, ISSN 0095-9901

Meng, J.; Muntoni, F.& Morgan, J.E. (2011a). Stem cells to treat muscular dystrophies - where are we? *Neuromuscular Disorders,* Vol.21, No.1, (Jan), pp. 4-12, ISSN 1873-2364

Meng, J.; Adkin, C.F.; Xu, S.W.; Muntoni, F. & Morgan, J.E. (2011b). Contribution of human muscle-derived cells to skeletal muscle regeneration in dystrophic host mice. *PloS One*, Vol.6, No.3, pp. e17454, ISSN 1932-6203

Meng, J.; Adkin, C.F.; Arechavala-Gomeza, V.; Boldrin, L.; Muntoni, F. & Morgan, J.E. (2010). The contribution of human synovial stem cells to skeletal muscle regeneration. *Neuromuscular Disorders*, Vol.20, No.1, (Jan), pp. 6-15, ISSN 1873-2364

Meregalli, M.; Farini, A. & Torrente, Y. (2008). Combining stem cells and exon skipping strategy to treat muscular dystrophy. *Expert Opinion in Biological Therapy*, Vol.8, No.8, (Aug), pp. 1051-61,

Miyazaki, D.; Nakamura, A.; Fukushima, K.; Yoshida, K.; Takeda, S. & Ikeda, S.I. (2011). Matrix metalloproteinase-2 ablation in dystrophin-deficient mdx muscles reduces angiogenesis resulting in impaired growth of regenerated muscle fibers. *Human Molecular Genetics*, Vol.20, No.9, (May 1), pp. 1787-99., ISSN 1460-2083

Monaco, A.P.; Bertelson, C.J.; Middlesworth, W.; Colletti, C.A.; Aldridge, J.; Fischbeck, K.H.; Bartlett, R.; Pericak-Vance, M.A.; Roses, A.D. & Kunkel, L.M. (1985). Detection of deletions spanning the Duchenne muscular dystrophy locus using a tightly linked DNA segment. *Nature*, Vol.316, No.6031, (Aug 29-Sep 4), pp. 842-5, ISSN 0028-0836

Montini, E.; Cesana, D.; Schmidt, M.; Sanvito, F.; Ponzoni, M.; Bartholomae, C.; Sergi Sergi, L.; Benedicenti, F.; Ambrosi, A.; Di Serio, C.; Doglioni, C.; von Kalle, C. & Naldini, L. (2006). Hematopoietic stem cell gene transfer in a tumor-prone mouse model uncovers low genotoxicity of lentiviral vector integration. *Nature Biotechnology*, Vol.24, No.6, (Jun), pp. 687-96,

Morgan, J.; Rouche, A.; Bausero, P.; Houssaini, A.; Gross, J.; Fiszman, M.Y. & Alameddine,H.S. (2010). MMP-9 overexpression improves myogenic cell migration and engraftment. *Muscle Nerve*, Vol.42, No.4, (Oct), pp. 584-95, ISSN 1097-4598

Morgan, J.E. & P.S. Zammit. (2010). Direct effects of the pathogenic mutation on satellite cell function in muscular dystrophy. *Experimental Cell Research*, Vol.316, No.18, pp. 3100-3108, ISSN 1090-2422

Morgan, J.E.; Hoffman, E.P. & Partridge, T.A. (1990). Normal myogenic cells from newborn mice restore normal histology to degenerating muscles of the mdx mouse. *The Journal of Cell Biology*, Vol.111, No.6 Pt 1, pp. 2437-49.,

Morgan, J.E.; Gross, J.G.; Pagel, C.N.; Beauchamp, J.R.; Fassati, A.; Thrasher, A.J.; Di Santo, J.P.; Fisher, I.B.; Shiwen, X.; Abraham, D.J.& Partridge,T.A. (2002). Myogenic cell proliferation and generation of a reversible tumorigenic phenotype are triggered by preirradiation of the recipient site. *The Journal of Cell Biology*, Vol.157, No.4, pp. 693-702, ISSN 0021-9525

Morrison, C.J.; Butler, G.S.; Rodriguez, D. & Overall, C.M. (2009). Matrix metalloproteinase proteomics: substrates, targets, and therapy. *Current Opinion in Cell Biology*, Vol.21, No.5, (Oct), pp. 645-53, ISSN 1879-0410

Morrison, J.; Lu, Q.L.; Pastoret, C.; Partridge T. & Bou-Gharios, G. (2000). T-cell-dependent fibrosis in the mdx dystrophic mouse. *Laboratory Investigation*, Vol.80, No.6, pp. 881-91.,

Murphy, G. (2010). Fell-Muir Lecture: Metalloproteinases: from demolition squad to master regulators. *International Journal of Experimental Pathology*, Vol.91, No.4, (Aug), pp. 303-13, ISSN 1365-2613

Nakamura, A. & Takeda, S. (2011). Mammalian models of Duchenne Muscular Dystrophy: pathological characteristics and therapeutic applications. *Journal of Biomedicine & Biotechnology,*Vol.2011, pp. 184393, ISSN 1110-7251

Negroni, E.; Vallese, D.; Vilquin, J.T.; Butler-Browne, G.; Mouly, V. & Trollet, C. (2011). Current advances in cell therapy strategies for muscular dystrophies. *Expert Opinion on Biological Therapy,* Vol.11, No.2, (Feb), pp. 157-76, ISSN 1744-7682

Negroni, E.; Riederer, I.; Chaouch, S.; Belicchi, M.; Razini, P.; Di Santo, J.; Torrente, Y.; Butler-Browne, G.S. & Mouly, V. (2009). In vivo myogenic potential of human CD133+ muscle-derived stem cells: a quantitative study. *Molecular Therapy,* Vol.17, No.10, (Oct), pp. 1771-8, ISSN 1525-0024

Niebroj-Dobosz, I.; Madej-Pilarczyk, A.; Marchel, M.; Sokolowska, B. & Hausmanowa-Petrusewicz, I. (2009). Matrix metalloproteinases in serum of Emery-Dreifuss muscular dystrophy patients. *Acta Biochimica Polonica,* Vol.56, No.4, pp. 717-22, ISSN 1734-154X

Nishimura, T.; Nakamura, K.; Kishioka, Y.; Kato-Mori, Y.; Wakamatsu, J. & Hattori, A. (2008). Inhibition of matrix metalloproteinases suppresses the migration of skeletal muscle cells. *Journal of Muscle Research and Cell Motility,* Vol.29, No.1, pp. 37-44, ISSN 0142-4319

Ohtake, Y.; Tojo, H. & Seiki, M. (2006). Multifunctional roles of MT1-MMP in myofiber formation and morphostatic maintenance of skeletal muscle. *Journal of Cell Science,* Vol.119, No Pt 18, (Sep 15), pp. 3822-32, ISSN 0021-9533

Pagel, C.N. & Partridge, T.A. (1999). Covert persistence of mdx mouse myopathy is revealed by acute and chronic effects of irradiation. *Journal of Neurological Science,* Vol.164, No.2, (Apr 1), pp. 103-16,

Pallafacchina, G.; Francois, S.; Regnault, B.; Czarny, B.; Dive, V.; Cumano, A.; Montarras, D. & Buckingham, M. (2010). An adult tissue-specific stem cell in its niche: a gene profiling analysis of in vivo quiescent and activated muscle satellite cells. *Stem Cell Research,* Vol.4, No.2, (Mar), pp. 77-91, ISSN 1876-7753

Palmieri, B.; Tremblay, J.P. & Daniele, L. (2010). Past, present and future of myoblast transplantation in the treatment of Duchenne muscular dystrophy. *Pediatric transplantation,* Vol.14, No.7, (Nov), pp. 813-9, ISSN 1399-3046

Palumbo, R.; Sampaolesi, M.; De Marchis, F.; Tonlorenzi, R.; Colombetti, S.; Mondino, A.; Cossu G. & Bianchi, M.E. (2004). Extracellular HMGB1, a signal of tissue damage, induces mesoangioblast migration and proliferation. *The Journal of Cell Biology,* Vol.164, No.3, (Feb 2), pp. 441-9, ISSN 0021-9525

Partridge, T.A.; Morgan, J.E.; Coulton, G.R.; Hoffman, E.P. & Kunkel, L.M. (1989). Conversion of mdx myofibers from dystrophin-negative to-positive by injection of normal myoblasts. *Nature,* Vol.337, pp. 176-179,

Pellegrini, K.L. & Beilharz, M.W. (2011). The survival of myoblasts after intramuscular transplantation is improved when fewer cells are injected. *Transplantation,* Vol.91, No.5, (Mar 15), pp. 522-6, ISSN 1534-6080

Piers, A.T.; Lavin, T.; Radley-Crabb, H.G.; Bakker, A.J.; Grounds ,M.D. & Pinniger, G.J. (2011). Blockade of TNF in vivo using cV1q antibody reduces contractile dysfunction of skeletal muscle in response to eccentric exercise in dystrophic mdx and normal mice. *Neuromuscular Disorders,* Vol.21, No.2, (Feb), pp. 132-41, ISSN 1873-2364

Pisani, D.F.; Clement, N.; Loubat, A.; Plaisant, M.; Sacconi, S.; Kurzenne, J.Y.; Desnuelle, C.; Dani C. &Dechesne, C.A. (2010). Hierarchization of myogenic and adipogenic progenitors within human skeletal muscle. *Stem Cells,* Vol.28, No.12, (Dec), pp. 2182-94, ISSN 1549-4918

Porreca, E.; Guglielmi, M.; Uncini, A.; Di Gregorio, P.; Angelini, A.; Di Febbo, C.; Pierdomenico, S.; Baccante G. & Cuccurullo,. F. (1999). Haemostatic abnormalities, cardiac involvement and serum tumor necrosis factor levels in X-linked dystrophic patients. *Thrombosis Haemostasis,* Vol.81, pp. 543–546.,

Porter, J.D.; Guo, W.; Merriam, A.P.; Khanna, S.; Cheng, G.; Zhou, X.; Andrade, F.H.; Richmonds, C. & Kaminski, H.J. (2003). Persistent over-expression of specific CC class chemokines correlates with macrophage and T-cell recruitment in mdx skeletal muscle. *Neuromuscular Disorders,* Vol.13, pp. 223–35,

Porter, J.D.; Khanna, S.; Kaminski, H.J.; Rao, J.S.; Merriam, A.; Richmonds, C.R.; Leahy, P.; Li, J.; Guo, W. & Andrade, F.H. (2002). A chronic inflammatory response dominates the skeletal muscle molecular signature in dystrophin-deficient mdx mice. *Human Molecular Genetics,* Vol.11, pp. 263–72,

Praud, C.; Montarras, D.; Pinset,C. & Sebille, A. (2003). Dose effect relationship between the number of normal progenitor muscle cells grafted in mdx mouse skeletal striated muscle and the number of dystrophin-positive fibres. *Neuroscience Letters,* Vol.352, No.1, (Nov 27), pp. 70-2,

Quenneville, S.P.; Chapdelaine, P.; Skuk, D.; Paradis, M.; Goulet, M.; Rousseau, J.; Xiao, X.; Garcia, L. & Tremblay, J.P. (2007). Autologous transplantation of muscle precursor cells modified with a lentivirus for muscular dystrophy: human cells and primate models. *Molecular Therapy,* Vol.15, No.2, (Feb), pp. 431-8,

Radley, H.G.; Davies, M.J. & Grounds,M.D. (2008). Reduced muscle necrosis and long-term benefits in dystrophic mdx mice after cV1q (blockade of TNF) treatment. *Neuromuscular Disorders,* Vol.18, No.3, (Mar), pp. 227-38, ISSN 0960-8966

Rahim, A.A.; Wong, A.M.; Howe, S.J.; Buckley, S.M.; Acosta-Saltos, A.D.; Elston, K.E.; Ward, N.J.; Philpott, N.J.; Cooper, J.D.; Anderson, P.N.; Waddington, S.N.; Thrashe, A.J. & Raivich,G. (2009). Efficient gene delivery to the adult and fetal CNS using pseudotyped non-integrating lentiviral vectors. *Gene Therapy,* Vol.16, No. 4, (Apr), pp. 509-20, ISSN 0969-7128

Rando, T.A. &Blau, H.M. (1994). Primary mouse myoblast purification, characterization, and transplantation for cell-mediated gene therapy. *The Journal of Cell Biology,* Vol.125, No.6, (Jun), pp. 1275-87, ISSN 0021-9525

Reznick, A.Z.; Menashe, O.; Bar-Shai, M.; Coleman, R. & Carmeli, E. (2003). Expression of matrix metalloproteinases, inhibitor, and acid phosphatase in muscles of immobilized hindlimbs of rats. *Muscle Nerve,* Vol.27, No.1, (Jan), pp. 51-9, ISSN 0148-639X

Rodriguez, D.; Morrison, C.J. & Overall, C.M. (2010). Matrix metalloproteinases: what do they not do? New substrates and biological roles identified by murine models and proteomics. *Biochimica Biophysica Acta,* Vol.1803, No.1, (Jan), pp. 39-54, ISSN 0006-3002

Rosenberg, G.A. (2009). Matrix metalloproteinases and their multiple roles in neurodegenerative diseases. *The Lancet Neurology,* Vol.8, No.2, pp. 205-216,

Sacco, A.; Doyonnas, R.; Kraft, P.; Vitorovic, S. & Blau,H.M. (2008). Self-renewal and expansion of single transplanted muscle stem cells. *Nature,* Vol.456, No.7221, (Nov 27), pp. 502-6,

Sacco, A.; Mourkioti, F.; Tran, R.; Choi, J.; Llewellyn, M.; Kraft, P.; Shkreli, M.; Delp, S.; Pomerantz, J.H.; Artandi, S.E. & Blau, H.M. (2010). Short telomeres and stem cell exhaustion model Duchenne muscular dystrophy in mdx/mTR mice. *Cell,* Vol.143, No.7, (Dec 23), pp. 1059-71, ISSN 1097-4172

Sampaolesi, M.; Torrente, Y.; Innocenzi, A.; Tonlorenzi, R.; D'Antona, G.; Pellegrino, M.A.; Barresi, R.; Bresolin, N.; De Angelis, M.G.; Campbell, K.P.; Bottinelli, R. & Cossu, G. (2003). Cell therapy of alpha-sarcoglycan null dystrophic mice through intra-arterial delivery of mesoangioblasts. *Science,* Vol.301, No.5632, (Jul 25), pp. 487-92, ISSN 1095-9203

Sampaolesi, M.; Blot, S.; D'Antona, G.; Granger, N.; Tonlorenzi,R.; Innocenzi, A.; Mognol, P.; Thibaud, J.L.; Galvez ,B.G.; Barthelemy, I.; Perani, L.; Mantero, S.; Guttinger, M.; Pansarasa, O.; Rinaldi, C.; Cusella De Angelis, M.G.; Torrente, Y.; Bordignon, C.; Bottinelli, R. & Cossu, G. (2006). Mesoangioblast stem cells ameliorate muscle function in dystrophic dogs. *Nature,* Vol.444, No.7119, (Nov 30), pp. 574-9,

Sancricca, C.; Mirabella, M.; Gliubizzi, C.; Broccolini, A.; Gidaro, T. & Morosetti, R. (2010). Vessel-associated stem cells from skeletal muscle: From biology to future uses in cell therapy. *World Journal of Stem Cells,* Vol.2, No.3, (Jun 26), pp. 39-49, ISSN 1948-0210

Sciorati, C.; Galvez, B.G.; Brunelli, S.; Tagliafico, E.; Ferrari, S.; Cossu G.& Clementi, E. (2006). Ex vivo treatment with nitric oxide increases mesoangioblast therapeutic efficacy in muscular dystrophy. *Journal of Cell Science,* Vol.119,.Pt 24, (Dec 15), pp. 5114-23,

Seale, P.;. Sabourin, L.A; Girgis-Gabardo, A.; Mansouri, A.; Gruss, P. & Rudnicki, M.A. (2000). Pax7 is required for the specification of myogenic satellite cells. *Cell,* Vol.102, No.6, (Sep 15), pp. 777-86,

Sharma, K. & Ziyadeh,F.N. (1994). The emerging role of transforming growth factor-beta in kidney diseases. *American Journal of Physiology Renal Physiology,* Vol.266, pp. F829–F842.,

Shiomi, T.; Lemaitre, V.; D'Armiento, J. & Okada, Y. (2010). Matrix metalloproteinases, a disintegrin and metalloproteinases, and a disintegrin and metalloproteinases with thrombospondin motifs in non-neoplastic diseases. *Pathology International,* Vol.60, No.7, (Jul), pp. 477-96, ISSN 1440-1827

Silva-Barbosa, S.D.; Butler-Browne, G.S.; Di Santo, J.P. & Mouly, V. (2005). Comparative analysis of genetically engineered immunodeficient mouse strains as recipients for human myoblast transplantation. *Cell Transplantation,* Vol.14, No.7, pp. 457-67,

Skuk, D. & Tremblay, J.P. (2011). Intramuscular cell transplantation as a potential treatment of myopathies: clinical and preclinical relevant data. *Expert Opinion on Biological Therapy,* Vol.11, No.3, (Mar), pp. 359-74, ISSN 1744-7682

Skuk, D.; Roy, B.; Goulet, M. & Tremblay, J.P. (1999). Successful myoblast transplantation in primates depends on appropriate cell delivery and induction of regeneration in the host muscle. *Experimental Neurology,* Vol.155, No.1, (Jan), pp. 22-30, ISSN 0014-4886

Skuk, D.; Caron, N.; Goulet, M.; Roy, B.; Espinosa, F. & Tremblay, J.P. (2002). Dynamics of the early immune cellular reactions after myogenic cell transplantation. *Cell Transplantation,* Vol.11, No.7, pp. 671-81,

Smythe, G.M.; Fan, Y. & Grounds, M.D. (2000). Enhanced migration and fusion of donor myoblasts in dystrophic and normal host muscle. *Muscle Nerve*, Vol.23, No.4, (Apr), pp. 560-74, ISSN 0148-639X

Springer, T.A. (1994). Traffic signals for lymphocyte recirculation and leukocyte emigration: the multistep paradigm. *Cell*, Vol.76, No.2, (Jan 28), pp. 301-14, ISSN 0092-8674

Sternlicht, M.D. & Werb, Z. (2001). How matrix metalloproteinases regulate cell behavior. *Annual Review of Cell and Developmental Biology*, Vol.17, pp. 463-516, ISSN 1081-0706

Stevenson, E.J.; Giresi, P.G.; Koncarevic, A. & Kandarian, S.C. (2003). Global analysis of gene expression patterns during disuse atrophy in rat skeletal muscle. *Journal of Physiology*, Vol.551, Pt 1, (Aug 15), pp. 33-48, ISSN 0022-3751

Sugita, H. & Takeda, S. (2010). Progress in muscular dystrophy research with special emphasis on gene therapy. *Proceedings of the Japan Academy. Series B, Physical and Biological sciences*, Vol.86, No.7, pp. 748-56, ISSN 1349-2896

Sun, G.; Haginoya, K.; Chiba, Y.; Uematsu, M.; Hino-Fukuyo, N.; Tanaka, S.; Onuma, A.; Iinuma, K. & Tsuchiya,S. (2010). Elevated plasma levels of tissue inhibitors of metalloproteinase-1 and their overexpression in muscle in human and mouse muscular dystrophy. *Journal of the Neurological Sciences*, Vol.297, No.1-2, pp. 19-28,

Sun, G.; Haginoya, K.; Wu, Y.; Chiba, Y.; Nakanishi, T.; Onuma, A.; Sato, Y.; Takigawa, M.; Iinuma, K. & Tsuchiya, S. (2008). Connective tissue growth factor is overexpressed in muscles of human muscular dystrophy. *Journal of Neurological Sciences*, Vol.267, No.1, (04/15), pp. 48-56,

Tedesco, F.S.; Dellavalle, A.; Diaz-Manera, J.; Messina G. & Cossu, G. (2010). Repairing skeletal muscle: regenerative potential of skeletal muscle stem cells. *The Journal of Clinical Investigation*, Vol.120, No.1, (Jan 4), pp. 11-9, ISSN 1558-8238

Torrente, Y.; El Fahime, E.; Caron, N.J.; Del Bo, R.; Belicchi, M.; Pisati, F.; Tremblay, J.P. & Bresolin, N. (2003). Tumor necrosis factor-alpha (TNF-alpha) stimulates chemotactic response in mouse myogenic cells. *Cell Transplantation*, Vol.12, No.1, pp. 91-100, ISSN 0963-6897

Torrente, Y.; Belicchi, M.; Sampaolesi, M.; Pisati, F.; Meregalli, M.; D'Antona, G.; Tonlorenzi, R.; Porretti, L.; Gavina, M.; Mamchaoui, K.; Pellegrino, M.A.; Furling, D.; Mouly, V.; Butler-Browne, G.S.; Bottinelli, R.; Cossu, G. & Bresolin, N. (2004). Human circulating AC133(+) stem cells restore dystrophin expression and ameliorate function in dystrophic skeletal muscle. *The Journal of Clinical Investigation*, Vol.114, No.2, (Jul), pp. 182-95,

Urso, M.L.; Szelenyi, E.R.; Warren, G. L. & Barnes, B. R. (2010). Matrix metalloprotease-3 and tissue inhibitor of metalloprotease-1 mRNA and protein levels are altered in response to traumatic skeletal muscle injury. *European Journal Applied Physiology*,Vol.109, No.5, pp. 963-72,

Vauchez, K.; Marolleau, J.P.; Schmid, M.; Khattar, P.; Chapel, A.; Catelain, C.; Lecourt, S.; Larghero, J.; Fiszman, M. & Vilquin, J.T. (2009). Aldehyde dehydrogenase activity identifies a population of human skeletal muscle cells with high myogenic capacities. *Molecular Therapy*, Vol.17, No.11, (Nov), pp. 1948-58, ISSN 1525-0024

Von Moers, A.; Zwirner, A.; Reinhold, A.; Bruckmann, O.; van Landeghem, F.; Stoltenburg-Didinger, G.; Schuppan, D.; Herbst, H. & Schuelke, M.. (2005). Increased mRNA expression of tissue inhibitors of metalloproteinase-1 and -2 in Duchenne muscular dystrophy. *Acta Neuropathologica*, Vol.109, No.3, (Mar), pp. 285-93, ISSN 0001-6322

Vu, T.H. & Werb, Z. (2000). Matrix metalloproteinases: effectors of development and normal physiology. *Genes & Development,* Vol.14, No.17, (Sep 1), pp. 2123-33, ISSN 0890-9369

Wakeford, S.; Watt, D.J. & Partridge, T.A. (1991). X-irradiation improves mdx mouse muscle as a model of myofiber loss in DMD. *Muscle Nerve,* Vol.14, No.1, (Jan), pp. 42-50,

Wang, W.; Pan, H.; Murray, K.; Jefferson, B.S. & Li, Y. (2009). Matrix metalloproteinase-1 promotes muscle cell migration and differentiation. *American Journal of Pathology,* Vol.174, No.2, (Feb), pp. 541-9, ISSN 1525-2191

Webster, C. & Blau, H.M. (1990). Accelerated age-related decline in replicative life-span of Duchenne muscular dystrophy myoblasts: implications for cell and gene therapy. *Somatic Cell Molecular Genetics,* Vol.16, No.6, (Nov), pp. 557-65, ISSN 0740-7750

Wells, D.J.; Ferrer, A. & Wells, K.E. (2002). Immunological hurdles in the path to gene therapy for Duchenne muscular dystrophy. *Expert Review Molecular Medicine,*Vol.4, No.23, (Nov), pp. 1-23, ISSN 1462-3994

Wilson, C.A. & Cichutek, K. (2009). The US and EU regulatory perspectives on the clinical use of hematopoietic stem/progenitor cells genetically modified ex vivo by retroviral vectors. *Methods in Molecular Biology,*Vol.506, pp. 477-88,

Wittwer, M.; Flück, M.; Hoppeler, H.; Müller, S.; Desplanches D. & Billeter, R. (2002). Prolonged unloading of rat soleus muscle causes distinct adaptations of the gene profile. *The FASEB Journal,* Vol.16, pp. 884-886,

Yokota, T.; Lu, Q.L.; Morgan, J.E.; Davies, K.E.; Fisher, R.; Takeda, S. & Partridge, T.A. (2006). Expansion of revertant fibers in dystrophic mdx muscles reflects activity of muscle precursor cells and serves as an index of muscle regeneration. *Journal of Cell Science,* Vol.119, Pt 13, (Jul 1), pp. 2679-87,

Zanotti, S.; Gibertini, S.; & Mora. M. (2010). Altered production of extra-cellular matrix components by muscle-derived Duchenne muscular dystrophy fibroblasts before and after TGF-β1 treatment. *Cell and Tissue Research,* Vol.339, No.2, pp. 397-410,

Zanotti, S.; Saredi, S.; Ruggieri, A.; Fabbri, M.; Blasevich, F.; Romaggi, S.; Morandi, L. & Mora, M. (2007). Altered extracellular matrix transcript expression and protein modulation in primary Duchenne muscular dystrophy myotubes. *Matrix Biology,* Vol.26, No.8, (Oct), pp. 615-24, ISSN 0945-053X

Zhang, F.; Thornhill, S.I.; Howe, S.J.; Ulaganathan, M.; Schambach, A.; Sinclair, J.; Kinnon, C.; Gaspar, H.B.; Antoniou, M. & Thrasher, A.J. (2007). Lentiviral vectors containing an enhancer-less ubiquitously acting chromatin opening element (UCOE) provide highly reproducible and stable transgene expression in hematopoietic cells. *Blood,* Vol.110, No.5, (Sep 1), pp. 1448-57,

Zheng, B.; Cao, B.; Crisan, M.; Sun, B.; Li, G.; Logar, A.; Yap, S.; Pollett, J.B.; Drowley, L.; Cassino, T.; Gharaibeh, B.; Deasy, B.M.; Huard, J. & Peault, B. (2007). Prospective identification of myogenic endothelial cells in human skeletal muscle. *Nature Biotechnology,* Vol.25, No.9, (Sep), pp. 1025-34,

Zhou, L.; Porter, J.D.; Cheng, G.; Gong, B.; Hatala, D.A.; Merriam, A.P.; Zhou, X.; Rafael, J.A. & Kaminski, H.J. (2006). Temporal and spatial mRNA expression patterns of TGF-[beta]1, 2, 3 and T[beta]RI, II, III in skeletal muscles of mdx mice. *Neuromuscular Disorders,* Vol.16, No.1, (Jan), pp. 32-38,

22

Genetic Therapy for Duchenne Muscular Dystrophy: Principles and Progress

Taeyoung Koo, Linda Popplewell,
Alberto Malerba and George Dickson
The Biomedical Sciences, Royal Holloway, University of London, Egham, Surrey, UK

1. Introduction

This chapter focuses on the gene therapy advances made in relation to Duchenne muscular dystrophy and discusses principles and perspectives of strategies currently being developed. The chapter explains the genetic mutations that cause Duchenne muscular dystrophy (DMD) and Becker muscular dystrophy (BMD) and the differences between the two are discussed in relation to disease severity. The histopathological features of DMD are explained and discussed in the context of available animal models for DMD. There are various genetic therapeutic options available for the treatment of DMD, and the progress of each therapeutic approach is promising. A number of specific areas for the treatment of DMD are comprehensively presented, alongside in-depth description of the genetic biology of muscular dystrophy.

2. Muscular dystrophies

Muscle-related proteins build the structural network of muscle, and disruption of this link can cause muscle wasting and progression of numerous types of muscular dystrophy. Muscular dystrophies are a heterogeneous group of genetic disorders caused by different forms of mutations in various genes related to muscles.

2.1 Duchenne and Becker muscular dystrophy

The most common forms of muscular dystrophy are Duchenne and Becker muscular dystrophy (DMD, BMD). DMD and BMD are X-linked recessive muscle-wasting disorders affecting the skeletal musculature, resulting from mutations in the gene encoding dystrophin, which is a cytoskeletal protein in muscle fibres. Dystrophin protein interacts with the intracellular and extracellular dystrophin associated protein (DAP) complexes. Mutations in dystrophin gene can cause severe muscular wasting.

Different mutation types in exon/ intron regions of dystrophin gene or promoters causes various forms of dystrophinopathies (Giliberto et al., 2004). Dystrophin deficiency leads to disruption of the dystrophin associated protein (DAP) complexes, as do mutations in DAP genes in other forms of congenital and autosomal muscular dystrophy.

DMD affects 1:3500 newborn males worldwide, and patients exhibit severe, progressive muscle weakening. From about the age of 4 years, youngsters affected by DMD suffer bouts of recurrent damage and regeneration of skeletal muscle, leading eventually to muscle wasting and weakness, wheelchair-dependence, and life-threatening cardiac and respiratory complications. This debilitating disease is associated with loss of dystrophin expression caused generally by frameshift gene deletions and duplications, or by nonsense point mutations in the dystrophin gene.

In BMD, muscle pathology is generally milder than in DMD, and can even be virtually asymptomatic. The milder BMD phenotype is caused by the continued expression of truncated but partially functional dystrophin proteins in the affected muscles. This phenotype commonly arises due to mutational events which delete central rod domain elements, but nevertheless maintain the open reading frame upstream and downstream of the mutation boundaries. Thus different mutation types across exon/intron regions of the dystrophin gene can give rise to either DMD or BMD, depending upon the deletion boundaries.

BMD can be related to large in-frame deletions, including examples where up to 46% of the dystrophin-coding sequence has been deleted (Acsadi et al., 1991). Despite the large gene deletion, BMD patients have a mild phenotype due to partial expression of an internally-deleted but highly functional dystrophin protein. Clinical phenotype of BMD pathology is discriminated by mild, intermediate and severe types resulting from different exon deletions (Chao et al., 1996). Around 20% of normal dystrophin expression is seen as the milder BMD phenotype (Beggs et al., 1991).

2.1.1 Histopathological features of DMD

Clinical symptoms of DMD become apparent in patients of three to five years of age, while fetal DMD muscle is histologically normal (Biggar, 2006). The lack of dystrophin causes DAP dissociation, followed by disruption of the transmembrane link between extracellular matrix and the cytoskeleton. This causes severe muscle damage along with progressive fibrosis and muscle fibre loss. Lack of dystrophin in DMD muscles is believed to compromise the integrity of the sarcolemma, leading to calcium influx and myofibre necrosis. Central nucleation and uneven size of fibres are observed in early stages of dystrophinopathies due to the muscle necrosis followed by muscle degeneration and regeneration (Bell et al., 1968, Bradley et al., 1972). In dystrophin-negative muscles, fibres are lost (necrosed) and degeneration of the fibres proceeds, and they are eventually replaced by adipose and fibrous connective tissue, followed by atrophy (**Figure** 1) (Blake et al., 2002).

In addition, an increased number of proteasomes is found in necrotic and regenerative muscles in DMD, leading to muscle fibre degradation (Kumamoto et al., 2000). Muscle membrane becomes abnormally permeable, leading to fragility and leakiness of the muscle cells. The muscle weakness results in loss of independent ambulation, usually by the age of 12 (Emery, 2001). DMD patients eventually die from intercostal muscle weakness and respiratory failure in their early twenties (Emery, 2001). DMD patients also develop cardiac dysfunction with cardiomyopathy, resulting in heart failure and progressive dilated cardiomyopathy (Emery, 2001).

There is also evidence that dystrophin deficiency is associated with aberrant signal transduction from influx of divalent cations such as calcium due to abnormal membrane permeability in DMD muscle cells (Ruegg et al., 2002). Abnormality of calcium homeostasis is found due to structural defects in the ryanodine receptor (RyR) 1, calcium release channel in the sarcoplasmic reticulum, leading to increase of intracellular Ca^{2+} in the dystrophic muscles (Bellinger et al., 2009). Increased intracellular Ca^{2+} can activate calpain, which has a role in proteolysis and increases reactive oxygen species (ROS). Calpain cleaves intracellular proteins including titin, nebulin, desmin, troponin, tropomyosin and many kinases and signalling molecules and it increases protein breakdown (Allen et al., 2005). This can cause protein and membrane damage (Whitehead et al., 2006).

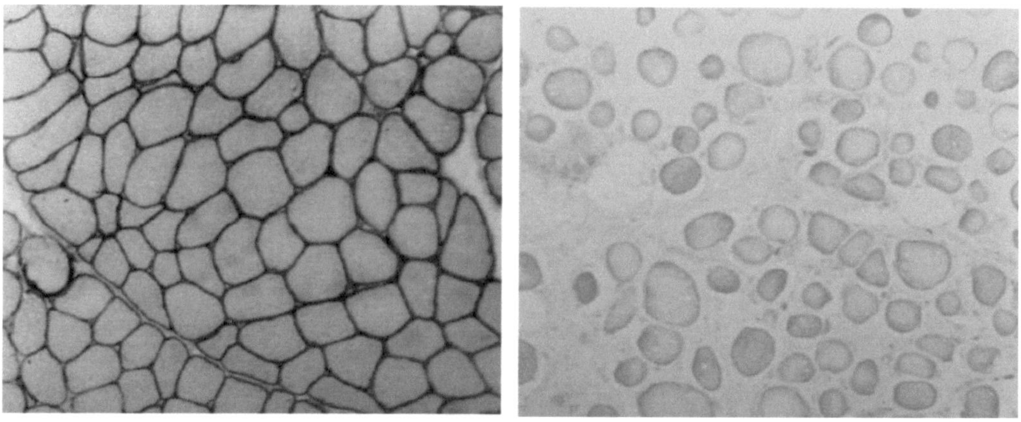

Normal muscle shows even size/diameter distribution of muscle fibres with dystrophin expression localised at the sarcolemma membrane. Lack of dystrophin protein expression in DMD causes muscle damage, which is accelerated by eccentric contraction of the muscle membrane. Eventually, muscle fibres are lost (necrosed) and replaced by adipose and fibrous connective tissue.

Fig. 1. Dystrophin immunohistochemistry in normal (left panel) and DMD muscle (right panel).

Damaged muscle membranes are demonstrated by staining with extracellulary applied labelled endogenous extracellular proteins such as albumin, immunoglobulin (Ig) G and IgM (Blake et al., 2002). The already permeable membrane in DMD becomes more permeable after mechanical stress or electric stimulation. Cardiomyopathies occur as a result of cardiac muscle damage in DMD. Myocardium is replaced by fat and connective tissue in dystrophinopathies. Clinical symptoms of cardiomyopathies appear after 10 years of age in DMD, and are present in all patients over 18 years (Finsterer et al, 2003). It has been currently reported that 20% of BMD and 50% of DMD patients eventually die due to cardiac failure (Finsterer et al., 2003). In the early stages of DMD, focal myofibre necrosis initially leads to muscle stem cell activity and tissue regeneration, via activation of so-called satellite cells. As the disease progresses, however, the capacity to regenerate muscle becomes impaired owing to depletion of stem cells and fibrosis of tissues, leading finally to severe muscle wasting. This leads to inflammation of DMD muscles, as a result of inflammatory cells such as CD4 and CD8, followed by muscle necrosis (Blake et al., 2002).

Creatine kinase (CK) level is one of the indicators for DMD pathology. CK level in DMD in affected boys is elevated at birth, to 50 to 100 times the novel level, and gradually declines in the late stages of the disease (Emery, 2001).

2.1.2 Animal models of DMD

The development of a treatment for any disease relies on the use of appropriate animal models to test the efficacy, deliverability, dosing regimen and toxicology *in vivo* having established the therapeutic potential *in vitro*.

2.1.2.1 Dystrophin deficient *mdx* model

The *mdx* mouse originates from the C57BL/10 colony and does not express the dystrophin protein due to a nonsense mutation (CAA to TAA) in exon 23 of the dystrophin gene (Sicinski et al., 1989). It shows similar pathological symptoms to human DMD patients. However the pathology of *mdx* mice is less severe compared to the human disease, because of effective regeneration of damaged muscles, which has not been observed in human DMD patients (Turk et al., 2005). In *mdx* mice, the event of degeneration/regeneration is ongoing throughout the life of the animal but peaks between the ages of 3-8 weeks (Tanabe et al., 1986). It has been demonstrated that the *mdx* mouse has a reduced life span and progressive dystrophic muscle histopathology compared to the wild-type C57BL/10 mouse (Chamberlain et al., 2007). Moreover, aged *mdx* mice are susceptible to muscle tumours, similar to human alveolar rhabdomyosarcoma (Chamberlain et al., 2007). Inflammatory cells such as CD4 and CD8 are found in dystrophin-deficient muscles followed by muscle necrosis, peaking at 4-8 weeks old of *mdx* mice (Blake et al., 2002). In dystrophic *mdx* mice, elevated CK level was also found in the serum (Bulfield et al., 1984).

2.1.2.2 Canine muscular dystrophy model

The golden retriever muscular dystrophy (*GRMD*) dog was the first characterized canine model of DMD (Cooper et al., 1988, Kornegay et al., 1988, Valentine et al., 1992). It has been reported that *GRMD* dogs eventually die due to cardiomyopathy. *GRMD* has been identified as complete dystrophin deficiency with higher genotypic/phenotypic similarity to human DMD disease than that of the *mdx* mouse model. Complete loss of dystrophin is the result of a nonsense mutation in the 3′ consensus splice site of intron 6, leading to skipping of exon 7 and alteration of the reading frame in exon 8, thereby inducing clinical symptoms similar to human DMD (Chamberlain et al., 2007). The Beagle-based *CXMD* canine model was also identified as a DMD model in Japan (Shimatsu et al., 2003). It has been reported that limb muscle abnormality appear after 2 months of age and the dogs eventually die mainly due to cardiomyopathy (Valentine et al., 1988). *CXMD* dog models show longer life span due to slower progression of muscle wasting compared to *GRMD* dogs (Willmann et al., 2009). Progress of cardiomyopathy in the *CXMD* dog is also milder than in *GRMD* (Yugeta et al., 2006).

2.1.2.3 Hypertrophic Feline muscular dystrophy model

Hypertrophic feline muscular dystrophy (*HFMD*) is exhibited in cats (Blake et al., 2002). The creatine kinase (CK) level is increased at the age of 4-5 weeks and development of severe muscle hypertrophy is shown resulting in muscle necrosis and regeneration. However, it is not considered to be a good model for human DMD since it does not induce muscle fibrosis and muscle wasting (Gaschen et al., 1992).

2.2 Other muscular dystrophies

2.2.1 Muscular disorders caused by mutations in membrane proteins

Mutations in integrin have been shown to cause congenital muscular dystrophies. Integrin, membrane protein, binds to laminin. Caveloin-3, which is localised to muscle cell membrane interacts with β-dystroglycan and mutations in Caveloin-3 cause the autosomal dominant form of Limb Girdle muscular dystrophy 1C (LGMD1C), rippling muscle disease and hyper CKemia (Betz et al., 2001, Carbone et al., 2000).

2.2.2 Muscular disorders caused by mutations in extracellular matrix proteins

Mutations in laminin α-2, one of the extracellular matrix proteins, can give rise to congenital muscular dystrophy 1A (MDC1A) (Helbling-Leclerc et al., 1995). α and β form of dystroglycan can interact with laminin and dystrophin, respectively. Mutations in α-dystroglycan have been reported in the muscle-eye-brain disease, Walker-Warburg syndrome (WWS) and a type of congenital MD (Longman et al., 2003). In mice, mutations in the dystroglycan gene can be embryonically lethal (Williamson et al., 1997). Disruption to the transmembrane related sarcoglycan-sarcospan complex leads to various types of LGMD. Sarcoglycan interacts with biglycan, which also binds to α-dystroglycan and as well as to collagen VI. Mutation in collagen VI gives rise to Ullrich syndrome and Bethlem myopathy (Camacho Vanegas et al., 2001).

2.2.3 Muscular disorders caused by mutations in intracellular proteins

Mutation in calpain 3, which is a calcium-dependent protease, gives rise to LGMD 2A. Mutations in several sarcomeric proteins lead to LGMD 2. Heterogeneous chromosomal mutations result in LGMD. There are two types of LGMD called type 1 and type 2, which have autosomal dominant or autosomal recessive mutations, respectively. The symptoms are not as severe as DMD or BMD, but weakness of proximal limb and trunk muscles is exhibited (Lovering et al., 2005). Mutations in syntrophin and dystrobrevin display mild forms of skeletal and cardiac muscle disease.

2.2.4 Muscular disorders caused by mutations in nuclear proteins

Laminopathies are caused by mutations in the LMNA gene, which encodes the inner nuclear envelope proteins lamin A and C, which interact with several proteins in the nucleus and inner nuclear membrane (Worman et al., 2000). Emery-Dreifuss muscular dystrophy (EDMD) has been identified due to a mutation in LMNA gene encoding A-type lamin, or in emerin gene encoding nuclear protein (Bione et al., 1994). Clinical symptoms are related to humero-peroneal weakness and dilated cardiomyopathy with conduction defects (Emery, 2000). Mutations in LMNA gene cause cardiomyocyte nuclear envelope abnormalities, leading to dilated cardiomyopathy in human patients (Gupta et al., 2010) and LGMD 1B (Muchir et al., 2000).

3. Pre-clinical & clinical approaches for DMD

Several pre-clinical research regimes have displayed that DMD pathology can be improved by functional expression of mini-or micro-dystrophin gene variants (Deconinck et al., 1996).

3.1 Recombinant adeno-associated virus vector (rAAV) mediated gene therapy

Gene therapy for DMD aims to compensate for dystrophin loss-of-function by different gene transfer approaches. To prevent muscle degeneration, around 30% of normal levels of dystrophin protein is likely to be required (Neri et al., 2007). Transfer of recombinant genes encoding full-length (~11 kb), mini- (>5 kb) or micro- (<5 kb) dystrophin recombinant gene into DMD-affected muscle is one of the proposed therapies to induce dystrophin protein expression. A Phase I clinical trial has been completed in which a eukaryotic expression plasmid encoding full length human dystrophin was injected directly into the muscles of DMD patients (Fardeau et al., 2005).

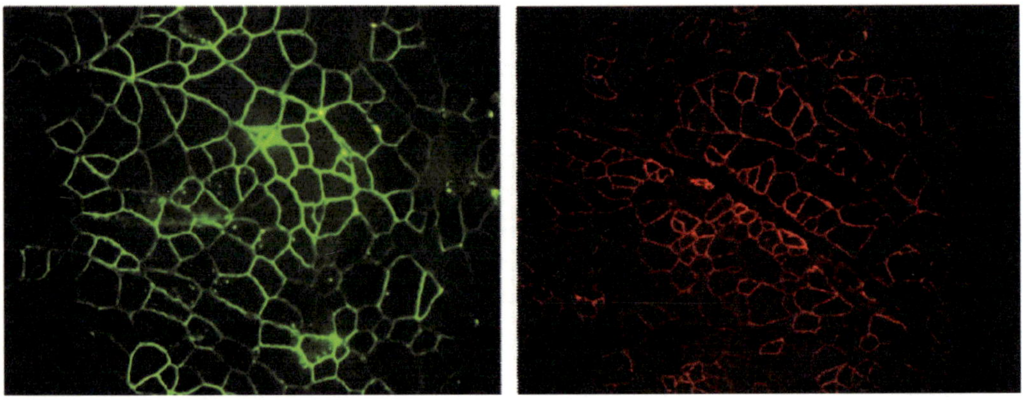

The mdx mice treated with AAV-mediated microdystrophin gene transfer (left-hand panel), or PMO antisense-induced skipping of the mutant exon 23 (right-hand panel) showed dystrophin expression at the sarcolemma in the TA muscle of mdx mouse.

Fig. 2. Dystrophin immunofluorescence staining of muscle.

Dystrophin expression at low levels was shown in all patients without any safety concerns and notably without a detectable immune response to dystrophin. A Phase I/II study is currently in preparation to evaluate this non-viral plasmid-mediated gene therapy using vascular systemic routes of administration to target multiple muscle groups. However, even with the aid of more sophisticated delivery strategies such as electrotransfer or even with enhanced vector configurations such as minicircles and episomes, effective plasmid gene therapy for DMD still has major hurdles to overcome to reach the gene-transfer efficiencies required for effectiveness. Therefore a range of replication-defective viral vectors have been evaluated as attractive delivery systems to mediated dystrophin gene transfer and DMD gene therapy.

In particular, gene transfer into the nuclei of muscle fibres using vectors based on adeno-associated virus (AAV) is one of the most promising delivery approaches for the therapy of muscle disease. AAV is a single-stranded non-pathogenic virus, and derived vectors of various serotypes can efficiently transduce, not only by local muscle injection, but also, notably, by vascular systemic delivery to widespread muscle groups and the heart. The tropism of various AAV vector serotypes for differentiated post-mitotic muscle tissues can be very high, reaching >90%.

However, there is a hurdle to AAV-mediated DMD gene therapy, since the full dystrophin coding sequence spans 14 kb mRNA with an open reading frame of >11 kb, and the packaging capacity of AAV virus vectors is generally thought to be <5 kb. Thus, on the basis of an understanding of the genotype-phenotype correlates in DMD and BMD, and based on structural knowledge of the dystrophin protein, recombinant dystrophin cDNAs have been engineered to produce, partially deleted, but highly functional microdystrophin products in both *mdx* mouse and *CXMD* dog models (Athanasopoulos et al., 2004, Foster et al., 2008, Koo et al., 2011). These genes can be packaged successfully inside AAV vector particles and can be delivered at high efficiency to skeletal muscles to rescue the dystrophin-deficient phenotype in animal models of DMD (**Figure** 2, left hand panel).

The life cycle of AAV vectors results in delayed expression, and it takes several weeks for full transcriptional activity to be established (Ferrari et al., 1996). Recently, self-complementary AAV (scAAV) vectors have been developed for fast expression by bypassing rate-limiting, second-strand DNA synthesis (McCarty 2008). However, scAAV can only retain smaller transgene cassettes compared to single stranded AAV (ssAAV). Moreover, high titres of rAAV are required for systemic delivery (Gregorevic et al., 2004).

AAV-mediated gene therapy has attractive characteristics and some advantages over other vector systems for several reasons. AAV vector particles are very stable and resistant to significant variation in pH and temperature. AAV vectors have an ability of long-term transgene expression without significant immune response. Therefore, it is a promising delivery vehicle for the transfer of therapeutic genes for the treatment of inherited diseases. Recombinant AAV-mediated gene therapy has been approved for use in over 40 clinical trials for various genetic diseases (Mueller at al., 2008). In order to generate recombinant AAV vector for the transfer of therapeutic genes, the genes for the capsid proteins and replication proteins are replaced with the gene of interest and packaged by ITRs. A Phase I clinical trial involving local intramuscular injection of AAV vectors to transfer a microdystrophin variant in DMD patients has been conducted by the groups of Mendel, Xiao and Samulski, in collaboration with Asklepios Biopharmaceuticals. However, microdystrophin expression was only detected in two of six patients treated at very low levels and two patients exhibited pre-existing dystrophin specific T cells (Mendell et al., 2010). Further work to enhance the expression and functionality of microdystrophins is still required due to reported failure of certain microdystrophin variants to protect muscle integrity in larger animal models (Sampaolesi et al., 2006).

3.2 Adenovirus-mediated gene therapy

Adenovirus is another vehicle which can be used to transfer dystrophin genes towards DMD mediated gene delivery applications. Due to the large gene capacity of the adenoviruses, large cDNA cassettes, up to 7 kb for E1/E3 deleted Ad vectors, can be transferred into the muscles. However, adenovirus is highly immunogenic and this may cause loss of transgene expression through immune responses. Moreover, the packaging capacity is still too small for the transfer of full length dystrophin (approximately 11 kb cDNA). To increase the packaging capacity of the viruses, helper dependent adenovirus vectors have been developed (Fisher et al., 1996). These vectors contain only ITR and capsid genes and so increase the packaging genome capacity of adenoviruses up to 36 kb; they are also less immunogenic compared to E1 gene-deleted adenovirus due to the lack of viral genes. Adenovirus-mediated full length dystrophin cDNAs have been successfully transferred to *mdx* mice leading to muscle improvement (Dudley et al., 2004). Cell transplantation of genetically corrected mesenchymal cells (MSCs) by adenovirus carrying microdystrophin gene was attempted and showed successful dystrophin expression in MSCs in *mdx* mice (Xiong et al., 2007).

3.3 Modulation of exon-splicing patterns with antisense oligonucleotides

About 70% of DMD and BMD cases are caused by genomic deletions, leading to the loss of one or more exons (Aartsma-Rus et al., 2006). Frameshift deletions, which juxtapose out-of-phase exons in the dystrophin gene, cause complete loss of expression of dystrophin and a DMD phenotype, whereas juxtaposition of in-phase exons leads to the milder BMD. Inhibition of the splicing of specific exons, by so called exon skipping, using antisense oligonucleotides (AONs) can induce exclusion of targeted exons and skipping of frame-shift exons, leading to restoration of disrupted reading frames and expression of BMD-type dystrophin molecules (**Figure** 2, right hand panel). AONs are designed to hybridize to consensus exon recognition or exonic splicing enhancer (ESE) sequences on dystrophin pre-mRNA, and antisense-induced exon skipping is thought to occur by interfering with binding of serine/arginine-rich (SR) proteins which play crucial roles in recruiting the splicing machinery (**Figure** 3).

AON-induced exon skipping to restore functional but truncated dystrophin protein expression has previously been demonstrated in animal models of DMD both *in vitro* (Graham et al., 2004) and *in vivo* (Yokota et al., 2009), and in DMD patient cells *in vitro* in culture (van Deutekom et al., 2001), and in DMD muscle explants (Arechavala-Gomeza et al., 2007). On the basis of these pre-clinical studies, a number of patient trials, phase I and more recently phase 2, have been undertaken. In the first of these, four DMD patients carrying appropriate deletions received a single intramuscular injection of a high dose of an AON with a 2'O-methylphosphorothioate backbone (PRO051), which targets exon 51. Each patient showed specific exon 51 skipping, myofibre expression of dystrophin protein, which was detectable at 3 to 12% of normal levels four weeks after injection. No clinically adverse events were detected (van Deutekom et al., 2007). In the second trial, the AON AVI-4658, which has a phosphorodiamidate morpholino (PMO) backbone and targets a slightly different intraexonic sequence (+68+95) of exon 51, has been injected intramuscularly in a dose-escalating trial into nine DMD boys. At the higher doses, this PMO AON produced good levels of local dystrophin protein production in treated muscles; the intensity of dystrophin staining was up to 42% of that seen in healthy muscle. The treatment had no adverse effects (Kinali et al., 2009). The clinical evaluation has been extended to 12 week systemic delivery of both exon 51 AONs and results have very recently been reported. Both chemistries showed no adverse effects and dose-dependent restoration of dystrophin production was clearly seen; functionality of this expressed dystrophin protein was established by the detection of other dystrophin-associated proteins at the sarcolemma (for AVI-4658), and by a modest but not statistically significant improvement in the patient six minute walk test after 12 weeks of extended treatment (for PRO051) (Goemans et al., 2011). On the basis of results seen in the mdx model using various dosing regimen over extended periods (Malerba et al., 2011), further clinical studies are required.

PMOs and 2'OMe AONs both have excellent safety profiles (van Deutekom et al., 2007), but PMOs have certain advantages over 2'OMe AONs. They give more sustained, consistent exon skipping in the animal mdx model in vivo (Heemskerk et al., 2009), and in human muscle explants (Arechavala-Gomeza et al., 2007). PMOs can be conjugated to cell-penetrating peptides (PPMO) that improve their deliverability and hence efficacy dramatically (Moulton et al., 2007, Yin et al., 2010).

The drug company AVI BioPharma has performed preclinical studies with AVI-5038 in collaboration with the charity Charley's fund. AVI-5038 is a PPMO targeted to skip exon 50 of the dystrophin gene. Repeated weekly intravenous bolus injection over four weeks at a low dose of this conjugated PMO was shown to be well-tolerated; however higher doses administered weekly for 12 weeks showed significant toxicological effects, particularly in relation to the kidney. As yet this problem has not been resolved, and an unconjugated version of the same PMO (AVI-4038) is being developed for clinical trial. There are a number of alternative peptide conjugates that show promise as enhancers of deliverability and are undergoing rapid pre-clinical development (Yin et al., 2010). The next planned UK phase I trial by the MDEX consortium will involve conjugation of a PPMO developed for the targeted skipping of exon 53 (Popplewell et al., 2010) and is supported by a Wellcome Trust. The Dutch are currently performing a phase I trial using a 2'OMe PS AON for the targeted skipping of exon 45. However, it should be noted that only 8%, 4%, 13% or 18% of DMD patient mutations should be convertible into a BMD phenotype by a single AON exon 45, 50, 51 or 53 skipping, respectively. Personalized molecular medicine for each skippable DMD deletion is necessary and this would require the optimization and clinical trial workup of many specific AONs. It has been suggested that multi-exon skipping, using cocktails of AONs or chemically linked AONs, around deletion hotspots (eg exons 45-55) may have the potential to treat approximately 65% of DMD patients (Adams et al., 2007). Such a strategy has been shown to work in mdx mice, but this has not yet been achieved in DMD patient cells.

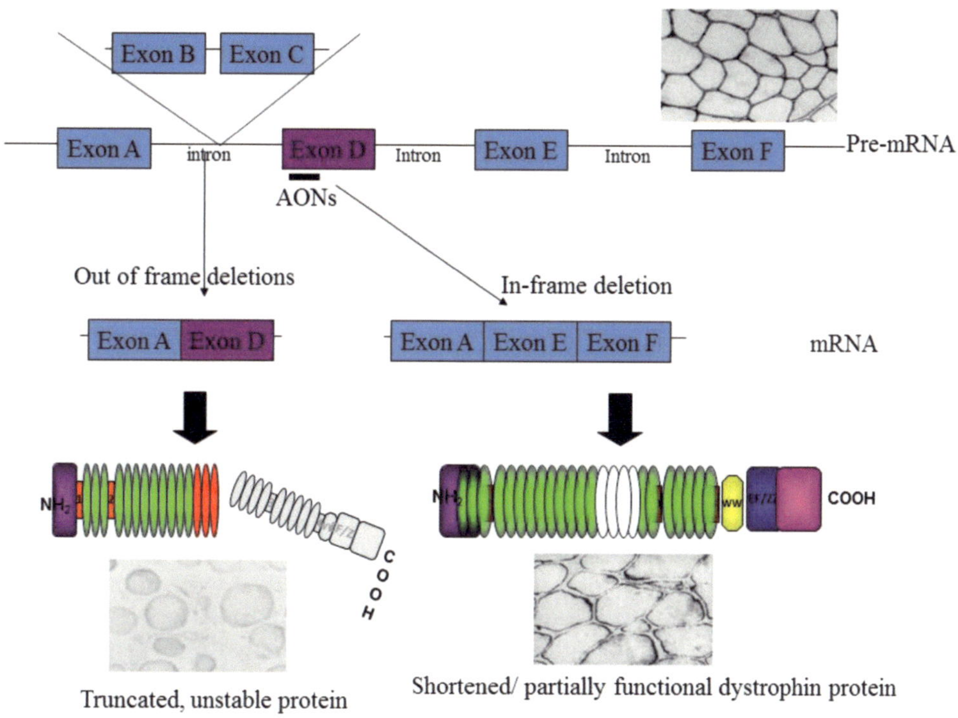

Fig. 3. AONs mediated exon skipping for Duchenne muscular dystrophy.

This gene therapy restores the open reading frame of the disrupted reading frame to allow synthesis of shortened dystrophin. The in-frame transcript contains both the N- and C-terminal domains of dystrophin and is partially functional since these domains have important signalling functions between the extracellular matrix and cytoskeleton. The in-frame transcript of dystrophin produced by AONs exon skipping ameliorates the severe muscle damage seen in *mdx* mice.

There are further obstacles to be overcome for AON-induced exon skipping to be a viable gene therapy for DMD. The cost implications may end up being prohibitive for many patients; since AONs are rapidly cleared from the circulation, regular administrations of high doses of AON would be required for therapeutic effect. Secondly, although deliverability, particularly to the heart, is enhanced with the use of conjugated PMOs, their potential toxicological and immunogenic problems need to be addressed. Lastly, the need for personalized medicine will require the completion of many expensive, lengthy clinical trials of many AONs.

3.4 Cell transplantation therapy

Cell-based gene therapy is another promising approach to treat DMD. Transplantation of genetically modified adult muscle stem cells or healthy wild-type donor cells has great potential to regenerate skeletal muscle cell tissues. For stem cell therapy, adult muscle stem cells, including mesoangioblasts, MDSCs (muscle derived stem cells), adult progenitor cells, AC133+ cells, bone marrow-derived stem cells and side population (SP) cells can be isolated from either muscle biopsies or blood (Farini et al., 2009). Isolated stem cells can be transduced *in vitro* by retroviral or lentiviral vectors to permanently introduce the micro- or mini-dystrophin gene. Retrovirus or lentiviral genome can integrate into the infected cell genome subsequent to cell divisions. Therefore this is a promising vehicle for the correction of muscle satellite stem cells. These genetically modified cells or healthy wild-type donor cells are expanded *ex vivo* and subsequently injected systemically to traffic and target to muscles. If taken from the patient themselves, transplantation of autologous gene-modified stem cells has the advantage to potentially avoid adverse immune responses and cell rejection.

Intramuscular myoblast transplantation in DMD yields dystrophin-positive myofibres at levels of 20-30% up to 18 months after transplantation (Skuk et al., 2007). However, intramuscular myoblasts transfer faces potential limitations in terms of cell migration, lack of systemic whole-body delivery and poor cell survival. There are currently two approaches using a cell transfer platform for systemic delivery of regenerative cell transplants to skeletal musculature, namely the mesoangioblast and the CD133+ stem cell systems. Following lentiviral vector-mediated gene transfer, dystrophin-expressing fibres have been shown in dystrophic dogs after transplantation of genetically modified mesoangioblasts which are vessel-associated progenitor cells. In this study, transplantation efficiency seemed higher in recipients treated with wild-type donor mesoangioblasts compared with autologous gene–modified mesoangioblasts (Sampaolesi et al., 2006), but uncontrolled effects of immune suppression regimes may complicate the interpretation. Even so, a clinical trial of mesoangioblast cells therapy for DMD using tissue –matched wild-type donor cells has been tried (Cossu et al., 2007). CD133+ stem cell therapy is another promising approach introduced recently, making systemic delivery and correction possible. CD133+ cells can be isolated from peripheral blood or skeletal muscle tissue, and differentiated into muscle, hematopoietic and endothelial cell lineages (Peault et al., 2007). A Phase I clinical trial of autologous transplantation of CD133+ stem cells in DMD boys has shown increased potential to contribute to muscle repair without adverse effects (Torrente et al., 2007). However, interaction between satellite cells and stem cells still remains largely unknown to date. Detailed understanding of the biological mechanism of interaction and structure/function relationship between muscle and the multiple components of these therapies can aid the search for an effective cure for DMD and other muscle diseases in the immediate future.

3.5 Muscle augmentation

Neuromuscular disorders, sarcopenia, cancer, AIDS and general insufficient energy intake can decrease the muscle mass with consequent irreversible loss of body weight (Matsakas et al., 2009). Several genetic based strategies have been tried to manipulate expression of specific molecules involved in muscle growth to counteract this muscle loss. One of the most promising approaches is based on the inactivation of the biological activity of myostatin or its receptor, Activin type 2b (ActRIIb). This strategy has a therapeutic potential to treat DMD by inhibiting the severe muscle loss.

3.5.1 Inactivation of Myostatin

Myostatin (named also GDF-8) is a member of transforming growth factor β superfamily of growth factors. Myostatin is initially synthesized as inactive pre-propeptide and it is cleaved to produce a smaller peptide (Thies et al., 2001, Hill et al., 2002) that is biologically active only after further post-translational processing including the formation of a homodimeric protein. Some animals carrying different types of mutations that inactive the functionality of myostatin, present a significant increase in muscle mass (Tobin et al., 2005). In myostatin mutant mice, individual muscles weigh twice as much compared to wild type mice (McPherron et al., 1997) due to hyperplasia and hypertrophy. Other identified mutations of myostatin gene have led to new breeds of cattle (e.g. Belgian blue or Piedmontese (McPherron et al., 1997) and dogs (Mosher et al., 2007). These findings have made myostatin the first target of a genetic approach to silence the gene expression and induce increase in muscle mass as therapeutic treatment for muscle wasting diseases. Indeed, even if the biodistribution of myostatin has not been conclusively clarified, the fact that skeletal muscle is the tissue with the highest expression of myostatin (Sharma et al., 1999, McPherron et al., 1997) means this protein is an appealing target for muscle augmentation strategies. Several strategies aiming to knock down myostatin to induce muscle mass augmentation have been preclinically tested: adeno-associated viral vectors have been used to deliver myostatin propeptide and so inactivate the growth factor by making it unavailable for binding its receptor (Foster et al., 2009; Matsakas et al., 2009). Follistatin-related gene (FLRG) and growth and differentiation factor association protein (GASP-1) are both able to bind to the homodimeric protein myostatin and inhibit its functionality even if the effect is less pronunciated compared to the use of a pro-peptide coded by viral vectors (Thies et al., 2001, Hill et al., 2002). Other strategies to inactivate myostatin are the use of antibodies raised against this growth factor in order to make it unavailable to the receptor. The antibodies JA16 or MYO-029 have been preclinically tested with the latter being also used for a clinical trial in humans where it demonstrated good tolerability and safety (Hill et al., 2002). A recent strategy to knock down myostatin is based on the use of antisense oligonucleotides to bind the pre-mRNA, skip the second exon of myostatin and induce the formation of an out of frame transcript unable of being translated in a functional protein (Kang et al., 2011). The systemic administration of antisense oligonucleotide in mouse showed encouraging results even if the effect was less pronunciated compared to the overexpression of pro-peptide or the myostatin specific antibody administration.

3.5.2 Inactivation of Activin receptor IIb

A second target used to significantly decrease the biological effect of myostatin is to inactivate its binding to the receptor, activin receptor IIb (ActRIIb). The overexpression of myostatin antagonist follistatin, which binds ActRIIb sterically, prevents the binding of myostatin (Rodino-Klapac et al., 2009) and induces an increase in muscle mass. Another study explored the possibility of inhibiting myostatin by using RNAi against ActRIIb and restore quasi dystrophin by AAV-U7 mediated exon skipping in a mouse model of muscular dystrophy (Dumonceaux et al., 2010). Recently in the same animal model the use of soluble ligands of ActRIIb as peptides, including the extracellular portion of the ActRIIb fused to the Fc portion of murine IgG (sActRIIb), has been shown to improve skeletal muscle mass and functional strength (Pistilli et al., 2011).

3.6 Drug-induced read-through of nonsense mutations

Although most DMD cases are caused by large intragenic deletions, 10-15% of DMD mutations are nonsense point mutations which cause premature termination codons (PTCs) in the dystrophin mRNA. PTC 124 is a drug designed to induce translational read through of PTCs, thus inducing expression of dystrophin and reducing nonsense-mediated mRNA decay. Because of the mechanistically structural differences between PTCs and natural stop codons, PTC 124 appears to preferentially recognize mutant nonsense codons without interfering strongly with native termination codons of unrelated genes. PTC 124 has been proven to enhance dystrophin expression in both primary DMD muscle cells and animal models (Welch et al., 2007). A Phase 2b clinical trial in subjects with nonsense-mutation-mediated DMD/BMD has been completed. Unfortunately, PTC 124 did not render any improvement in the six minute walk distance.

4. Conclusion

Preclinical and clinical genetic and cell-based therapy trials are currently progressing rapidly, with the interaction of multiple research units, biotechnology companies and patient groups. Several studies in the clinic are now reporting promising results with restoration of dystrophin expression in local muscle fibres. Future perspectives of the current strategies will be to overcome obstacles in the way of them becoming therapeutic treatments for DMD

5. References

AARTSMA-RUS, A., VAN DEUTEKOM, J.C., FOKKEMA, I.F., VAN OMMEN, G.J. and DEN DUNNEN, J.T. (2006). Entries in the Leiden Duchenne muscular dystrophy mutation database: an overview of mutation types and paradoxical cases that confirm the reading-frame rule. *Muscle & nerve,* 34(2), pp. 135-144.

ACSADI, G., DICKSON, G., LOVE, D.R., JANI, A., WALSH, F.S., GURUSINGHE, A., WOLFF, J.A. and DAVIES, K.E. (1991). Human dystrophin expression in mdx mice after intramuscular injection of DNA constructs. *Nature,* 352(6338), pp. 815-818.

ADAMS, A.M., HARDING, P.L., IVERSEN, P.L., COLEMAN, C., FLETCHER, S. and WILTON, S.D. (2007). Antisense oligonucleotide induced exon skipping and the dystrophin gene transcript: cocktails and chemistries. *BMC molecular biology,* 8, pp. 57.

ALLEN, D.G., WHITEHEAD, N.P. and YEUNG, E.W. (2005). Mechanisms of stretch-induced muscle damage in normal and dystrophic muscle: role of ionic changes. *The Journal of physiology,* 567(Pt 3), pp. 723-735.

ARECHAVALA-GOMEZA, V., GRAHAM, I.R., POPPLEWELL, L.J., ADAMS, A.M., AARTSMA-RUS, A., KINALI, M., MORGAN, J.E., VAN DEUTEKOM, J.C., WILTON, S.D., DICKSON, G. and MUNTONI, F. (2007). Comparative analysis of antisense oligonucleotide sequences for targeted skipping of exon 51 during dystrophin pre-mRNA splicing in human muscle. *Human Gene Therapy,* 18(9), pp. 798-810.

ATHANASOPOULOS, T., GRAHAM, I.R., FOSTER, H. and DICKSON, G. (2004). Recombinant adeno-associated viral (rAAV) vectors as therapeutic tools for Duchenne muscular dystrophy (DMD). *Gene therapy,* 11 Suppl 1, pp. S109-21.

BEGGS, A.H., HOFFMAN, E.P., SNYDER, J.R., ARAHATA, K., SPECHT, L., SHAPIRO, F., ANGELINI, C., SUGITA, H. and KUNKEL, L.M. (1991). Exploring the molecular basis for variability among patients with Becker muscular dystrophy: dystrophin gene and protein studies. *American Journal of Human Genetics,* 49(1), pp. 54-67.

BELL, C.D. and CONEN, P.E. (1968). Histopathological changes in Duchenne muscular dystrophy. *Journal of the neurological sciences,* 7(3), pp. 529-544.

BELLINGER, A.M., REIKEN, S., CARLSON, C., MONGILLO, M., LIU, X., ROTHMAN, L., MATECKI, S., LACAMPAGNE, A. and MARKS, A.R. (2009). Hypernitrosylated ryanodine receptor calcium release channels are leaky in dystrophic muscle. *Nature medicine,* 15(3), pp. 325-330.

BETZ, R.C., SCHOSER, B.G., KASPER, D., RICKER, K., RAMIREZ, A., STEIN, V., TORBERGSEN, T., LEE, Y.A., NOTHEN, M.M., WIENKER, T.F., MALIN, J.P., PROPPING, P., REIS, A., MORTIER, W., JENTSCH, T.J., VORGERD, M. and KUBISCH, C. (2001). Mutations in CAV3 cause mechanical hyperirritability of skeletal muscle in rippling muscle disease. *Nature genetics,* 28(3), pp. 218-219.

BIGGAR, W.D. (2006). Duchenne muscular dystrophy. *Pediatrics in review / American Academy of Pediatrics,* 27(3), pp. 83-88.

BIONE, S., MAESTRINI, E., RIVELLA, S., MANCINI, M., REGIS, S., ROMEO, G. and TONIOLO, D. (1994). Identification of a novel X-linked gene responsible for Emery-Dreifuss muscular dystrophy. *Nature genetics,* 8(4), pp. 323-327.

BLAKE, D.J., WEIR, A., NEWEY, S.E. and DAVIES, K.E. (2002). Function and genetics of dystrophin and dystrophin-related proteins in muscle. *Physiological Reviews,* 82(2), pp. 291-329.

BRADLEY, W.G., HUDGSON, P., LARSON, P.F., PAPAPETROPOULOS, T.A. and JENKISON, M. (1972). Structural changes in the early stages of Duchenne muscular dystrophy. *Journal of neurology, neurosurgery, and psychiatry,* 35(4), pp. 451-455.

BULFIELD, G., SILLER, W.G., WIGHT, P.A. and MOORE, K.J. (1984). X chromosome-linked muscular dystrophy (mdx) in the mouse. *Proceedings of the National Academy of Sciences of the United States of America,* 81(4), pp. 1189-1192.

CAMACHO VANEGAS, O., BERTINI, E., ZHANG, R.Z., PETRINI, S., MINOSSE, C., SABATELLI, P., GIUSTI, B., CHU, M.L. and PEPE, G. (2001). Ullrich scleroatonic muscular dystrophy is caused by recessive mutations in collagen type VI. *Proceedings of the National Academy of Sciences of the United States of America,* 98(13), pp. 7516-7521.

CARBONE, I., BRUNO, C., SOTGIA, F., BADO, M., BRODA, P., MASETTI, E., PANELLA, A., ZARA, F., BRICARELLI, F.D., CORDONE, G., LISANTI, M.P. and MINETTI, C. (2000). Mutation in the CAV3 gene causes partial caveolin-3 deficiency and hyperCKemia. *Neurology,* 54(6), pp. 1373-1376.

CHAMBERLAIN, J.S., METZGER, J., REYES, M., TOWNSEND, D. and FAULKNER, J.A. (2007). Dystrophin-deficient mdx mice display a reduced life span and are susceptible to spontaneous rhabdomyosarcoma. *The FASEB journal : official publication of the Federation of American Societies for Experimental Biology,* 21(9), pp. 2195-2204.

CHAO, D.S., GOROSPE, J.R., BRENMAN, J.E., RAFAEL, J.A., PETERS, M.F., FROEHNER, S.C., HOFFMAN, E.P., CHAMBERLAIN, J.S. and BREDT, D.S. (1996). Selective loss of sarcolemmal nitric oxide synthase in Becker muscular dystrophy. *The Journal of experimental medicine,* 184(2), pp. 609-618.

COOPER, B.J., WINAND, N.J., STEDMAN, H., VALENTINE, B.A., HOFFMAN, E.P., KUNKEL, L.M., SCOTT, M.O., FISCHBECK, K.H., KORNEGAY, J.N. and AVERY, R.J. (1988). The homologue of the Duchenne locus is defective in X-linked muscular dystrophy of dogs. *Nature,* 334(6178), pp. 154-156.

COSSU, G. and SAMPAOLESI, M. (2007). New therapies for Duchenne muscular dystrophy: challenges, prospects and clinical trials. *Trends in molecular medicine,* 13(12), pp. 520-526.

DECONINCK, N., RAGOT, T., MARECHAL, G., PERRICAUDET, M. and GILLIS, J.M. (1996). Functional protection of dystrophic mouse (mdx) muscles after adenovirus-mediated transfer of a dystrophin minigene. *Proceedings of the National Academy of Sciences of the United States of America,* 93(8), pp. 3570-3574.

DUDLEY, R.W., LU, Y., GILBERT, R., MATECKI, S., NALBANTOGLU, J., PETROF, B.J. and KARPATI, G. (2004). Sustained improvement of muscle function one year after full-length dystrophin gene transfer into mdx mice by a gutted helper-dependent adenoviral vector. *Human Gene Therapy,* 15(2), pp. 145-156.

DUMONCEAUX, J., MARIE, S., BELEY, C., TROLLET, C., VIGNAUD, A., FERRY, A., BUTLER-BROWNE, G. and GARCIA, L. (2010). Combination of myostatin pathway interference and dystrophin rescue enhances tetanic and specific force in dystrophic mdx mice. *Molecular therapy : the journal of the American Society of Gene Therapy,* 18(5), pp. 881-887.

EMERY, A.E. (2000). Emery-Dreifuss muscular dystrophy - a 40 year retrospective. *Neuromuscular disorders : NMD,* 10(4-5), pp. 228-232.

EMERY, A.E.H. (2001). *The muscular dystrophies.* Oxford: Oxford University Press.

FARDEAU, M., BRAUN, S., ROMERO, N.B., HOGREL, J.Y., ROUCHE, A., ORTEGA, V., MOUROT, B., SQUIBAN, P., BENVENISTE, O. and HERSON, S. (2005). About a phase I gene therapy clinical trial with a full-length dystrophin gene-plasmid in Duchenne/Becker muscular dystrophy. *Journal de la Societe de biologie,* 199(1), pp. 29-32.

FARINI, A., RAZINI, P., ERRATICO, S., TORRENTE, Y. and MEREGALLI, M. (2009). Cell based therapy for Duchenne muscular dystrophy. *Journal of cellular physiology,* 221(3), pp. 526-534.

FERRARI, F.K., SAMULSKI, T., SHENK, T. and SAMULSKI, R.J. (1996). Second-strand synthesis is a rate-limiting step for efficient transduction by recombinant adeno-associated virus vectors. *Journal of virology,* 70(5), pp. 3227-3234.

FINSTERER, J. and STOLLBERGER, C. (2003). The heart in human dystrophinopathies. *Cardiology,* 99(1), pp. 1-19.

FISHER, K.J., CHOI, H., BURDA, J., CHEN, S.J. and WILSON, J.M. (1996). Recombinant adenovirus deleted of all viral genes for gene therapy of cystic fibrosis. *Virology,* 217(1), pp. 11-22.

FOSTER, H., SHARP, P.S., ATHANASOPOULOS, T., TROLLET, C., GRAHAM, I.R., FOSTER, K., WELLS, D.J. and DICKSON, G. (2008). Codon and mRNA sequence optimization of microdystrophin transgenes improves expression and physiological outcome in dystrophic mdx mice following AAV2/8 gene transfer. *Molecular therapy* 16(11), pp. 1825-1832.

GASCHEN, F.P., HOFFMAN, E.P., GOROSPE, J.R., UHL, E.W., SENIOR, D.F., CARDINET, G.H.,3RD and PEARCE, L.K. (1992). Dystrophin deficiency causes lethal muscle hypertrophy in cats. *Journal of the neurological sciences,* 110(1-2), pp. 149-159.

GILIBERTO, F., FERREIRO, V., DALAMON, V. and SZIJAN, I. (2004). Dystrophin deletions and cognitive impairment in Duchenne/Becker muscular dystrophy. *Neurological research,* 26(1), pp. 83-87.

GOEMANS, N.M., TULINIUS, M., VAN DEN AKKER, J.T., BURM, B.E., EKHART, P.F., HEUVELMANS, N., HOLLING, T., JANSON, A.A., PLATENBURG, G.J., SIPKENS, J.A., SITSEN, J.M., AARTSMA-RUS, A., VAN OMMEN, G.J., BUYSE, G., DARIN, N., VERSCHUUREN, J.J., CAMPION, G.V., DE KIMPE, S.J. and VAN DEUTEKOM, J.C. (2011). Systemic administration of PRO051 in Duchenne's muscular dystrophy. *The New England journal of medicine,* 364(16), pp. 1513-1522.

GRAHAM, I.R., HILL, V.J., MANOHARAN, M., INAMATI, G.B. and DICKSON, G. (2004). Towards a therapeutic inhibition of dystrophin exon 23 splicing in mdx mouse muscle induced by antisense oligoribonucleotides (splicomers): target sequence optimisation using oligonucleotide arrays. *The journal of gene medicine,* 6(10), pp. 1149-1158.

GREGOREVIC, P., BLANKINSHIP, M.J., ALLEN, J.M., CRAWFORD, R.W., MEUSE, L., MILLER, D.G., RUSSELL, D.W. and CHAMBERLAIN, J.S. (2004). Systemic delivery of genes to striated muscles using adeno-associated viral vectors. *Nature medicine,* 10(8), pp. 828-834.

GUPTA, P., BILINSKA, Z.T., SYLVIUS, N., BOUDREAU, E., VEINOT, J.P., LABIB, S., BOLONGO, P.M., HAMZA, A., JACKSON, T., PLOSKI, R., WALSKI, M., GRZYBOWSKI, J., WALCZAK, E., RELIGA, G., FIDZIANSKA, A. and TESSON, F.

(2010). Genetic and ultrastructural studies in dilated cardiomyopathy patients: a large deletion in the lamin A/C gene is associated with cardiomyocyte nuclear envelope disruption. *Basic research in cardiology,* 105(3), pp. 365-377.

HEEMSKERK, H.A., DE WINTER, C.L., DE KIMPE, S.J., VAN KUIK-ROMEIJN, P., HEUVELMANS, N., PLATENBURG, G.J., VAN OMMEN, G.J., VAN DEUTEKOM, J.C. and AARTSMA-RUS, A. (2009). In vivo comparison of 2'-O-methyl phosphorothioate and morpholino antisense oligonucleotides for Duchenne muscular dystrophy exon skipping. *The journal of gene medicine,* 11(3), pp. 257-266.

HELBLING-LECLERC, A., ZHANG, X., TOPALOGLU, H., CRUAUD, C., TESSON, F., WEISSENBACH, J., TOME, F.M., SCHWARTZ, K., FARDEAU, M. and TRYGGVASON, K. (1995). Mutations in the laminin alpha 2-chain gene (LAMA2) cause merosin-deficient congenital muscular dystrophy. *Nature genetics,* 11(2), pp. 216-218.

HILL, J.J., DAVIES, M.V., PEARSON, A.A., WANG, J.H., HEWICK, R.M., WOLFMAN, N.M. and QIU, Y. (2002). The myostatin propeptide and the follistatin-related gene are inhibitory binding proteins of myostatin in normal serum. *The Journal of biological chemistry,* 277(43), pp. 40735-40741.

KANG, J.K., MALERBA, A., POPPLEWELL, L., FOSTER, K. and DICKSON, G. (2011). Antisense-induced myostatin exon skipping leads to muscle hypertrophy in mice following octa-guanidine morpholino oligomer treatment. *Molecular therapy* 19(1), pp. 159-164.

KINALI, M., ARECHAVALA-GOMEZA, V., FENG, L., CIRAK, S., HUNT, D., ADKIN, C., GUGLIERI, M., ASHTON, E., ABBS, S., NIHOYANNOPOULOS, P., GARRALDA, M.E., RUTHERFORD, M., MCCULLEY, C., POPPLEWELL, L., GRAHAM, I.R., DICKSON, G., WOOD, M.J., WELLS, D.J., WILTON, S.D., KOLE, R., STRAUB, V., BUSHBY, K., SEWRY, C., MORGAN, J.E. and MUNTONI, F. (2009). Local restoration of dystrophin expression with the morpholino oligomer AVI-4658 in Duchenne muscular dystrophy: a single-blind, placebo-controlled, dose-escalation, proof-of-concept study. *Lancet neurology,* 8(10), pp. 918-928.

KOO, T., MALERBA, A., ATHANASOPOULOS, T., TROLLET, C., BOLDRIN, L., FERRY, A., POPPLEWELL, L., FOSTER, H., FOSTER, K. and DICKSON, G. (2011). Delivery of AAV2/9-microdystrophin genes incorporating helix 1 of the coiled-coil motif in the C-terminal domain of dystrophin improves muscle pathology and restores the level of alpha1-syntrophin and alpha-dystrobrevin in skeletal muscles of mdx mice. *Human Gene Therapy,* 22(11), pp. 1379-1388.

KOO, T., OKADA, T., ATHANASOPOULOS, T., FOSTER, H., TAKEDA, S. and DICKSON, G. (2011). Long-term functional adeno-associated virus-microdystrophin expression in the dystrophic CXMDj dog. *The journal of gene medicine,* 13(9), pp. 497-506.

KORNEGAY, J.N., TULER, S.M., MILLER, D.M. and LEVESQUE, D.C. (1988). Muscular dystrophy in a litter of golden retriever dogs. *Muscle & nerve,* 11(10), pp. 1056-1064.

KUMAMOTO, T., FUJIMOTO, S., ITO, T., HORINOUCHI, H., UEYAMA, H. and TSUDA, T. (2000). Proteasome expression in the skeletal muscles of patients with muscular dystrophy. *Acta Neuropathologica,* 100(6), pp. 595-602.

LONGMAN, C., BROCKINGTON, M., TORELLI, S., JIMENEZ-MALLEBRERA, C., KENNEDY, C., KHALIL, N., FENG, L., SARAN, R.K., VOIT, T., MERLINI, L.,

SEWRY, C.A., BROWN, S.C. and MUNTONI, F. (2003). Mutations in the human LARGE gene cause MDC1D, a novel form of congenital muscular dystrophy with severe mental retardation and abnormal glycosylation of alpha-dystroglycan. *Human molecular genetics,* 12(21), pp. 2853-2861.

LOVERING, R.M., PORTER, N.C. and BLOCH, R.J. (2005). The muscular dystrophies: from genes to therapies. *Physical Therapy,* 85(12), pp. 1372-1388.

MALERBA, A., SHARP, P.S., GRAHAM, I.R., ARECHAVALA-GOMEZA, V., FOSTER, K., MUNTONI, F., WELLS, D.J. and DICKSON, G. (2011). Chronic systemic therapy with low-dose morpholino oligomers ameliorates the pathology and normalizes locomotor behavior in mdx mice. *Molecular therapy : the journal of the American Society of Gene Therapy,* 19(2), pp. 345-354.

MATSAKAS, A., FOSTER, K., OTTO, A., MACHARIA, R., ELASHRY, M.I., FEIST, S., GRAHAM, I., FOSTER, H., YAWORSKY, P., WALSH, F., DICKSON, G. and PATEL, K. (2009). Molecular, cellular and physiological investigation of myostatin propeptide-mediated muscle growth in adult mice. *Neuromuscular disorders : NMD,* 19(7), pp. 489-499.

MCCARTY, D.M. (2008). Self-complementary AAV vectors; advances and applications. *Molecular therapy : the journal of the American Society of Gene Therapy,* 16(10), pp. 1648-1656.

MCPHERRON, A.C., LAWLER, A.M. and LEE, S.J. (1997). Regulation of skeletal muscle mass in mice by a new TGF-beta superfamily member. *Nature,* 387(6628), pp. 83-90.

MCPHERRON, A.C. and LEE, S.J. (1997). Double muscling in cattle due to mutations in the myostatin gene. *Proceedings of the National Academy of Sciences of the United States of America,* 94(23), pp. 12457-12461.

MENDELL, J.R., CAMPBELL, K., RODINO-KLAPAC, L., SAHENK, Z., SHILLING, C., LEWIS, S., BOWLES, D., GRAY, S., LI, C., GALLOWAY, G., MALIK, V., COLEY, B., CLARK, K.R., LI, J., XIAO, X., SAMULSKI, J., MCPHEE, S.W., SAMULSKI, R.J. and WALKER, C.M. (2010). Dystrophin immunity in Duchenne's muscular dystrophy. *The New England journal of medicine,* 363(15), pp. 1429-1437.

MOSHER, D.S., QUIGNON, P., BUSTAMANTE, C.D., SUTTER, N.B., MELLERSH, C.S., PARKER, H.G. and OSTRANDER, E.A. (2007). A mutation in the myostatin gene increases muscle mass and enhances racing performance in heterozygote dogs. *PLoS genetics,* 3(5), pp. e79.

MOULTON, H.M., FLETCHER, S., NEUMAN, B.W., MCCLOREY, G., STEIN, D.A., ABES, S., WILTON, S.D., BUCHMEIER, M.J., LEBLEU, B. and IVERSEN, P.L. (2007). Cell-penetrating peptide-morpholino conjugates alter pre-mRNA splicing of DMD (Duchenne muscular dystrophy) and inhibit murine coronavirus replication in vivo. *Biochemical Society transactions,* 35(Pt 4), pp. 826-828.

MUCHIR, A., BONNE, G., VAN DER KOOI, A.J., VAN MEEGEN, M., BAAS, F., BOLHUIS, P.A., DE VISSER, M. and SCHWARTZ, K. (2000). Identification of mutations in the gene encoding lamins A/C in autosomal dominant limb girdle muscular dystrophy with atrioventricular conduction disturbances (LGMD1B). *Human molecular genetics,* 9(9), pp. 1453-1459.

MUELLER, C. and FLOTTE, T.R. (2008). Clinical gene therapy using recombinant adeno-associated virus vectors. *Gene therapy,* 15(11), pp. 858-863.

NERI, M., TORELLI, S., BROWN, S., UGO, I., SABATELLI, P., MERLINI, L., SPITALI, P., RIMESSI, P., GUALANDI, F., SEWRY, C., FERLINI, A. and MUNTONI, F. (2007). Dystrophin levels as low as 30% are sufficient to avoid muscular dystrophy in the human. *Neuromuscular disorders : NMD,* 17(11-12), pp. 913-918.

PEAULT, B., RUDNICKI, M., TORRENTE, Y., COSSU, G., TREMBLAY, J.P., PARTRIDGE, T., GUSSONI, E., KUNKEL, L.M. and HUARD, J. (2007). Stem and progenitor cells in skeletal muscle development, maintenance, and therapy. *Molecular therapy : the journal of the American Society of Gene Therapy,* 15(5), pp. 867-877.

PISTILLI, E.E., BOGDANOVICH, S., GONCALVES, M.D., AHIMA, R.S., LACHEY, J., SEEHRA, J. and KHURANA, T. (2011). Targeting the activin type IIB receptor to improve muscle mass and function in the mdx mouse model of Duchenne muscular dystrophy. *The American journal of pathology,* 178(3), pp. 1287-1297.

POPPLEWELL, L.J., ADKIN, C., ARECHAVALA-GOMEZA, V., AARTSMA-RUS, A., DE WINTER, C.L., WILTON, S.D., MORGAN, J.E., MUNTONI, F., GRAHAM, I.R. and DICKSON, G. (2010). Comparative analysis of antisense oligonucleotide sequences targeting exon 53 of the human DMD gene: Implications for future clinical trials. *Neuromuscular disorders : NMD,* 20(2), pp. 102-110.

RODINO-KLAPAC, L.R., HAIDET, A.M., KOTA, J., HANDY, C., KASPAR, B.K. and MENDELL, J.R. (2009). Inhibition of myostatin with emphasis on follistatin as a therapy for muscle disease. *Muscle & nerve,* 39(3), pp. 283-296.

RUEGG, U.T., NICOLAS-METRAL, V., CHALLET, C., BERNARD-HELARY, K., DORCHIES, O.M., WAGNER, S. and BUETLER, T.M. (2002). Pharmacological control of cellular calcium handling in dystrophic skeletal muscle. *Neuromuscular disorders : NMD,* 12 Suppl 1, pp. S155-61.

SAMPAOLESI, M., BLOT, S., D'ANTONA, G., GRANGER, N., TONLORENZI, R., INNOCENZI, A., MOGNOL, P., THIBAUD, J.L., GALVEZ, B.G., BARTHELEMY, I., PERANI, L., MANTERO, S., GUTTINGER, M., PANSARASA, O., RINALDI, C., CUSELLA DE ANGELIS, M.G., TORRENTE, Y., BORDIGNON, C., BOTTINELLI, R. and COSSU, G. (2006). Mesoangioblast stem cells ameliorate muscle function in dystrophic dogs. *Nature,* .

SHARMA, M., KAMBADUR, R., MATTHEWS, K.G., SOMERS, W.G., DEVLIN, G.P., CONAGLEN, J.V., FOWKE, P.J. and BASS, J.J. (1999). Myostatin, a transforming growth factor-beta superfamily member, is expressed in heart muscle and is upregulated in cardiomyocytes after infarct. *Journal of cellular physiology,* 180(1), pp. 1-9.

SHIMATSU, Y., KATAGIRI, K., FURUTA, T., NAKURA, M., TANIOKA, Y., YUASA, K., TOMOHIRO, M., KORNEGAY, J.N., NONAKA, I. and TAKEDA, S. (2003). Canine X-linked muscular dystrophy in Japan (CXMDJ). *Experimental animals / Japanese Association for Laboratory Animal Science,* 52(2), pp. 93-97.

SICINSKI, P., GENG, Y., RYDER-COOK, A.S., BARNARD, E.A., DARLISON, M.G. and BARNARD, P.J. (1989). The molecular basis of muscular dystrophy in the mdx mouse: a point mutation. *Science (New York, N.Y.),* 244(4912), pp. 1578-1580.

SKUK, D., GOULET, M., ROY, B., PIETTE, V., COTE, C.H., CHAPDELAINE, P., HOGREL, J.Y., PARADIS, M., BOUCHARD, J.P., SYLVAIN, M., LACHANCE, J.G. and TREMBLAY, J.P. (2007). First test of a "high-density injection" protocol for myogenic cell transplantation throughout large volumes of muscles in a Duchenne muscular dystrophy patient: eighteen months follow-up. *Neuromuscular disorders : NMD,* 17(1), pp. 38-46.

TANABE, Y., ESAKI, K. and NOMURA, T. (1986). Skeletal muscle pathology in X chromosome-linked muscular dystrophy (mdx) mouse. *Acta Neuropathologica,* 69(1-2), pp. 91-95.

THIES, R.S., CHEN, T., DAVIES, M.V., TOMKINSON, K.N., PEARSON, A.A., SHAKEY, Q.A. and WOLFMAN, N.M. (2001). GDF-8 propeptide binds to GDF-8 and antagonizes biological activity by inhibiting GDF-8 receptor binding. *Growth factors (Chur, Switzerland),* 18(4), pp. 251-259.

TOBIN, J.F. and CELESTE, A.J. (2005). Myostatin, a negative regulator of muscle mass: implications for muscle degenerative diseases. *Current opinion in pharmacology,* 5(3), pp. 328-332.

TORRENTE, Y., BELICCHI, M., MARCHESI, C., DANTONA, G., COGIAMANIAN, F., PISATI, F., GAVINA, M., GIORDANO, R., TONLORENZI, R., FAGIOLARI, G., LAMPERTI, C., PORRETTI, L., LOPA, R., SAMPAOLESI, M., VICENTINI, L., GRIMOLDI, N., TIBERIO, F., SONGA, V., BARATTA, P., PRELLE, A., FORZENIGO, L., GUGLIERI, M., PANSARASA, O., RINALDI, C., MOULY, V., BUTLER-BROWNE, G.S., COMI, G.P., BIONDETTI, P., MOGGIO, M., GAINI, S.M., STOCCHETTI, N., PRIORI, A., D'ANGELO, M.G., TURCONI, A., BOTTINELLI, R., COSSU, G., REBULLA, P. and BRESOLIN, N. (2007). Autologous transplantation of muscle-derived CD133+ stem cells in Duchenne muscle patients. *Cell transplantation,* 16(6), pp. 563-577.

TURK, R., STERRENBURG, E., DE MEIJER, E.J., VAN OMMEN, G.J., DEN DUNNEN, J.T. and 'T HOEN, P.A. (2005). Muscle regeneration in dystrophin-deficient mdx mice studied by gene expression profiling. *BMC genomics,* 6, pp. 98.

VALENTINE, B.A., COOPER, B.J., DE LAHUNTA, A., O'QUINN, R. and BLUE, J.T. (1988). Canine X-linked muscular dystrophy. An animal model of Duchenne muscular dystrophy: clinical studies. *Journal of the neurological sciences,* 88(1-3), pp. 69-81.

VALENTINE, B.A., WINAND, N.J., PRADHAN, D., MOISE, N.S., DE LAHUNTA, A., KORNEGAY, J.N. and COOPER, B.J. (1992). Canine X-linked muscular dystrophy as an animal model of Duchenne muscular dystrophy: a review. *American Journal of Medical Genetics,* 42(3), pp. 352-356.

VAN DEUTEKOM, J.C., BREMMER-BOUT, M., JANSON, A.A., GINJAAR, I.B., BAAS, F., DEN DUNNEN, J.T. and VAN OMMEN, G.J. (2001). Antisense-induced exon skipping restores dystrophin expression in DMD patient derived muscle cells. *Human molecular genetics,* 10(15), pp. 1547-1554.

VAN DEUTEKOM, J.C., JANSON, A.A., GINJAAR, I.B., FRANKHUIZEN, W.S., AARTSMA-RUS, A., BREMMER-BOUT, M., DEN DUNNEN, J.T., KOOP, K., VAN DER KOOI, A.J., GOEMANS, N.M., DE KIMPE, S.J., EKHART, P.F., VENNEKER, E.H., PLATENBURG, G.J., VERSCHUUREN, J.J. and VAN OMMEN, G.J. (2007). Local dystrophin restoration with antisense oligonucleotide PRO051. *The New England journal of medicine,* 357(26), pp. 2677-2686.

WELCH, E.M., BARTON, E.R., ZHUO, J., TOMIZAWA, Y., FRIESEN, W.J., TRIFILLIS, P., PAUSHKIN, S., PATEL, M., TROTTA, C.R., HWANG, S., WILDE, R.G., KARP, G., TAKASUGI, J., CHEN, G., JONES, S., REN, H., MOON, Y.C., CORSON, D., TURPOFF, A.A., CAMPBELL, J.A., CONN, M.M., KHAN, A., ALMSTEAD, N.G.,

HEDRICK, J., MOLLIN, A., RISHER, N., WEETALL, M., YEH, S., BRANSTROM, A.A., COLACINO, J.M., BABIAK, J., JU, W.D., HIRAWAT, S., NORTHCUTT, V.J., MILLER, L.L., SPATRICK, P., HE, F., KAWANA, M., FENG, H., JACOBSON, A., PELTZ, S.W. and SWEENEY, H.L. (2007). PTC124 targets genetic disorders caused by nonsense mutations. *Nature,* 447(7140), pp. 87-91.

WHITEHEAD, N.P., YEUNG, E.W. and ALLEN, D.G. (2006). Muscle damage in mdx (dystrophic) mice: role of calcium and reactive oxygen species. *Clinical and experimental pharmacology & physiology,* 33(7), pp. 657-662.

WILLIAMSON, R.A., HENRY, M.D., DANIELS, K.J., HRSTKA, R.F., LEE, J.C., SUNADA, Y., IBRAGHIMOV-BESKROVNAYA, O. and CAMPBELL, K.P. (1997). Dystroglycan is essential for early embryonic development: disruption of Reichert's membrane in Dag1-null mice. *Human molecular genetics,* 6(6), pp. 831-841.

WILLMANN, R., POSSEKEL, S., DUBACH-POWELL, J., MEIER, T. and RUEGG, M.A. (2009). Mammalian animal models for Duchenne muscular dystrophy. *Neuromuscular disorders : NMD,* 19(4), pp. 241-249.

WORMAN, H.J. and COURVALIN, J.C. (2000). The inner nuclear membrane. *The Journal of membrane biology,* 177(1), pp. 1-11.

XIONG, F., ZHANG, C., XIAO, S.B., LI, M.S., WANG, S.H., YU, M.J. and SHANG, Y.C. (2007). Construction of recombinant adenovirus including microdystrophin and expression in the mesenchymal cells of mdx mice. *Sheng wu gong cheng xue bao = Chinese journal of biotechnology,* 23(1), pp. 27-32.

YIN, H., MOULTON, H.M., BETTS, C., MERRITT, T., SEOW, Y., ASHRAF, S., WANG, Q., BOUTILIER, J. and WOOD, M.J. (2010). Functional rescue of dystrophin-deficient mdx mice by a chimeric peptide-PMO. *Molecular therapy : the journal of the American Society of Gene Therapy,* 18(10), pp. 1822-1829.

YOKOTA, T., LU, Q.L., PARTRIDGE, T., KOBAYASHI, M., NAKAMURA, A., TAKEDA, S. and HOFFMAN, E. (2009). Efficacy of systemic morpholino exon-skipping in Duchenne dystrophy dogs. *Annals of Neurology,* 65(6), pp. 667-676.

YUGETA, N., URASAWA, N., FUJII, Y., YOSHIMURA, M., YUASA, K., WADA, M.R., NAKURA, M., SHIMATSU, Y., TOMOHIRO, M., TAKAHASHI, A., MACHIDA, N., WAKAO, Y., NAKAMURA, A. and TAKEDA, S. (2006). Cardiac involvement in Beagle-based canine X-linked muscular dystrophy in Japan (CXMDJ): electrocardiographic, echocardiographic, and morphologic studies. *BMC cardiovascular disorders,* 6, pp. 47.

Section 5

Current Advances and Future Promises

23

From Basic Research to Clinical Trials: Preclinical Trial Evaluation in Mouse Models

Sasha Bogdanovich[1,3] and Emidio E. Pistilli[2]
[1]*University of Pennsylvania School of Medicine and Pennsylvania Muscle Institute, Department of Physiology, Philadelphia, Pennsylvania*
[2]*West Virginia University School of Medicine, Division of Exercise Physiology, Morgantown, West Virginia*
[3]*Current address: University of Kentucky College of Medicine, Department of Ophthalmology and Visual Sciences, Lexington, Kentucky*
USA

1. Introduction

Duchenne Muscular Dystrophy (DMD) is a fatal, X chromosome-inherited disease which affects the whole world population equally and has an incidence of 1 in 3500 boys. The disease is progressive in nature with the first signs of muscle wasting appearing as early as age 3 (Dubowitz 1975; Jennekens et al. 1991). The disease slowly weakens the skeletal muscles of the arms and legs (mostly muscles of shoulder and pelvic girdles) and abdomen. By the early teens, heart and respiratory muscles may also become affected. Nearly all children with DMD lose the ability to walk between the age of 7 and the early teen years, with activities involving the arms, legs or trunk requiring assistance or mechanical support. Patients are typically confined to a wheelchair and they rarely survive the fourth decade of their life. Most DMD patients die due to respiratory or cardiac failure because of the progressive damage to the diaphragm or cardiac myopathy. A milder form of muscular dystrophy, termed Becker Muscular Dystrophy (BMD), has been characterized with a milder clinical presentation (Becker 1955). Children with this variation remain physically active and independent later in life compared to DMD patients. Symptoms begin to appear after 20 years of age and patients live longer compared to DMD patients.

Histologically, muscles from DMD patients are characterized by increased variation in muscle fiber size, necrosis of individual muscle fibers and replacement of necrotic fibers by fibrofatty tissue (Emery 1995; Engel 1994). In addition, an increase in serum Creatine Kinase (CK), derived from degenerating muscle fibers, has been recognized as one of the main diagnostic characteristics of the disease (Engel 1994; Guyton 1995). In 1983, Kay Davies of London, England found linkage between a DNA marker and the DMD gene located on the short arm of the X chromosome (Xp21) (Davies et al. 1983). This discovery finally confirmed the long time theory that DMD inheritance is through the X chromosome and explained Duchenne's notes of affected boys while girls remained without symptoms.

The culmination of DMD research occurred in 1986 when Louis Kunkel of Boston, United States of America (USA) isolated and cloned the gene which caused DMD / BMD (Kunkel et al. 1986). One year later (1987) Eric Hoffman from the same laboratory identified the protein product of the DMD / BMD gene (Hoffman et al. 1987). This protein was called dystrophin. The discovery of the dystrophin gene mutation as the cause of DMD opened the door for diagnostic development and therapeutic strategies for this disease (Bogdanovich et al. 2004).

1.1 Dystrophin

Disease symptoms are progressive and characterized by quantitative and qualitative changes in dystrophin protein (Brown 1997; Khurana et al. 1990). The dystrophin gene is located on the short arm of chromosome Xp21 and is a large gene comprised of 79 exons. With a total size of 3Mb, the gene represents about 0.1% of the entire human genome. The dystrophin protein consists of 3645 amino acids (AA) and has a molecular mass of 426 kDa (Coffey et al. 1992; Monaco et al. 1986). The molecule can be divided into 4 parts: an N-terminal actin binding domain, a central rod, a cysteine rich segment and a C-terminal end (Einbond & Sudol 1996; Koenig et al. 1988; Ponting et al. 1996; Roberts et al. 1996;). Dystrophin forms a link between the extra and intra-cellular cytoskeleton, and it is hypothesized that dystrophin acts to neutralize stressful events that come from outside the cell toward the intracellular matrix, although the full function of dystrophin is still unknown. With a lack of dystrophin protein, the sarcolemma is susceptible to contraction-induced ruptures and permanent cell damage is inevitable (Wrogemann & Pena 1976). Previous experiments have demonstrated an influx of extracellular Ca^{2+} or sarcoplasmatic reticulum leakage due to membrane disruption, which can result in proteolitic activities by Ca^{2+} dependent proteases. This cycle leads to necrosis, inflammatory cell infiltration, and phagocytosis. Additionally, the presence of mast cells can stimulate the release of basic fibroblast growth factor (bFGF) which contributes to fibrotic changes in dystrophic muscle.

The clinical presentation of DMD depends on the nature of the *dystrophin* gene mutation mutation. Nonsense mutations in the *DMD* gene lead to a premature stop codon that blocks dystrophin translation (Hoffman et al. 1987). In the case of a frame shift mutation, there is an exchange of one nucleotide base with another, resulting in the synthesis of shorter or longer dystrophin variants. These mutations result in a milder clinical presentation, namely BMD, where expression of dystrophin protein is present but reduced (Monaco et al. 1988). Dystrophin mutations can be localized in any of its 4 parts and the mutation localization is in direct correlation with the severity of clinical disease presentation. The most severe cases of DMD are described with mutations in the cystein rich component because of its multiple functions (Beggs et al. 1991; Koenig et al. 1989), while mutations in the other 3 parts result in milder clinical presentation.

Disease diagnosis starts with taking a careful history of the disease as well as laboratory testing. The level of CK in the blood is significantly higher in DMD patients, especially at the beginning of the disease, where it can often be 10 times higher compared to normal (Engel 1994). Many advantages are achieved by genetic analysis of DMD mutations. It is possible to discover mutations in the DMD gene using polymerase chain reaction (Flanigan et al. 2003; White et al. 2002). These methods are used routinely in prenatal diagnosis of male fetuses. Typically, DMD patients become wheelchair bound before 13 years of age, while BMD patients can remain physically active after 16 years of age. More invasive methods such as electrodiagnostics and muscle biopsy are used in cases of negative genetic analysis, for the differential diagnosis between DMD and BMD, and especially in autosomal disorders such as Limb-Girdle Muscular Dystrophy, where big differences between clinical presentations and laboratory testing do not exist (Laval & Bushby 2004). In such cases, muscle biopsy samples are used for histopathology and immunohistochemistry examination.

2. Mouse models of DMD

The identification and utilization of animal models in biomedical research is a necessary step in evaluating disease pathology and designing effective therapies for that disease (Table 1). In 1984, a mouse model of DMD was identified and has been termed the *mdx* mouse (*mdx* = muscular disease x-chromosome). The identification of a mouse model for DMD proved to be useful for further understanding of both the normal function of dystrophin and the pathology of the disease (Petrof et al. 1993; Stedman et al. 1991), and the *mdx* mouse currently remains the most widely used mouse model of DMD (Brockdorff et al. 1987; Cavanna et al. 1988). *Mdx* mice have a natural mutation in the dystrophin gene, caused by a point mutation. Compared to human DMD patients, *mdx* mice have a relatively mild disease presentation, characterized by periods of muscle fiber degeneration and regeneration starting approximately 2 weeks after birth although not all muscles are similarly affected. Despite the milder disease phenotype in these mice, the characteristic cycles of muscle fiber degeneration and regeneration provide a variable to evaluate therapies in this mouse model. In addition, biochemical analyses have demonstrated that there is a consistent increase in serum CK in the *mdx* mouse, mirroring an important biomarker in human patients (Bulfield et al. 1984; Moens et al. 1993). Inasmuch as there are recognized limitations of this mouse model, the *mdx* mouse remains a widely used animal in biomedical research.

The *mdx* mouse is very suitable for experiments designed to elucidate function and causality of the disease, as well as for gene and pharmaceutical therapy. It is in fact proving to be useful for furthering our understanding on both the normal function of dystrophin and the pathology of the disease. Experiments using *mdx* mice have provided us with invaluable information regarding the function of the gene product involved in DMD as well as the dystrophin-associated proteins (DAP) and the dystroglycan/sarcoglycan complex (DGC/SGC).

Additional allelic variants of the original *mdx* mouse mutation were created by treating mice with the mutagen, N-ethylnitrosourea (Rafael et al. 2000). This resulted in the formation of 4 new mouse models with specific mutations in the dystrophin gene and relevant increases in circulating CK levels in the blood. These mouse models have been described previously (Chapman et al. 1989; Cox et al. 1993; Im et al. 1996). Briefly, the mdx^{2cv} mouse has a mutation in intro 42; the mdx^{3cv} mouse has a mutant splice acceptor site in nintron 65; the mdx^{4cv} mouse has a "C" to "T" substitution in exon 53; and mdx^{5cv} has an "A" to "T" transition in exon 10. Due to the different sites of these point mutations, different dystrophin isoforms can be expressed in the form of revertant fibers. It has been proposed that these strains of *mdx* mice may be usefule to elucidate the role of these various dystrophin isoforms, although the original *mdx* variant remains the mouse model most utilized (Banks & Chamberlain 2008).

The mild phenotype of *mdx* mice is a recognized limitation of this mouse model. For example, *mdx* mice maintain cage activity and do not have significant exercise limitations (De Luca et al. 2003). Indeed, forced treadmill exercise has been used as a way to increase the degree of muscle pathology present in these mice (Fraysse et al. 2004). Also, there is only approximately a 20% difference in the lifespan of the *mdx* mouse compared to wild-type, thus limiting the ability to detect a therapy-based improvement on lifespan (Chamberlain et al. 2007). For these reasons, a more severe mouse model was developed that introduced the knockout of the utrophin gene into the *mdx* mouse; thus creating the dystrophin:utrophin double knockout mouse (DKO) (Deconinck et al. 1997, 1998; Grady et al. 1997; Huang et al. 2011). These mice have a severely limited lifespan coupled with severe impairments in muscle function (Chamberlain et al. 2007).

Most commonly used mouse models in muscular dystrophies		
Muscular Dystrophy	**Gene product**	**Mouse model**
Duchenne/Becker MD	Dystrophin	*mdx*, $mdx^{2\text{-}5cv}$, $mdx{:}utr^{-/-}$
Limb-Girdle MD		
Type 1C	Caveolin 3	$cav3^{-/-}$
Type 2A	Calpain 3	$capn3^{-/-}$
Type 2B (Miyoshi myopathy)	Dysferlin	SJL, A/J
Type 2C	γ-Sarcoglycan	$Sgcg^{-/-}$
Type 2D	α-Sarcoglycan (Adhalin)	$sgca^{-/-}$
Type 2E	β-Sarcoglycan	$sgcb^{-/-}$
Type 2F	δ-Sarcoglycan	$sgcd^{-/-}$
Congenital MD (CMD)		dy, dy^{2J}, dy^{3k}, dy^{w}, dy^{PAS}

Table 1. Mouse models in MDs

3. Current progress and evaluation

It has recently been proposed that a set of standard operating procedures be established for evaluating pre-clinical testing data in *mdx* mice (Grounds et al. 2008; Nagaraju & Willmann 2009; Spurney et al. 2009; Willmann et al. 2011). Through the universal adoption of standardized laboratory assays, the results of multiple pre-clinical trials performed in independent laboratories could be evaulated. The laboratory assays that we have employed in designing our new scaling system have been identified as robust tests for evaluating endpoints in the *mdx* mouse (Spurney et al. 2009). Before introducing the new scaling methodology, we will review the results of a number of preclinical trials performed in the *mdx* mouse. The data from these trials will then be utilized in presenting and evaulating the new scaling system, we call the Multiparametric Muscle Improvement Score (MMIS). These preclinical trials use a variety of parameters to establish the beneficial effect of the administered compound, and can be catogorized as either functional, morphological, or biochemical. Functional evaluation was done using a specially designed system to quantify *ex vivo* isometric and eccentric contractions (ECC) in freshly dissected muscle. Morphologic measures were quantified from hematoxylin and eosin (H&E) or immuno-stained muscle sections, and included counting of total muscle fibers, single fiber cross-sectional area, and the percentage of centrally nucleated fibers. Determination of serum creatine kinase and up-regulation of utrophin constituted the biochemical evaluation. Improvement in any of these individual parameters would suggest a therapy-based improvement in the dystrophic phenotype in *mdx* mice. However, some parameters are suggestive of more significant clinical improvement (i.e. greater muscle force, lower serum CK) and are therefore given more weight in our scaling system.

Preclinical trials were performed to determine the extent that small molecule therapies could up-regulate utrophin, and therefore functionally compensate for the loss of dystrophin in the muscles of *mdx* mice. These small moleculaes included heregulin (Krag et al. 2004) and biglycan (Amenta et al. 2011). In general, these utrophin-based up-regulation strategies resulted in very similar benefits in the *mdx* mouse. Parameters that were improved included isometric force following ECC, increased regenerative capacities of *mdx* muscle (i.e. greater number of regenerative fibers), and less necrotic areas in the diaphragm muscle. However, these strategies did not show improvements isometric force producing capacity of limb muscles or the levels of serum creatine kinase. The improvements in the ECC force coupled with the up-regulation of utrophin demonstrate that utrophin can functionally substitute for the loss of dystrophin. However, the incomplete amelioration of the dystrophic phenotype suggests that these therapies have limitations when administered individually.

A number of preclinical studies were performed to analyze the effects of blocking the activity of myostatin, a negative regulator of muscle growth and member of the TGF-β family (McPherron et al. 1997; McPherron & Lee 1997). Strategies included using antibodies directed against myostatin and administration of the myostatin propeptide, to sequester circulating myostatin and neutralize its activity. Administration of these compounds to *mdx* mice resulted in significant improvements in overall body and skeletal muscle mass. Muscle mass increases were greater in response to the myostatin propeptide, and may be due to a higher binding affinity for myostatin compared to the myostatin antibody (Bogdanovich et al. 2002, 2005). In addition, muscle function was improved as evidenced by greater absolute forces in muscles from treated mice in both trials. However, the propeptide-based strategy also resulted in improvements in specific force (i.e. force normalized to muscle cross-sectional area). Both strategies demonstrated improvements in overall muscle histopathology and the levels of serum creatine kinase, suggesting an improvement in the sarcolemma by a utrophin independent mechanism. Collectively, these myostatin blockade strategies were effective in stimulating increases in muscle mass and muscle function, along with measures of muscle histopathology and serum CK. However, complete amelioration of the dystrophic phenotype was not accomplished due to the fact that no improvements were noted in the force loss following eccentric lengthening contractions.

Furthermore, we wanted to determine whether myostatin blockade would be beneficial to additional mouse models of muscular dystrophy. We utilized the myostatin-antibody strategy in gamma sarcoglycan (*Sgcg*$^{-/-}$) knockout mice, a model of Limb-Girdle 2C muscular dystrophy (LGMD 2C) (Bogdanovich et al. 2008). Interestingly, myostatin antibody blockade did not show desired improvement in this mouse model. Improvement was minimal and evident in body and muscle weight increases. Physiological improvement was notable only in one parameter, absolute force improvement. Histopathological and biochemical parameters were unchaged when compared to control mice. Therefore, unique disease charactersitics of LGMD 2C compared to DMD in mouse models may have led to these differing results and a preferential benefit in the *mdx* mouse.

Recently, we tested the efficacy of a novel myostatin blockade strategy using a soluble form of the activin type IIB receptor (ActRIIB) (Pistilli et al. 2011). The ActRIIB is the receptor for myostain as well as other member of the TGF-β superfamily. The solubilized form of the receptor (sActRIIB) would be able to bind to and sequester multiple TGF-β superfamily members, thereby potentially providing a greater therapeutic effect. In this preclinical trial, two doses of sActRIIB were utilized, a low dose of 1,0 mg/kg bodyweight and a high dose 10,0 mg/kg bodyweight. Notable differences were observed when comparing these two dosing strategies. The high dose of sActRIIB resulted in dramatic increases in body weight and lean muscle mass, while minimal changes in overall body mass were noted in the response to the low dose. Both doses of sActRIIB improved absolute forces produced by limb muscles. However, the low dose significantly improved specific force, indicating an improvement in force producing capacity independent of muscle size. Serum CK levels were also lower in sActRIB treated mice. Unfortunately, force loss follwing eccentric lengthening contractions and muscle histopathology were not significantly improved in these trials. Therefore, as with the myostatin antibody and the myostatin propeptide, complete amelioration of the dystrophic phenotype was not observed with sActRIIB therapy.

The results of these trials demonstrate that small molecule-based therapies have the potential to improve a number of paremeters related to the dystrophic phenotype in *mdx* mice. However, as noted, no therapy has been able to completely ameliorate the phenotype and rescue the *mdx* mouse. Also, evaluating the therapeutic efficacy of drugs identified through preclinical trials is inefficient, due to the large number of preclinical trials published

Multiparametric Muscle Improvement Score -MMIS	
	Bogdanovich / Khurana points
Body weight (g)	1
Muscle weights (mg)	2
Absolute force, twitch (mN)	1
Specific force, twitch (mN/mm^2)	3
Absolute force, tetanus (mN)	4
Specific force, tetanus (mN/mm^2)	5
Eccentric contractions improvement	5
Centrally nucleated fibers	5
Loss of fibrotic changes	3
Decreased CK value	5
Total score	**34**

Total umeric score: 34
01-08 no improvement
09-22 intermediate
23-34 optimal

Table 2. Multiparametric Muscle Improvement Score

in animal models, and the differential methodology used to evaluate the data. Therefore, a scaling system that can evaluate the therapeutic efficacy of independent preclinical trials would be useful to identify those compounds with the most therapeutic promise. The purpose of this research was to formulate a single, objective scoring system to evaluate preclinical trial data arising from multiple laboratories. More detailed and precise quantification of different therapies can be obtained by utilizing the Multiparametric Muscle Improvement Score (MMIS) system (Bogdanovich 2009).

4. Methods

The authors have complied preclinical trial data acquired during the last 10 years, and evaluated the data using the MMIS scoring system (Bogdanovich 2009). This system consists of ten of the most important anatomical, physiological and biochemical elements directly related to improvement of the dystrophic phenotype in mouse models of muscular dystrophy. These include: body and muscle weight changes, muscle force production during isometric and lengthening contractions, evidence of histological improvement, and reductions in circulating creatine kinase (see Table 2). These elements are weighted with one single numerical value from 1 (least important) to 5 (most important). Only statistically significant improvements in measured parameters can be scored. Scoring is done in such a way that every parameter receives maximal value if there is improvement. Scored elements are summarized at the end and the final number is the improvement score.

Comparison of possible therapeutic strategies for muscular dystrophies (before MMIS system)

Mice	*mdx*	*mdx*	*Sgcg*$^{-/-}$	*mdx*		*mdx*	*mdx*
Treatment	**Myostatin blockade or inhibition**					**Utrophin upregulation**	
	Antibody	*Propeptide*	*Antibody*	*sActRIIB* 1mg/kg	*sActRIIB* 10mg/kg	Heregulin	*Biglycan*
	Bogdanovich *et al.* 2002 (Nature)	Bogdanovich *et al.* 2005 (FASEB J)	Bogdanovich *et al.* 2007 (Muscle&Nerve)	Pistilli *et al.* 2011 (Am. J. Pathol.)		Krag *et al.* 2004 (PNAS)	Amenta *et al.* 2010 (PNAS)
Body weight (g)	+	+	+	-	+	-	-
Muscle weights (mg)	+	+	+	+	+	-	-
Absolute force, twitch (mN)	+	+	+	+	+	-	-
Specific force, twitch (mN/mm^2)	-	-	-	+	-	-	-
Absolute force, tetanus (mN)	+	+	+	+	+	-	-
Specific force, tetanus (mN/mm^2)	-	+	-	+	-	-	-
Eccentric contractions	-	-	-	-	-	+	+
Centrally nucleated fibers	+	-	-	-	-	+	+
Loss of fibrotic changes	+	+	-	-	-	+	+
Decreased CK value	+	+	-	+	+	-	-

Legend: Sgcg$^{-/-}$, gamma sarcoglycan (LGMD 2C mouse model); -, no improvement; +, positive improvement

Table 3. Evaluation of possible therapeutic stratagies for muscular dystrophy (before MMIS system)

5. Results

The scoring system is objective and excludes human error. It is possible to review and rank therapies based on a final single numeric score using the MMIS scale. With the MMIS scale, we have objectively assessed the therapeutic efficacy of multiple drug therapies in mouse models of muscular dystrophy (*mdx* mouse, *Sgcg-/-* mouse) (Table 3, 4). However, the limitations of these promising methods were identified objectively using the MMIS scale. Despite significant effects on muscle mass and muscle force production, neither strategy completely ameliorated the dystrophic phenotype with regards to eccentric lenghtening contractions or histological improvement as identified using the MMIS scale.

Comparison of possible therapeutic strategies for muscular dystrophies (MMIS system)

Mice	*mdx*	*mdx*	*Sgcg-/-*	*mdx*		*mdx*	*mdx*
Treatment	**Myostatin blockade or inhibition**					**Utrophin upregulation**	
	Antibody	*Propeptide*	*Antibody*	*sActRIIB* 1mg/kg	*sActRIIB* 10mg/kg	Heregulin	*Biglycan*
	Bogdanovich *et al.* 2002 (Nature)	Bogdanovich *et al.* 2005 (FASEB J)	Bogdanovich *et al.* 2007 (Muscle&Nerve)	Pistilli *et al.* 2011 (Am. J. Pathol.)		Krag *et al.* 2004 (PNAS)	Amenta *et al.* 2010 (PNAS)
Body weight (g)	1	1	1	0	1	0	0
Muscle weights (mg)	2	2	2	2	2	0	0
Absolute force, twitch (mN)	1	1	1	1	1	0	0
Specific force, twitch (mN/mm^2)	0	0	0	3	0	0	0
Absolute force, tetanus (mN)	4	4	4	4	4	0	0
Specific force, tetanus (mN/mm^2)	0	5	0	5	0	0	0
Eccentric contractions	0	0	0	0	0	5	5
Centrally nucleated fibers	5	0	0	0	0	5	5
Loss of fibrotic changes	3	3	0	0	0	3	3
Decreased CK value	5	5	0	5	5	0	0
Total score	**21**	**21**	**8**	**20**	**13**	**13**	**13**

Legend: Sgcg-/-, gamma sarcoglycan (LGMD 2C mouse model) ; Total numeric score: 34; 01-08 no improvement; 09-22 intermediate; 23-34 optimal

Table 4. Possible therapeutic stratagies for muscular dystrophy (MMIS system)

6. Conclusion

Currently, there is a need for standardization of measurement and objective evaluation of different preclinical studies of the muscular dystrophies, which would allow for a better understanding of the disease and its response to potential therapies. We suggest that the MMIS provides a single numeric value useful for cross-comparing different preclinical studies and prioritizing drug development for muscular dystrophy therapy. We suggest that the use of the MMIS scale will allow for precise and rigorous evaluation of functional improvements of therapeutic interventions performed in preclinical trials.

7. Acknowledgment

We would like to thank to Dr. T. S. Khurana (University of Pennsylvania, USA) for helpful discussion on this topic.

8. References

Amenta, A. R.; Yilmaz, A., et al. (2011). Biglycan recruits utrophin to the sarcolemma and counters dystrophic pathology in mdx mice. *Proc Natl Acad Sci U S A*, Vol.108, No.2, (Jan 11 2011), pp. 762-767, ISSN 1091-6490 (Electronic); 0027-8424 (Linking)

Banks, G. B. & Chamberlain, J. S. (2008). The value of mammalian models for duchenne muscular dystrophy in developing therapeutic strategies. *Curr Top Dev Biol*, Vol.84, 2008), pp. 431-453, ISSN 0070-2153 (Print); 0070-2153 (Linking)

Becker, P. E., Kiener, F (1955). [A new x-chromosomal muscular dystrophy]. *Arch. Psychiatr. Nervenkr Z Gesamte Neurol Psychiatr.*, Vol.193 (n.d.) No.4, pp. 427-448, PMID 13249581

Beggs, A. H.; Hoffman, E. P., et al. (1991). Exploring the molecular basis for variability among patients with Becker muscular dystrophy: dystrophin gene and protein studies. *Am J Hum Genet*, Vol.49, No.1, (Jul 1991), pp. 54-67, ISSN 0002-9297 (Print) 0002-9297 (Linking)

Bogdanovich, S. (2009). *Myostatin blockade for functional improvement of Duchenne's dystrophic phenotype.* Doctoral dissertation. University of Novi Sad Faculty of Medicine. UCK 616.8-009.5-08:612.085, Novi Sad, Serbia.

Bogdanovich, S.; Krag, T. O., et al. (2002). Functional improvement of dystrophic muscle by myostatin blockade. *Nature*, Vol.420, No.6914, (Nov 28 2002), pp. 418-421, ISSN 0028-0836 (Print); 0028-0836 (Linking)

Bogdanovich, S.; McNally, E. M., et al. (2008). Myostatin blockade improves function but not histopathology in a murine model of limb-girdle muscular dystrophy 2C. *Muscle Nerve*, Vol.37, No.3, (Mar 2008), pp. 308-316, ISSN 0148-639X (Print); 0148-639X (Linking)

Bogdanovich, S.; Perkins, K. J., et al. (2004). Therapeutics for Duchenne muscular dystrophy: current approaches and future directions. *J Mol Med (Berl)*, Vol.82, No.2, (Feb 2004), pp. 102-115, ISSN 0946-2716 (Print); 0946-2716 (Linking)

Bogdanovich, S.; Perkins, K. J., et al. (2005). Myostatin propeptide-mediated amelioration of dystrophic pathophysiology. *FASEB J*, Vol.19, No.6, (Apr 2005), pp. 543-549, ISSN 1530-6860 (Electronic); 0892-6638 (Linking)

Brockdorff, N.; Cross, G. S., et al. (1987). The mapping of a cDNA from the human X-linked Duchenne muscular dystrophy gene to the mouse X chromosome. *Nature*, Vol.328, No.6126, (Jul 9-15 1987), pp. 166-168, ISSN 0028-0836 (Print); 0028-0836 (Linking)

Brown, S. C. & Lucy, J. A. (Ed.) (1997) *Dystrophin Gene, Protein and Cell Biology*. Cambridge University Press, ISBN 0-521-55033-5, Cambridge, United Kingdom

Bulfield, G.; Siller, W. G., et al. (1984). X chromosome-linked muscular dystrophy (mdx) in the mouse. *Proc Natl Acad Sci U S A*, Vol.81, No.4, (Feb 1984), pp. 1189-1192, ISSN 0027-8424 (Print); 0027-8424 (Linking)

Cavanna, J. S.; Coulton, G., et al. (1988). Molecular and genetic mapping of the mouse mdx locus. *Genomics*, Vol.3, No.4, (Nov 1988), pp. 337-341, ISSN 0888-7543 (Print); 0888-7543 (Linking)

Chamberlain, J. S.; Metzger, J., et al. (2007). Dystrophin-deficient mdx mice display a reduced life span and are susceptible to spontaneous rhabdomyosarcoma. *FASEB J*, Vol.21, No.9, (Jul 2007), pp. 2195-2204, ISSN 1530-6860 (Electronic); 0892-6638 (Linking)

Chapman, V. M.; Miller, D. R., et al. (1989). Recovery of induced mutations for X chromosome-linked muscular dystrophy in mice. *Proc Natl Acad Sci U S A*, Vol.86, No.4, (Feb 1989), pp. 1292-1296, ISSN 0027-8424 (Print); 0027-8424 (Linking)

Coffey, A. J.; Roberts, R. G., et al. (1992). Construction of a 2.6-Mb contig in yeast artificial chromosomes spanning the human dystrophin gene using an STS-based approach. *Genomics*, Vol.12, No.3, (Mar 1992), pp. 474-484, ISSN 0888-7543 (Print); 0888-7543 (Linking)

Cox, G. A.; Phelps, S. F., et al. (1993). New mdx mutation disrupts expression of muscle and nonmuscle isoforms of dystrophin. *Nat Genet*, Vol.4, No.1, (May 1993), pp. 87-93, ISSN 1061-4036 (Print); 1061-4036 (Linking)

Davies, K. E.; Jackson, J., et al. (1983). Linkage analysis of myotonic dystrophy and sequences on chromosome 19 using a cloned complement 3 gene probe. *J Med Genet*, Vol.20, No.4, (Aug 1983), pp. 259-263, ISSN 0022-2593 (Print); 0022-2593 (Linking)

De Luca, A.; Pierno, S., et al. (2003). Enhanced dystrophic progression in mdx mice by exercise and beneficial effects of taurine and insulin-like growth factor-1. *J Pharmacol Exp Ther*, Vol.304, No.1, (Jan 2003), pp. 453-463, ISSN 0022-3565 (Print); 0022-3565 (Linking)

Deconinck, A. E.; Rafael, J. A., et al. (1997). Utrophin-dystrophin-deficient mice as a model for Duchenne muscular dystrophy. *Cell*, Vol.90, No.4, (Aug 22 1997), pp. 717-727, ISSN 0092-8674 (Print); 0092-8674 (Linking)

Deconinck, N.; Rafael, J. A., et al. (1998). Consequences of the combined deficiency in dystrophin and utrophin on the mechanical properties and myosin composition of some limb and respiratory muscles of the mouse. *Neuromuscul Disord*, Vol.8, No.6, (Aug 1998), pp. 362-370, ISSN 0960-8966 (Print); 0960-8966 (Linking)

Dubowitz, V. (1975). Neuromuscular disorders in childhood. Old dogmas, new concepts. *Arch Dis Child*, Vol.50, No.5, (May 1975), pp. 335-346, ISSN 1468-2044 (Electronic); 0003-9888 (Linking)

Einbond, A. & Sudol, M. (1996). Towards prediction of cognate complexes between the WW domain and proline-rich ligands. *FEBS Lett*, Vol.384, No.1, (Apr 8 1996), pp. 1-8, ISSN 0014-5793 (Print); 0014-5793 (Linking)

Emery, A. H. E., Emery, M.L.H (1995) *The History of a Gentic Disease*. Royal Society of Medicine Press, ISBN 978-0-19-959147-3, London, United Kingdom

Engel, A. G., Franzini-Armstrong, C (2004) *Myology*. McGraw-Hill, ISBN 0-07-137180-X, New York, USA

Flanigan, K. M.; von Niederhausern, A., et al. (2003). Rapid direct sequence analysis of the dystrophin gene. *Am J Hum Genet*, Vol.72, No.4, (Apr 2003), pp. 931-939, ISSN 0002-9297 (Print); 002-9297 (Linking)

Fraysse, B.; Liantonio, A., et al. (2004). The alteration of calcium homeostasis in adult dystrophic mdx muscle fibers is worsened by a chronic exercise in vivo. *Neurobiol Dis*, Vol.17, No.2, (Nov 2004), pp. 144-154, ISSN 0969-9961 (Print); 0969-9961 (Linking)

Grady, R. M.; Teng, H., et al. (1997). Skeletal and cardiac myopathies in mice lacking utrophin and dystrophin: a model for Duchenne muscular dystrophy. *Cell*, Vol.90, No.4, (Aug 22 1997), pp. 729-738, ISSN 0092-8674 (Print); 0092-8674 (Linking)

Grounds, M. D.; Radley, H. G., et al. (2008). Towards developing standard operating procedures for pre-clinical testing in the mdx mouse model of Duchenne muscular dystrophy. *Neurobiol Dis*, Vol.31, No.1, (Jul 2008), pp. 1-19, ISSN 1095-953X (Electronic); 0969-9961 (Linking)

Guyton, A. (2011) *Textbook of Medical Physiology*. Saunders ISBN 978-1-4160-4574-8, New York, USA

Hoffman, E. P.; Brown, R. H., Jr., et al. (1987). Dystrophin: the protein product of the Duchenne muscular dystrophy locus. *Cell*, Vol.51, No.6, (Dec 24 1987), pp. 919-928, ISSN 0092-8674 (Print); 0092-8674 (Linking)

Huang, P.; Cheng, G., et al. (2011). Impaired respiratory function in mdx and mdx/utrn(+/-) mice. *Muscle Nerve*, Vol.43, No.2, (Feb 2011), pp. 263-267, ISSN 1097-4598 (Electronic); 0148-639X (Linking)

Im, W. B.; Phelps, S. F., et al. (1996). Differential expression of dystrophin isoforms in strains of mdx mice with different mutations. *Hum Mol Genet*, Vol.5, No.8, (Aug 1996), pp. 1149-1153, ISSN 0964-6906 (Print); 0964-6906 (Linking)

Jennekens, F. G.; ten Kate, L. P., et al. (1991). Diagnostic criteria for Duchenne and Becker muscular dystrophy and myotonic dystrophy. *Neuromuscul Disord*, Vol.1, No.6, 1991), pp. 389-391, ISSN 0960-8966 (Print); 0960-8966 (Linking)

Khurana, T. S.; Hoffman, E. P., et al. (1990). Identification of a chromosome 6-encoded dystrophin-related protein. *J Biol Chem*, Vol.265, No.28, (Oct 5 1990), pp. 16717-16720, ISSN 0021-9258 (Print); 0021-9258 (Linking)

Koenig, M.; Beggs, A. H., et al. (1989). The molecular basis for Duchenne versus Becker muscular dystrophy: correlation of severity with type of deletion. *Am J Hum Genet*, Vol.45, No.4, (Oct 1989), pp. 498-506, ISSN 0002-9297 (Print); 0002-9297 (Linking)

Koenig, M.; Monaco, A. P., et al. (1988). The complete sequence of dystrophin predicts a rod-shaped cytoskeletal protein. *Cell*, Vol.53, No.2, (Apr 22 1988), pp. 219-228, ISSN 0092-8674 (Print); 0092-8674 (Linking)

Krag, T. O.; Bogdanovich, S., et al. (2004). Heregulin ameliorates the dystrophic phenotype in mdx mice. *Proc Natl Acad Sci U S A*, Vol.101, No.38, (Sep 21 2004), pp. 13856-13860, ISSN 0027-8424 (Print); 0027-8424 (Linking)

Kunkel, L. M.; Monaco, A. P., et al. (1986). Molecular genetics of Duchenne muscular dystrophy. *Cold Spring Harb Symp Quant Biol*, Vol.51 Pt 1, 1986), pp. 349-351, ISSN 0091-7451 (Print); 0091-7451 (Linking)

Laval, S. H. & Bushby, K. M. (2004). Limb-girdle muscular dystrophies--from genetics to molecular pathology. *Neuropathol Appl Neurobiol*, Vol.30, No.2, (Apr 2004), pp. 91-105, ISSN 0305-1846 (Print); 0305-1846 (Linking)

McPherron, A. C.; Lawler, A. M., et al. (1997). Regulation of skeletal muscle mass in mice by a new TGF-beta superfamily member. *Nature*, Vol.387, No.6628, (May 1 1997), pp. 83-90, ISSN 0028-0836 (Print); 0028-0836 (Linking)

McPherron, A. C. & Lee, S. J. (1997). Double muscling in cattle due to mutations in the myostatin gene. *Proc Natl Acad Sci U S A*, Vol.94, No.23, (Nov 11 1997), pp. 12457-12461, ISSN 0027-8424 (Print); 0027-8424 (Linking)

Moens, P.; Baatsen, P. H., et al. (1993). Increased susceptibility of EDL muscles from mdx mice to damage induced by contractions with stretch. *J Muscle Res Cell Motil*, Vol.14, No.4, (Aug 1993), pp. 446-451, ISSN 0142-4319 (Print); 0142-4319 (Linking)

Monaco, A. P.; Bertelson, C. J., et al. (1988). An explanation for the phenotypic differences between patients bearing partial deletions of the DMD locus. *Genomics*, Vol.2, No.1, (Jan 1988), pp. 90-95, ISSN 0888-7543 (Print); 0888-7543 (Linking)

Monaco, A. P.; Neve, R. L., et al. (1986). Isolation of candidate cDNAs for portions of the Duchenne muscular dystrophy gene. *Nature*, Vol.323, No.6089, (Oct 16-22 1986), pp. 646-650, ISSN 0028-0836 (Print); 0028-0836 (Linking)

Nagaraju, K. & Willmann, R. (2009). Developing standard procedures for murine and canine efficacy studies of DMD therapeutics: report of two expert workshops on "Pre-clinical testing for Duchenne dystrophy": Washington DC, October 27th-28th 2007 and Zurich, June 30th-July 1st 2008. *Neuromuscul Disord*, Vol.19, No.7, (Jul 2009), pp. 502-506, ISSN 1873-2364 (Electronic); 0960-8966 (Linking)

Petrof, B. J.; Shrager, J. B., et al. (1993). Dystrophin protects the sarcolemma from stresses developed during muscle contraction. *Proc Natl Acad Sci U S A*, Vol.90, No.8, (Apr 15 1993), pp. 3710-3714, ISSN 0027-8424 (Print); 0027-8424 (Linking)

Pistilli, E. E.; Bogdanovich, S., et al. (2011). Targeting the activin type IIB receptor to improve muscle mass and function in the mdx mouse model of Duchenne muscular dystrophy. *Am J Pathol*, Vol.178, No.3, (Mar 2011), pp. 1287-1297, ISSN 1525-2191 (Electronic); 0002-9440 (Linking)

Ponting, C. P.; Blake, D. J., et al. (1996). ZZ and TAZ: new putative zinc fingers in dystrophin and other proteins. *Trends Biochem Sci*, Vol.21, No.1, (Jan 1996), pp. 11-13, ISSN 0968-0004 (Print); 0968-0004 (Linking)

Rafael, J. A.; Nitta, Y., et al. (2000). Testing of SHIRPA, a mouse phenotypic assessment protocol, on Dmd(mdx) and Dmd(mdx3cv) dystrophin-deficient mice. *Mamm Genome*, Vol.11, No.9, (Sep 2000), pp. 725-728, ISSN 0938-8990 (Print); 0938-8990 (Linking)

Roberts, R. G.; Freeman, T. C., et al. (1996). Characterization of DRP2, a novel human dystrophin homologue. *Nat Genet*, Vol.13, No.2, (Jun 1996), pp. 223-226, ISSN 1061-4036 (Print); 1061-4036 (Linking)

Spurney, C. F.; Gordish-Dressman, H., et al. (2009). Preclinical drug trials in the mdx mouse: assessment of reliable and sensitive outcome measures. *Muscle Nerve*, Vol.39, No.5, (May 2009), pp. 591-602, ISSN 0148-639X (Print); 0148-639X (Linking)

Stedman, H. H.; Sweeney, H. L., et al. (1991). The mdx mouse diaphragm reproduces the degenerative changes of Duchenne muscular dystrophy. *Nature*, Vol.352, No.6335, (Aug 8 1991), pp. 536-539, ISSN 0028-0836 (Print); 0028-0836 (Linking)

White, S.; Kalf, M., et al. (2002). Comprehensive detection of genomic duplications and deletions in the DMD gene, by use of multiplex amplifiable probe hybridization. *Am J Hum Genet*, Vol.71, No.2, (Aug 2002), pp. 365-374, ISSN 0002-9297 (Print); 0002-9297 (Linking)

Willmann, R.; De Luca, A., et al. (2011). Enhancing translation: Guidelines for standard pre-clinical experiments in mdx mice. *Neuromuscul Disord*, Vol.(Jul 5 2011), pp. 1873-2364 ISSN 0960-8966 (Linking)

Wrogemann, K. & Pena, S. D. (1976). Mitochondrial calcium overload: A general mechanism for cell-necrosis in muscle diseases. *Lancet*, Vol.1, No.7961, (Mar 27 1976), pp. 672-674, ISSN 0140-6736 (Print); 0140-6736 (Linking)

24

A Two Stage Model of Skeletal Muscle Necrosis in Muscular Dystrophy – The Role of Fiber Branching in the Terminal Stage

Stewart Head
Department of Physiology, School of Medical Sciences, University of New South Wales, Sydney, Australia

1. Introduction

Branched fibers are a well-documented phenomenon of regenerating dystrophic skeletal muscle. They are found in the muscles of boys with Duchenne muscular dystrophy (DMD) and in the muscles of *mdx* "aged" mice, an animal model of DMD. However, only a handful of studies have investigated how the contractile properties of these morphologically deformed fibers differ from those of normal fibers in aged muscle. These studies have found an association between the extent of fiber branching and susceptibility to damage from eccentric contractions. They have also found that branched muscle fibers cannot sustain maximal contractions and that branch points are sites of increased mechanical stress. New imaging techniques like second harmonic imaging have revealed that the sub-cellular myofibrillar structure is greatly disturbed at branch points. These findings have important implications for understanding the function of dystrophin. It is commonly thought that dystrophin's role is to mechanically stabilise the sarcolemma, as numerous studies have shown that eccentric contractions damage dystrophic muscle more than normal muscle. However, the finding that branched fibers are mechanically weakened raises the question: Is it the lack of dystrophin, or is it the fiber branching, that leads to the vulnerability of dystrophic muscle to contractile damage? The other question is how the presence of these branched fibers alters the contractile properties of "aged" dystrophic muscle. Throughout this chapter I will use the term branched to describe the malformed fibers. Most earlier studies use the terminology "split fiber", but because it conjures up images of a Y-shaped bifurcation, with one adult fiber giving rise to two daughter fibers it is somewhat misleading as we now know many fibers, if not most display a complex syncytia of interconnecting branches. Some branches do not originate from the main fiber but are results of incomplete regeneration with myotubes fusing to repair the damaged adult fiber. Branching, I feel, is a more accurate description of the malformed fiber morphology. With respect to the branching terminology I am following the lead of Ontell & Feng, 1981 where they state "the term branched has been preferred because it describes an existing condition while the term split implies a mode formation. Unfortunately there is no immediate apparent substitute the terms parent and daughter". Readers can make up their own mind on the split verse branched question by examining morphology of fibers in the following chapter.

2. Evolutionary aspects of fiber branching

2.1 Fiber branching in crustacean proprioceptors

Even though in mammalian skeletal muscle fiber branching occurs during the regenerative process, there are a group of muscles that normally show fiber branching. These are the intrafusal muscle fibers found in muscle proprioceptors, muscle fibers specialized for their role of proprioception. In crustaceans, using confocal laser scanning and conventional light microscopy, the morphology and organization of the muscle fibers in a proprioceptor, the thoracic coxal muscle receptor organ (TCMRO), and the associated 'extrafusal' promoter muscle were investigated in two species of decapod crustacean, the crayfish *Cherax destructor* and the mud crab *Scylla serrata*. The diameter of the TCMROs was shown to increase distally, with an increase up to 350% recorded for the crayfish. The tapered shape of the crayfish TCMRO was demonstrated to amplify movements mechanically at the transducer region where the afferent nerves attach. Serial sectioning of the TCMROs, showed that the fiber number increased in the proximal to distal direction from 14 to 30 fibers in the crayfish and from 7 to 20 in the crab. Optical sectioning with laser scanning confocal microscope revealed that the increase in fiber numbers was the result of muscle fibers branching in the distal third section of the TCMRO Fig. 1.

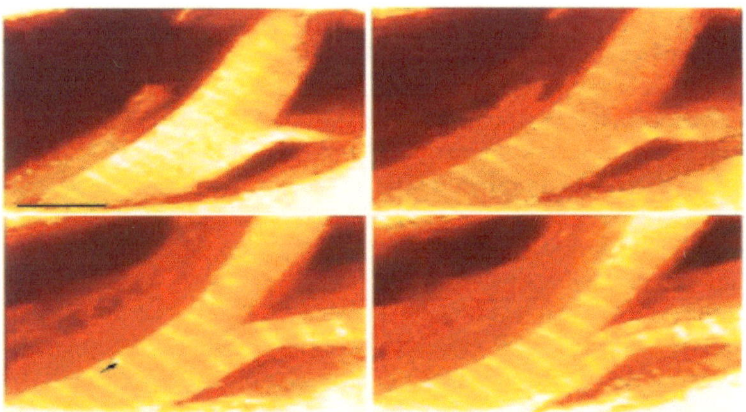

Fig. 1. Laser scanning confocal longitudinal sections of TCMROs from *Cherax destructor*. Fibers were stained with the F-actin binding dye phalloidin, conjugated with rhodamine, BODIPY, or fluorescein. —A. Preparation of a macerated crayfish TCMRO, showing a series of sections from the top of a single branched fiber stained with phalloidin/rhodamine through to the bottom section of the branch. Modified from Parkinson et al., 2001.

2.2 Fiber branching in mammalian proprioceptors

In the mammalian muscle spindle the intrafusal muscle fibers also exhibit branching, although it should be stressed that the evidence for this is not as strong as the case for crustacean propriorceptors. Vertebrate muscle spindle intrafusal fibers have been demonstrated to have the unique morphologies of the nuclear bag and nuclear chain fibers (Boyd, 1962). They are striated except for their central regions and branching has been reported in the central regions close to the area where the afferent nerve fibers originate (Barker & Gidumal, 1961). In the muscle spinal the branching of a small or intermediate fibers takes place over a distance of 60-90 micrometers. This largely occurs in the proximal pole or in the proximal part of the equatorial region of the muscle spindle. The two fibers produced may either taper off, or reunite in the distal pole or distal part of the equatorial region. The process of branching or reuniting is distinct from the condition where one fiber branches into two over a length of several hundred microns. Fig. 2 is a serial section from a mammalian muscle spindle and it clearly shows one fiber branching into two.

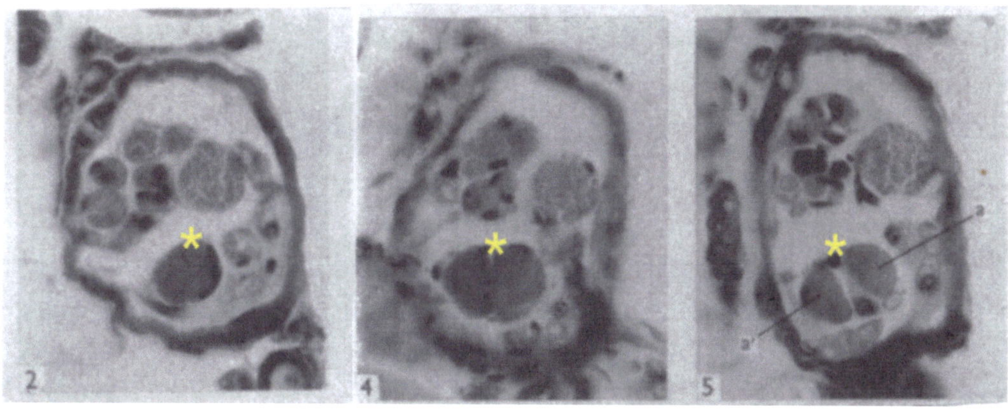

Fig. 2. Serial section through a single spindle from cat rectus femoris, the yellow * marks the position of a single intrafusal fiber as it branches into 2, in the first panel the diameter of the fiber is 11 micrometers. Serial transverse 12 micrometer paraffin sections stained with haematoxylin and eosin; numbers in the bottom left indicate the interval between segments. Modified from plate 2 in Barker & Gidumal, 1961.

2.2.1 What is the role of fiber branching in these systems?

In the crustacean receptor the tapered shape that results from fiber branching serves to amplify small movements, fine tuning the proprireceptor to respond to minor perturbations of its leg. However, overall it is tempting to speculate that fiber branching is protective and helps to protect the proprocepor intrafusal muscles from eccentric damages that occurs as a result of repeated eccentric length changes during locomotion.

3. What is a branched fiber?

A branched fiber is a skeletal muscle fiber composed of two or more cytoplasmically continuous strands. Some examples are shown in Fig.3 *B–F* and Fig.4. Branched fibers are demonstrable either by enzymatic muscle digestion (Head *et al.* 1990) or by reconstruction of serial cross-sections (Isaacs *et al.* 1973). Branching patterns vary greatly (Blaivas&Carlson, 1991;Tamaki *et al.* 1993), ranging from simple bifurcations (e.g. Fig. 3B) to complex, intertwining syncytia (e.g. Fig. 3E and Fig.4). Branched fibers have been found in muscular dystrophy (Swash & Schwartz, 1977; Ontell & Feng, 1981), in whole muscle transplants Fig.4 (Bourke & Ontell, 1984; Blaivas & Carlson, 1991), in muscles subjected to chemical or physical injury (Sadeh *et al.* 1985; Guti´errez *et al.* 1991) and in overloaded muscles undergoing hypertrophy (Hall-Craggs, 1970; Eriksson *et al.* 2006).

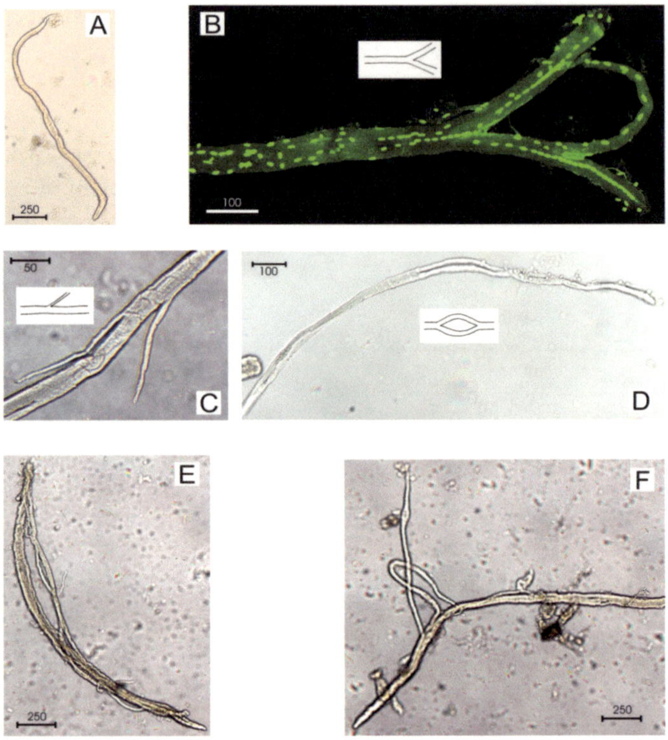

Fig. 3. **Examples of branched fibers.** Low power images of enzymatically dispersed single muscle fibers from EDL muscles of *mdx* mice. A, a morphologically normal, unbranched fiber. B, a branched fiber with bifurcations, imaged with confocal laser scanning microscopy and stained with ethidium bromide to highlight nuclei. Note the centrally located nuclei within the branches. C, a fiber with two small branches. D, a fiber that branches, then recombines. E, a fiber with highly complex branching patterns, forming an intertwining syncytium. F, another fiber with complex branching. Scale bar units are in microns. Modified from Chan *et al.*,2007.

3.1 How does branching occur?

Branching is most likely to result from the imperfect fusion of myogenic cells as they attempt to regenerate a fiber segment or complete fiber that has become necrotic (Schmalbruch, 1976; Ontell *et al.*1982). The association of branching with regeneration is evidenced by the frequent occurrence of centrally located nuclei in branched fibers (e.g. Fig. 3*B*; and see Schmalbruch, 1976; Ontell *et al.* 1982). Regenerating muscle has different functional characteristics from uninjured muscle. During regeneration, muscles display contractile differences such as reduced isometric force (Beitzel *et al.* 2004; Stupka *et al.* 2007; Iwata *et al.* 2010), longer twitch contraction and relaxation times (Beitzel *et al.* 2004; Stupka *et al.* 2007) and a dependence of contractility upon the extracellular Ca^{2+} concentration (Louboutin *et al.* 1996). Although branched fibers are a well-documented phenomenon of regenerating muscle, only a handful of studies have examined how their physiological properties may differ from those of morphologically normal fibers (Head *et al.* 1990, 1992, 2004; Chan *et al.* 2007; Lovering *et al.* 2009; Friedrich *et al.* 2010; Head, 2010).

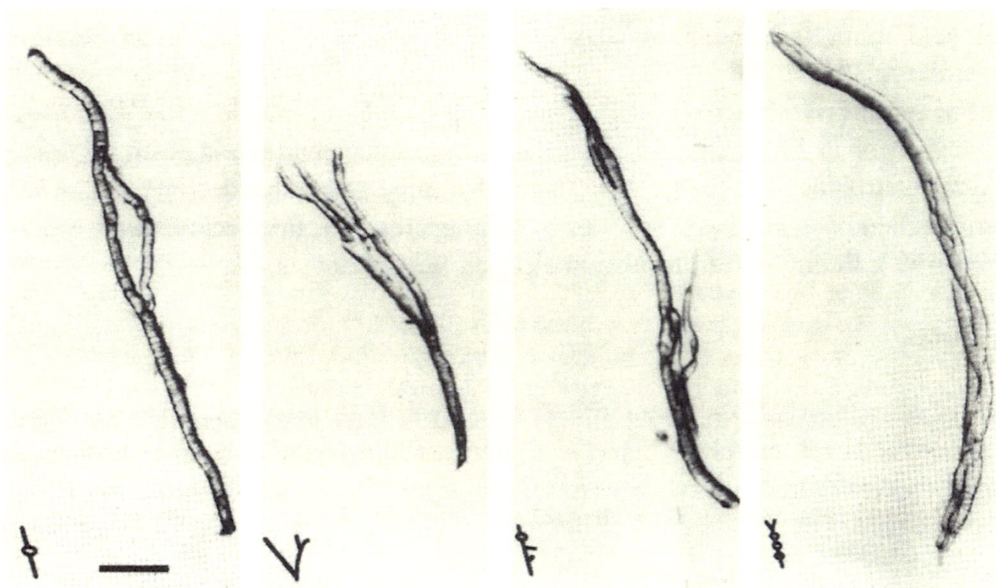

(a)

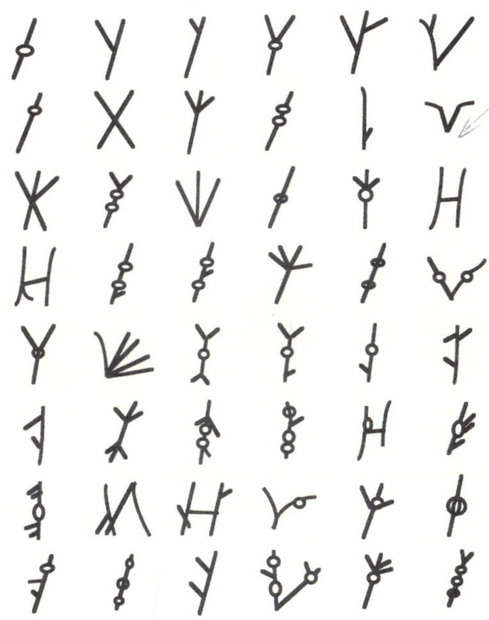

(b)

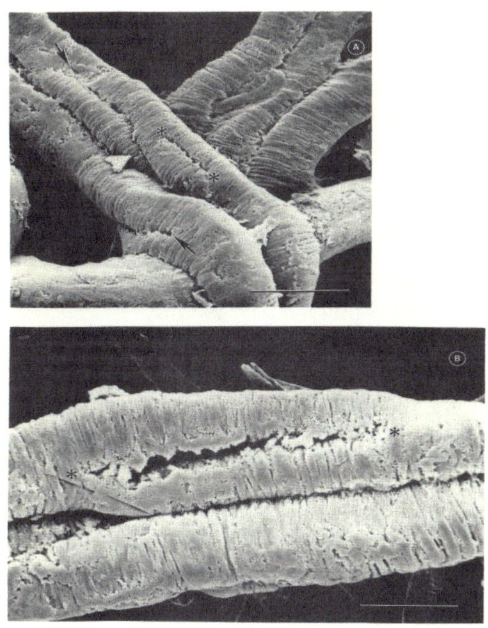

(c)

Fig. 4 A. LM pictures of dystrophin positive branched fibers form grafted rat muscle, the stick drawing in the bottom left of each panel represents the branch pattern. scale bar 100 micrometers. B. Patterns of branching encountered in the dystrophin positive grafted muscle. C. SEM of branched fibers, top panel arrows indicates branch points, * show a loop scale bar 100 micrometers. Bottom panel high magnification of loop shown by * in both panels Scale bar 50 micrometeres. Taken from Blaivas & Carlson, 1991.

3.1.1 Assessing intracellular continuity of branched fibers

It is essential to determine the actual boundaries of a single functional fiber to establish that these complex structures were not simply strong structural associations between more than one discrete cells. Intracellular continuity between the main body of the fibers and various appendages was assessed by a number of physiological techniques. The fluorescent dye, Lucifer Yellow, was ionophoresed into the intracellular environment of fibers (n = 9) of varying complexity at a single focal point. As is apparent in Fig. 5, Lucifer Yellow was able to diffuse from the point of injection to occupy the cytoplasm of all appendages of deformed fibers indicating that no barrier existed, at any junction within the fiber, to the internal diffusion of this dye. It was also possible to measure the resting membrane potential with an intracellular microelectrode at a number of locations in branches of deformed fibers. All values recorded from individual segments of a single, complex fiber were within a few millivolts, fiber depolarization, which was initiated with the impalement electrode, always lead to the contraction of all branches which constituted part of a single fiber. It was apparent, however, that the contraction of individual branches within a single fiber, as detected by video frame-by-frame analysis, was often unsynchronized, with some branches distal to the impalement electrode shortening before proximal branches (Head et al., 1990).

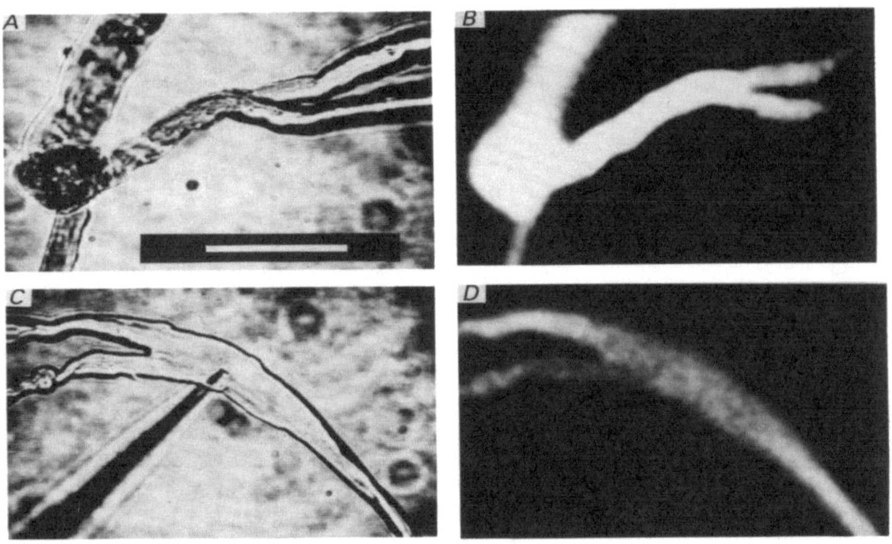

Fig. 5. Fluorescence images (B and D) of single intact dystrophic soleus muscle fibers (A and C). In each case in A & C an intracellular microelectrode was used to inject the dye just above the branch point, In C the tapering shadow of the electrode can be seen delivering dye. Scale bar 80 micrometers. From Head et al., 1990.

3.2 Do branched fibers exist in the intact muscle?

The early evidence for the presence of branched fibers within the skeletal muscle relied on reconstructing serial sections. In recent times collagenase has been used to digest the muscle so that entire isolated single fibers can be viewed, Head *et al.*, 1990 were among the first groups to apply this to mouse muscle, where it is now a key physiological tool worldwide. This has advanced our understanding of branched fiber physiology because it has allowed the visualisation from tendon to tendon of the entire extent of branching in a fiber. It has also enabled contractile physiology experiments to be carried out on branched fibers. It has been suggested that fiber branching may be an artefact of the enzyme digestion technique, although it is hard to explain why we do not see branching in normal muscle! Given the importance of this point a study was undertaken in my laboratory using confocal laser scanning microscopy to examine branched fibers *in situ*, as they lay within the muscle. This involves fixing the muscle in formalin and then dehydrating the muscle in an alcohol series, before finally clearing the tissue with methyl salicylate. Before fixation a micro electrode had been used to fill 2 to 3 fibers within the muscle with the marker dye Lucifer yellow. The auto-fluorescence of the fibers was such that it was possible to imaging all muscle fibers *in situ* in the muscle Fig 6. Interestingly in fibers with simple Y-shaped bifurcating branches, both branches are aligned along the longitudinal axis of the muscle Fig. 6 B&D. These *in situ* pictures of dystrophic muscle fibers are also interesting because with they have caught branched fibers which have been damaged and are undergoing necrosis Fig 6. E&F. (from Head et al., 1992)

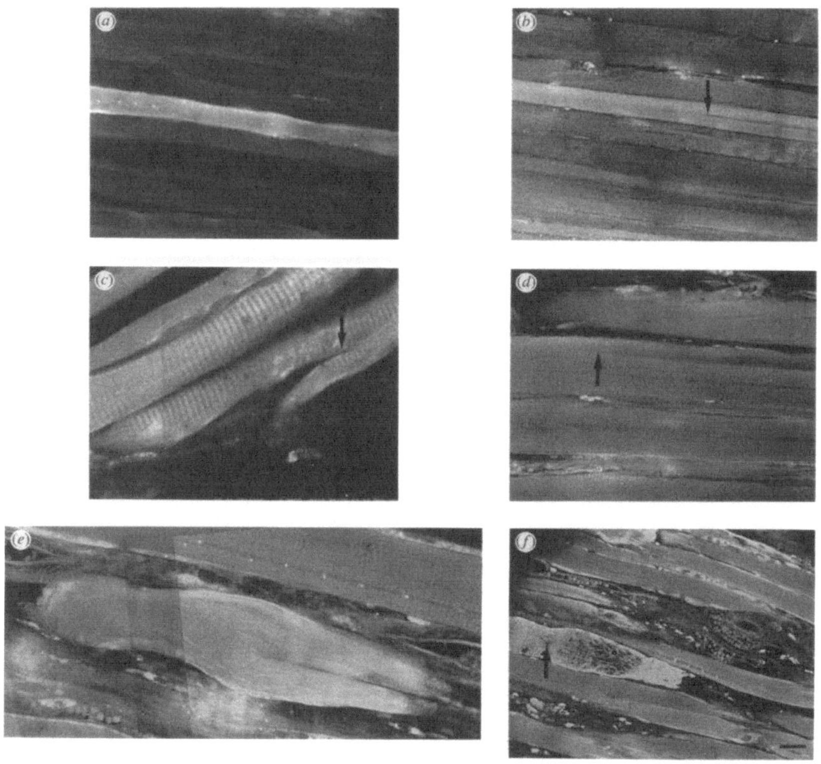

Fig. 6. Confocal laser scanning micrographs showing muscle fibers in the muscle. (a). A single EDL fiber filled with Lucifer Yellow, note the surrounding fibers are visible because they are auto-fluorescence. (b) Further along this same fiber a clear branch is evident (arrow). (c) Auto-fluorescence image from an FDB muscle showing a fiber branching at the at the attachment to the tendon(arrow). (d). A soleus fiber which branches into 2 asymmetrically with a large and small daughter branch (arrow). (e) A deformed EDL muscle fiber which is in the process of pathologically hyper-contracting and has detached from the tendons.(f) a necrotic soleus muscle fiber. Scale bar (all are scaled in relation to the bar bottom right on panel (f)) in micrometers: (a,b), 30; (c), 10; (d), 15; (e),15; (f), 30. From Head et al., 1992.

3.2.1 Myofibrillar micro branching within a muscle fiber

Friedrichs group has utilised a novel biological imaging technique which allows the microarchitecture of the myofibers in single muscle fibers to be visualised. Using their recently developed technique of second harmonic imaging they have elegantly demonstrated that in old *mdx* mice the myofibrils within muscle fibers are deformed, bifurcating into Y shaped branches which they term verniers Fig.7. Even in dystrophic fibers which appear to be macroscopically unbranched i.e. are straight fibers similar to those seen in control animals, the myofibrils branch into Y shaped verniers which are misaligned with the longitudinal axis of the fiber. The myofibril malformations in branched fibers are even more marked. Friedrich *et al.* 2010 have calculated that this alteration in the microarchitecture of the dystrophic fibers has a deleterious effect on the force output. From a biophysical standpoint because neighbouring sarcomere activation would be unsynchronized, myofibril misorientations in single mdx fibers can partly explain the decreased force in *mdx* muscle. Their image analysis provides the first quantitative estimate of an ultrastructure relate force deficit in *mdx* fibers. This deficit will vary among individual fibers, depending on the degree of myofibril twisting and local angle deviations. The force deficit is also inhomogeneous within fibers, depending on whether additional branches are present or not. They found normalized cosine angle deviations of up to 20% from the long axis that would not contribute to force output from the dystrophic muscle fiber (Friedrich et al., 2010).

3.2.2 Friedrich summarised

In the dystrophinopathies it is apparent that all the myofibrils are not pulling together and this worsens as the animal ages. As the force vectors are not aligned along the longitudinal axis the tendon doesn't get all the tension you would expect from the cross section of myofibrils. In effect the muscle is wasting energy because the cross bridges are working, burning up ATP, but the force is not being transmitted to the tendons.

4. Do branched fibers occur in human muscle disease especially DMD?

In recent years my laboratory and several others around the world, have used the *mdx* mouse model of DMD to demonstrate the importance of branched muscle fibers in the pathophysiology of dystrophic muscle function. One of the critiques of this work has been "YES, but does this phenomenon occur in boys with DMD, and also does it occur in other human myopathies?" The answer to these questions is a resounding "YES"!

4.1 Evidence for branched fibers in human dystrophy

In the 1970s and 1980s there was a large amount of detailed histological work carried out on human tissue. This work demonstrated unequivocally that branched fibers are present in DMD and other human myopathies. In fact the importance of fiber branching in human muscle diseases was the subject of an editorial in the Lancet in March 25, 1978 pp.646; *Muscle Fiber Splitting_ A Reappraisal*. Because of the importance of this question, i.e. does the *mdx* mouse model of fiber branching makes a good model for human DMD, in this section I am going to review the evidence that demonstrates that fiber branching is a major factor in DMD and also other human myopathies.

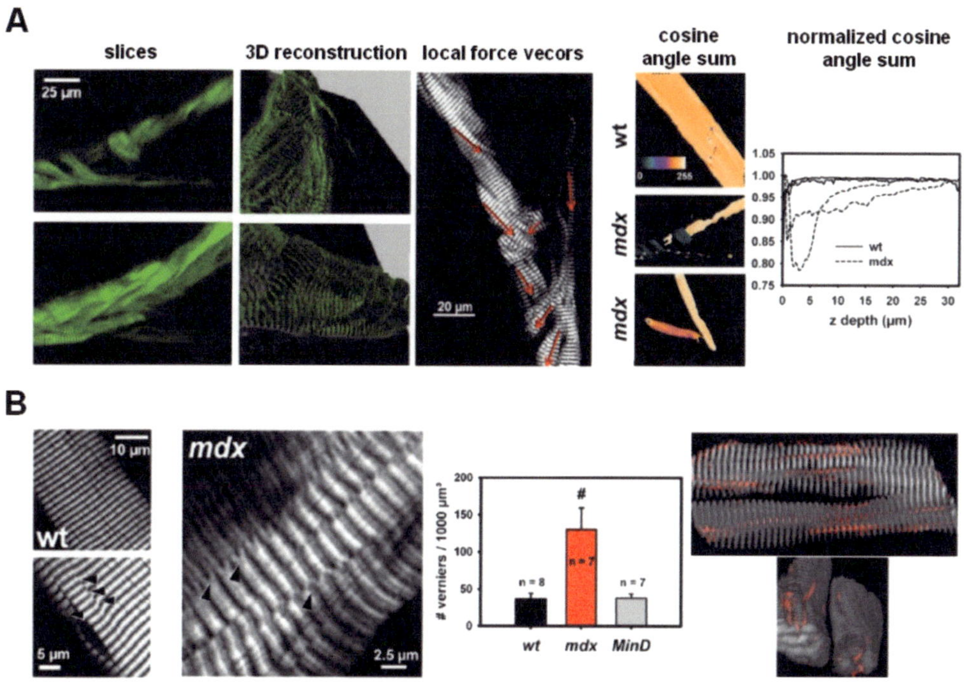

Fig. 7. SHG-microscopy reveals vastly altered sarcomere ultrastructure in intact single mdx fibers. **A,** example slices and 3D reconstruction of an *mdx* fiber (12 mo) show tilted myofibril geometry suggesting misorientated local force vectors. The degree of force drop from the geometry was quantified with gradient filter masks. The cosine angle sum is close to unity within wt single fibers (myofibrils run parallel) and reduced ~20 % in *mdx* fibers. **B,** magnified images show local disruptions of the sarcomere pattern ('verniers'). Their number is vastly increased in *mdx* but close to wt levels in minidystrophin (MinD) fibers. In *mdx* fibers, verniers run in streaks through the fiber centre (From Friedrich et al., 2010.).

4.1.1 The long history of branched fiber reports in human dystrophies

In humans fiber branching was first reported in boys with DMD by Erb in 1891, closely followed by Krosing in 1892. In the 20th century there have been reports by Greenfield *et al.* 1957; Adams *et al.* 1962; Pearce & Walton 1962; Bell and Conen 1968; Schwartz *et al.* 1976; Swash *et al.* 1977; Schmalbruch 1984 and Hamida *et al.* 1992.

4.2 Regenerated fibers in DMD: A serial section study by Schmalbruch (1984)

Fig. 8 shows a cross-section from two patients with Duchenne muscular dystrophy. Due to the importance of this result the 2 figures have been scanned and retain their orininal figure numbers and legend. They will be referred to as Figure1'and Figure 2'. In each case a sample cross-section from each patient is shown in the first panel while the second panel shows a reconstruction 6 mm long and from these cross-sections. In order to produce this very detailed reconstruction, 1200 sections were obtained from the 6 mm biopsy. Then every 10th section was photographed at X350. From these prints he reconstructed the fibers shown in the second panels. This rigorous approach allows the reconstruction of branched fibers and shows how they positioned *in situ* in the human muscle. This elegant study was one of the

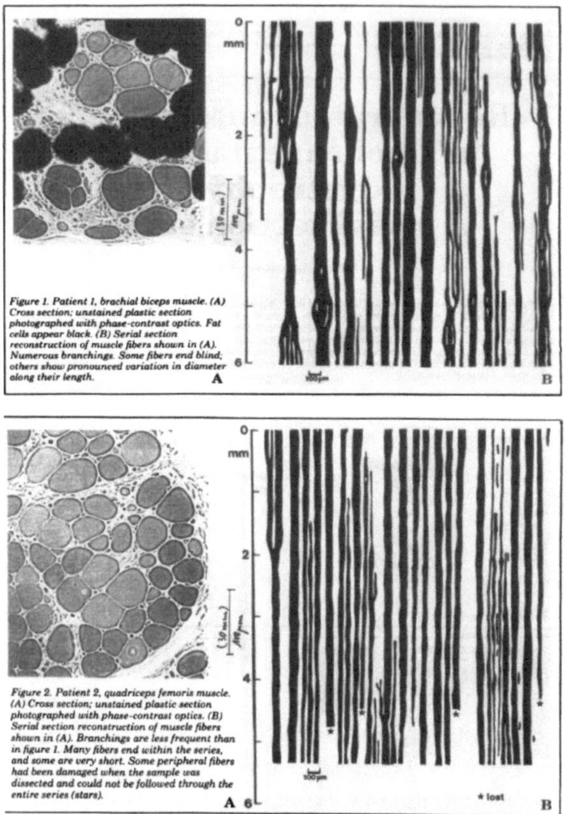

Fig. 8. Copied from Schmalbruch (1984) Figure 1 & 2.

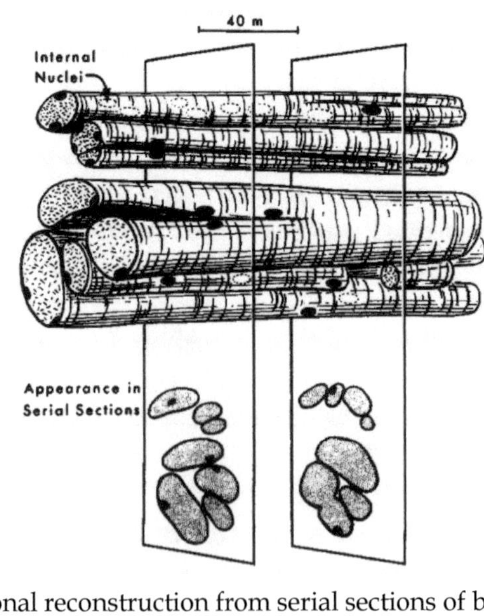

Fig. 8. A three-dimensional reconstruction from serial sections of branched fibers in DMD copied from Bell & Conen 1968.

first to link the degree of fiber branching to the severity of the disease. Patient one Figure 1′ was clinically more severely affected than patient two Figure 2′, the creating kinase level was higher and the biopsy specimen was heavily infiltrated with fat. As can clearly be seen patient one Figure 1B′had a much higher degree of fiber branching.

4.2.1 Branched fibers in samples from 84 boys with Ducehenne muscular dystrophy

In another landmark study Bell & Conen 1968, obtained muscle biopsies from 84 DMD patients and control samples from a further 72 children. All of the control fibers showed predominantly normal histological features. All of the samples from the 84 DMD boys showed branching. Fig.8. illustrates branched fibers serially reconstructed from cross-sections.

4.2.2 branched fibers occur in other human muscle diseases

It's not only in DMD that we see branched fibers, they are present in many other myopathies (Swash & Schwartz 1977). demonstrates. Fig. 9 is taken from that paper to show some serial sections taken from the quadriceps of a patient suffering from Kugelberg-Welander disease of at least 10 years duration. This is a very nice illustration in humans of a large fiber separating into three apparently separate fibers, but of course we know that the three separate "daughter" fibers actually branch from a common trunk. Interestingly this panel also illustrates a commonly observed phenomena associated with fiber branching that is the presence of a "sentinel" nuclei near the membrane invagination at the stem of the branch

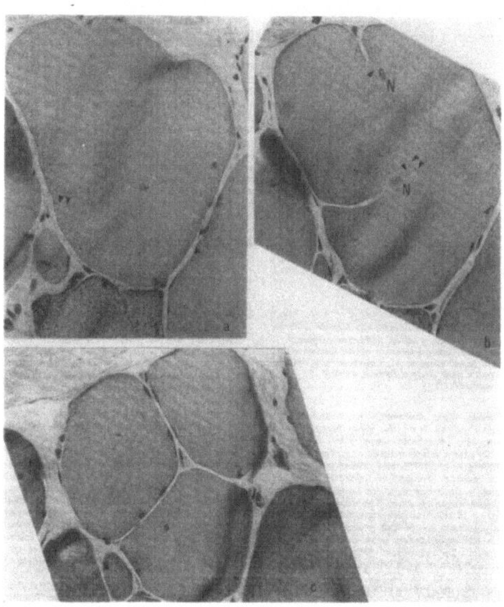

Fig. 9. Serial section of quadriceps. Arrows=branch formation, Kugelberg-Welander disease H&E X 560.(a) One complete large fiber 250 micrometer in diameter.(b) 22 micrometers from (a) two clefts associated with central nuclei (N); (C) 70 micrometers from (a) the fiber has branched into three daughter fibers. From Swash & Schwartz 1977.

In this paper they also demonstrated fiber branching in Charcot-Marie-Tooth syndrome. In humans fiber branching has also been reported in poliomyelitis, motor neuron disease and limb girdle dystrophies.

4.2.3 Is fiber branching a compensatory respose to muscle loss?

Swash and Schwartz 1977 proposed that fiber branching represents a compensatory mechanism whereby the number of fibers and the overall mass of the diseased muscle is increased. This is a very teleological explanation and nowadays one I think that can be discounted in light of new information we have regarding the fact that fiber branching represents misguided skeletal muscle regeneration.

4.2.4 Some observations on branch formation in human myopahties

The paper by Schwartz *et al.*, 1976, throws further light on the role of the nucleus in fiber branching. They used the electron microscope to look at early phase fiber branching and found that a zone of separation of myofibrils was often in close relation to a central nucleus. This zone consisted of granular cytoplasm containing glycogen granules and myofibrillar debris. Present, in nearly all cases, near the boundary of the dividing edge were large mitochondria and pinocytotic vesicles. In fact the membrane forming the dividing branch point seemed to be derived from the membrane formed during the extrusion of material by these pinocytotic vesicles. These observations require further investigation in order to understand the mechanisms involved.

4.2.5 Is there a fiber type bias for branching?

Several of these human studies have noted that the branching appears to affect type slow I fibers more commonly than their fast type II cousins. Studies on the *mdx* mouse also show that fiber branching is most prevalent in slow muscle (Head *et al.*,1992). This is an area which merits more investigation.

4.3 Microneurography studies on single human dystrophic muscle fibers

In humans branched fibers have complicated the interpretation of microneurography results obtained from patients with dystrophinopathies. Studies in Duchenne and Becker dystrophy by Stalberg 1977 and Hilton-Brown & Stalberg, 1983 have shown substantially increased fiber density. While typical multiple spike potentials have greatly increased duration there is also an increase in the duration of the mean interspike interval, these findings reflect an increased fiber size variation. Also there are occurrences of simultaneous blocking of two or more single muscle fiber action potentials in a multiple spike potential which is thought to be due to transmission failure at a neuromuscular junction of a muscle fiber branch. The increased fiber density reported in DMD and Becker dystrophy is at first site an apparent contradiction to the known loss of muscle fibers from the motor units in these conditions. However, the contradiction is resolved because the increased fiber density was interpreted to arise as a result of fiber branching. Each branch of a multiply branched fiber gives rise to a separate action potential, indistinguishable from true single muscle fiber action potentials; however, they are identified by a low jitter between action potentials. Thus the split fibers may account for a significant part of the increase fiber density in muscular dystrophy (Hilton-Brown et al., 1985).

5. Whole muscle and skinned fibers experiments show the susceptibility of branch points to damage

Enzymatically digesting soleus and EDL muscles from old *mdx* mice revealed that > 90% of fibers had some degree of branching, confirming numerous previous studies on dystrophic muscle (Isaacs 1973; Ontell & Feng, 1981; Bourke & Ontell, 1984; Schmalbruch 1984; Head et al 1990;1992; Tamaki et al. 1993; Pastoret & Sebille1995; Lefaucheur et al. 1995; Schafer et al. 2005; Bockhold et al. 1998; Chan et al. 2007; Lovering et al. 2009; Friedrich et al. 2010, Head, 2010). It seems clear that these branches occur as part of the regenerative process in *mdx* muscles (Blaveri et al 1999). If the enzymatically isolated branched fibers are suspended in a high relaxing solution (50mM EGTA) then they can be manipulated under a dissecting microscope so that they can be attached to a force transducer in various configurations; i.e. with or without a branch between the attachment points. It is also possible to liberate single fibers from eccentrically damaged muscle and probe them with the membrane impermeable dye, Evans blue, to see where the membrane integrity has been compromised. In skinned fiber experiments the absence of the sarcolemma removes any contribution played by the presence or absence of dystrophin to the stability of the surface sarcolemma. This is because dystrophin, if present on the inner surface of the sarcolemma, is removed with the membrane. When a fiber was activated (>50% of max) with a branch point between the attachment points, in the majority of cases it broke: when the unbranched portion of the same fiber was reattached to the transducer, the unbranched segment could generate a normal force/pCa curve Fig. 10Ai/ii. (and see; Head et al.,1990; 2010)

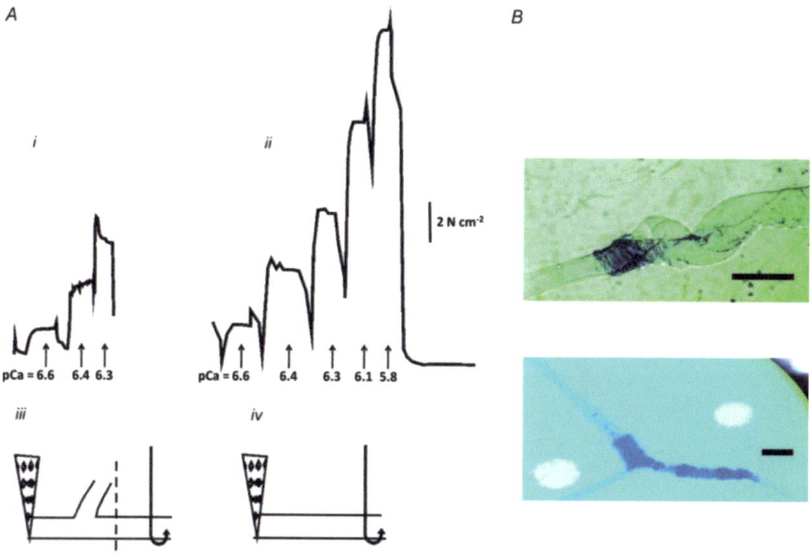

Fig. 10. *A*, generation of force-pCa curves in a branched EDL fiber from an *mdx* mouse. Top traces are the force-pCa curves, with each peak representing the force developed by the fiber at a certain value of pCa (i.e. $-\log10[Ca^{2+}]$). The $[Ca^{2+}]$ was progressively increased until maximal force was reached or until the fiber broke. The schematic drawings below each force-pCa curve indicate how the fiber was tied when generating that curve. When the fiber was tied as shown in *Aiii*, with a branch point between the sites of attachment, the fiber broke before reaching maximal activation (*Ai*). When the main trunk was retied as shown in *Aiv*, with no intervening branches, a full force-pCa curve was obtained (*Aii*). *B*, two fibers from eccentrically contracted EDL muscle from an *mdx* mouse, showing uptake of Evans Blue dye at branch points. Scale bar represents 50 μm in upper picture, 30 μm in lower picture.(From Head, 2010).

When old *mdx* muscles were subjected to a moderate eccentric contraction (a contraction which caused no damage in age matched controls or young mdx with less than 10% branched fibers) the branched fibers were damaged at a branch point, fig. 10B shows examples of two branched enzymatically liberated fibers from the eccentrically contracted muscle. Evans blue will only penetrate damaged membrane and it is clear in this figure that the Evans blue uptake is in the vicinity of the branch points. These experiments support the hypothesis that it is the mechanical architecture of the fiber branches which weakens the fiber Fig. 10.

6. Reduced life span of mdx mice

Surprisingly there has been a misrepresentation in the literature to the effect that *mdx* mice have a normal lifespan. It's time to put this myth to rest, there have been several publications clearly demonstrating that *mdx* mice have a significantly reduced lifespan (Pastoret & Sebille 1995a,b; Lefaucheur, *et al.*, 1995). Most recently Chamberlain *et al.*, 2007 looking very old mice demonstrated a significantly reduced lifespan in both male and female *mdx* mice Fig. 11.

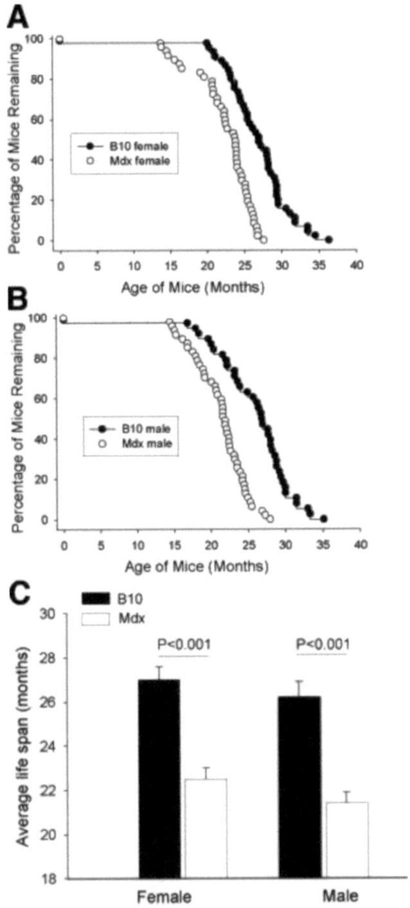

Fig. 11. Life span analysis for wild-type and mdx male and female mice. Graphs showing the age at death for the female (A) and male (B) mice. Circles denote the age at which each animal died. C) Histogram showing the average age at death of male and female wild-type (C57BL/10) and *mdx* mice. The average life span between wild-type and *mdx* males and between wild-type and *mdx* females was highly significant, as shown. From Chamberlain *et al.*, 2007.

They also noted as might be expected, that 24 month wild-type diaphragm muscles displayed no morphological abnormalities while aged matched *mdx* diaphragm showed a large degree of fibrotic infiltration and loss of muscle fibers. It is commonly accepted in the field that the diaphragm is the muscle with clinical features most similar to DMD. However, importantly and in direct contradiction to publications reporting that *mdx* muscle limb muscle do not display a DMD morphology, they noted they the *mdx* muscles displayed typical dystrophic features at each age examined. The dystrophic features included centrally located myofibers, necrotic fibers, small calibre regenerating fibers, moderate amounts of fibrosis, and some fatty infiltration. By 26 months of age fibrosis and fatty ill filtration were extreme. For example, they note increased necrosis fibrosis and adipocyte accumulation in the 26 months soleus compared with the same muscle group at 4 months. Interestingly they highlight the slow-twitch soleus as the most morphologically dystrophic limb muscle in the *mdx* mouse at any age. This correlates with early findings from my laboratory that the soleus muscle is the first to display extensive branching in the *mdx* mouse and reports (see section 4.2.5) that it is type I slow-twitch muscle fibers in humans which are most likely to be branched.

6.1 Aged mdx mice are an excellent model for Duchenne muscular dystrophy

Aged *mdx* mice represent the most advanced dystrophic condition that can be generated as a result of dystrophin deficiency in a small mammal model. The aged mouse phenotype resembles late stage DMD (Gregorevic et al., 2008). As detailed in this section the assumption that *mdx* skeletal muscle does not show dystrophic changes is because most of these studies were carried out on young animals of less than three months of age, when the dystrophic phenotype has not fully developed.

6.2 The main age related dystrophic change in the *mdx* mouse is the formation of branched fibers

The major skeletal muscle changes that you see with age in the *mdx* mouse is an increase in the number of branched fibers, both in the number of branched fibers present within the muscle and the number of branches on an individual muscle fiber (Head *et al.*, 1992; Tamaki *et al.*, 1993; Bockhold *et al.*, 1998; Chan *et al.*, 2007; Lovering *et al.*, 2009; Friedrich *et al.*, 2010; Head 2010). Since branched mature myofibers are not present at the time of onset of clinical symptoms, they must be formed as a secondary consequence of the absence of dystrophin Fig. 12.

6.2.1 Contractile abnormalities of aged muscles with branched fibers

Numerous studies have shown that old *mdx* dystrophin deficient skeletal muscles resembles the DMD phenotype, due to space constraints only a selection is given here, (Pastoret & Sebille,1995; Lefaucheur *et al.*, 1995; Lynch *et al.*, 2001; Chan *et al.*, 2007; Claflin & Brooks, 2008; Lovering *et al.*, 2009; Friedrich *et al.*, 2010; Head,2010; Mouisel *et al.*, 2010; Wooddell *et al.*, 2010; Hakim *et al.*, 2011). Old *mdx* muscles generate less specific force and are more easily damaged by mild eccentric contractions when compared with young *mdx* dystrophin deficient muscles.

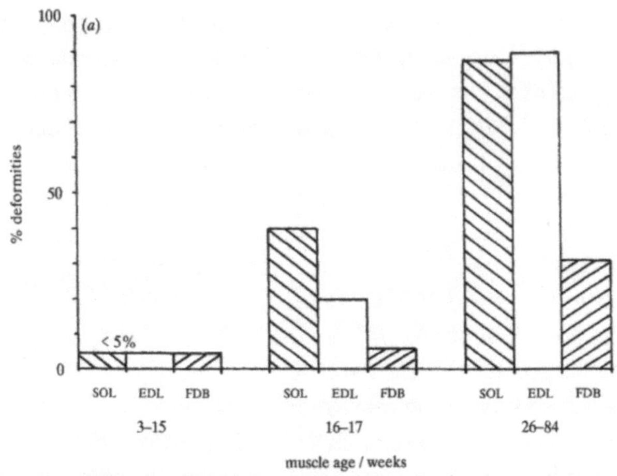

Fig. 12. Percentage of fibers with branched in different age groups of mdx mice, From Head et al., 1992.

6.2.2 Both young and old mdx muscle lack dystrophin so why should old mdx be more susceptible to damage? We know its not aging per se

So the primary question is; given dystrophin is absent from both young and old muscles, why is absence of dystrophin linked to major membrane damage only in old muscles? My laboratory has carried out a key study in this field (Chan *et al.,* 2007). We developed a mild eccentric contraction protocol which had no significant effect on normal muscle. When this contraction protocol was carried out on young *mdx*, there was no difference compared to young age matched controls. When the same contraction protocol was given to aged *mdx* where over 80% of the muscle fibers were extensively branched then there was a massive 60% drop in force. My thesis and the theme of this chapter is: The drop of force is not due to an absence of dystrophin, but is due to the presence of branched fibers. Wooddell *et al.,* 2010 exercised young and old *mdx* mice and compare the degree of muscle damage by the use of the membrane impermeable dye Evans blue. Evans blue is only taken up by damaged cells. There was significant threefold increase of dye uptake only in old *mdx* mice 12 to 19 month of age. Young *mdx* mice were not affected and there was little dye uptake. They also confirm this finding by measuring the creating kinase levels (a marker of muscle damage) which was only significantly elevated in old *mdx* mice. Once again it has been shown branched fibers are mechanically weak and more easily damaged when they contract (Chan *et al.,* 2007; Friedrich *et al.,* 2010; Head *et al.,* 1990,1992; Head 2010; Lovering *et al.,* 2009;). So it is reasonable to conclude that Wooddell *et al.,* 2010 results are explained by the presence of branched fibers in the old *mdx*. It must be emphasised that other factors such as age and absence of dystriophin have been taken into account and do not play a major role.

6.2.3 Even when not damaged old mdx muscles generate less force and power

Lynch *et al.,* 2001 showed differences in the effect of age on structure-function relationships of limb muscles of *mdx* mice compared to control mice. They demonstrated that limb muscles from 24- to 28-month-old *mdx* mice are smaller and weaker with lower normalised force and power; once again age matched studies showed that this was not an ageing phenomenon but was due to the disease process. These findings were supported and extended by Mouisel *et al.*, 2010. Given that both young and old *mdx* lack dystrophin I propose that the force and power deficits are due to the presence of branched fibers. It has been shown that the architecture of the branched fiber compromises the coordinated activation of the fiber in the longitudinal axis of the muscle fiber (Friedrich et al., 2010; Head, 2010)

7. Branched fibers in other systems are also susceptible to damage: Lamininopathies and regeneration in normal tissue

The129/ReJ dy/dy mouse lacks laminin-alpha-2 and has a severe muscular dystrophy phenotype. It shares three fundamental characteristics with Duchenne muscular dystrophy; progressive and severe muscle weakness, progressive degeneration and disappearance of skeletal muscle with a massive degree of fibrosis and increased serum activity of sarcoplasmic enzymes (Rowland, 1985). In some respects it is a superior functional mouse model for DMD. By three months of age animals are unable to use their hind legs. Enzyme digests have demonstrated the presence of extensive complexed fiber branching in limb muscles in the laminopathies (Head *et al.*, 1990, 2004).

7.1 Skinned fiber studies in the dy/dy mouse show branched fiber weakness

In an early study we utilised the skin fiber technique to tie up single branched fibers on the force transducer, such that a branch was between the connection points, the large majority of cases the these fibers broke at a branch point. Importantly the muscle fiber was not itself intrinsically weak in itself because when the same broken fiber was retied with no branch between the points of attachment fibers could sustain maximal force development (Head et al., 1990).

7.1.1 Intact dy/dy muscles cannot sustain isometric stimulation and the subsequent force drop is directly connected to the number of branched fibers lost

When these branched fibers were present in the intact muscle and the isolated muscle stimulated repeatedly with maximal isometric contractions then the muscle force loss was around 35% (after allowing for the effects of fatigue and in comparison to age matched controls). Because of large amounts of connective tissue present in the dy/dy mouse enzyme digests were particularly successful and it proved possible to view almost the entire population of fibers after digestion. This facilitated the very important discovery that after repeated isometric stimulation there was a 35% drop of force and this force loss was correlated with a 40% loss of branched fibers (Head et al., 1990)!

8. Passive properties of mdx mice, if you stretch an old mdx muscle it pulls apart

In the most recent publication on the effect of age on the *mdx* mouse Hakim *et al.*, 2011 looked at the passive properties of fast-twitch edl muscle in two month old mice compared with 20 months old *mdx* mice. What they did to the EDL was to passively stretch it, i.e. the muscle was not contracting actively, and look at the effect on muscle integrity. Surprisingly when they gave the muscle a very large stretch from 110% Lo to 160% Lo; in 2 month old mdx mice a partial tear was observed only at the proximal end of the muscle, at 6 months of age there was some separation across the entire muscle belly, although there were still substantial attachment and finally in 14 and 20 month old *mdx* mice the muscle simply pulled apart. The important point here is that the damage in age matched control was minimal! It is instructive to compare this finding with results from my laboratory which show a strong correlation in the degree of eccentric contraction damage and the age related increase in branched fibers and the increased complexity of the branching (Chan *et al.* 2007). Once again it is important to bear in mind that both the young and old *mdx* mouse lack dystrophin, and the age matched control animals demonstrated age in itself is not a significant factor. So logically it is reasonable to infer that some other disease process, which increases with age, is causing the muscle weakness in the aged dystrophin deficient *mdx* mouse. The branched fibers are the obvious, and I would suggest, the only candidate to account for the age related increase in susceptibility to damage in dystrophinopathies.

9. Young muscles are not unaffected by the absence of dystrophin

This chapter focuses on old *mdx* muscle and branched fibers, however, I do not wish to imply that young dystrophin deficient non-branched muscle fibers are normal. As I detail in the final section of this chapter the hypothesis is that muscular dystrophy is a two-stage process. In the first stage in the dystrophinopathies, around the time when the animal starts to use their skeletal muscles, there is a rise in cytosolic calcium which acts as a trigger for fiber necrosis. This starts the cycle of degeneration and regeneration which produces the branched fiber phenotype. Initially it was thought absence of dystrophin weakened the sarcolemma and when the muscle was activated micro-tears appeared allowing a pathological influx of calcium. Most current research shows that this explanation was too simplistic and not supported by experimental data. It now seems clear that dystrophin plays a role in organizing and aggregating ion channels in the membrane.

9.1 The role of free radicals, stretched activated ion channels and calcium in dystrophic damage

Eccentric contraction studies on non-branched dystrophic fibers showed that there was a long time delay between the contraction and subsequent increase in intracellular calcium (see Allen & Whitehead, 2010 for a review). If the muscle membrane simply ripped then the calcium would go up immediately, as is the case in branched fibers, where the contraction induced damage leads to an almost instantaneous explosive rise in intracellular calcium (Head, 2010). A similar argument applies to the proposal that the dystrophic membrane contains population of abnormal stretch activated channels, in this case you would predict that the calcium would rise as soon as the muscle is stretched, the significant delay allows this mechanism to be discounted. However, blocking the stretch activated channel does prevent he delayed rise in intracellular calcium, so clearly they do have a role to play (see Allen *et al.*, 2010 for a review). So what's happening? It seems stretching the dystrophic muscle causes a higher than normal free radical oxygen production and it is these free ROS molecules that activated the stretch activated channels allowing the delayed influx of calcium to occur (Whitehead *et al.*, 2006). This calcium triggers fiber necrosis, followed by regeneration producing branched fibers. The branched fibers are mechanically weak and as mentioned before strong activation will directly allow calcium to rush in through membrane ruptures.

10. Dystrophinopatheis a 2 stage pathology: The importance of branched fibers in the aetiology of muscular dystrophy

I propose that the skeletal muscle pathophysiology of the dystrophinopathies is a twofold process see Fig. 13. Initially, before the animal becomes mobile the muscle fibers are normal in appearance, although the plasma creating kinase is elevated. There are several studies on the *mdx* mouse which show that if muscles are immobilised either by denervation or mechanically using rods or a cast, dystrophic changes do not occur in the muscle (see for example; Mokhtarian et al., 1999). So the absence of dystrophin is thought to either weaken the membrane and/or alter the activity of membrane ion channels. The alteration of stretch activated ion channels is mediated by abnormal free radical formation that occurs during dystrophic muscle contraction. This first stage leads to muscle fiber degeneration and initiates a cycle of degeneration and regeneration which results in the accumulation branched fibers. Branched fibers are mechanically compromised and cannot sustain the normal stresses and strains of everyday contraction. It is the presence of these branched fibers which terminally weaken the muscle.

10.1 Implications for the pathogenesis of Duchenne muscular dystrophy

The fact that fiber branching in itself can increase muscle damage during eccentric contractions challenges our current understanding of dystrophin's function as a mechanical and ion channel stabiliser of the sarcolemma. It has important implications for our understanding of the progression of dystrophin-deficient muscular dystrophy.

10.2 The branch initiating dystrophic event in straight fibers

The initiating event that triggers fiber necrosis in *mdx* mice must occur while the fibers are still unbranched, as branching results from regeneration following necrosis. Hence, to ascertain the function of dystrophin, it is necessary to study fibers before they become branched. The studies mentioned in this chapter which found greater force deficits for *mdx* mice compared with wild-types all used mice which were older than 6-8 weeks, at which age it is known that 17% of fibers are already branched (Chan *et al.*, 2007). Thus not clear whether they are examining the primary pathological event, or the downstream consequences, resulting from a loss of dystrophin. Any supposed mechanical weakness resulting from an absence of dystrophin is confounded by the mechanical weakness resulting from fiber branching. It is just as likely that the initiating event is an influx of Ca^{2+} through malfunctioning ion channels (Carlson, 1998), rather than contraction-induced damage to a mechanically compromised sarcolemma. Several classes of ion channels, reviewed in Allard, 2006, have been observed to function abnormally in mdx muscle fibers. It has been proposed that Ca^{2+} entering through these channels activates enzyme mediated cell damage pathways, leading to fiber necrosis. Another class of ion channel that may allow excessive Ca^{2+} influx is stretch-activated channels, which may be abnormally activated in *mdx* fibers through mechanisms involving reactive oxygen species (ROS) (Allen *et al.*, 2010; Allen & Whitehead, 2010).

My argument may be summarised in the flowchart in Fig. 13. We envisage dystrophinopathy in the *mdx* mouse as a two-stage process. The immediate consequences of losing dystrophin's normal functions might be referred to for simplicity as a "primary stage" in which the loss of dystrophin initiates muscle damage, in the absence of any pre-existing fiber deformity. The regenerated fibers formed during the primary stage are branched. It is the progressive increase of branching which initiates the secondary stage. In the secondary stage the branched fibers are mechanically weak and damage in this terminal phase enters into a positive feedback loop.

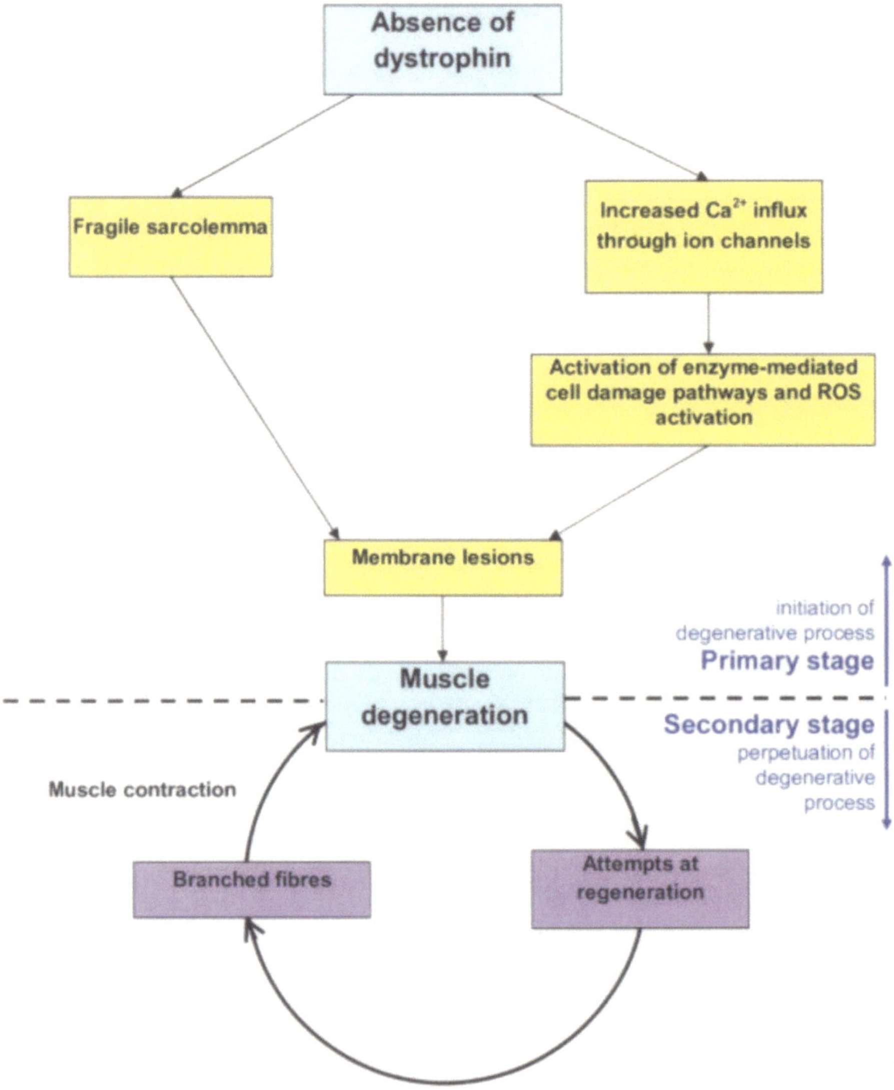

Fig. 13. **Proposed pathogensis of dystrophinopathy in *mdx* mice.** The primary effects of dystrophin's absence could be either a mechanical weakening of the sarcolemma (*left*) or an influx of Ca^{2+} through malfunctioning ion channels (*right*). Whatever the mechanism, muscle degeneration ensues. The secondary stage is a cycle in which attempted regeneration produces branched fibers, which are structurally compromised and easily damaged by contractile activity, resulting in further degeneration. In this scheme, research into dystrophin's function would be best directed at the primary stage, before fiber branching contributes to any observed susceptibility to contraction-induced damage in dystrophin-deficient muscle.

11. Conclusion and clinical implications of the two stage model

The two stage dystrophic process explains why there is a loss of muscle function over time, i.e. why the muscles are not simply destroyed on first use. Clinically this is potentially a very important point because it means if the initial pathological increase in calcium is prevented the disease process will be halted before it enters the 2nd stage degeneration/ regeneration cycle and the mechanically compromised branched fibers will not form. Research suggests the unbranched dystrophin-negative fibers are relatively normal in regard to their contractile properties (Williams *et al.,* 1993; Lynch *et al.,* 2001; Chan *et al.,* 2007). Thus if the initial calcium influx is prevented the dystrophin-negative muscle fibers will serve for day to day activities possibly for a normal life span.

12. References

Allen, D.G.; Gervasio, O.L., Yeung, E.W. & Whitehead, N.P. (2010). Calcium and the damage pathways in muscular dystrophy. *Can J Physiol Pharmacol* Vol., 88, pp. 83-91.

Allen, D.G. & Whitehead, N.P. (2010). Duchenne muscular dystrophy - What causes the increased membrane permeability in skeletal muscle? *Int J Biochem Cell Biol,* doi: 10.1016/ j.biocel .2010.11.005.

Barker, D. and Gidumal, J. L. (1961). The morphology of intrafusal muscle fibres in the cat. *Journal of Physiology,* Vol., 157: pp.513–528.

Beitzel, F; Gregorevic, P., Ryall, J.G., Plant, D.R., Sillence, M.N. & Lynch, G.S. (2004). β2-Adrenoceptor agonist fenoterol enhances functional repair of regenerating rat skeletal muscle after injury. *J Appl Physiol,* Vol., 96, pp. 1385–1392.

Bell, C.D. & Conen, P.E. (1968). Histopathological changes in Duchenne muscular dystrophy. *Journal of the Neurological Sciences,* Vol., 7, pp. 529-544.

Blaivas, M. & Carlson, B.M. (1991). Muscle fiber branching -- difference between grafts in old and young rats. *Mechanisms of Ageing and Development,* Vol.,60 pp. 43-53.

Blaveri, K.; Heslop, L., Yu, D.S., Rosenblatt, J.D., Gross, J.G., Partridge, T.A. & Morgan, J.E. (1999). Patterns of repair of dystrophic mouse muscle: studies on isolated fibers. *Dev Dyn.,* Vol., 216, pp. 244-56.

Bockhold, K.J.; Rosenblatt, J.D. & Partridge, T.A. (1998). Aging normal and dystrophic mouse muscle: analysis of myogenicity in cultures of living single fibers. *Muscle Nerve,* Vol., 21, pp. 173-83.

Bourke, D.L. & Ontell, M. (1984). Branched myofibers inlong-term whole muscle transplants: a quantitative study. *Anat Rec,* Vol., 209, pp. 281–288.

Boyd, I. A. (1962). The structure and innervation of the nuclear bag muscle fibre system and the nuclear chain muscle fibre system in mammalian muscle spindles. *Proc. R. Soc.,* B Vol., 245, pp. 81-136.

Chamberlain, J. S.; Metzger, J., Reyes, M., Townsend, D. &. Faulkner, J.A. (2007). Dystrophin-deficient mdx mice display a reduced life span and are susceptible to spontaneous rhabdomyosarcoma. *FASEB J.,* Vol.,21, pp. 2195–2204.

Chan, S. & Head, S. I., (2010). The role of branched fibres in the pathogenesis of Duchenne muscular dystrophy. *Exp Physiol* Vol., 96.6 pp. 564–571.

Chan, S.; Head S. I. & Morley, J. W. (2007). Branched fibers in dystrophic mdx muscle are associated with a loss of force following lengthening contractions. *Am J Physiol Cell Physiol,* Vol., 293, pp. C985–C992.

Claflin, D.R. & Brooks, S.V. (2008). Direct observation of failing fibers in muscles of dystrophic mice provides mechanistic insight into muscular dystrophy. *Am J Physiol Cell Physiol,* Vol., 294, pp. C651-658.

Eriksson, A.; Lindström, M., Carlsson, L. & Thornell, L.E. (2006). Hypertrophic muscle fibers with fissures in power-lifters; fiber splitting or defect regeneration? *Histochem Cell Biol.,* Vol.,126, pp. 409-417.

Friedrich, O.; Both, M., Weber, C., Schurmann, S., Teichmann, M.D.H., von Wegner, F., Fink, R.H.A., Vogel, M., Chamberlain, J.S. & Garbe, C. (2010). Microarchitecture is severely compromised but motor protein function is preserved in dystrophic mdx skeletal muscle. *Biophys J* Vol., 98, pp. 606-616.

Gregorevic, P.; Blankinship, M.J., Allen, J.M. & Chamberlain JS. (2008). Systemic microdystrophin gene delivery improves skeletal muscle structure and function in old dystrophic mdx mice. *Mol Ther.,* Vol., 16, pp. 657-64.

Gutiérrez, J.M.; Núñez, J., Díaz, C., Cintra, A.C., Homsi-Brandeburgo, M.I. & Giglio, J.R. (1991). Skeletal muscle degeneration and regeneration after injection of bothropstoxin-II, a phospholipase A2 isolated from the venom of the snake Bothrops jararacussu. *Exp Mol Pathol* Vol., 55, pp. 217-229.

Hakim, C.H.; Grange, R.W. & Duan, D. (2011). The passive mechanical properties of the extensor digitorum longus muscle are compromised in 2- to 20-mo-old mdx mice. *J Appl Physiol.,* Vol., 110, pp. 1656-63.

Hall-Craggs, E.C. (1970). The longitudinal division of fibres in overloaded rat skeletal muscle. *J Anat* Vol., 107, pp. 459-470.

Head, S.I. (2010). Branched fibres in old dystrophic mdx muscle are associated with mechanical weakening of the sarcolemma, abnormal Ca2+ transients and a breakdown of Ca2+ homeostasis during fatigue. *Exp Physiol* Vol., 95, pp. 641-656.

Head, S.I.; Bakker, A.J. & Liangas, G. (2004). EDL and soleus muscles of the C57BL6J/dy2j laminin-a2-deficient dystrophic mouse are not vulnerable to eccentric contractions. *Exp Physiol* Vol., 89, pp. 531-539.

Head, S.I.; Stephenson, D.G. & Williams, D.A. (1990). Properties of enzymatically isolated skeletal fibres from mice with muscular dystrophy. *J Physiol* Vol., 422, pp. 351-367.

Head, S.I.; Williams, D.A. & Stephenson, D.G. (1992). Abnormalities in structure and function of limb skeletal muscle fibres of dystrophic mdx mice. *Proceedings of the Royal Society of London - Series B: Biological Sciences* Vol., 248, pp. 163-169.

Hilton-Brown, P. & Stålberg, E. (1983). *Electroencephalography and Clinical Neurophysiology ,* Vol., 56, pp.S99-S99.

Hilton-Brown, P.; Stålberg, E., Trontelj, J. & Mihelin, M. (1985). Causes of the increased fiber density in muscular dystrophies studied with single fiber EMG during electrical stimulation. Muscle Nerve. Vol., 8, pp. 383-388.

Isaacs, E.R.; Bradley, W.G. & Henderson, G. (1973). Longitudinal fibre splitting in muscular dystrophy: a serial cinematographic study. *J Neurol Neurosurg Psychiatry* Vol., 36 pp. 813-819.

Iwata, A.; Fuchioka, S., Hiraoka, K., Masuhara, M. & Kami, K. (2010). Characteristics of locomotion, muscle strength, and muscle tissue in regenerating rat skeletal muscles. *Muscle Nerve* Vol., 41, pp. 694–701.

Lefaucheur, J.P.; Pastoret, C. & Sebille, A. (1995). Phenotype of dystrophinopathy in old mdx mice. *Anat Rec,* Vol., 242, pp.70–76.

Louboutin, J.P.; Fichter-Gagnepain, V. & Noireaud, J. (1996). External calcium dependence of extensor digitorum longusmuscle contractility during bupivacaine-inducedregeneration. *Muscle Nerve* Vol., 19, pp. 994–1002.

Lovering, R.M.; Michaelson, L. & Ward, C.W. (2009). Malformed mdx myofibers have normal cytoskeletal architecture yet altered EC coupling and stress-induced Ca2+ signaling. *Am J Physiol Cell Physiol* Vol., 297, pp. C571-580.

Lynch, G.S.; Hinkle, R.T., Chamberlain, J.S, Brooks, S.V., & Faulkner, J.A. (2001). Force and power output of fast and slow skeletal muscles from mdx mice 6-28 months old. *J Physiol,* Vol., 535, pp. 591-600.

Mokhtarian, A.; Lefaucheur, J. P., Even, P. C. & Sebille, A. (1999). Hindlimb immobilization applied to 21-day-oldmdx mice prevents the occurrence of muscle degeneration. *Journal of Applied Physiology,* Vol. 86, pp. 924-931.

Mouisel, E.; Vignaud, A., Hourdé, C., Butler-Browne G. & Ferry, A. (2010). Muscle weakness and atrophy are associated with decreased regenerative capacity and changes in mTOR signaling in skeletal muscles of venerable (18-24-month-old) dystrophic mdx mice. *Muscle Nerve.,* Vol., 41, pp. 809-18.

Ontell, M. & Feng, K.C. (1981). The three-dimensional cytoarchitecture and pattern of motor innervation of branched striated myotubes. *Anat Rec.,* Vol., 200 No.1, pp. 11-31.

Ontell ,M.; Hughes, D. & Bourke, D. (1982). Secondary myogenesis of normal muscle produces abnormal myotubes. *Anat Rec* Vol., 204, pp. 199-207.

Parkinson, A.L.; Bakker, A.J. & Head, S.I. (2001). Morphology and organization of muscle fibres in the thoracic coxal muscle receptor organ and the associated promoter muscle, in a crayfish, Cherax destructor , and mud crab, Scylla serrata. *Acta Zoologica* (Stockholm) Vol., 82, pp. 251–260.

Pastoret, C. & Sebille, A. (1995a). Age-related differences in regeneration of dystrophic (mdx) and normal muscle in the mouse. *Muscle Nerve,* Vol., 18, pp. 1147-54.

Pastoret, C. & Sebille, A. (1995b). mdx mice show progressive weakness and muscle deterioration with age. *J Neurol Sci,* Vol., 129, pp. 97-105.

Sadeh, M.; Czyewski, K. & Stern, L.Z. (1985). Chronic myopathy induced by repeated bupivacaine injections. *J Neurol Sci* Vol., 67, pp. 229-238.

Stalberg, E. (1977) A course in Single Fibre Electromyography, Uppsala, Sweden.

Schäfer, R.; Zweyer, M., Knauf, U., Mundegar, R.R. & Wernig A. (2005). The ontogeny of soleus muscles in mdx and wild type mice. *Neuromuscul Disord,* Vol.,15, pp. 57-64.

Schmalbruch, H. (1976). The morphology of regeneration of skeletal muscles in the rat. *Tissue Cell* Vol., 8, pp. 673-692.

Schmalbruch, H. (1984). Regenerated muscle fibers in Duchenne muscular dystrophy: a serial section study. *Neurology,* Vol., 34, pp. 60-65.

Schwartz M. S.; Sargeant, M. & Swash, M. (1976). Longitudinal fibre splitting in neurogenic muscular disorders—its relation to the pathogenesis of 'myopathic' change. *Brain* vol., 99, pp. 617-636.

Stupka, N.; Schertzer, J.D., Bassel-Duby, R., Olson, E.N. & Lynch, G.S. (2007). Calcineurin-Aα activation enhances the structure and function of regenerating muscles after myotoxic injury. *Am J Physiol Regul Integr Comp Physiol* Vol., 293, pp. R686–R694.

Swash, M. & Schwartz, M.S. (1977). Implications of longitudinal muscle fibre splitting in neurogenic and myopathic disorders. *J Neurol Neurosurg Psychiatry* Vol., 40, pp. 1152-1159.

Tamaki, T.; Sekine, T., Akatsuka, A., Uchiyama, S. & Nakano, S. (1993). Three-dimensional cytoarchitecture of complex branched fibers in soleus muscle from *mdx* mutant mice. *Anat Rec.*, Vol.,237, pp. 338-344.

Whitehead, N.P.; Streamer, M., Lusambili, L.I., Sachs, F. & Allen, D.G. (2006). Streptomycin reduces stretch-induced membrane permeability in muscles from mdx mice. *Neuromuscul Disord*, Vol., 16, pp. 845-54.

Williams, D.A.; Head, S.I., Lynch, G. & Stephenson, D.G. (1993). Contractile properties skinned muscle fibres from young and adult normal and dystrophic mdx mice. *Journal of Physiology*, Vol., 460, pp, 51-67.

Wooddell, .CI.; Zhang, G., Griffin, J.B., Hegge, J.O., Huss, T. & Wolff, J.A. (2010). Use of Evans blue dye to compare limb muscles in exercised young and old mdx mice. *Muscle Nerve.*, Vol., 41, pp. 487-99.

25

Myotonic Dystrophy Type 1: Focus on the RNA Pathology and Therapy

Nikolaos P. Mastroyiannopoulos,
Andrie Koutsoulidou and Leonidas A. Phylactou*
Department of Molecular Genetics, Function & Therapy,
The Cyprus Institute of Neurology & Genetics,
Cyprus

1. Introduction

Almost 100 years ago, Steinert (1909), Batten and Gibb (1909), independently described Myotonic Dystrophy type 1 (DM1) that is now recognized as the most common form of muscular dystrophies in adults and the second most common type of muscular dystrophy after Duchenne Muscular Dystrophy, affecting 1 in 8000 individuals globally (Harper, 1989). DM1 is a genetic disorder, which is inherited in an autosomal dominant fashion (the mutation in one copy of the affected allele is enough to cause the disease). Although the disease affects mainly the skeletal muscle, it is considered a multi-systemic disorder with variable clinical symptoms affecting skeletal muscle, heart, and the central nervous system (CNS) (Larkin & Fardaei, 2001). Individual patients with DM1 are often identified as having congenital, juvenile or adult-onset disease based on the age of symptom onset. Congenital cases display the most severe phenotype and face a neonatal mortality rate of 25% (Harper, 1989).

The involvement of skeletal muscle in DM1 is highly characteristic and largely unwavering. Skeletal muscle in DM1 displays progressive weakness and wasting, myotonia and pain. Moreover, at the early stages of the disease, DM1 patients exhibit facial and neck flexion muscle weaknesses. Also, ptosis and weakness of eye and mouth closure are classical facial changes observed in DM1 patients. Weakness of neck flexion is an early sign, and patients may notice difficulty in lifting their heads from the pillow or experience tendency for the head to fall backwards during acceleration of the vehicle in which they are traveling (Machuca-Tzili et al., 2005). At a later stage in the course of the disease, distal weakness in the limbs, affecting particularly the finger flexors causes substantial disability. Less marked but often occurring, the weakness of ankle dorsiflexion causes foot drop. The combination of facial muscle weakness (with ptosis) and distal muscle weakness in DM1, even in the absence of myotonia, does not occur in any other disease (Ranum & Day, 2002). Respiratory failure due to the weakness of the respiratory muscles can also occur. This may be lethal in some cases, and is presented mainly in DM1 patients that experienced anesthesia or suffered from various chest infections (Machuca-Tzili et al., 2005). Myotonia is demonstrable in most

* Corresponding Author

symptomatic adults, whatever their symptoms. The commonest symptom of myotonia is difficulty in relaxing the grip. Myotonia can also affect the facial muscles, tongue, and other bulbar muscles, causing problems when talking, chewing and swallowing. Muscle pain is clearly independent to myotonia and more common in the lower limbs, where myotonia is usually not observed (Machuca-Tzili et al., 2005; Ranum & Day, 2002). Biopsies of DM1 muscle show a markedly increased variation in fibre diameter that ranges from 10μm to greater than 100μm. Severely atrophic fibres have pygnotic nuclei with minimal remaining contractile elements. DM1 muscle observations also showed ring fibre and central nuclear chains. Moreover, ATPase staining of the affected muscle sections showed atrophy of type 1 fibres. Finally, basophilic regenerating fibres, splitting fibres, fibrosis and adipose deposition are common muscle abnormalities of DM1, always depending on the extent of muscle involvement (Vihola et al., 2003).

Antrioventricular and intraventricular conduction abnormalities are very common in DM1 and require regular monitoring. DM1 patients were shown to be more vulnerable to cardiac conduction abnormalities than impaired myocardial function. Atrial fibrillation, ventricular arrhythmias and cardiomyopathy are also very common abnormalities in DM1 affected individuals (Phillips & Harper, 1997). Sudden death, due to heart block, is not common in DM1, but does occur in severe DM1 patients, as a result of extreme sinus bradycardia or tachyarrhythmia, necessitating the use of pacemakers and implantable defibrillators by these patients (Colleran et al., 1997). There is extensive evidence for CNS involvement in DM1. Cognitive impairment / mental retardation, specific patterns of psychological dysfunction and personality traits, are widely recognized features of congenital and juvenile DM1 affected patients. In addition to the above, DM1 patients develop CNS white matter and cerebral blood flow abnormalities (Ogata et al., 1998). Central hypersomnia, another recognized CNS effect of DM1, appears to occur in adulthood. Excessive daytime sleepiness is very common and in some cases very disabling. Apathy, epilepsy, stroke and parkinsonism are rarely observed in adult DM1 patients, but are fairly common in congenitally affected patients (Rubinsztein et al., 1997). Posterior capsular, iridescent, multicoloured opacities are regularly seen in DM1 patients. Cataracts can be detected in DM1 patients at a very early stage in the course of the disease by slit-lamp examination. When vision is significantly impaired, surgical intervention is required (Klesert et al., 2000). Irritable bowel-like symptoms such as constipation, diarrhea, colicky abdominal pain and pseudo-obstruction are extremely common in DM1. The upper gastrointestinal tract is affected in later stages of the disease and can cause dysphagia and aspiration resulting in serious chest infections that can cause morbidity and mortality of DM1 patients. DM1 patients display a large variety of endocrine abnormalities. Testicular failure, hypotestosteronism and oligospermia are associated with the reduced fertility of these patients. Laboratory observations have also shown a reduction in the serum levels of IgG and IgM and as a result, hypogammaglobulinemia can affect these patients. Insulin resistance is also seen in DM1 patients, but even in severe cases, type 2 diabetes clinical symptoms are not linked with the disease, whilst recent evidence supports that there is alteration in the normal functioning of the insulin receptor (Moxley et al., 1984).

DM1 is caused by an unstable expansion of CTG repeats in the 3′-untranslated region (3′ UTR) of the *dystrophia myotonica protein kinase (DMPK)* gene on chromosome 19q13.3 (Aslanidis et al., 1992; Brook et al., 1992; Davies et al., 1983). The number of CTG repeats is in the range of 5-35 in the normal population and increases to between 50 and several thousand in DM1 patients. The variation in the number of CTG repeats is closely related to the phenomenon of 'anticipation': The number of CTG repeats can increase through successive generations, due to mitotic and meiotic instabilities (Martorell et al., 1999; Monckton et al., 1995). Interesting is also the fact that DM1 patients might show difference in the number of CTG repeats from one cell to another (genetic heterogeneity). 3'UTR is a region that is transcribed into RNA but not translated into protein therefore the CTG expansion at the DM1 locus does not alter the protein sequence encoded by DMPK. The mechanism of pathogenesis in DM1 is different from other genetic disorders. Three different mechanisms of pathogenesis have been proposed to explain how repeat expansions in the *DMPK* gene result in DM1 (Tapscott & Thornton, 2001):

i. The mutant RNA accumulates in discrete foci in the cell nucleus rather than being transported to the cytoplasm (Davis et al., 1997; Taneja et al., 1995), where translation of mRNA into protein normally takes place. According to experimental evidence this causes deficiency in the production of DMPK (DMPK Haploinsufficiency) (Jansen et al., 1996; Reddy et al., 1996).
ii. The second mechanism of pathogenesis, involves the disruption of the expression and function of DMPK neighboring genes. Scientific evidence showed that the expanded CTG repeats interfere with the nucleosome assembly and therefore on the total chromatin structure. This process disrupts and prevents the binding of necessary factors for the expression of neighboring genes (Klesert et al., 1997; Wang & Griffith, 1995; Westerlaken et al., 2003).
iii. Lastly, evidence suggests that the molecular pathogenesis of DM1 is to a great extent due to the downstream effects of the retention of the mutant DMPK transcripts in the nucleus. Some of these include the inhibition of myogenesis and the defective splicing of cellular RNA molecules (Mankodi et al., 2000; Miller et al., 2000; Timchenko et al., 1996).

This book chapter will focus mainly on the pathology which arises from nuclear RNA retention and the therapeutic approaches against it. The correlation between the CTG repeat size and the severity of the disease, suggests that the repeats represent the major cause of DM1 pathogenesis. After investigations of the mutant DMPK transcripts, it was found that these form nuclear foci that are enclosed within the nucleus of the affected cells (Amack & Mahadevan, 2001; Taneja et al., 1995). Moreover, it was postulated that these nuclear foci might contribute to DM1 pathogenesis, perhaps by disrupting the transport of mRNA from DMPK and/or other genes to the cytoplasm (Alwazzan et al., 1999; Klesert et al., 1997; Otten & Tapscott, 1995; Taneja et al., 1995). Further on, cell models expressing the CTG repeat expansion, showed also nuclear localization of mutant RNA foci and extended myogenic defects (Amack & Mahadevan, 2004). These nuclear RNA foci were also shown to interact with nuclear RNA binding proteins and subsequently alter the regulation or localization (Fardaei et al., 2002; Philips et al., 1998). Mutant DMPK RNA foci were found to interact with the CUG-binding protein (Timchenko et al., 1996) and three different forms of the muscleblind binding protein (MBNL) (Ho et al., 2005). Scientific evidence, using knockout MBNL or CUGBP animal models revealed similarities to the DM1 pathophysiology, including cardiac, endocrine system and muscle abnormalities (Kanadia et al., 2003; Kanadia et al., 2003; Roberts et al., 1997).

2. RNA pathogenesis

2.1 RNA nuclear retention

Mutant DMPK alleles are transcribed in the nucleus to produce RNA molecules containing expanded CUG repeats. The expanded CUG transcript folds back on itself to form stable duplex hairpin structures. Napierala and Kryzosiak provided evidence that hairpins indeed exist in the DMPK RNA fragments containing 11–49 CUG repeats and that the stability of these structures increases with the repeat length (Napierala & Krzyzosiak, 1997). Koch and Leffert, generated secondary structures of partial and full-length DMPK mRNAs carrying variable numbers of CUG triplet repeats (up to 500) (Koch & Leffert, 1998). They suggested that CUG hairpins are the most stable structures formed and also that the DMPK mRNAs are sterically impeded from transport through nuclear pores, by giant hairpins or hairpin clusters formed by CUG repeats above a limit size (44 or less) (Koch & Leffert, 1998). Further thermal melting and nuclease mapping studies indicated that CUG repeats form highly stable hairpins (Tian et al., 2000). Michalowski et al., used electron microscopy to provide the first visual evidence that the DMPK mRNA expansion forms an RNA hairpin structure (Michalowski et al., 1999). Visualization of large RNAs containing up to 130 CUG repeats revealed perfect double-stranded RNA segments whose lengths were that expected for duplex RNA (Michalowski et al., 1999). The duplex segments were highly stable, since the hairpin structures reformed rapidly during the electron microscopy mounting procedures when the RNAs were boiled and quickly cooled, even under low salt conditions (Michalowski et al., 1999).

RNA harboring CUG repeat expansion impose dominant-negative effects by aberrantly interacting and recruiting RNA-binding proteins thus leading to nuclear retention of the mutant transcript and the formation of ribonuclear inclusions known as RNA foci. Taneja et al., used fluorochrome-conjugated and digoxigenin-conjugated oligonucleotide probes to analyze the intracellular localization of DMPK transcripts in fibroblasts derived from DM patients and normal individuals and showed a striking difference in the nuclear distribution of the DMPK transcripts, a difference that was verified in a muscle biopsy from an affected individual (Taneja et al., 1995). Davis et al., generated "myoblasts" by *MyoD* retroviral infection of DM1 fibroblast lines and showed that mutant *DMPK* transcripts were abundant in myoblasts, but could not contribute to kinase production, as the transcripts were quantitatively retained within myoblast nuclei (Davis et al., 1997). Terminally differentiated myoblasts contained no cytoplasmic mutant transcripts; instead, they formed stable, long-lived clusters that were tightly linked to the nuclear matrix (Davis et al., 1997). Myoblasts and myotubes isolated from patients with congenital myotonic dystrophy (CDM1) also showed abnormal retention of mutant RNA in nuclear foci (Furling et al., 2001).

2.2 CUG binding protein 1 (CUGBP1)

Proteins of the CELF family are a group of proteins extensively studied for their implication in DM1 pathogenesis. CELF (CUGBP and ETR-3-like factors) proteins are a family of structurally related RNA-binding proteins involved in various aspects of RNA processing including alternative splicing, translation and mRNA stability. The first member of the CELF family, CELF1/CUGBP1, was identified in investigating the molecular mechanisms of DM1 (Gallo & Spickett, 2010). Timchenko et al. reported that CUG binding protein 1

(CUGBP1) binds specifically to CUG triplet repeated sequences (Timchenko et al., 1996; Timchenko et al., 1996). Electron microscopy studies showed that CUGBP1 is primarily a single-stranded RNA-binding protein that has a binding preference for CUG-rich RNA elements but not double-stranded CUG hairpins (Michalowski et al., 1999). Moreover, CUGBP1 was visualized to localize to the base of the RNA hairpin and not along the stem (Michalowski et al., 1999). In a yeast three-hybrid system CUGBP1 was found to associate with long CUG trinucleotide repeats ($(CUG)_{(11)}(CUG)_{(12)}$), but not with short repeats ($(CUG)_{(12)}$) (Takahashi et al., 2000). However, using a combination of indirect immunofluorescence to detect endogenous proteins and overexpression of proteins with green fluorescent protein (GFP) tags it has been shown that CUGBP1 does not co-localise with triplet repeat foci in DM1 fibroblast cell lines (Fardaei et al., 2001).

Experiments in tissue culture and analysis of DM1 patients demonstrated that RNA CUG repeats directly affect expression and activity of CUGBP1 in DM1 myoblasts, heart, and skeletal muscle tissues (Timchenko et al., 2001). Specifically, the formation of CUGBP1 · CUG RNA complexes is accompanied by increased CUGBP1 protein stability and subsequent elevation of CUGBP1 (Timchenko et al., 2001). Furthermore, nuclear CUGBP1 levels have been found increased in DM1 patients, compared to normal subjects (Timchenko et al., 2001). These observations suggest that abnormal activation of CUGBP1 is related to DM1 pathogenesis. Furthermore, in a transgenic mice model, overexpression of CUGBP1 in heart and skeletal muscle, produced DM1-like symptoms such as central nuclei, chains of nuclei, centralized nicotinamide adenine dinucleotide (NADH) reactivity and mis-splicing (Ho et al., 2005). De Haro et al., generated a *Drosophila* model of DM1 that showed degenerative phenotypes in muscle and eye tissue and key histopathological features of the DM1, including accumulation of the expanded transcripts in nuclear foci (de Haro et al., 2006). Using this model they showed that by increasing the levels of CUGBP1 degeneration is deteriorated even though CUGBP1 distribution is not altered by the expression of the expanded triplet repeat (de Haro et al., 2006). Wang et al., generated an inducible and heart-specific DM1 mouse model expressing expanded CUG RNA in the context of DMPK 3' UTR that recapitulated pathological and molecular features of DM1 including dilated cardiomyopathy, arrhythmias, systolic and diastolic dysfunction, and mis-regulated alternative splicing (Wang et al., 2007). Combined *in situ* hybridization and immunofluorescent staining for CUGBP1 protein expressed in heart, showed increased protein levels specifically in nuclei containing foci of CUG repeat RNA (Wang et al., 2007).

Although the molecular mechanisms for increased CUGBP1 is not completely understood, Kuyumcu-Martinez et al. reported that the expression of mutant DMPK-CUG-repeat RNA results in hyperphosphorylation and stabilization of CUGBP1 through the inappropriate activation of the protein kinase C (PKC) pathway, in DM1 tissues, cells, and a DM1 mouse model (Kuyumcu-Martinez et al., 2007). Experiments performed in C2C12 mouse cell line showed that expression of a mutant DMPK 3'-UTR containing 960 CUG repeats is sufficient to increase expression and stability of an mRNA encoding the potent proinflammatory cytokine, tumor necrosis factor (TNF), which was found elevated in DM1 patients serum (Mammarella et al., 2002; Zhang et al., 2008). Moreover, activation of the protein kinase C (PKC) pathway also stabilized the TNF transcript. These results suggest that the elevated serum TNF seen in DM1 patients may be derived from muscle where it is induced by expression of toxic DMPK RNA (Zhang et al., 2008). In a more recent study, Koshelev et al.

used tetracycline-inducible CUGBP1 and heart-specific reverse tetracycline trans-activator transgenes in order to express human CUGBP1 in adult mouse heart (Koshelev et al., 2010). Up-regulation of CUGBP1 was sufficient to reproduce molecular, histopathological and functional changes observed in DM1 patients and in a DM1 mouse model thus supporting a role for CUGBP1 up-regulation in DM1 pathogenesis (Koshelev et al., 2010). In another mouse model, Ward et al. overexpressed CUGBP1 and showed that mice reproduced molecular and physiological defects of DM1 tissue, suggesting that CUGBP1 has a major role in DM1 skeletal muscle pathogenesis (Ward et al., 2010).

2.3 Muscleblind (MBNL) family proteins

Muscleblind (MBNL) family proteins, initially identified by Miller et al. were selectively associated with CUG repeat expansions and named as triplet repeat expansion (EXP) double-stranded (ds) RNA-binding proteins (Miller et al., 2000). Human EXP proteins are found to be orthologous to the *Drosophila* MBNL proteins, which are required for terminal differentiation of photoreceptors and muscle cells (Artero et al., 1998; Begemann et al., 1997). The alternative splicing factor MBNL1 binds to pyrimidine-rich pre-mRNAs containing YGCY motifs and promotes either the inclusion or the exclusion of alternative exons depending on the 5′ or 3′ localization of *cis*-regulatory elements (Goers et al., 2010). All three isoforms of MBNL family proteins (MBNL/MBNL1, MBLL/MBNL2 and MBXL/MBNL3) co-localize with the nuclear mutant RNA foci in DM1 cells, presumably diverting them from their normal cellular functions (Wojciechowska & Krzyzosiak, 2011). The biological significance of the interaction between mutant RNA and MBNL-family proteins has been manifested through the disruption of alternative splicing which is a characteristic feature of DM1 pathogenesis (Wojciechowska & Krzyzosiak, 2011). Fardaei et al. investigated for the first time the localization of MBNL (EXP) protein with mutant DMPK transcripts (Fardaei et al., 2001). Using indirect immunofluorescence to detect endogenous proteins and overexpression of GFP-tagged MBNL, they showed that MBNL forms foci in DM1 fibroblast cell lines and co-localises with the foci of expanded repeat transcripts in the nuclei of DM1 cells (Fardaei et al., 2001). The binding of MBNL1 with expanded CUG repeats was further verified in DM1 muscle biopsy tissues (Mankodi et al., 2003) and in a yeast three-hybrid system (Kino et al., 2004). Overexpression of MBNL1 *in vivo* using a recombinant adeno-associated viral vector rescued disease-associated muscle myotonia and aberrant splicing of specific gene transcripts, characteristic of DM1 skeletal muscle supporting the hypothesis that loss of MBNL1 activity is a primary pathogenic event in the development of the disease (Kanadia et al., 2006).

Analysis of the expression pattern of the mouse *Mbnl1*, *Mbnl2*, *Mbnl3* and *Dmpk* genes during embryonic development revealed a striking overlap between the expression of *Dmpk* and the *Mbnl* genes during development of the limbs, nervous system and various muscles, including the diaphragm and tongue (Kanadia et al., 2003). In 2003, Kanadia et al. generated the first MBNL knockout mouse model for DM1 (Kanadia et al., 2003). The disruption of the mouse *Mbnl1* gene led to muscle, eye and RNA splicing abnormalities which are characteristics of DM1 disease (Kanadia et al., 2003). Examination of DM1 post-mortem brain tissue by FISH indicated that the mutant DMPK mRNA is widely expressed in cortical and subcortical neurons and accumulated in discrete foci within neuronal nuclei (Jiang et al., 2004). Moreover, MBNL family proteins were recruited into the RNA foci and a subset of neuronal pre-mRNAs showed abnormal regulation of alternative splicing suggesting that central nervous system impairment in DM1 may result from a deleterious gain-of-function by mutant DMPK mRNA (Jiang et al., 2004). In 2005, Mankodi et al. provided evidence that accumulation of expanded CUG repeats in nuclear foci was associated with sequestration of MBNL proteins and abnormal regulation of alternative splicing in cardiac muscle tissue from DM1 patients (Mankodi et al., 2005).

In a *Drosophila* model of DM1 expressing CTG repeats in the 3'-UTR of a marker gene CUG repeats form discrete ribonuclear foci in muscle cells that co-localize with MBNL (Houseley et al., 2005). Moreover, MBNL was also revealed as having a previously unrecognized role in stabilizing CUG transcripts (Houseley et al., 2005). In another *Drosophila* model of DM1 that shows degenerative phenotypes in muscle and eye tissue as well as key histopathological features of the DM1, including accumulation of the expanded transcripts in nuclear foci and their co-localization with MBNL1 protein, reduced levels of MBNL1 aggravate the muscle and eye phenotypes of DM1 flies whereas MBNL1 overexpression suppresses the degenerative phenotypes (de Haro et al., 2006). *Mbnl2*-deficient mice developed myotonia, skeletal muscle pathology consistent with human DM1 and defective CLCN1 mRNA splicing in skeletal muscle, supporting the hypothesis that MBNL proteins and specifically MBNL2 contribute to the pathogenesis of human DM1 (Hao et al., 2008). These results are consistent with the notion that *Mbnl1* deficiency alone is not sufficient to fully replicate the human DM1 phenotype (Kanadia et al., 2003). An additional mouse DM1 model with inducible and skeletal muscle-specific expression of 960 CTG repeats in the context of DMPK exon 15 recapitulated many findings associated with DM1 skeletal muscle, such as nuclear foci with MBNL1 protein co-localization, mis-splicing, myotonia, characteristic histological abnormalities, and increased CUGBP1 protein levels (Orengo et al., 2008). Importantly, this DM1 mouse model exhibited severe muscle wasting, which has not been reported previously in models in which MBNL1 depletion was the main feature (Orengo et al., 2008). More recently, Machuca-Tzili et al. generated an *mbnl2* knockdown zebrafish model, which exhibits features of DM (Machuca-Tzili et al., 2011). They showed that loss of zebrafish mbnl2 function causes muscle defects and splicing abnormalities of clcn1 and tnnt2 transcripts, similar to those observed in DM1 patients (Machuca-Tzili et al., 2011).

Wheeler et al., showed that CUG expanded RNA is also expressed in subsynaptic nuclei of muscle fibers and in motor neurons in DM1 patients, causing sequestration of MBNL1 protein in both locations (Wheeler et al., 2007). Additionally, in a transgenic mouse model, expression of CUG expanded RNA at high levels in extrajunctional nuclei replicates many features of DM1, including myotonia, spliceopathy, internal nuclei, ring fibers, and sarcoplasmic masses, but the toxic RNA is poorly expressed in subsynaptic nuclei and mice fail to develop denervation-like features of DM1 myopathology (Wheeler et al., 2007). These findings suggest that subsynaptic nuclei and motor neurons are at risk for DM1-induced mis-splicing, which may affect function or stability of the neuromuscular junction (Wheeler et al., 2007). MBNL1 protein was also found in the human brain, and consists of several isoforms, as shown by RT-PCR and sequencing. In the brain tissue of DM1 patients, a fetal isoform of MBNL1 was found overexpressed (Dhaenens et al., 2008). The expression of this fetal isoform can also be reproduced by the ectopic expression of long CUG repeats *in vitro* (Dhaenens et al., 2008).

2.4 Mis-regulation of alternative splicing

At the molecular level, one of the best-characterized trans-dominant effects induced by the mutant *DMPK* RNAs in DM1 is the mis-regulation of alternative splicing of a subset of pre-mRNAs. Alternative splicing is a process by which the exons of the transcribed pre-mRNA are reconnected in multiple ways to give rise to different mRNAs which are in turn translated into different protein isoforms. To date, more than twenty transcripts have been found to be mis-spliced in different tissues of DM1 patients (Klein et al., 2011).

2.4.1 CUGBP1 and MBNL1 significance in alternative splicing mis-regulation

Mis-splicing events observed in DM1 result from an inappropriate regulation of alternative splicing due to altered activities of splicing regulators such as CUGBP1 and MBNL1. The biological significance of CUGBP1 overexpression and MBNL family proteins sequestration to nuclear RNA foci has been manifested through the disruption of alternative splicing, which is a characteristic feature of DM1 pathogenesis. Muscle wasting and weakness, heart problems and insulin resistance are associated with aberrant alternative splicing of a range of pre-mRNAs.

2.4.1.1 Cardiac troponin T (cTNT)

The first mis-regulation of alternative splicing described in DM1 was the abnormal inclusion of exon 5 in cardiac troponin T (cTNT) in cardiac muscle (Philips et al., 1998). CUGBP1 was found to bind to the human cTNT pre–mRNA and regulate its alternative splicing. Splicing of cTNT was disrupted in DM1 striated muscle and in normal cells expressing CUG expanded RNAs (Philips et al., 1998). Transgenic mice with a targeted deletion of *Mbnl1* exon 3 (E3) (*Mbnl1*$^{\Delta E3/\Delta E3}$) in adult heart showed abnormal retention of the *cTNT* "fetal" exon 5, as was observed in DM1 (Kanadia et al., 2003; Philips et al., 1998). Ho et al., involved for the first time all three MBNL family members with mis-regulation of alternative splicing in DM1 (Ho et al., 2004). MBNL proteins were found to act antagonistically to CELF proteins on the human and chicken cTNT pre-mRNAs (Ho et al., 2004). MBNL1 binds a common motif near the human and chicken cTNT alternative exons within intronic regions, which appear to be single stranded (Ho et al., 2004). Furthermore, CELF and MBNL proteins bind to distinct *cis*-elements and minigenes containing CELF- or MBNL-binding site mutations thus showing that regulation by one family does not require responsiveness to the other (Ho et al., 2004). However, modified cTNT minigenes made nonresponsive to the *trans*-dominant effects of CUG repeat RNA still respond to MBNL depletion, suggesting that CUG repeat RNA affects splicing by a mechanism more complex than MBNL depletion alone (Ho et al., 2004).

2.4.1.2 Insulin receptor (IR)

Three years after the discovery of the first pre-mRNA that is mis-spliced in DM1, Savkur et al., described the second pre-mRNA that undergoes mis-regulation of alternative splicing in DM1 skeletal tissue (Savkur et al., 2001). Alternative splicing of the insulin receptor (IR) pre-mRNA was aberrantly regulated in DM1, resulting in predominant expression of the lower-signaling non-muscle isoform (IR-A) of the receptor (Savkur et al., 2001). IR-A also predominates in DM1 skeletal muscle cultures, which exhibit a reduced responsiveness to the metabolic effects of insulin (Savkur et al., 2001). Furthermore, the aberrant regulation of

IR alternative splicing was reproduced in normal cells by the expression of CUG-repeat RNA (Savkur et al., 2001). Additionally, overexpression of CUGBP1 also induced a switch to IR-A in normal cells (Savkur et al., 2001). The CUGBP1 protein mediates this switch through an intronic element located upstream of the alternatively spliced exon 11, and specifically binds within this element *in vitro* (Savkur et al., 2001). The research group suggested a model in which increased expression CUGBP1 splicing regulator contributes to insulin resistance observed in DM1 by affecting IR alternative splicing (Savkur et al., 2001).

In addition to CUGBP1, IR alternative splicing was found to be regulated by MBNL1 (Ho et al., 2004). Down-regulation of MBNL1 and MBNL2 in normal myoblasts resulted in abnormal splice pattern observed in DM1 (Dansithong et al., 2005). Moreover, CUGBP1 was found to regulate the equilibrium of splice site selection by antagonizing the facilitatory activity of MBNL1 and MBNL2 on IR exon 11 splicing in a dose-dependent manner (Dansithong et al., 2005). Rescued experiments in DM1 myoblasts demonstrated that loss of MBNL1 function is the critical event, whereas CUGBP1 overexpression plays a secondary role in the aberrant alternative splicing of IR RNA in DM1 (Dansithong et al., 2005). Therefore, these experiments demonstrated that MBNL1 sequestration is the primary determinant of the IR pre-mRNA abnormal splicing in DM1 myoblasts (Dansithong et al., 2005).

2.4.1.3 Chloride channel - 1 (ClC-1)

In a transgenic mouse model of DM1, the expression of expanded CUG repeats reduced the transmembrane chloride conductance to an extent sufficient to account for myotonia (Mankodi et al., 2002). These mice showed abnormal splicing of pre-mRNA encoding chloride channel - 1 (ClC-1), the main chloride channel in skeletal muscle, resulting in loss of ClC-1 protein from the surface membrane (Mankodi et al., 2002). Furthermore, the induction of abnormal ClC-1 splicing, the corresponding loss of ClC-1 protein from the muscle membrane, and the development of myotonia were tightly correlated with the level of expanded CUG repeats in different transgenic lines (Mankodi et al., 2002). Additional to the mice models, similar effects on CLC-1 splicing and protein accumulation in muscle tissue from patients with DM1 (Mankodi et al., 2002). These findings suggest that mis-regulation of ClC-1 pre-mRNA alternative splicing is an important factor that leads to myotonia observed in DM1 patients. In an additional study, loss of ClC-1 mRNA and protein due to aberrant splicing of the ClC-1 pre-mRNA was detected in DM1 skeletal muscle tissue (Charlet et al., 2002). Specifically, the majority of ClC-1 mRNAs contained premature termination codons due to retention of intron 2 or inclusion of two novel exons between exons 6 and 7 (Charlet et al., 2002). CUGBP1, which is found elevated in DM1 striated muscle, bound to the ClC-1 pre-mRNA, and overexpression of CUGBP1 in normal cells reproduced the aberrant pattern of ClC-1 splicing observed in DM1 skeletal muscle (Charlet et al., 2002). In particular, CUGBP1 induced retention of intron 2 by binding to a U/G-rich motif common to other pre-mRNA targets of CUGBP1 thus suggesting that increased CUGBP1 activity in DM1 causes aberrant regulation of ClC-1 alternative splicing (Charlet et al., 2002).

2.4.1.4 Tau

Tau protein belongs to the family of microtubule-associated proteins whose transcript undergoes complex regulated splicing in the mammalian nervous system. They are essentially expressed in neurons where their essential function is to regulate the microtubule network. In the adult human central nervous system, alternative splicing of exons 2, 3 and 10 of the single *tau* gene transcript gives six tau isoforms (Sergeant et al., 2001). The tau isoforms aggregated in DM1 brain lesions consists mainly of the shortest human tau isoform suggesting that the $(CTG)_n$ expansion is altering the processing of tau pre-mRNA splicing and gives rise to symptoms such as dementia (Sergeant et al., 2001).

2.4.1.5 Myotubularin-related 1 (MTMR1)

The *myotubularin-related 1 (MTMR1)* gene belongs to a highly conserved family of phosphatases with at least 11 isoforms in humans (Buj-Bello et al., 2002). One of the transcripts resulting from MTMR1 alternative slicing is muscle-specific and is induced during myogenesis both *in vitro* and *in vivo*, and represents the major isoform in adult skeletal muscle (Buj-Bello et al., 2002). *MTMR1* splicing pattern was found strikingly altered in cultured muscle cells, in skeletal muscle from patients with congenital myotonic dystrophy (CDM1) and in DM1 muscle biopsies (Buj-Bello et al., 2002; Santoro et al., 2010).

2.4.1.6 Ryanodine receptor 1 (RyR1) and sarcoplasmic/endoplasmic reticulum Ca2+-ATPase (SERCA) 1 or 2

Ryanodine receptor 1 (RyR1) and sarcoplasmic/endoplasmic reticulum Ca2+-ATPase (SERCA) 1 or 2 which are the main sarcoplasmic reticulum regulators of intracellular Ca^{2+} homeostasis in skeletal muscle cells (Kimura et al., 2005). The fetal variants, ASI(-) of RyR1 which lacks residue 3481-3485, and SERCA1b which differs at the C-terminal were found significantly increased in skeletal muscles from DM1 patients and a transgenic mouse model of DM1 thus suggesting that aberrant splicing of RyR1 and SERCA1 mRNAs might contribute to impaired Ca^{2+} homeostasis in DM1 muscle (Kimura et al., 2005).

2.4.1.7 Myocyte enhancer factor 2 (Mef2)

MBNL3 regulates the splicing pattern of the muscle transcription factor myocyte enhancer factor 2 (Mef2) (Lee et al., 2010). MBNL3 antagonizes muscle differentiation by disrupting the expression of (+)β isoform of Mef2D which is transcriptionally more active (Lee et al., 2010). Using a DM1 cell culture model and DM1 patient tissue, they provided evidence that expression of CUG expanded RNAs can lead to an increase in MBNL3 expression accompanied by a decrease in Mef2D β-exon splicing (Lee et al., 2010). These studies suggest that an increase in MBNL3 activity may play a role in the skeletal muscle degeneration experienced by DM1 patients (Lee et al., 2010).

2.4.1.8 Bridging integrator-1 (BIN1)

Bridging integrator-1 (BIN1) is a myc box-dependent-interacting protein involved in tubular invaginations of membranes and is required for the biogenesis of muscle T tubules, which are specialized skeletal muscle membrane structures essential for excitation-contraction coupling (Fugier et al., 2011). Mutations in the *BIN1* gene cause centronuclear myopathy, which shares some histopathological features with myotonic dystrophy (Jungbluth et al., 2008). BIN1's function is regulated by alternative splicing which was found altered in skeletal muscle samples of people with CDM1 and DM1 (Fugier et al., 2011). Particularly, MBNL1 was detected to bind the BIN1 pre-mRNA and regulate the alternative splicing of the exon 11 (Fugier et al., 2011). Sequestration of MBNL1 by expanded CUG repeats in DM1 patients resulted in expression of an inactive form of BIN1 lacking phosphatidylinositol 5-

phosphate-binding and membrane-tubulating activities (Fugier et al., 2011). Consistent with a defect of BIN1, muscle T tubules found altered in DM1 patients, and membrane structures were restored upon expression of the normal splicing form of BIN1 in muscle cells of such individuals (Fugier et al., 2011). Finally, reproducing BIN1 splicing alteration in mice was sufficient to promote T tubule alterations and muscle weakness, a predominant feature of DM1 (Fugier et al., 2011).

2.4.1.9 Myomesin 1 (MYOM1)

Myomesin 1 (MYOM1) is a constituent of the M band of the sacromere which is the basic unit of a muscle (Lange et al., 2005). The fact that MYOM1 is a structural constituent of muscle suggests that it could be involved in muscle impairment in patients with DM1. Koebis et al. used exon array and identified aberrant inclusion of *MYOM1* exon 17a as a novel splicing abnormality in DM1 muscle (Koebis et al., 2011). A cellular splicing assay using a *MYOM1* minigene revealed that MBNL and CELF family proteins function as *trans*-acting factors in the alternative splicing of *MYOM1* exon 17a (Koebis et al., 2011). Expression of expanded CUG repeat impeded MBNL1 activity but did not affect CUGBP1 activity on the splicing of *MYOM1* minigene (Koebis et al., 2011). These results suggested that the downregulation of MBNL proteins should lead to the abnormal splicing of *MYOM1* exon 17a in DM1 muscle (Koebis et al., 2011).

2.5 Myogenic defects

DM1-associated molecular events, such as abberant recruitment of RNA-binding proteins into ribonuclear foci and mis-splicing, could eventually provoke alterations in global cell function. Notably, a critical disorder of DM1 that distinguishes it from other muscular dystrophies is the defects observed in muscle differentiation. Fetal muscle development is affected in fetuses with congenital myotonic dystrophy whereas muscle regeneration is compromised in adult patients (Amack & Mahadevan, 2004).

Initial experiments performed in the mouse myoblast cell line C2C12 showed that overexpression of the mouse *dmpk* gene leads to markedly inhibition of both fusion and terminal differentiation of the cell line (Okoli et al., 1998). Further experiments performed on C2C12 cell line showed that overexpression of human DMPK mRNA caused a marked inhibition of terminal differentiation accompanied by a reduction of myogenin mRNA levels (Sabourin et al., 1997). These results suggest that overexpression of the DMPK 3'-UTR may interfere with the expression of muscle-specific mRNAs leading to a delay in muscle terminal differentiation (Sabourin et al., 1997). Amack et al. used reporter assays to provide unambiguous evidence that the expression of the mutant *DMPK* 3'-UTR mRNA with $(CUG)_{200}$ selectively inhibited myogenic differentiation of C2C12 myoblasts (Amack et al., 1999). In agreement, overexpression of DMPK 3'-UTR including either wild-type or expanded CTG repeats resulted in aberrant and delayed muscle development in fetal transgenic mice and displayed muscle atrophy at 3 months of age. Moreover, primary myoblast cultures from both wild-type and expanded CTG repeat mice showed reduced fusion potential with greater reduction observed in the expanded repeat cultures (Storbeck et al., 2004). Interestingly, the differentiation defect was confirmed in muscle cell cultures derived from DM1 fetuses and patients (Furling et al., 2001; Timchenko et al., 2001).

Molecular studies have begun to uncover the effect of the mutant DMPK mRNA on myogenesis inhibition. Various studies implicate CUGBP1 protein with myogenic impairment in DM1, since it is a key regulator of translation of proteins that are involved in muscle development and differentiation. Timchenko et al. reported that cultured myoblasts isolated from DM1 patients failed to permanently withdraw from the cell cycle when stimulated to differentiate (Timchenko et al., 2001). Skeletal muscle cells from DM1 patients failed to induce cytoplasmic levels of CUGBP1, while normal differentiated cells accumulate CUGBP1 in the cytoplasm (Timchenko et al., 2001). In normal cells, CUGBP1 up-regulates p21 translation during differentiation by binding to a GC-rich sequence located within the 5' region of p21 mRNA (Timchenko et al., 2001). DM1 cultured cells failed to accumulate CUGBP1 in the cytoplasm thus leading to a significant reduction of p21 and to alterations of other proteins responsible for the cell cycle withdrawal (Timchenko et al., 2001). In normal cells, activity of cdk4 declines during differentiation, whereas in DM1 cells cdk4 is highly active during all stages of differentiation (Timchenko et al., 2001). Furthermore, DM1 cells do not form Rb/E2F repressor complexes that are abundant in differentiated cells from normal individuals (Timchenko et al., 2001). These data provide evidence for an impaired cell cycle withdrawal in DM1 muscle cells and suggest that alterations in the CUGBP1 activity causes disruption of p21-dependent control of cell cycle arrest (Timchenko et al., 2001). Another study showed that CUGBP1 is phosphorylated by different kinases during myoblast proliferation and differentiation and that phosphorylation of CUGBP1 at different sites directs CUGBP1 to different mRNA targets (Salisbury et al., 2008). Specifically, Akt kinase and cyclinD3-cdk4/6 phosphorylate CUGBP1 during proliferation and differentiation, respectively (Salisbury et al., 2008). Cyclin D3-cdk4-mediated phosphorylation of CUGBP1 increases the interactions of CUGBP1 with eIF2 during normal myogenesis, a pathway found to be reduced in DM1 cells (Salisbury et al., 2008). Moreover, ectopic expression of cyclin D3 in DM1 cells enhances fusion of DM1 myoblasts and leads to the correction of differentiation (Salisbury et al., 2008). A more recent study, showed that human skeletal muscle satellite cells isolated from fetal congenital DM1 patients bearing large CTG expansions (>3000) secrete prostaglandin E2 (PGE(2)) that inhibits the fusion of normal myoblasts in culture by decreasing the intracellular levels of calcium (Beaulieu et al., 2011). Authors suggest that the delay in muscle maturation observed in congenital DM1 patients may result, at least in part, from an altered autocrine mechanism (Beaulieu et al., 2011).

3. Therapeutic approaches for DM1

3.1 Restoring MBNL1 and CUGBP1 protein activity

It is widely accepted that MBNL and CUGBP play a major role in the pathogenesis of DM1 and are therefore targets for the reversal of the defective splicing and subsequent alleviation of symptoms in the disease. MBNL activity is compromised due to its sequestration in RNA foci. Therefore an approach to increase its expression levels and hence its activity could serve as a potential route for restoring alternative splicing. Kanadia et al. used intramuscular injection with an AAV (adeno-associated virus) expressing MBNL1 protein in a transgenic mouse model of DM1. This transgenic mouse model carries the human skeletal *α-actin (HSA)* gene modified by insertion of 250 CTG repeats within the 3′ untranslated region. These mice develop severe myotonia and dystrophic muscle features characteristic of DM1 disease. Overexpression of MBNL1 saturated the expanded CUG binding sites of the mutant DMPK transcripts and free MBNL1 was able to cause the reversal of muscle hyperexcitability, myotonia and spliceopathy (Kanadia et al., 2006). These results, demonstrated that the elevated expression of MBNL1 alone was sufficient to rescue myotonia, a key pathological feature of DM1, and aberrant splicing of specific gene transcripts, characteristic of the DM1 skeletal muscle. In a parallel study, de Haro et al. used a *Drosophila* model of DM1 expressing mRNA transcripts containing 480 CUG repeats, which accumulate in nuclear foci and show degenerative phenotypes in muscle (muscle wasting) and eye tissue (disorganization and fusion of the ommatidia as well as loss and duplication of inter-ommatidial bristles) as well as other key histopathological features of DM1. Furthermore, this DM1 model shows altered levels of MBNL1 and CUGBP1, as observed in DM1 pathogenesis. Overexpression of MBNl1 in this DM1 model showed to suppress the muscle and eye phenotypes of DM1. Interestingly, expanded RNA transcripts that accumulated in nuclear foci within muscle cells were decreased in flies expressing the mutant RNA transcripts that also overexpress MBNL1 (de Haro et al., 2006).

CUGBP1 has been shown to be up-regulated in DM1 as a result of PKC activation and subsequent CUGBP1 protein hyperphosphorylation and stabilization (Kuyumcu-Martinez et al., 2007). Wang et al. created a heart specific Tamoxifen-inducible mouse model containing 960 CTG repeats within the last exon of the DMPK. These mice exhibited high mortality, conduction abnormalities, and systolic and diastolic dysfunction as well as molecular changes seen in DM1 patients, such as increased levels of CUGBP1, colocalization of MBNL1 with RNA foci and reversion of splicing to embryonic patterns. Blocking of PKC activity, using a specific PKC inhibitor (Ro-31-8220), in this heart-specific DM1 mouse model ameliorated several DM1 symptoms, including cardiac conduction defects and contraction abnormalities (Wang et al., 2009). The inhibitor also reduced the splicing defects regulated by CUGBP1, but not those regulated by MBNL1, suggesting distinct roles for these proteins in DM1 cardiac pathogenesis (Wang et al., 2009). As previously described, DM1 mouse models showed elevated levels of CUGBP1 that leads to a delay of muscle development and differentiation. Salisbury et al. presented evidence that two signal transduction pathways regulate CUGBP1 activity in normal muscle and that these pathways are altered in DM1 cells. CUGBP1 was found to be phosphorylated by different kinases, during myoblast proliferation and differentiation and that phosphorylation of CUGBP1 at different sites directs CUGBP1 to different mRNA targets. Moreover, cyclin D3-cdk4-mediated phosphorylation of CUGBP1 increases the interactions of CUGBP1 with eIF2 during normal myogenesis. Furthermore, it was found that cyclin D3-cdk4 pathway is reduced in DM1 cells and that the normalization of cyclin D3 expression in DM1 cells leads to the correction of differentiation (Salisbury et al., 2008).

Overexpression of MBNL1 and downregulation of CUGBP1 or modulation of their counterparts showed encouraging results towards the development of rational therapies for DM1. These two key proteins play a major role in the pathogenesis of the disease and any attempt to normalize their function will be beneficial.

3.2 Targeting the mutant DMPK transcripts

A promising gene therapy approach is to target the mutant DMPK transcripts. Most of the attempts to eliminate toxic *DMPK* transcripts in DM1 cells and animal models used catalytic

RNA (ribozymes) (Langlois et al., 2003; Phylactou et al., 1998), chemically modified antisense oligonucleotides (Furling et al., 2003; Mulders et al., 2009) and siRNA duplexes (Langlois et al., 2005).

Ribozymes are RNA molecules that adopt a tertiary structure and function as catalysts. The hammerhead, hairpin and hepatitis delta virus (HDV) ribozyme motifs can be characterized by their ability for self-cleavage of a particular phosphodiester bond. Hammerhead ribozymes have the ability to suppress gene expression through specific cleavage of RNA molecules (Phylactou et al., 1998; Tedeschi et al., 2009). Langlois et al. designed a hammerhead ribozyme with significant accessibility to a specific target site within the 3′ UTR of the DMPK mRNA. Utilizing this system, a significant reduction of mutant and normal DMPK 3′ UTR transcripts was observed. Furthermore, these human DM1 myoblasts showed a significant reduction of nuclear RNA foci and a partial restoration of insulin receptor isoform B expression. This study demonstrated for the first time intracellular ribozyme-mediated cleavage of nuclear-retained mutant DMPK mRNAs, providing a potential gene therapy agent for the treatment of myotonic dystrophy (Langlois et al., 2003). Beside degradation of their targets, ribozymes can lead to splicing events that replace target RNA with embedded sequences. Group I Intron ribozymes can be characterized by their capacity for self-splicing by cleavage and ligation of phosphodiester bonds (Cech, 1990; Fiskaa & Birgisdottir, 2010). Group I intron ribozymes can be designed to act in *trans* by recognition and separation of RNA molecules in a sequence specific manner, and ligation of a new RNA sequence to the separated RNA molecules. In their 1998 study, Phylactou et al. created a group I intron ribozyme to cleave, *in vitro*, a DMPK RNA containing 12 repeats and replace them with 5 repeats. Furthermore, it was shown that similar splicing was able to be achieved in human cultured fibroblasts (Phylactou et al., 1998). Another promising approach is to target the mutant DMPK transcripts with antisense oligonucleotides. In 2003, Furling et al. showed that by infecting DM1 cells in culture with an adenoviral vector expressing an antisense RNA to the CUG repeat sequence, the mutant DMPK mRNA was significantly reduced. In addition, effective restoration of human DM1 myoblast functions such as myoblast fusion and the uptake of glucose was achieved (Furling et al., 2003). Furthermore, DM1 cells expressing the antisense RNA indicated a correction of CUGBP1 expression in infected DM1 cells. Muscle differentiation and insulin resistance in DM1 were found to be in close proximity with the misregulation of CUGBP1 protein levels.

Alternative approaches towards targeting the mutant DMPK transcripts in DM1, include the use of chemically modified antisense oligonucleotides. A recent report showed convincingly the therapeutic effect of 2-*O*-methyl phosphorothioate modified $(CAG)_7$ oligonucleotides in DM1 mouse models and in patient myoblast cultures (Mulders et al., 2009). The addition of 2-O-methyl groups to a phosphorothioate-modified oligonucleotide confirms increased stability of binding and reduced nonspecific effects. Local administration of the modified oligonucleotide in skeletal muscle resulted in approximately 50% reduction of expanded *DMPK* RNA. As a result, RNA foci were also reduced and defective splicing corrected. Such findings demonstrate that a low (CUG) *n* RNA dosage can still be beneficial to patients and be an attractive therapeutic approach. Myotonia is one of the key features of DM1 and is associated with abnormal alternative splicing of the muscle-specific chloride channel (ClC-1) and reduced conductance of chloride ions in the sarcolemma. Wheeler et al. developed a morpholino antisense oligonucleotide targeting the 3′ splice site of ClC-1 exon 7a and reversed the defect of ClC-1 alternative splicing in two mouse models of

DM1. The levels of ClC-1 mRNA and eventually protein were found to be upregulated. Moreover, treated mice had a fully functional chloride channel and lack myotonia (Wheeler et al., 2007).

In one approach to inhibit the sequestration of MBNL1 with the expanded CUG repeats, Wheeler et al. used a $(CAG)_{25}$ antisense oligonucleotide morpholino. Antisense morpholinos are unable to cause the cleavage of their target RNAs. *In vitro*, these morpholinos were able to bind to the expanded CUG repeats forming a stable RNA-morpholino heteroduplex that was able to block the formation of MBNL1-RNA complexes and disrupt complexes that had already formed. *In vivo*, intramuscular injection and electroporation of the $(CAG)_{25}$ antisense oligonucleotide morpholino in a transgenic mouse model that accumulate expanded CUG RNA and MBNL1 protein in nuclear foci in skeletal muscle, caused the reduction of nuclear foci and redistribution of MBNL1 protein. 14 weeks after treatment, myotonia was significantly reduced and ClC-1 function restored. The same approach was used to test the effect of this morpholino in an mbnl-1 deficient mouse, which mimics most of the splicing abnormalities of DM1. The morpholino had no effect, confirming that the morpholino specifically acts on the expanded repeats, which are not present in the mbnl1 knockout model (Wheeler et al., 2009).

RNAi has also been used successfully to degrade mutant *DMPK* transcripts. SiRNA duplexes induce the specific cleavage of target RNAs in mammalian cells. Although most of the RNAi applications rely on the cytoplasmic effect of these molecules, it has been shown that RNAi phenomena can occur in the nucleus of primary DM1 cells by targeting nuclear retained *DMPK* mRNAs (Langlois et al., 2005). Krol et al. attempted to target particularly long hairpin structures formed from the interactions of CUG repeats rather than the targeting of nascent RNA in general. In this study it was demonstrated that these long CUG repeat hairpins are under the control of a ribonuclease Dicer, involved in the RNA interference pathway whose main function is to induce the fragmentation of double-stranded RNA duplexes into shorter duplexes, which then act as endogenous siRNAs and trigger the downstream silencing effect. Furthermore, it was shown that the transduction of synthetic $(CAG)_7$ siRNAs into DM1 patient fibroblasts, leads towards a selective reduction of mutant transcripts containing long CUG repeats (Krol et al., 2007).

An alternative approach to confront the toxicity of nuclear RNA retention is to block the binding of RNA-binding proteins to mutant *DMPK* transcripts using small chemical molecules with high affinity towards the mutant *DMPK* transcripts. The binding of these molecules on the mutant *DMPK* transcripts should prevent the binding and therefore the sequestration of RNA-binding proteins, such as MBNL1, and restore aberrant splicing (Mastroyiannopoulos et al., 2010). Several approaches have been performed with the most promising of these being the use of pentamidine, a small molecule that binds to the expanded CUG RNA sequence with high affinity and specificity causing reduction of CUG repeat foci formation and relieves MBNL1 sequestration (Warf et al., 2009). Moreover, pentamidine reversed the mis-splicing of 4 different pre-mRNAs affected in DM1 (Warf et al., 2009). Gareiss et al. used resin-bound dynamic combinatorial chemistry in order to identify the compounds that are able to inhibit MBNL1 binding to expanded CUG RNA. Screening of 11,325 members yielded several molecules with significant selectivity for binding to CUG repeat RNA. These compounds were also able to inhibit the interaction of expanded CUG with MBNL1 *in vitro* (Gareiss et al., 2008). In another report, the design of high affinity ligands that bind to expanded CUG and CAG repeats and inhibit the formation of RNA-protein complexes that are implicated in DM1 was described (Pushechnikov et al., 2009). Similarly, Garcia-Lopez et al. identified molecules that aim to target toxic CUG RNA transcripts when applied on a *Drosophila* model of DM1. By performing a positional scanning combinatorial peptide library screen, a D-amino acid hexapeptide (ABP1) that reduced CUG-induced toxicity in fly eyes and muscles was identified. Furthermore, ABP1 reversed muscle histopathology and splicing misregulation of MBNL1 targets in DM1 model mice. *In vitro*, ABP1 was found bound to CUG hairpins and induced a switch to a single-stranded conformation (Garcia-Lopez et al., 2011). In another study, Arambula et al. created a ligand with high nanomolar affinity to CUG RNA or CTG DNA repeats. This ligand is a triaminotriazine-acridine conjugate designed to hydrogen bond to both U's or T's in the U-U or T-T mismatch, interactions observed between binding of multi CUG and CTG repeats. This ligand was found to destabilize the interactions of MBNL1 with multi CUG repeats (Arambula et al., 2009).

3.3 Induction of mutant DMPK transcripts nuclear export

Few studies have attempted to determine whether the export of mutant DMPK transcripts is beneficial for the disease. The export of mutant DMPK RNA transcripts from the nucleus to the cytoplasm will have as a result the recovery of these cells from DM1 pathogenic events. The export of mRNA from the nucleus is a highly ordered and complicated procedure that implicates several molecules. As previously described, mutant DMPK RNA carrying long CUG repeats form haipin structures which then interact with proteins such as MBNL1 and CUGBP1. These interactions most possibly prohibit the export of these transcripts to the cytoplasm and cause nuclear retention in the form of foci.

Mastroyiannopoulos et al. have demonstrated nuclear export of mutant DMPK 3′-UTR transcripts by introducing a viral post-transcriptional regulatory element. The WPRE (Woodchuck post-transcriptional regulatory element) has been widely used as an enhancer during transgene expression (Lee et al., 2005). It is also known to enhance gene expression through stimulation of nuclear RNA export (Donello et al., 1998). WPRE was inserted downstream of the 3′-end of a mutant DMPK 3′-UTR sequence and was shown to bypass nuclear entrapment. With the use of fluorescence *in situ* hybridization it was shown that the mutant DMPK transcripts that carried the WPRE sequence were localized mainly in the cytoplasm of C2C12 cells in the form of foci. WPRE mediated nuclear export enhanced muscle cell differentiation (Mastroyiannopoulos et al., 2005) and more specifically initial fusion of myoblasts (Mastroyiannopoulos et al., 2008). In another study, cardiac cells, identified from a transgenic mouse in which 400 CTG repeats were positioned downstream of the reporter *LacZ* gene and upstream of the bovine growth hormone polyadenylation signal, localized CUG aggregates exclusively in the cytoplasm of cells (Dansithong et al., 2005). Aggregation of CUG RNAs within the cytoplasm resulted both in MBNL1 sequestration and in approximately 2-fold increase in both nuclear and cytoplasmic CUGBP1 levels. Significantly, and despite these changes, RNA splice defects were not observed, and functional analysis revealed only subtle cardiac dysfunction. These results demonstrate that the presence of mutant DMPK transcripts in the cytoplasm in the form of foci is insufficient to elicit DM1 defects. Interestingly, Garcia-Lopez et al. described a transgenic *Drosophila* model expressing expanded CTG repeats which exhibit an extended

DM1 phenotype. Such as, muscle degeneration, ribonuclear formation, interactions with muscleblinds including misregulated alternative splicing of muscle genes and CUG depended central nervous system alterations. Genetic screens and functional assays on this *Drosophila* model identified the RNA export factor Aly as one of the causes of the phenotype. It has been shown that the Aly phenotype has a close relationship to mRNA export factors and EJC (exon junction complex) components. Mutations in Aly were shown to be associated with nuclear accumulation of CUG repeats. It is therefore important to study further the mRNA export pathway implicated in DM1 and identify candidate targets for repairing nuclear retention of the DMPK transcripts (Garcia-Lopez et al., 2008). Finally, a report proved in a very convincing way the benefit of exporting mutant DMPK transcripts to the cytoplasm. Wheeler et al. attempted to reverse the myotonic dystrophy symptoms in a well-studied animal model by interfering with the MBNL1 and CUG RNA hairpins interaction. The authors used a 25-nt antisense molecule, composed of CAG repeats, in order to prevent the interaction between MBNL1 and expanded CUG repeats by forming a heteroduplex with the hairpins. The oligonucleotide caused elimination of foci and released the trapped transcripts to the cytoplasm. Moreover, the antisense oligonucleotide repaired the defect of mis-splicing and restored the CLCN1 function and myotonia. This paper provided proof-of concept about the therapeutic potential of molecules that prevent the deleterious interactions between proteins and RNA in diseases.

4. Discussion / conclusions

In conclusion, almost 20 years after the discovery of DM1 mutation there is a very good understanding of the pathogenic mechanisms involved in DM1. As previously stated, the mutant DM1 RNA transcripts generate most of the pathological aspects of DM1. The retention of DMPK transcripts as ribonuclear inclusions in the nucleus of DM1 cells is considered to be an important pathogenic mechanism of the disease (Mankodi et al., 2000). A growing body of evidence showed that pleiotropic effects of aberrant interactions between mutant DMPK 3' UTR transcripts and RNA-binding proteins alter the metabolism of 'target' messenger RNAs (Ho et al., 2005; Jiang et al., 2004; Timchenko et al., 1996; Timchenko et al., 2001; Timchenko et al., 2004). Members of the muscleblind family (MBNL, MBXL and MBLL), which usually regulate mRNA splicing, have been shown to colocalize with the ribonuclear inclusions. The nuclear interactions of the MBNL proteins with the mutant DMPK 3' UTR transcripts, have shown to affect the splicing of various mRNAs, such as the insulin receptor (IR), troponin T (cTNT) and the muscle-specific chloride channel (ClC-1). Another RNA-binding protein, implicated in DM1 mechanism of pathogenesis, is CUGBP1. Extensive investigations have shown that CUGBP1 activity is increased in DM cells, and results in a trans-dominant effect on gene splicing.

Although there is very good understanding of the consequences of the genetic mutation that causes DM1, the exact mechanisms responsible for the DM1 phenotype is not completely understood. DM1 pathogenesis is very complex and therefore, different potential approaches and multiple targets can be used for the development of DM1 therapies. To date, several attempts have been described as potential approaches for the therapy of the disease, either by restoring the levels of CUGBP1 and MBNL proteins, by targeting the mutant DMPK 3′ UTR transcripts or by the export of this toxic RNA from the nucleus to the cytoplasm of DM1 cells. All of the above approaches hold a great promise for the future treatment of myotonic dystrophy, nevertheless it is also certain that more therapeutic approaches will be unveiled in the near future, which may be variations of the existing methods or novel ways to tackle the pathogenesis of the disease. Further research in DM1 needs to be done in order to move these therapies forward into clinical trials for the cure of DM1 disease.

5. Acknowledgements

Work carried out in the authors' laboratory and described in this chapter was supported by a grant to L.A.P. by A.G. Leventis Foundation.

6. References

Alwazzan, M., E. Newman, M. G. Hamshere & J. D. Brook (1999). "Myotonic dystrophy is associated with a reduced level of RNA from the DMWD allele adjacent to the expanded repeat." *Hum Mol Genet* 8(8): 1491-1497.

Amack, J. D. & M. S. Mahadevan (2001). "The myotonic dystrophy expanded CUG repeat tract is necessary but not sufficient to disrupt C2C12 myoblast differentiation." *Hum Mol Genet* 10(18): 1879-1887.

Amack, J. D. & M. S. Mahadevan (2004). "Myogenic defects in myotonic dystrophy." *Dev Biol* 265(2): 294-301.

Amack, J. D., A. P. Paguio & M. S. Mahadevan (1999). "Cis and trans effects of the myotonic dystrophy (DM) mutation in a cell culture model." *Hum Mol Genet* 8(11): 1975-1984.

Arambula, J. F., S. R. Ramisetty, A. M. Baranger & S. C. Zimmerman (2009). "A simple ligand that selectively targets CUG trinucleotide repeats and inhibits MBNL protein binding." *Proc Natl Acad Sci U S A* 106(38): 16068-16073.

Artero, R., A. Prokop, N. Paricio, G. Begemann, I. Pueyo, M. Mlodzik, M. Perez-Alonso & M. K. Baylies (1998). "The muscleblind gene participates in the organization of Z-bands and epidermal attachments of Drosophila muscles and is regulated by Dmef2." *Dev Biol* 195(2): 131-143.

Aslanidis, C., G. Jansen, C. Amemiya, G. Shutler, M. Mahadevan, C. Tsilfidis, C. Chen, J. Alleman, N. G. Wormskamp, M. Vooijs, J. Buxton, K. Johnson, H. J. M. Smeets, G. G. Lennon, A. V. Carrano, R. G. Korneluk, B. Wieringa & P. J. de Jong (1992). "Cloning of the essential myotonic dystrophy region and mapping of the putative defect." *Nature* 355(6360): 548-551.

Beaulieu, D., P. Thebault, R. Pelletier, P. Chapdelaine, M. Tarnopolsky, D. Furling & J. Puymirat (2011). "Abnormal prostaglandin E2 production blocks myogenic differentiation in myotonic dystrophy." *Neurobiol Dis.*

Begemann, G., N. Paricio, R. Artero, I. Kiss, M. Perez-Alonso & M. Mlodzik (1997). "muscleblind, a gene required for photoreceptor differentiation in Drosophila, encodes novel nuclear Cys3His-type zinc-finger-containing proteins." *Development* 124(21): 4321-4331.

Brook, J. D., M. E. McCurrach, H. G. Harley, A. J. Buckler, D. Church, H. Aburatani, K. Hunter, V. P. Stanton, J. P. Thirion, T. Hudson, R. Sohn, B. Zemelman, R. G. Snell, S. A. Rundle, S. Crow, J. Davies, P. Shelbourne, J. Buxton, C. Jones, V. Juvonen, K. Johnson, P. S. Harper, D. J. Shaw & D. E. Housman (1992). "Molecular basis of myotonic dystrophy: expansion of a trinucleotide (CTG) repeat at the 3' end of a transcript encoding a protein kinase family member." *Cell* 68(4): 799-808.

Buj-Bello, A., D. Furling, H. Tronchere, J. Laporte, T. Lerouge, G. S. Butler-Browne & J. L. Mandel (2002). "Muscle-specific alternative splicing of myotubularin-related 1 gene is impaired in DM1 muscle cells." *Hum Mol Genet* 11(19): 2297-2307.

Cech, T. R. (1990). "Self-splicing of group I introns." *Annu Rev Biochem* 59: 543-568.

Charlet, B. N., R. S. Savkur, G. Singh, A. V. Philips, E. A. Grice & T. A. Cooper (2002). "Loss of the muscle-specific chloride channel in type 1 myotonic dystrophy due to misregulated alternative splicing." *Mol Cell* 10(1): 45-53.

Colleran, J. A., R. J. Hawley, E. E. Pinnow, P. F. Kokkinos & R. D. Fletcher (1997). "Value of the electrocardiogram in determining cardiac events and mortality in myotonic dystrophy." *Am J Cardiol* 80(11): 1494-1497.

Dansithong, W., S. Paul, L. Comai & S. Reddy (2005). "MBNL1 is the primary determinant of focus formation and aberrant insulin receptor splicing in DM1." *J Biol Chem* 280(7): 5773-5780.

Davies, K. E., J. Jackson, R. Williamson, P. S. Harper, S. Ball, M. Sarfarazi, L. Meredith & G. Fey (1983). "Linkage analysis of myotonic dystrophy and sequences on chromosome 19 using a cloned complement 3 gene probe." *J Med Genet* 20(4): 259-263.

Davis, B. M., M. E. McCurrach, K. L. Taneja, R. H. Singer & D. E. Housman (1997). "Expansion of a CUG trinucleotide repeat in the 3' untranslated region of myotonic dystrophy protein kinase transcripts results in nuclear retention of transcripts." *Proc Natl Acad Sci U S A* 94(14): 7388-7393.

de Haro, M., I. Al-Ramahi, B. De Gouyon, L. Ukani, A. Rosa, N. A. Faustino, T. Ashizawa, T. A. Cooper & J. Botas (2006). "MBNL1 and CUGBP1 modify expanded CUG-induced toxicity in a Drosophila model of myotonic dystrophy type 1." *Hum Mol Genet* 15(13): 2138-2145.

Dhaenens, C. M., S. Schraen-Maschke, H. Tran, V. Vingtdeux, D. Ghanem, O. Leroy, J. Delplanque, E. Vanbrussel, A. Delacourte, P. Vermersch, C. A. Maurage, H. Gruffat, A. Sergeant, M. S. Mahadevan, S. Ishiura, L. Buee, T. A. Cooper, M. L. Caillet-Boudin, N. Charlet-Berguerand, B. Sablonniere & N. Sergeant (2008). "Overexpression of MBNL1 fetal isoforms and modified splicing of Tau in the DM1 brain: two individual consequences of CUG trinucleotide repeats." *Exp Neurol* 210(2): 467-478.

Donello, J. E., J. E. Loeb & T. J. Hope (1998). "Woodchuck hepatitis virus contains a tripartite posttranscriptional regulatory element." *J Virol* 72(6): 5085-5092.

Fardaei, M., K. Larkin, J. D. Brook & M. G. Hamshere (2001). "In vivo co-localisation of MBNL protein with DMPK expanded-repeat transcripts." *Nucleic Acids Res* 29(13): 2766-2771.

Fardaei, M., M. T. Rogers, H. M. Thorpe, K. Larkin, M. G. Hamshere, P. S. Harper & J. D. Brook (2002). "Three proteins, MBNL, MBLL and MBXL, co-localize in vivo with nuclear foci of expanded-repeat transcripts in DM1 and DM2 cells." *Hum Mol Genet* 11(7): 805-814.

Fiskaa, T. & A. B. Birgisdottir (2010). "RNA reprogramming and repair based on trans-splicing group I ribozymes." *N Biotechnol* 27(3): 194-203.

Fugier, C., A. F. Klein, C. Hammer, S. Vassilopoulos, Y. Ivarsson, A. Toussaint, V. Tosch, A. Vignaud, A. Ferry, N. Messaddeq, Y. Kokunai, R. Tsuburaya, P. de la Grange, D. Dembele, V. Francois, G. Precigout, C. Boulade-Ladame, M. C. Hummel, A. L. de Munain, N. Sergeant, A. Laquerriere, C. Thibault, F. Deryckere, D. Auboeuf, L. Garcia, P. Zimmermann, B. Udd, B. Schoser, M. P. Takahashi, I. Nishino, G. Bassez, J. Laporte, D. Furling & N. Charlet-Berguerand (2011). "Misregulated alternative splicing of BIN1 is associated with T tubule alterations and muscle weakness in myotonic dystrophy." *Nat Med* 17(6): 720-725.

Furling, D., L. Coiffier, V. Mouly, J. P. Barbet, J. L. St Guily, K. Taneja, G. Gourdon, C. Junien & G. S. Butler-Browne (2001). "Defective satellite cells in congenital myotonic dystrophy." *Hum Mol Genet* 10(19): 2079-2087.

Furling, D., G. Doucet, M. A. Langlois, L. Timchenko, E. Belanger, L. Cossette & J. Puymirat (2003). "Viral vector producing antisense RNA restores myotonic dystrophy myoblast functions." *Gene Ther* 10(9): 795-802.

Furling, D., D. Lemieux, K. Taneja & J. Puymirat (2001). "Decreased levels of myotonic dystrophy protein kinase (DMPK) and delayed differentiation in human myotonic dystrophy myoblasts." *Neuromuscul Disord* 11(8): 728-735.

Gallo, J. M. & C. Spickett (2010). "The role of CELF proteins in neurological disorders." *RNA Biol* 7(4): 474-479.

Garcia-Lopez, A., B. Llamusi, M. Orzaez, E. Perez-Paya & R. D. Artero (2011). "In vivo discovery of a peptide that prevents CUG-RNA hairpin formation and reverses RNA toxicity in myotonic dystrophy models." *Proc Natl Acad Sci U S A* 108(29): 11866-11871.

Garcia-Lopez, A., L. Monferrer, I. Garcia-Alcover, M. Vicente-Crespo, M. C. Alvarez-Abril & R. D. Artero (2008). "Genetic and chemical modifiers of a CUG toxicity model in Drosophila." *PLoS One* 3(2): e1595.

Gareiss, P. C., K. Sobczak, B. R. McNaughton, P. B. Palde, C. A. Thornton & B. L. Miller (2008). "Dynamic combinatorial selection of molecules capable of inhibiting the (CUG) repeat RNA-MBNL1 interaction in vitro: discovery of lead compounds targeting myotonic dystrophy (DM1)." *J Am Chem Soc* 130(48): 16254-16261.

Goers, E. S., J. Purcell, R. B. Voelker, D. P. Gates & J. A. Berglund (2010). "MBNL1 binds GC motifs embedded in pyrimidines to regulate alternative splicing." *Nucleic Acids Res* 38(7): 2467-2484.

Hao, M., K. Akrami, K. Wei, C. De Diego, N. Che, J. H. Ku, J. Tidball, M. C. Graves, P. B. Shieh & F. Chen (2008). "Muscleblind-like 2 (Mbnl2) -deficient mice as a model for myotonic dystrophy." *Dev Dyn* 237(2): 403-410.

Harper, P. S. (1989). "Gene mapping and the muscular dystrophies." *Prog Clin Biol Res* 306: 29-49.

Ho, T. H., D. Bundman, D. L. Armstrong & T. A. Cooper (2005). "Transgenic mice expressing CUG-BP1 reproduce splicing mis-regulation observed in myotonic dystrophy." *Hum Mol Genet* 14(11): 1539-1547.

Ho, T. H., B. N. Charlet, M. G. Poulos, G. Singh, M. S. Swanson & T. A. Cooper (2004). "Muscleblind proteins regulate alternative splicing." *EMBO J* 23(15): 3103-3112.

Ho, T. H., R. S. Savkur, M. G. Poulos, M. A. Mancini, M. S. Swanson & T. A. Cooper (2005). "Colocalization of muscleblind with RNA foci is separable from mis-regulation of alternative splicing in myotonic dystrophy." *J Cell Sci* 118(Pt 13): 2923-2933.

Houseley, J. M., Z. Wang, G. J. Brock, J. Soloway, R. Artero, M. Perez-Alonso, K. M. O'Dell & D. G. Monckton (2005). "Myotonic dystrophy associated expanded CUG repeat muscleblind positive ribonuclear foci are not toxic to Drosophila." *Hum Mol Genet* 14(6): 873-883.

Jansen, G., P. J. Groenen, D. Bachner, P. H. Jap, M. Coerwinkel, F. Oerlemans, W. van den Broek, B. Gohlsch, D. Pette, J. J. Plomp, P. C. Molenaar, M. G. Nederhoff, C. J. van Echteld, M. Dekker, A. Berns, H. Hameister & B. Wieringa (1996). "Abnormal myotonic dystrophy protein kinase levels produce only mild myopathy in mice." *Nat Genet* 13(3): 316-324.

Jiang, H., A. Mankodi, M. S. Swanson, R. T. Moxley & C. A. Thornton (2004). "Myotonic dystrophy type 1 is associated with nuclear foci of mutant RNA, sequestration of muscleblind proteins and deregulated alternative splicing in neurons." *Hum Mol Genet* 13(24): 3079-3088.

Jungbluth, H., C. Wallgren-Pettersson & J. Laporte (2008). "Centronuclear (myotubular) myopathy." *Orphanet J Rare Dis* 3: 26.

Kanadia, R. N., K. A. Johnstone, A. Mankodi, C. Lungu, C. A. Thornton, D. Esson, A. M. Timmers, W. W. Hauswirth & M. S. Swanson (2003). "A muscleblind knockout model for myotonic dystrophy." *Science* 302(5652): 1978-1980.

Kanadia, R. N., J. Shin, Y. Yuan, S. G. Beattie, T. M. Wheeler, C. A. Thornton & M. S. Swanson (2006). "Reversal of RNA missplicing and myotonia after muscleblind overexpression in a mouse poly(CUG) model for myotonic dystrophy." *Proc Natl Acad Sci U S A* 103(31): 11748-11753.

Kanadia, R. N., C. R. Urbinati, V. J. Crusselle, D. Luo, Y. J. Lee, J. K. Harrison, S. P. Oh & M. S. Swanson (2003). "Developmental expression of mouse muscleblind genes Mbnl1, Mbnl2 and Mbnl3." *Gene Expr Patterns* 3(4): 459-462.

Kimura, T., M. Nakamori, J. D. Lueck, P. Pouliquin, F. Aoike, H. Fujimura, R. T. Dirksen, M. P. Takahashi, A. F. Dulhunty & S. Sakoda (2005). "Altered mRNA splicing of the skeletal muscle ryanodine receptor and sarcoplasmic/endoplasmic reticulum Ca2+-ATPase in myotonic dystrophy type 1." *Hum Mol Genet* 14(15): 2189-2200.

Kino, Y., D. Mori, Y. Oma, Y. Takeshita, N. Sasagawa & S. Ishiura (2004). "Muscleblind protein, MBNL1/EXP, binds specifically to CHHG repeats." *Hum Mol Genet* 13(5): 495-507.

Klein, A. F., E. Gasnier & D. Furling (2011). "Gain of RNA function in pathological cases: Focus on myotonic dystrophy." *Biochimie.*

Klesert, T. R., D. H. Cho, J. I. Clark, J. Maylie, J. Adelman, L. Snider, E. C. Yuen, P. Soriano & S. J. Tapscott (2000). "Mice deficient in Six5 develop cataracts: implications for myotonic dystrophy." *Nat Genet* 25(1): 105-109.

Klesert, T. R., A. D. Otten, T. D. Bird & S. J. Tapscott (1997). "Trinucleotide repeat expansion at the myotonic dystrophy locus reduces expression of DMAHP." *Nat Genet* 16(4): 402-406.

Koch, K. S. & H. L. Leffert (1998). "Giant hairpins formed by CUG repeats in myotonic dystrophy messenger RNAs might sterically block RNA export through nuclear pores." *J Theor Biol* 192(4): 505-514.

Koebis, M., N. Ohsawa, Y. Kino, N. Sasagawa, I. Nishino & S. Ishiura (2011). "Alternative splicing of myomesin 1 gene is aberrantly regulated in myotonic dystrophy type 1." *Genes Cells.*

Koshelev, M., S. Sarma, R. E. Price, X. H. Wehrens & T. A. Cooper (2010). "Heart-specific overexpression of CUGBP1 reproduces functional and molecular abnormalities of myotonic dystrophy type 1." *Hum Mol Genet* 19(6): 1066-1075.

Krol, J., A. Fiszer, A. Mykowska, K. Sobczak, M. de Mezer & W. J. Krzyzosiak (2007). "Ribonuclease dicer cleaves triplet repeat hairpins into shorter repeats that silence specific targets." *Mol Cell* 25(4): 575-586.

Kuyumcu-Martinez, N. M., G. S. Wang & T. A. Cooper (2007). "Increased steady-state levels of CUGBP1 in myotonic dystrophy 1 are due to PKC-mediated hyperphosphorylation." *Mol Cell* 28(1): 68-78.

Lange, S., I. Agarkova, J. C. Perriard & E. Ehler (2005). "The sarcomeric M-band during development and in disease." *J Muscle Res Cell Motil* 26(6-8): 375-379.

Langlois, M. A., C. Boniface, G. Wang, J. Alluin, P. M. Salvaterra, J. Puymirat, J. J. Rossi & N. S. Lee (2005). "Cytoplasmic and nuclear retained DMPK mRNAs are targets for RNA interference in myotonic dystrophy cells." *J Biol Chem* 280(17): 16949-16954.

Langlois, M. A., N. S. Lee, J. J. Rossi & J. Puymirat (2003). "Hammerhead ribozyme-mediated destruction of nuclear foci in myotonic dystrophy myoblasts." *Mol Ther* 7(5 Pt 1): 670-680.

Larkin, K. & M. Fardaei (2001). "Myotonic dystrophy--a multigene disorder." *Brain Res Bull* 56(3-4): 389-395.

Lee, K. S., Y. Cao, H. E. Witwicka, S. Tom, S. J. Tapscott & E. H. Wang (2010). "RNA-binding protein Muscleblind-like 3 (MBNL3) disrupts myocyte enhancer factor 2 (Mef2) {beta}-exon splicing." *J Biol Chem* 285(44): 33779-33787.

Lee, Y. B., C. P. Glover, A. S. Cosgrave, A. Bienemann & J. B. Uney (2005). "Optimizing regulatable gene expression using adenoviral vectors." *Exp Physiol* 90(1): 33-37.

Machuca-Tzili, L., D. Brook & D. Hilton-Jones (2005). "Clinical and molecular aspects of the myotonic dystrophies: a review." *Muscle Nerve* 32(1): 1-18.

Machuca-Tzili, L. E., S. Buxton, A. Thorpe, C. M. Timson, P. Wigmore, P. K. Luther & J. D. Brook (2011). "Zebrafish deficient for Muscleblind-like 2 exhibit features of myotonic dystrophy." *Dis Model Mech* 4(3): 381-392.

Mammarella, A., P. Ferroni, M. Paradiso, F. Martini, V. Paoletti, S. Morino, G. Antonini, P. P. Gazzaniga, A. Musca & S. Basili (2002). "Tumor necrosis factor-alpha and myocardial function in patients with myotonic dystrophy type 1." *J Neurol Sci* 201(1-2): 59-64.

Mankodi, A., X. Lin, B. C. Blaxall, M. S. Swanson & C. A. Thornton (2005). "Nuclear RNA foci in the heart in myotonic dystrophy." *Circ Res* 97(11): 1152-1155.

Mankodi, A., E. Logigian, L. Callahan, C. McClain, R. White, D. Henderson, M. Krym & C. A. Thornton (2000). "Myotonic dystrophy in transgenic mice expressing an expanded CUG repeat." *Science* 289(5485): 1769-1773.

Mankodi, A., M. P. Takahashi, H. Jiang, C. L. Beck, W. J. Bowers, R. T. Moxley, S. C. Cannon & C. A. Thornton (2002). "Expanded CUG repeats trigger aberrant splicing of ClC-1 chloride channel pre-mRNA and hyperexcitability of skeletal muscle in myotonic dystrophy." *Mol Cell* 10(1): 35-44.

Mankodi, A., P. Teng-Umnuay, M. Krym, D. Henderson, M. Swanson & C. A. Thornton (2003). "Ribonuclear inclusions in skeletal muscle in myotonic dystrophy types 1 and 2." *Ann Neurol* 54(6): 760-768.

Martorell, L., M. A. Pujana, J. Valero, J. Joven, V. Volpini, A. Labad, X. Estivill & E. Vilella (1999). "Anticipation is not associated with CAG repeat expansion in parent-offspring pairs of patients affected with schizophrenia." *Am J Med Genet* 88(1): 50-56.

Mastroyiannopoulos, N. P., E. Chrysanthou, T. C. Kyriakides, J. B. Uney, M. S. Mahadevan & L. A. Phylactou (2008). "The effect of myotonic dystrophy transcript levels and location on muscle differentiation." *Biochem Biophys Res Commun* 377(2): 526-531.

Mastroyiannopoulos, N. P., M. L. Feldman, J. B. Uney, M. S. Mahadevan & L. A. Phylactou (2005). "Woodchuck post-transcriptional element induces nuclear export of myotonic dystrophy 3' untranslated region transcripts." *EMBO Rep* 6(5): 458-463.

Mastroyiannopoulos, N. P., C. Shammas & L. A. Phylactou (2010). "Tackling the pathogenesis of RNA nuclear retention in myotonic dystrophy." *Biol Cell* 102(9): 515-523.

Michalowski, S., J. W. Miller, C. R. Urbinati, M. Paliouras, M. S. Swanson & J. Griffith (1999). "Visualization of double-stranded RNAs from the myotonic dystrophy protein kinase gene and interactions with CUG-binding protein." *Nucleic Acids Res* 27(17): 3534-3542.

Miller, J. W., C. R. Urbinati, P. Teng-Umnuay, M. G. Stenberg, B. J. Byrne, C. A. Thornton & M. S. Swanson (2000). "Recruitment of human muscleblind proteins to (CUG)(n) expansions associated with myotonic dystrophy." *EMBO J* 19(17): 4439-4448.

Monckton, D. G., L. J. Wong, T. Ashizawa & C. T. Caskey (1995). "Somatic mosaicism, germline expansions, germline reversions and intergenerational reductions in myotonic dystrophy males: small pool PCR analyses." *Hum Mol Genet* 4(1): 1-8.

Moxley, R. T., A. J. Corbett, K. L. Minaker & J. W. Rowe (1984). "Whole body insulin resistance in myotonic dystrophy." *Ann Neurol* 15(2): 157-162.

Mulders, S. A., W. J. van den Broek, T. M. Wheeler, H. J. Croes, P. van Kuik-Romeijn, S. J. de Kimpe, D. Furling, G. J. Platenburg, G. Gourdon, C. A. Thornton, B. Wieringa & D. G. Wansink (2009). "Triplet-repeat oligonucleotide-mediated reversal of RNA toxicity in myotonic dystrophy." *Proc Natl Acad Sci U S A* 106(33): 13915-13920.

Napierala, M. & W. J. Krzyzosiak (1997). "CUG repeats present in myotonin kinase RNA form metastable "slippery" hairpins." *J Biol Chem* 272(49): 31079-31085.

Ogata, A., S. Terae, M. Fujita & K. Tashiro (1998). "Anterior temporal white matter lesions in myotonic dystrophy with intellectual impairment: an MRI and neuropathological study." *Neuroradiology* 40(7): 411-415.

Okoli, G., N. Carey, K. J. Johnson & D. J. Watt (1998). "Over expression of the murine myotonic dystrophy protein kinase in the mouse myogenic C2C12 cell line leads to inhibition of terminal differentiation." *Biochem Biophys Res Commun* 246(3): 905-911.

Orengo, J. P., P. Chambon, D. Metzger, D. R. Mosier, G. J. Snipes & T. A. Cooper (2008). "Expanded CTG repeats within the DMPK 3' UTR causes severe skeletal muscle wasting in an inducible mouse model for myotonic dystrophy." *Proc Natl Acad Sci U S A* 105(7): 2646-2651.

Otten, A. D. & S. J. Tapscott (1995). "Triplet repeat expansion in myotonic dystrophy alters the adjacent chromatin structure." *Proc Natl Acad Sci U S A* 92(12): 5465-5469.

Philips, A. V., L. T. Timchenko & T. A. Cooper (1998). "Disruption of splicing regulated by a CUG-binding protein in myotonic dystrophy." *Science* 280(5364): 737-741.

Phillips, M. F. & P. S. Harper (1997). "Cardiac disease in myotonic dystrophy." *Cardiovasc Res* 33(1): 13-22.

Phylactou, L. A., C. Darrah & M. J. Wood (1998). "Ribozyme-mediated trans-splicing of a trinucleotide repeat." *Nat Genet* 18(4): 378-381.

Phylactou, L. A., M. W. Kilpatrick & M. J. Wood (1998). "Ribozymes as therapeutic tools for genetic disease." *Hum Mol Genet* 7(10): 1649-1653.

Pushechnikov, A., M. M. Lee, J. L. Childs-Disney, K. Sobczak, J. M. French, C. A. Thornton & M. D. Disney (2009). "Rational design of ligands targeting triplet repeating transcripts that cause RNA dominant disease: application to myotonic muscular dystrophy type 1 and spinocerebellar ataxia type 3." *J Am Chem Soc* 131(28): 9767-9779.

Ranum, L. P. & J. W. Day (2002). "Myotonic dystrophy: clinical and molecular parallels between myotonic dystrophy type 1 and type 2." *Curr Neurol Neurosci Rep* 2(5): 465-470.

Reddy, S., D. B. Smith, M. M. Rich, J. M. Leferovich, P. Reilly, B. M. Davis, K. Tran, H. Rayburn, R. Bronson, D. Cros, R. J. Balice-Gordon & D. Housman (1996). "Mice lacking the myotonic dystrophy protein kinase develop a late onset progressive myopathy." *Nat Genet* 13(3): 325-335.

Roberts, R., N. A. Timchenko, J. W. Miller, S. Reddy, C. T. Caskey, M. S. Swanson & L. T. Timchenko (1997). "Altered phosphorylation and intracellular distribution of a (CUG)n triplet repeat RNA-binding protein in patients with myotonic dystrophy and in myotonin protein kinase knockout mice." *Proc Natl Acad Sci U S A* 94(24): 13221-13226.

Rubinsztein, J. S., D. C. Rubinsztein, P. J. McKenna, S. Goodburn & A. J. Holland (1997). "Mild myotonic dystrophy is associated with memory impairment in the context of normal general intelligence." *J Med Genet* 34(3): 229-233.

Sabourin, L. A., K. Tamai, M. A. Narang & R. G. Korneluk (1997). "Overexpression of 3'-untranslated region of the myotonic dystrophy kinase cDNA inhibits myoblast differentiation in vitro." *J Biol Chem* 272(47): 29626-29635.

Salisbury, E., K. Sakai, B. Schoser, C. Huichalaf, C. Schneider-Gold, H. Nguyen, G. L. Wang, J. H. Albrecht & L. T. Timchenko (2008). "Ectopic expression of cyclin D3 corrects differentiation of DM1 myoblasts through activation of RNA CUG-binding protein, CUGBP1." *Exp Cell Res* 314(11-12): 2266-2278.

Santoro, M., A. Modoni, M. Masciullo, T. Gidaro, A. Broccolini, E. Ricci, P. A. Tonali & G. Silvestri (2010). "Analysis of MTMR1 expression and correlation with muscle pathological features in juvenile/adult onset myotonic dystrophy type 1 (DM1) and in myotonic dystrophy type 2 (DM2)." *Exp Mol Pathol* 89(2): 158-168.

Savkur, R. S., A. V. Philips & T. A. Cooper (2001). "Aberrant regulation of insulin receptor alternative splicing is associated with insulin resistance in myotonic dystrophy." *Nat Genet* 29(1): 40-47.

Sergeant, N., B. Sablonniere, S. Schraen-Maschke, A. Ghestem, C. A. Maurage, A. Wattez, P. Vermersch & A. Delacourte (2001). "Dysregulation of human brain microtubule-associated tau mRNA maturation in myotonic dystrophy type 1." *Hum Mol Genet* 10(19): 2143-2155.

Storbeck, C. J., S. Drmanic, K. Daniel, J. D. Waring, F. R. Jirik, D. J. Parry, N. Ahmed, L. A. Sabourin, J. E. Ikeda & R. G. Korneluk (2004). "Inhibition of myogenesis in transgenic mice expressing the human DMPK 3'-UTR." *Hum Mol Genet* 13(6): 589-600.

Takahashi, N., N. Sasagawa, K. Suzuki & S. Ishiura (2000). "The CUG-binding protein binds specifically to UG dinucleotide repeats in a yeast three-hybrid system." *Biochem Biophys Res Commun* 277(2): 518-523.

Taneja, K. L., M. McCurrach, M. Schalling, D. Housman & R. H. Singer (1995). "Foci of trinucleotide repeat transcripts in nuclei of myotonic dystrophy cells and tissues." *J Cell Biol* 128(6): 995-1002.

Tapscott, S. J. & C. A. Thornton (2001). "Biomedicine. Reconstructing myotonic dystrophy." *Science* 293(5531): 816-817.

Tedeschi, L., C. Lande, A. Cecchettini & L. Citti (2009). "Hammerhead ribozymes in therapeutic target discovery and validation." *Drug Discov Today* 14(15-16): 776-783.

Tian, B., R. J. White, T. Xia, S. Welle, D. H. Turner, M. B. Mathews & C. A. Thornton (2000). "Expanded CUG repeat RNAs form hairpins that activate the double-stranded RNA-dependent protein kinase PKR." *RNA* 6(1): 79-87.

Timchenko, L. T., J. W. Miller, N. A. Timchenko, D. R. DeVore, K. V. Datar, L. Lin, R. Roberts, C. T. Caskey & M. S. Swanson (1996). "Identification of a (CUG)n triplet repeat RNA-binding protein and its expression in myotonic dystrophy." *Nucleic Acids Res* 24(22): 4407-4414.

Timchenko, L. T., N. A. Timchenko, C. T. Caskey & R. Roberts (1996). "Novel proteins with binding specificity for DNA CTG repeats and RNA CUG repeats: implications for myotonic dystrophy." *Hum Mol Genet* 5(1): 115-121.

Timchenko, N. A., Z. J. Cai, A. L. Welm, S. Reddy, T. Ashizawa & L. T. Timchenko (2001). "RNA CUG repeats sequester CUGBP1 and alter protein levels and activity of CUGBP1." *J Biol Chem* 276(11): 7820-7826.

Timchenko, N. A., P. Iakova, Z. J. Cai, J. R. Smith & L. T. Timchenko (2001). "Molecular basis for impaired muscle differentiation in myotonic dystrophy." *Mol Cell Biol* 21(20): 6927-6938.

Timchenko, N. A., R. Patel, P. Iakova, Z. J. Cai, L. Quan & L. T. Timchenko (2004). "Overexpression of CUG triplet repeat-binding protein, CUGBP1, in mice inhibits myogenesis." *J Biol Chem* 279(13): 13129-13139.

Vihola, A., G. Bassez, G. Meola, S. Zhang, H. Haapasalo, A. Paetau, E. Mancinelli, A. Rouche, J. Y. Hogrel, P. Laforet, T. Maisonobe, J. F. Pellissier, R. Krahe, B. Eymard & B. Udd (2003). "Histopathological differences of myotonic dystrophy type 1 (DM1) and PROMM/DM2." *Neurology* 60(11): 1854-1857.

Wang, G. S., D. L. Kearney, M. De Biasi, G. Taffet & T. A. Cooper (2007). "Elevation of RNA-binding protein CUGBP1 is an early event in an inducible heart-specific mouse model of myotonic dystrophy." *J Clin Invest* 117(10): 2802-2811.

Wang, G. S., M. N. Kuyumcu-Martinez, S. Sarma, N. Mathur, X. H. Wehrens & T. A. Cooper (2009). "PKC inhibition ameliorates the cardiac phenotype in a mouse model of myotonic dystrophy type 1." *J Clin Invest* 119(12): 3797-3806.

Wang, Y. H. & J. Griffith (1995). "Expanded CTG triplet blocks from the myotonic dystrophy gene create the strongest known natural nucleosome positioning elements." *Genomics* 25(2): 570-573.

Ward, A. J., M. Rimer, J. M. Killian, J. J. Dowling & T. A. Cooper (2010). "CUGBP1 overexpression in mouse skeletal muscle reproduces features of myotonic dystrophy type 1." Hum Mol Genet 19(18): 3614-3622.

Warf, M. B., M. Nakamori, C. M. Matthys, C. A. Thornton & J. A. Berglund (2009). "Pentamidine reverses the splicing defects associated with myotonic dystrophy." *Proc Natl Acad Sci U S A* 106(44): 18551-18556.

Westerlaken, J. H., C. E. Van der Zee, W. Peters & B. Wieringa (2003). "The DMWD protein from the myotonic dystrophy (DM1) gene region is developmentally regulated and is present most prominently in synapse-dense brain areas." *Brain Res* 971(1): 116-127.

Wheeler, T. M., M. C. Krym & C. A. Thornton (2007). "Ribonuclear foci at the neuromuscular junction in myotonic dystrophy type 1." *Neuromuscul Disord* 17(3): 242-247.

Wheeler, T. M., J. D. Lueck, M. S. Swanson, R. T. Dirksen & C. A. Thornton (2007). "Correction of ClC-1 splicing eliminates chloride channelopathy and myotonia in mouse models of myotonic dystrophy." *J Clin Invest* 117(12): 3952-3957.

Wheeler, T. M., K. Sobczak, J. D. Lueck, R. J. Osborne, X. Lin, R. T. Dirksen & C. A. Thornton (2009). "Reversal of RNA dominance by displacement of protein sequestered on triplet repeat RNA." *Science* 325(5938): 336-339.

Wojciechowska, M. & W. J. Krzyzosiak (2011). "Cellular toxicity of expanded RNA repeats: focus on RNA foci." *Hum Mol Genet.*

Zhang, L., J. E. Lee, J. Wilusz & C. J. Wilusz (2008). "The RNA-binding protein CUGBP1 regulates stability of tumor necrosis factor mRNA in muscle cells: implications for myotonic dystrophy." *J Biol Chem* 283(33): 22457-22463.

26

Duchenne Muscular Dystrophy: Experimental Models on Physical Therapy

Thais Gaiad[1], Karla Araujo[2],
Fátima Caromano[3] and Carlos Eduardo Ambrosio[4]
[1]*Department of Physical Therapy, University of Jequitinhonha and Mucuri Valley - UFVJM,*
[2]*Department of Surgery, Sector of Anatomy, University of São Paulo - USP,*
[3]*Department of Physical Therapy, University of São Paulo - USP,*
[4]*Department of Basic Science, University of São Paulo - USP,*
Brazil

1. Introduction

Neuromuscular disorders are a heterogeneous group of genetic diseases. Nowadays, more than 30 genetically defined forms are recognized and, in the last decade, mutations in several genes have been reported to result in the deficiency or loss of function of a variety of important muscle proteins (Shelton & Engvall, 2005). Defects in components of the dystrophin-glycoprotein complex (DGC) are known to be an important cause of different forms of muscular dystrophies (Ervasti & Campbell 1993; Yoshida & Ozawa 1990). Lack of dystrophin protein in muscle cells is characteristic of Duchenne muscular dystrophy (DMD), which is a progressive and fatal X-linked genetic disorder. Many animal models have been studied to identify an efficient treatment for this disease in humans. Two mammalian models of DMD have been widely used in preclinical trials to understand the pathogenesis of the disease and development of efficient therapeutic strategies for humans. *Mdx*-mouse is the most used animal model for DMD, followed by the Golden Retriever Muscular Dystrophy (GRMD) canine model. *Mdx*-mouse morphology displays some features of muscle degeneration, but the pathogenesis of the disease is comparatively mild. This model has a slightly shorter life spam as compared to wild-type controls (Banks & Chamberlain, 2008) and muscle degeneration is different from the one seen in DMD patients. An important degeneration and regeneration of muscle fibers is observed at a young age in the *mdx*-mouse (2 to 4 weeks), which results in the muscle morphological changes of centralized nuclei and heterogeneity of fiber size. Necrosis is also observed at this early age but decreases around sixty days. Loss of muscle tissue is slow and muscle weakness is not evident until later in life. Fibrosis, a marked feature of DMD muscle, is less pronounced in *mdx*-mouse, with the exception of diaphragm muscle (Hueber et al., 2008). Dystrophin deficiency has also been reported in cats as hypertrophic feline muscular dystrophy (HFMD), in which diaphragmatic hypertrophy is often fatal (Shelton & Engvall, 2005). Similar to *mdx* pathology, the skeletal muscle of the HFMD cats undergoes repeated cycles of degeneration and regeneration but does not develop the debilitating fibrosis that is characteristic of both DMD and the canine GRMD model (Hoffman & Gorospe, 1991). The GRMD model has been widely studied (Collins & Morgan, 2003) since it presents muscle abnormalities that are closest to the ones seen in humans: increased creatine kinase (CK) activity, muscle hypotrophy associated with contractures, muscle necrosis, degeneration, endomysial and perimysial fibrosis and cardiomyopathy (Howell et al., 1997). This model also presents repeated cycles of muscular necrosis and regeneration, muscle wasting, postural abnormalities, respiratory or heart failure and premature death, as seen in DMD patients (Valentine et al., 1988). Despite the phenotype variability of this model, it has been used due to the strong similarities of body weight and pathological expression of the disease in human (Collins & Morgan, 2003). Since the coding sequence of the dystrophin gene was discovered in 1987, no treatment has been found to stop DMD progression. To improve quality of life and prevent complications of this progressive disease, patients have access to supportive therapies such as motor and respiratory physical therapy, occupational therapy, psychology, nutritional supplements and corticosteroids. Although these therapies cannot cure DMD, they should be well investigated as they intend to lead these patients to a better quality of life and to decrease the complications of their degenerative and progressive illness. Physical therapy (PT) has been used to reduce muscular, cardiac and vascular abnormalities which develop in association with muscle strength loss (Gaiad et al., 2009). The main objective of such motor physical therapy is the prevention of muscle contractures and bone deformities (Strober, 2006). However, motor PT approaches have yielded controversial recommendations (Carter et al., 2002) and there is no consensus regarding the type and intensity of PT (Cup et al., 2007). Just as other muscular dystrophies, DMD is a progressive disorder which causes death by cardiac or respiratory failure. Nevertheless, the absence of dystrophin in the sarcolema of muscle cells makes DMD a special illness regarding therapeutic exercise prescription. Research using animal models can answer questions regarding which are the best type, frequency, and intensity of therapeutic exercise, as well as highlight a beneficial approach of PT for DMD patients. This chapter aims to detail some actual studies using *mdx* and GRMD models which reported new insights in this subject contributing to future research designs of therapeutic exercise on dystrophic muscle.

2. Duchenne muscular dystrophy (DMD)

Dystrophin is located beneath the sarcolemma and is part of a large dystroglycan complex termed the dystrophin-glycoprotein complex (DGC), which includes the dystroglican complex (α and β), sarcoglycan complex (α, β, γ and δ) and syntrophin/dystrobrevin subcomplexes (Ervasti & Campbell, 1991). DGC forms a critical link for force transmission between the contractile machinery of the muscle fiber and the extracellular matrix. Where dystrophin is defective or absent, the myofiber is fragile and the sarcolemma is readily damaged in response to exercise, leading to myofiber necrosis (Hoffman et al., 1987; Sharp et al., 1989). The absence of dystrophin in dystrophic muscles leads to altered myofiber integrity, perturbed calcium homeostasis, and activation of the calcium-dependent calpain proteases and necrosis (Straub et al., 1997). The other consequence of the loss of dystrophin is the absence or great reduction of components of the DGC, as described for skeletal muscle fibers from DMD patients and the *mdx* mouse (Ervasti et al., 1990; Ohlendieck & Campbell, 1991). Loss of dystrophin leads to membrane leakiness as a result of mechanical or hypoosmotic stress. Consequently, Ca^{2+} permeability is increased and various Ca^{2+} dependent proteases such as calpain are activated under conditions of dystrophin deficiency. It has also been proposed that alteration of the expression or function of plasma membrane proteins associated with dystrophin such as neuronal nitric oxide synthase (nNOS) and various ion channels are involved in the molecular mechanisms of muscle degeneration (Straub et al., 1997). Although the defective gene of dystrophin was identified in 1987, there is still no effective treatment for DMD patients. While cell or gene therapy to replace the defective dystrophin is the ideal solution, the clinical application of such therapies has yet to become a reality (Davies & Grounds, 2006; Foster et al., 2006). The existing treatment for DMD is administration of corticosteroids, broad-based anti-inflammatory drugs that decrease inflammatory cell populations in dystrophic muscle and increase myofiber mass. However, their precise mechanism of action in DMD is not yet known and is under intense investigation (Griggs et al., 1993; Connolly et al., 2002). Disadvantages of steroid treatment include their association with severe adverse side effects such as weight gain and osteoporosis and the variable response by the individuals undergoing treatment (Muntoni et al., 2002; Moxley et al., 2005).

3. Animal models for neuromuscular diseases

Several animal models that have been identified in nature or generated in laboratory present the phenotypes observed in neuromuscular diseases. These models generally present physiological symptoms observed in human patients and can be used as important tools for genetic, clinic, and histopathological studies (Vainzof et al., 2008). Animal models are essential for elucidation of the disease pathogenicity and for assessment of efficacy and toxicity during therapy development. Two mammalian models of DMD have been widely used in preclinical trials to understand the pathogenesis of the disease and to develop efficient therapeutic strategies for humans. *Mdx*-mouse is the most used animal model for DMD, followed by the Golden Retriever Muscular Dystrophy (GRMD) canine model.

3.1 Mouse model (*mdx*-mouse)

A mouse X-chromosome mutant (*mdx*) was first discovered in 1984 due to the observations of elevated plasma levels of muscle creatine kinase and pyruvate kinase enzymes and histological lesions characteristic of muscular dystrophy. In the *mdx* model the mutations cause a premature stop codon in exon 23 due a single base substitution (Sicinski et al., 1989). *Mdx*-mouse shows a mild non-progressive phenotype associated with comparatively moderate muscle pathology and muscle degeneration followed by subsequent significant regeneration (Dangain & Vrbova, 1984). Though the mouse models have slightly shorter life spans compared to wild-type controls (Banks & Chamberlain, 2008), they are indispensable for elucidation of the pathogenic mechanism and for development of therapeutic approaches, since they can be easily and reliably reproduced (Nakamura & Takeda, 2011).

3.1.1 Pathogenesis in the *mdx* mouse

Muscle degeneration in the *mdx* mouse is different from that seen in DMD patients. The progression of pathology in the *mdx* mouse is influenced by growth (Grounds, 2008) and may be divided into three main phases: (1) the pre-weaning phase (0–3 weeks of age), which is strongly influenced by growth and corresponds roughly to the first 6 months of human patients, (2) the post-weaning phase, with an acute onset of pathology around 3 weeks, followed at about 8 weeks by (3) the adult phase with a reduced low level of chronic damage that persists throughout life (Willmann et al., 2011). An important degeneration and regeneration of muscle fibers is observed at a young age of *mdx*-mouse (2 to 4 weeks) which results in the muscle morphological changes such as centralized nuclei and heterogeneity of fiber size. In mature limb muscle, the murine model is characterized by successive degeneration/regeneration processes and does not exhibit the progressive muscle wasting and accumulation of connective tissue observed during development of the human disease (Coulton et al., 1988). Necrosis is also observed at this early age but decreases around sixty days. Loss of muscle tissue is slow and muscle weakness is not evident until later in life. Fibrosis, a marked feature of DMD muscle, is less pronounced in *mdx*-mouse, with the exception of diaphragm muscle (Hueber et al., 2008). For this reason, histological analysis of the diaphragm, one of the most severely affected muscles of the *mdx*, is often used as a marker of weakness progression, once it reproduces the degenerative changes of muscular dystrophy.

3.2 Feline muscular dystrophy

Dystrophin deficiency has also been reported in cats, called hypertrophic feline muscular dystrophy (HFMD). The HFMD cat has a large deletion of muscle and Purkinje promoters resulting in a lack of dystrophin in the skeletal and cardiac muscle. These animals have a unique phenotypic expression of hypertrophy of the tongue, neck, and shoulder muscles, lingual calcification, excessive salivation, megaesophagus, gait disturbance manifesting as bunny hopping, dilated cardiomyopathy, hepatosplenomegaly, and kidney failure (Winand et al., 1994). Diaphragmatic hypertrophy is the principal cause of death in these animals (Shelton & Engvall, 2005). Similar to *mdx* pathology, the skeletal muscle of the HFMD cat undergoes repeated cycles of degeneration and regeneration but does not develop the debilitating fibrosis that is characteristic of both DMD and GRMD (Hoffman & Gorospe, 1991). Muscular dystrophy associated with absence of Merosin (laminin α2) was described in cats that presented muscle atrophy and marked weakness or progressive spasticity and contractions, as well as the serum creatine kinase (CK) at moderate levels (O'Brien et al., 2001). Other muscular dystrophies that have been reported are α-dystroglycan deficiency in Sphynx and Devon Rex cats (Martin et al., 2008) and reduced β- sarcoglycan in a shorthair male cat (Salvadori et al., 2009).

3.3 Canine muscular dystrophy

Numerous sporadic cases of canine muscular dystrophy have been recognized in the last two decades, but the Golden Retriever Muscular Dystrophy (GRMD) has been the most extensively examined and characterized (Cooper et al., 1988). GRMD is a degenerative myopathy homologue to Duchenne muscular dystrophy (DMD) in humans. A frame-shift point mutation in the dystrophin gene is responsible for the GRMD phenotype (Sharp et al., 1992), whereas deletions are the most frequent mutations in DMD patients. Nevertheless, in both DMD and GRMD patients, dystrophin protein is lacking (Hoffman et al., 1987; Cooper et al., 1988). Canine dystrophinopathies have also been reported in many other purebred and mixed breed dogs. In addition to the Golden Retriever (Kornegay et al., 1988), genetic mutations have also been characterized in Labrador Retriever (Bergman et al., 2002; Cosford et al., 2008), Irish Terrier (Wentink et al., 1972), German shorthaired pointer (Schatzberg et al., 1999), Samoieda (Presthus & Nordstoga, 1993), Japanese Spitz (Jones et al., 2004), English Spaniel (Van Ham et al., 1995), Old English Sheepdog (Wieczorek et al., 2006), Schnauzer miniature (Paola et al.,1993), Weimaraner (Baltzer et al., 2007), and Boston Terrier (Deitz et al., 2008). GRMD dogs closely resemble DMD patients in terms of both body weight and in the pathological expression of the disease (Collins & Morgan, 2003). However, their phenotype is variable (Banks & Chamberlain, 2008), as some pups survive only for a few days, while others are ambulant for months or even years (Ambrosio et al, 2008). Animal trials employing these dogs have substantial animal welfare implications and high costs associated with both maintenance and treatment (Nakamura & Takeda, 2011).

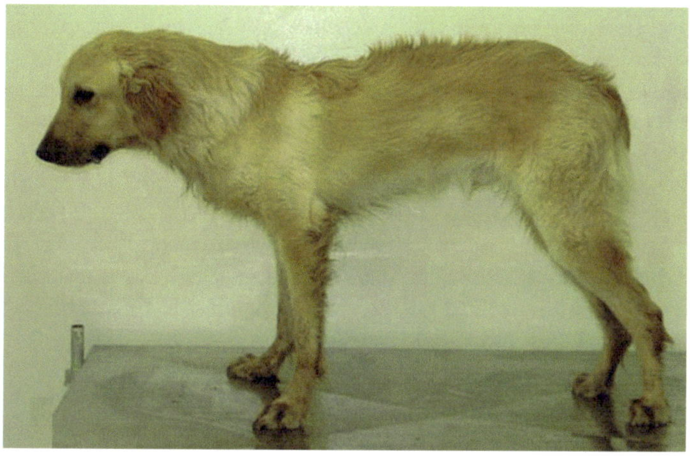

Fig. 1. Golden Retriever muscular dystrophy dog (GRMD model). (Ambrosio et al. 2009)

Researchers have developed a strain of medium sized dystrophic Beagles, designated as canine X-linked muscular dystrophy in Japan (CXMDj). They show atrophy and weakness of limb muscles which appear at 2-3 months, followed by development of macroglossia, dysphasia, gait disturbance, and joint contracture around 4 months of age. These symptoms rapidly progress until around 10 months of age, after which the progression of the disease is retarded (Shimatsu et al., 2005). The GSHPMD (German shorthaired pointer muscular dystrophy) is a spontaneous canine dystrophin 'knockout' model with complete lack of dystrophin immune reactivity. These dogs have been useful for dystrophin gene therapy trials, myoblast transfer, and in combination of the two. Any dystrophin transcripts or protein detected in GSHP skeletal muscle after therapeutic intervention could therefore only be produced by the dystrophin delivery vehicle (Schatzberg et al., 1999). Due to the common genetic basis of the disease in dog and human, the GRMD and other inbred dystrophic dog lines descended from animals with spontaneous mutations have been extensively used in preclinical settings, particularly for cell and gene therapy studies. An interesting Becker-like dystrophy with a truncated form of dystrophin was recently identified in a family of Japanese Spitz dogs (Jones et al., 2004). In these dogs, a 70–80 kDa protein on immunoblots that reacted with antibodies to the C-terminal domain of dystrophin was found, but not with antibodies to the rod domain. Canine models with deficient sarcoglycan (SG) proteins have been identified in Boston Terriers and Cocker Spaniels. The phenotype includes failure to thrive and exercise intolerance. Serum CK is highly elevated, and muscle histopathology shows a dystrophic pattern and a variable degree of loss of SG proteins staining (Shelton & Engvall 2005). A dystrophic myopathy should be considered in any young dog or cat (male or female, mixed breed or purebred) with persistent muscle weakness, muscle atrophy or hypertrophy, gait abnormality, or contractures beginning in the first few months of life

(Shelton & Engvall, 2002). The breed of an affected animal is one of the most useful distinguishing diagnostic criteria. A DNA-based test is commercially available for the dystrophin mutation in Golden Retrievers, but not yet for mutations in dystrophin or related proteins in other breeds. Diagnosis of Muscular Dystrophy (MD) in companion animals has been based on clinical presentation, markedly elevated serum creatine kinase concentration, and the presence of a dystrophic phenotype based on histopathological evaluation of muscle biopsy specimens (Shelton, 2010). Such analysis can be done by immunohistochemical localizations of dystrophin, dystrophin-associated proteins, laminin and other proteins. This is a cost-effective and sensitive method which can be performed directly on fresh-frozen biopsy specimens. Results of immunohistochemical staining using various monoclonal and polyclonal antibodies against skeletal muscle proteins involved in the muscular dystrophies can guide the direction of mutational analyses and development of diagnostic tests for specific mutations (Shelton, 2004). Serum CK activity should be part of every neuromuscular minimum database, most importantly for preneuter evaluations in young dogs because increased activity may be an early indicator of underlying muscle disease. Marked or persistent increases of CK activity may be indicative of a congenital or inherited muscle disease even if the animal is clinically asymptomatic (Shelton, 2010). The most marked increases in serum CK activity (420,000 U/L) are associated with necrotizing myopathies or MD (Kornegay et al., 1988; Bergman et al., 2002).

3.3.1 Pathogenesis in the GRMD dog

Mutations in the dystrophin protein result in membrane damage allowing massive infiltration of immune cells, chronic inflammation, necrosis, and severe muscle degeneration (Valentine et al., 1990b). The histopathological changes in the muscle are similar to the ones seen in humans and include muscle fiber degeneration and regeneration, fiber splitting, numerous fibers with centralized myonuclei, and intense connective tissue replacement. Myofiber hypertrophy and variability in myofiber size are likely to be an early change associated with dystrophin deficiency rather than a compensatory mechanism related to muscle impairment (Hoffman & Gorospe, 1991). Dystrophin deficiency in *mdx* mice and HFMD cats does not lead to significant muscle weakness (Hoffman & Gorospe, 1991). GRMD dogs, as well as DMD patients, suffer from repeated cycles of muscular necrosis and regeneration, muscle wasting and fibrosis, postural abnormalities, respiratory or heart failure, and premature death (Valentine et al, 1988). The clinical signs in GRMD dogs include the gradual loss of muscle mass and the development of contractures that often lead to skeletal deformities (Cooper et al., 1988). A prominent feature in dystrophic dogs is enlargement of the base of the tongue due to muscle fiber hypertrophy and pseudohypertrophy. Dysphagia, regurgitation and drooling associated with pharyngeal and esophageal dysfunction can be observed (Shelton and Engvall, 2005). GRMD dogs can present difficulty in opening the mouth, exercise intolerance, and atrophy of the trunk, limbs and *temporallis* muscle (Valentine et al., 1988). Elevation of serum CK is a feature of both canine and human muscular dystrophies (Cooper et al., 1998; Valentine et al., 1988). CK values were significantly elevated in GRMD dogs and increased with exercise. Serum ALT activity was also elevated, a finding which has been identified in Duchenne-like muscular dystrophy in dogs. The degree of elevation of the CK and ALT did not correlate with the severity of the clinical signs in any dog (Valentine et al, 1990a, Ambrosio et al., 2009). Gaiad et al. (2011) have found no correlation between clinical features or premature death in GRMD dogs and CK levels. Female dogs present a variety of clinical signs including generalized weakness, muscle wasting, tremors, exercise intolerance, gait abnormalities, and limb deformity. Elevation of serum creatine kinase activity may vary (Shelton et al., 2001). The gait abnormalities in GRMD dogs during growth and disease progression using an ambulatory gait analyzer (3D-accelerometers) showed that speed, stride length, total power and force had already significantly decreased ($p < 0.01$) at the age of 2 months. The decrease of stride frequency was a later event, secondarily contributing to the reduction of speed (Barthélémy et al., 2011).

3.3.2 Therapeutic approaches using canine model of muscular dystrophy

Papers have been recently published using the canine model of muscular dystrophy to develop various therapeutic approaches such as gene therapy, cell therapy, and pharmaceutical agents. As an animal model for DMD therapy, GRMD dogs were used in preclinical trials examining the transfer of dystrophin gene (Howell et al., 1998), utrophin gene (Cerletti et al., 2003) or oligonucleotides (Bartlett et al., 2000). These therapeutic strategies were all applied to a single muscle after local intramuscular injection. However, dystrophin deficiency appears as a generalized muscle defect, therefore achieving clinically relevant improvement may likely require intravascular delivery of genetic material. Gene therapy using viral vectors has been extensively investigated. Adeno-associated virus (AAV) vectors are the most appropriate tools for viral vector gene therapy because they are nonpathogenic due to a replication defect and have low immunogenicity as well as an effective ability to infect non dividing cells (Nakamura & Takeda, 2011). The intravenous administration of a dystrophin cDNA plasmid in the dystrophin-deficient *mdx* mouse resulted in significant dystrophin expression (Liu et al., 2001). This gene transfer was carried out on 5-week-old *mdx* mice diaphragm muscles, in which fibrosis is still minimal. It is not certain that similar gene transfer efficiency would be achieved in heavily compromised muscles, such as those occurring in GRMD and DMD. However, the treatment using myoblast or mesenchymal stem cell implantation in GRMD dogs during the early 1990s did not show improvement of muscle condition, even though other studies had demonstrated success in the mdx mouse. Similarly, hematopoietic stem cell transplantation did not restore dystrophin expression in affected dogs despite promising results in mdx mice (Dell'Agnola et al., 2004). In older GRMD dogs, fibrosis seems to be the major factor influencing microvascular architecture in skeletal muscles. Increasing extent of connective tissue correlated with lower microvessel density and longer intercapillary distance. The fibrosis might create a physical barrier between the capillary contour and the myofiber membrane. Thus, endomysial fibrosis, the hallmark of muscle pathology in DMD patients and GRMD dogs, may compromise intravascular therapeutic trials performed in the late stage of the dystrophic process. Anti-fibrotic treatment may be a necessary prerequisite to systemic genetic transfer in dystrophin-deficient canine and human muscles (Nguyen et al., 2005). Among these therapeutic strategies, exon skipping using antisense oligonucleotides (AOs) is considered to be one of the most promising therapies for the restoration of dystrophin expression at the sarcolemma in dystrophin-deficient muscle. The therapy involves a multiexon-skipping technique for targeting exons 6 and 8 to convert an out-of-frame mutation into an in-frame mutation using PMOs (Yokota et al., 2009). Kerkis et al. (2008) have reported the transplantation of human immature dental pulp stem cells from baby teeth to GRMD dogs by local and systemic via. Moreover, they have analyzed the efficiency of single and consecutive early transplantation of these cells. Their results show that Human Immature Dental Pulp Stem Cells (hIDPSC) presented significant engraftment in GRMD dog muscles, although human dystrophin expression was modest and limited to several muscle fibers. Better clinical condition was also observed in the dog which received monthly arterial injections and was still clinically stable at 25 months of age. Systemic myostatin inhibition in GRMD dogs by liver directed gene transfer of a vector designed to express a secreted negative myostatin peptide showed increase in muscle mass in these dogs assessed by MRI (Magnetic Resonance Imaging) and confirmed by muscle histology (Bish et al., 2011).

4. Pre-clinical therapeutic studies using animal models

The availability of standardized operating procedures (SOPs) to unify experimental protocols used to test the effects of new treatment in animal models is a step that will undoubtedly improve the comparability of studies from different laboratories (http://www.treat-nmd.eu/research/preclinical/dmd-sops/). To date, the main attempt to evaluate the relative translational benefit from an animal species to human subjects has focused on the minimal levels of dystrophin protein required for functional stabilization of dystrophic myofibers. Many factors need to be considered. This protective effect will depend not only on the amount of dystrophin protein within an individual myofibers, but also on the extent of distribution within all myofibers, the size of the nuclear domain (how far dystrophin protein extends along the sarcolema from the myonuclei where the mRNA is generated) and on when during development the dystrophin must be produced (Willmann et al., 2011). This situation was considered by Chamberlain (1997) who concluded from analysis of mosaic transgenic mice and viral vector delivery with suboptimal doses into *mdx* mice, that >50% of myofibers need to express dystrophin, and that these must accumulate approximately 20% of wild-type levels of dystrophin for a significant correction of the muscle pathology in mice. Factors to consider in the selection of outcome measurements (Determination and evaluation of the results of an activity, plan, process, or program and their comparison with the intended or projected results) for pre-clinical therapeutic studies using mouse model include reproducibility, objectivity, blind assessment, relevance to disease biology (e.g. muscle histology), and similarity of measures in the *mdx* mice (e.g. locomotion and in vivo muscle strength) to human clinical trials endpoints (e.g. ability to walk and muscle strength testing). Depending on the presumed mechanism of action and the intended target of the experimental agent, additional outcome measures (e.g. to assess cardiac function) may be appropriate (Willmann et al., 2011). Standardized protocols for the assessment of most of the recommended parameters have already been produced by specialized working groups of experts and are reported in brackets (PDFs available http://www.treat-nmd.eu/research/preclinical/dmd-models/). Based on the mechanism of action, different drugs may be more or less effective depending on the age at which treatment is initiated and the time period over which the drug is administered (i.e. treatment duration). Due to the ultimate translational aim of the pre-clinical experiments, it is important to consider the relationship between the age of the *mdx* mice and possible equivalence in DMD patients. A comparison of developmental stages in mice and humans is described in details elsewhere (Grounds et al., 2008). The recovery score is a tool that can be used to compare different therapies applied to mice or results obtained by different laboratories with the same therapy.

$$\text{Recovery score } (\%) \frac{[\text{treated}\,mdx] - [\text{untreated}\,mdx]}{[\text{wild type}] - [\text{untreated}\,mdx]} \times 100$$

A score of 100% indicates that the parameter in treated *mdx* mice is equal to that of control wild type mice, and 0% indicates that no improvement was obtained relative to untreated *mdx* mice (Gillis et al., 2002) Therefore, this calculation represents a tool to evaluate the effective recovery achieved by the treatment tested. Although this implies the need to include a wild type group of mice in any pre-clinical therapeutic study, we encourage the calculation of the recovery score in all studies where this effort is feasible (Willmann et al., 2011). Measurements of muscle strength, joint contractures, and timed function tests were made in dogs to evaluate recovery of muscular function after drugs or gene therapy. The evaluation of muscle by magnetic resonance imaging (MRI) was performed by Kornegay et al. (2010) after single intravenous injection of an AAV9 vector (1.5 × 1014 vector genomes/kg) carrying a human codon-optimized human mini-dystrophin gene under control of the cytomegalovirus (CMV) promoter. Earlier, the same research group performed analysis of muscle strength by measuring isometric force decrement after eccentric contraction (Childers et al., 2002) and by measuring the titanic isometric force at the tibiotarsal joint in vivo (Kornegay et al., 1994). The MRI evaluation has several strengths that include studying distribution of pathology, pathophysiology, monitoring of therapies, assessment of heart and diaphragm, and morphometry (Bish et al., 2011).

5. What's new on exercise training that can guide physical therapy for DMD related to *mdx* and GRMD models?

The coding sequence of the dystrophin gene in DMD was discovered and deciphered in 1987 (Koenig et al., 1987). Its discovery has brought hope for a cure of DMD through gene therapy, although it has not happened yet. Several therapeutic strategies are being investigated in developing a cure for this disease. Nowadays, DMD patients have access to therapeutic and supportive care aiming to prevent complications and improve their quality of life. Among them, drug therapy with corticosteroids has been widely studied in DMD and there is some controversy in its use mainly due to its multiple side effects. Nutritional supplements, psychology, occupational and physical therapy are the most used supportive therapies.

Although these therapies cannot lead to a cure of DMD, they should be well investigated because they intend to lead these patients to a better quality of life and to decrease complications of their degenerative and progressive illness. Physical therapy (PT) has been used to reduce muscular, skeletal, cardiac, and vascular abnormalities which develop in association with muscle strength loss (Gaiad et al., 2009). The main objective of such motor therapy is the prevention of muscle contractures and bone deformities (Strober, 2006). However, motor PT approaches have yielded controversial recommendations (Carter et al., 2002) and there is no consensus regarding the type and intensity of physical therapy (Cup et al., 2007). The recommendations often include exercise therapy to improve or preserve muscle strength or endurance and aerobic capacity to prevent the secondary problems of contractures, pain and fatigue. According to the review published by Grange & Call (2007) the same exercise used to increase muscle strength and endurance in normal individuals can exacerbate muscle damage in a dystrophic muscle. The authors suggested that a threshold must be defined to guide suitable exercise prescription for DMD patients (Grange & Call, 2007; Cup et al., 2007). Kimura et al. (2006) showed in a case report that immobility could reduce muscle fiber necrosis in muscular dystrophy cases. They reported a case of a three-year-old boy with a diagnosis of spina bifida and DMD. A muscle biopsy on this patient showed that necrosis and regeneration of muscle fiber was more prevalent in the biceps brachii (with normal movement) than in the gastrocnemius muscle (without movement). The authors suggest that immobility reduces muscle fiber necrosis in dystrophin-deficient muscle and attribute this characteristic to the movement restriction in the lower extremity of this patient. Reduced physical activity by *mdx* mice could theoretically be a muscle sparing strategy (Landisch et al., 2008). On the other hand, authors suggest that patients should undergo some physical activity in order to avoid muscle disuse associated with the intrinsic loss of muscle mass related to the disease progression (Ansved, 2005; Eagle, 2002, McDonald, 2002 and Caromano, 1999). Once physical therapies display an important role on DMD patients' quality of life, the prescription of its parameters must be evidence-based and well documented. In the last few years, some researchers have brought some insights into the subject of therapeutic exercise using experimental animal models for DMD. There are many publications on gene, cellular and pharmacological therapies using the DMD animal models, *mdx*-mice and GRMD dogs, but these models also have much remaining to contribute to the therapeutic exercise approach (Mercuri et al., 2008). The contribution of animal models, mainly the GRMD model, on prescription of type, frequency and modality of PT was also suggested by Grange & Call (2007).

According to Markert et al. (2011) the effect of exercise on DMD has poorly researched parameters (frequency, intensity, time and type) and until now it is unknown whether therapeutic exercise is beneficial or detrimental to dystrophic skeletal muscle. Despite the difference between *mdx*-mice and humans DMD patients in terms of regenerative ability and compensatory protein expression, this model is still the most used one to investigate exercise prescription for this population. Reasons for the wide use of *mdx*-mouse, despite its limitations, are well detailed in the first topic of this chapter.

In 2002, Eagle published a consensus about exercise recommendations for patients with neuromuscular disorders. Among them, they suggest maintenance or improvement of muscle stretch, improvement of functional ability and use of nocturnal orthesis to avoid contractures. More recently, Bushby et al. (2010) have brought some recommendations for management of rehabilitation of DMD patients. Regarding stretching, authors suggested that during ambulatory and non-ambulatory phases a regular active, active-assisted and/or passive stretching to prevent or minimize contractures should be performed a minimum of 4–6 days per week for any specific joint or muscle group. The authors agree that only limited research has been carried out on type, frequency and intensity of exercise for DMD. Although, their recommendations are in accordance with the known pathophysiology and animal studies which show contraction-induced muscle injury in dystrophinopathies. According to these authors, PT should avoid high-resistance strength training and eccentric exercise due to the knowing contraction-induced muscle fiber injury. They recommend that patients should undergo regular submaximum functional strengthening activity, including a combination of swimming-pool exercises and recreation-based exercises in the community. Based on these questions and recommendations of exercise prescription on DMD, some recent publications using animal models will be detailed in order to highlight the contribution of these models to PT prescription and recommendations.

5.1 PT exercise prescription

Kumar & Boriek (2003) studied the effects of passive mechanical stretch on the activation of nuclear factor-kappaB (NF-kB) pathways in skeletal muscles from normal and *mdx* mouse. Nuclear factor-kappaB (NF-kB) is a transcription factor which regulates genes involved in the inflammatory and acute stress response. They found that this factor in the diaphragm muscle was increased by the application of mechanical stress in a time-dependent manner. Their results show that one of the stretch exercises, mechanical stretch, activates the classical NF-kB pathway and it seems to be more active in DMD muscle than control muscle. Another study investigated the morphological effect of two different protocols of passive stretch on the immobilized soleus mucle of healthy rats (Gomes et al., 2007). They have analyzed the morphology and the proportion of fibers types (I, II and C) of four groups: control, immobilized, immobilized and stretched every 3 days, and immobilized and stretched every 7 days. The passive stretch was 40 minutes long. They found that signs of cell degeneration were more intense in the group immobilized and stretched three times a week. The authors suggest that the passive stretching applied to the soleus muscle during immobilization induce muscle fiber injury, suggesting that this therapeutic tool should be applied carefully to disused muscles, such as dystrophic ones. Even if stretch exercises are widely used in PT, its real implication on muscle structure and morphology must be better investigated, especially on dystrophic muscle. Exercise-induced muscle injury in healthy humans occurs mainly after unaccustomed exercise, particularly if the exercise involves a large amount of eccentric (muscle lengthening) contractions (Clarkson & Hubal, 2002). The exact mechanism of this injury remains unknown, but it has been ascribed to mechanical disruption of the fiber, and subsequent damage is linked to inflammatory processes and to changes in excitation-contraction coupling within the muscle. According to Childers et al. (2002) a cycle of weakness, stretch, damage, and further weakness might explain observations of selective involvement of eccentric-contraction in dystrophic muscles. This mode of exercise has not been widely recommended for DMD patients (de Araujo Leitão et al., 1995; Eagle, 2002; Ansved, 2005; Cup et al., 2007; Bushby et al., 2010). This exercise-induced dystrophic muscle damage due to eccentric contraction was also attested in the *mdx*-mouse and GRMD models (Childers et al., 2002; Tegeler et al., 2010; Mathur et al., 2010) and humans DMD patients (Marqueste et al., 2008). Childers et al. (2002) have investigated the eccentric injury in dystrophic GRMD dogs. They have found that dystrophic canine flexor muscles of hindlimbs are more susceptible than normal ones to eccentric contraction-induced injury analyzing muscle torque three days after the eccentric contraction. Clinical implications of this study show that dystrophic muscle is preferentially injured by mechanical stress. Another study by the same group of Childers and co-authors (Tegeler et al., 2010) has shown that dystrophic muscles of GRMD dogs undergo damage immediately after the eccentric contraction. Mathur et al. (2010) studied the effects of downhill and horizontal running on the magnetic resonance imaging (MRI) in *mdx*-mouse. A higher percentage of pixels with elevated T_2 were observed in *mdx*-mouse compared with controls pre-exercise, which suggest muscle damage. Moreover, downhill running which is dependent on lengthening muscle contraction induced acute changes in *mdx*-mouse muscle after exercise. Also using the MRI technique, Marqueste et al. (2008) investigated the effect of acute and successive bouts of downhill running on muscle performance of healthy rats. Their results show less muscle injury effect due to repetition of exercise bouts at a low frequency (one session per week) probably due to muscle adaptation and to the inflammatory phase occurring for a week after a single eccentric exercise bout. Another interesting result of this study is the specificity of the stimulated muscle. Soleus and gastrocnemius muscle have shown different responses to lengthening contractions on MRI analysis. The author suggested that this muscle specificity might be linked to different anatomical properties, such as fiber pennation angles, typology and/or exhausting nature of the downhill running sessions. This last result is quite interesting because in PT sessions it is more difficult to isolate a single muscle as it is possible in an experimental model. So, care must be taken when translating experimental data to human therapy. On the other hand, it is important to keep in mind that a single therapeutic exercise can influence different muscles of the same limb in different manners. In agreement with the results presented by Kimura et al. (2006) that immobility can lead to preservation of dystrophic muscle in humans DMD Mokhtarian et al. (1999) investigated whether immobilization of the hindlimbs of the *mdx*-mice would prevent the occurrence of muscle degeneration. The authors clarify that dystrophin-deficient skeletal muscle of *mdx*-mice undergo their first rounds of degeneration-regeneration at the age of 14-28 days. They have mechanically immobilized the hindlimbs of 3 week old *mdx*-mice to restrain the *Soleus* and *Extensor digitorum longus* muscles in the stretched or shortened position. The position had no influence in the final result that showed low percentage of regenerated myofibers in Soleus and Extensor digitorum longus muscles when compared to the same muscles of the contralateral limb. Regenerated myofibers was attested by the presence of central nuclei in dystrophic fibers. According to these authors (Mokhtarian et al. 1999), limb immobilization prevents the occurrence of the first round of myofibers necrosis in *mdx*-mice and reinforces the idea that muscle contractions play a role in the skeletal muscle degeneration of dystrophin-deficient muscles. Even though some authors have suggested that restriction of movement prevent cycles of degeneration and regeneration in dystrophic muscle, we should consider that restriction of movement leads to muscle disuse and has drastic consequences to the patients, e.g. contractures, bone deformities, cardiovascular disease, obesity, and osteoporosis over time. It is imperative that a balanced threshold of therapeutic exercise must be well-defined and that more research on this subject is necessary. Over the last ten years, the number of papers aiming to define the threshold of PT prescription has grown. Outcome measurements of these investigations generally use morphological features of dystrophic muscle, enzymatic, protein localization and quantification, and/or biomechanical analyses. Podhorska-Okolow et al. (1998) have studied apoptosis of myofibers and the presence of satellite cells in skeletal muscle of healthy mice after spontaneous exercise wheel running. Exercised mice have run for sixteen hours and were sacrificed after a period of 6 or 96 hours. For analysis, the authors have counted the numbers of myofibers with central nuclei, (indicative of regenerated myofibers), performed immune histochemistry, quantified by Western blot proteins related to cell death, and used electron microscopy to find satellite cells. Their results show that spontaneous running in sedentary mice increases the number of apoptotic nuclei in adult muscle fibers and in endothelial cells. These results suggested that voluntary exercise plays an important and detrimental role on disused muscle, which can be applied to dystrophic muscle. In general, any study that used voluntary wheel running detrimentaly affected the hindlimbs of *mdx* mice (Landisch et al., 2008). Studies that have investigated non-voluntary exercise have shown muscle injury in *mdx* model mainly when animals are running downhill. Landisch et al. (2008) investigated whether a voluntary endurance type of exercise could be beneficial to dystrophic muscle;

assessing cellular adaptations that typically occur in response to endurance exercise. They hypothesized that a voluntary endurance type of exercise would improve *mdx* mouse muscle to the same extent that exercise improves healthy muscle. They analyzed the histological features by counting the central nuclei, fiber types, capillarity and mitochondrial enzymes activity. In part their hypothesis was true, except that mitochondrial adaptations did not occur in *mdx* mouse muscles. They suggest that this type of exercise can improve skeletal muscle weakness and fatigue as well as prevent secondary consequences of the inactivity. In 2009, Gaiad et al. reported the effect of the free walking activity during 24weeks/3 times perweek during 45 minutes in GRMD dogs. Muscle collagen area was quantified by histomorphometry and collagen types I, III and IV were localizated by immunohistochemistry. Passive joint range of motion (ROM) was measured to investigate the secondary consequences of the exercise on the muscle skeletal system. There was an improvement on tarsal ROM in dogs of the treated group. Muscle collagen area was different between the groups after treatment, and an increasing trend in these values was observed in non-treated group. This suggests a higher muscle fibrosis in dogs that have not undergone exercise. Collagen types I and III were observed in both groups. The authors suggest that the modality of free walking activity can improve ROM without increasing muscle fibrosis in dystrophic dogs. Studying markers of oxidative stress in skeletal muscle of *mdx*-mouse, Kacsor et al. (2007) applied low intensity training through treadmill running 30 minutes per day, 2 times per week during 8 weeks. They considered 9 meters perminute as a training of low intensity based on previous studies with the same animal model. This intensity of training has not been able to provoke any adaptation on healthy mice (wild type). In *mdx*-mouse, low intensity training has lead to physiologic adaptations evidenced by decrease of markers of oxidative stress. New studies should be conducted following this same intensity of training for new analyses. The investigation of creatine quinase (CK) enzyme, muscle fibrosis and morphology, as well as clinical and behavioral features of these animals can elucidate aspects of the best threshold of exercise for DMD patients. With this focus, van Putten and co-authors (2010) have investigated some functional tools on the disease progression of 4-week-old mdx mice using CK analysis and muscle morphology (measuring percentage of fibrotic/necrotic area). They suggest four functional tests (forelimb grip strength, rotarod analysis, and two and four limb hanging wire) that may be suitable for short-term functional evaluation of therapeutic approaches in the *mdx* mouse without affecting dystrophy progression. Aiming to validate parameters of functional evaluation on pre-clinical trials for DMD, Gaiad et al. (2011) investigated the use of PT assessment tools to evaluate disease progression and phenotype variability in GRMD dogs. In this study the outcome measurements were passive joint range of motion, limb and thorax circumferences, weight, CK analysis, and physical features of each of the dogs using a physical exam score previously described by Thibaud et al. (2007). The author have described the physical and behavioral features of 11 dystrophic dogs during 9 months and these PT measurements tools were considered reliable and useful to evaluate disease progression in GRMD dogs.

6. Conclusion

In the last ten years, research on exercise prescription using *mdx* mouse and GRMD dogs has increased and much of the research were discussed here. We have much to discover about the effects of type, frequency, and intensity of therapeutic exercise on DMD.

Regarding the type of exercise, it is possible to say that eccentric/lengthening contraction has no beneficial effects on dystrophic muscle, and that concentric or aerobic training should be better investigated. Free or voluntary activities seem to prevent secondary consequences of disuse while not leading to detrimental effects. The morphological and clinical effects of the intensity of exercise must be well investigated once it seems near the threshold that must still be defined. Low intensity training leads to beneficial effects though the parameters of this intensity must also be well defined and afterwards, translated to human patients. The harmonization of assessment tools for exercise research with both animal models is another important point on this subject. The definition of assessment tools to pre-clinical trials on animal models will enable the advancement of research on this subject and bring knowledge to the prescription of beneficial therapeutic exercise to DMD patients.

7. References

Ambrosio, CE; Fadel, L.; Gaiad, TP; Martins, DS; Araújo, KPC; Zucconi, E.; Brolio, MP; Giglio, RF; Morini, AC; Jazedje, T; Froes, TR; Feitosa, MLT; Valadares, MC; Beltrão-Braga, PCB; Meirelles, FV & Miglino, MA. (2009). Identification of three distinguishable phenotypes in golden retriever muscular dystrophy. *Genetics and Molecular Research*, v: 8, n: 2, pp. 389-396.

Ambrosio, CE; Valadares, MC; Zucconi, E; Cabral, R; Pearson, PL; Gaiad TP; Canovas, M; Vainzof, M; Miglino, MA & Zatz, M. (2008). Ringo, a golden retriever muscular dystrophy (grmd) dog with absent dystrophin but normal strength. *Neuromuscular Disorders*, v. 18, n. 11, pp. 892-3.

Baltzers, WI; Calise, DV; Levine, J M; Shelton, GD; Edwards, JF & Steiner, JM. (2007). Dystrophin-deficient muscular dystrophy in Weimaraner. *Journal of the American Hospital Association*, v. 43, pp. 227-232.

Banks, GB. & Chamberlain, J.S. (2008). The value of mammalian models for Duchenne Muscular Dystrophy in developing therapeutic strategies. In: *Current Topics in Developmental Biology*, Krauss, R.S. (Ed.). 431-453, Burlington: Academic Press.

Barthélémy, I; Barrey, E; Aguilar, P; Uriarte, A; Le Chevoir, M; Thibaud J; Voit, T; Blot, S & Hogrel, J. (2011). Longitudinal ambulatory measurements of gait abnormality in dystrophin-deficient dogs. *Musculoskeletal Disorders*, v.12, pp. 75 (http://www.biomedcentral.com/1471-2474/12/75).

Bartlett, RJ; Stockinger, S; Denis, MM; Bartlett, WT; Inverardi, L; Le, TT; thi Man, N; Morris, GE; Bogan, DJ; Metcalf-Bogan, J & Kornegay, JN. (2000). In vivo targeted repair of a point mutation in the canine dystrophin gene by a chimeric RNA/DNA oligonucleotide. *Nature Biotechnology*, v. 18, pp. 615–22.

Bergman, RL; Inzana, KD; Monroe, WE; Shell, LG; Liu, LA; Engvall, E & Shelton, GD. (2002). Dystrophin-deficient muscular dystrophy in Labrador retriever. *Journal of the American Animal Hospital Association*, v. 38, pp. 255-261.

Bish, TB; Sleeper, MM; Forbes, SC; Morine, KJ; Reynolds, C.; Singletary, GE; Trafny, D; Pham, J; Bogan, J; Kornegay, JN; Vandenborne, K; Walter, GA & Sweeney, HL. (2011). Long-term systemic myostatin inhibition via liver-targeted gene transfer in Golden Retriever Muscular Dystrophy. *Human gene Therapy*, [Epub ahead of print].

Carter, GT; Abresch, RT; Fowler, WM Jr. (2002). Adaptations to exercise training and contraction-induced muscle injury in animal models of muscular dystrophy. *American Journal of Physical Medicine and Rehabilitation*,v. 81, Suppl 11, pp.151-61.

Cerletti, M; Negri, T; Cozzi, F; Colpo, R; Andreetta, F; Croci, D; Davies, KE; Cornelio, F; Pozza, O; Karpati, G; Gilbert, R & Mora, M. (2003). Dystrophic phenotype of canine X-linked muscular dystrophy is mitigated by adenovirus-mediated utrophin gene transfer. *Gene Therapy*, v.10, pp. 750–7.

Chakkalakal, JV; Thompson, J; Parks, RJ &Jasmin, BJ. (2005). Molecular, cellular, and pharmacological therapies for Duchenne/Becker muscular dystrophies. *The FASEB Journal*, v. 19, pp. 880-895.

Chamberlain, JS. (1997). Dystrophin levels required for genetic correction of duchenne muscular dystrophy. *Basic and Applied Myology*, v. 7, pp. 251–5.

Childers, MK; Okamura, CS; Bogan, DJ; Bogan, JR; Petroski, GF; McDonald, K. & Kornegay, JN. Eccentric contraction injury in dystrophic canine muscle (2002). *Archives of Physical Medicine and Rehabilitation*, vol.83, pp. 1572-1578.

Clarkson, PM. & Hubal, MJ.(2002). Exercised-induced muscle damage in humans. *American Journal of Physical Medicine and Rehabilitation*, v.81(Suppl.), pp. S52-69.

Collins, CA & Morgan, JE. (2003). Duchenne's muscular dystrophy: animal models used to investigate pathogenesis and develop therapeutic strategies. *International Journal of Experimental Pathology*, v. 84, pp. 165-172.

Connolly, AM; Schierbecker, J; Renna, R & Florence, J. (2002). High dose weekly oral prednisone improves strength in boys with Duchene muscular dystrophy. *Neuromuscular Disorders*, v. 12, pp. 917-925.

Cosford, KL; Taylor, SM; Thompson, L; Shelton, GD. (2008). A possible new inherited myopathy in young Labrador retriever. *Canadian Veterinary Journal*, v. 49, p. 393-397.

Coulton, GR.; Morgan, JE.; Partridge, TA & Sloper, JC. (1988). The *mdx* mouse skeletal muscle myopathy: I. A histological, morphometric and biochemical investigation. *Neuropathology and Applied Neurobiology*, v. 14, n. 1, pp. 53–70.

Cup, EH; Pieterse, AJ; Broek-Pastoor, JM; Munneke, M; van Engelen, BG; Hendricks, HT; van der Wilt, G. & Oostendorp, RA. (2007). Exercise therapy and other types of physical therapy for patients with neuromuscular diseases: A Systematic review. *Archives of Physical Medicine and Rehabilitation*, v. 88, pp. 1452-64.

Dangain, J & Vrbova, G. (1984). Muscle development in (*mdx*) mutant mice. *Muscle & Nerve*, v. 7, pp. 700–704.

Davies, KE & Grounds, MD. (2006). Treating Muscular Dystrophy with stem cells? *Cell*, v. 127, n. 7, pp. 1304-1306.

Dell'Agnola, C; Want, Z; Storb, R; Tapscott, SJ; Kuhr, CS; Hauschka, SD; Lee, RS; Sale, GE; Zellmer, E; Gisburne, S; Bogan, J; Kornegay, JN; Cooper, BJ; Gooley, TA & Little, MT. (2004). Hematopoietic stem cell transplantation does not restore dystrophin expression in Duchenne muscular dystrophy dogs. *Blood*, v. 104, pp. 4311-4318.

Deitz, K; Morrison, JA; Kline, K; Guo, LT & Shelton, GD. (2008). Sarcoglycan-Deficient Muscular Dystrophy in a Boston Terrier. *Journal of Veterinary Intern Medicine, v.*22, pp. 476–480.

Ervasti, JM; Ohlendieck, K; Kahl, SD; Gaver, MG & Campbell, KP. (1990). Deficiency of glycoprotein component of the dystrophin complex in dystrophic muscle. *Nature*, v. 345, p. 315-319.

Ervasti, JM &Campbell, KP. (1991). Membrane organization of the dystrophin glycoprotein complex. *Cell*, v. 66, pp. 1121-1131.

Foster, K; Foster, H & Dickson, JG. (2006). Gene therapy progress and prospects: Duchenne muscular dystrophy. *Gene Therapy*, v.13, pp. 1677–1685,

Gaiad, TP; Silva, MB; Silva, GCA; Caromano, FA; Miglino, MA. & Ambrosio, CE. (2011). Physical therapy assessment tools to evaluate disease progression and phenotype variability in Golden Retriever Muscular Dystrophy. *Research in Veterinary Science*, v. 9, [Epub ahead of print].

Gaiad, TP; Miglino, MA; Zatz, M; Hamlett, WC & Ambrosio, CE. (2009). Effect of physical therapy on joint range of motion and muscle collagen deposition in the Golden Retriever Muscular Dystrophy (GRMD) model. *Brazilian Journal of Physical Therapy*, v.13, n. 3, pp. 244-51.

Gillis, JM. (2002). Multivariate evaluation of the functional recovery obtained by the overexpression of utrophin in skeletal muscles of the *mdx* mouse. *Neuromuscular Disorders*, v. 12(Suppl 1), pp. S90–94.

Griggs, RC; Mendell, JR; Fenichel, GM; Brooke, MH; Pestronk, A; Miller, JP; Cwik, VA; Pandya, S & Robison, J. (1993). Duchenne dystrophy: randomized, controlled trial of prednisone (18 months) and azathioprine (12 months). *Neurology*, v. 43, pp. 520-527.

Gomes, AR; Cornachione, A; Salvini, TF & Mattiello-Sverzuti, AC. (2007). Morphological effects of two protocols of passive stretch over the immobilized rat soleus muscle. *Journal of Anatomy*, v. 210, n. 3, p. 328-335.

Grange, RW & Call, JA. (2007). Recommendations to define exercise prescription for Duchenne Muscular Dystrophy. *Exercise and Sport Sciences Review*, v. 35, n. 1, pp. 12-7.

Grounds, M.D., Radley, H.G., Lynch, G.S., Nagaraju, K, de Luca, A. (2008). Towards developing standard operating procedures for pre-clinical testing in the mdx mouse model of Duchenne muscular dystrophy. *Neurobiology of Disease*, v. 31, pp. 1–19.

Hoffman, EP &, Gorospe, JRM. (1991). The animal-models of duchenne muscular-dystrophy - windows on the pathophysiological consequences of dystrophin deficiency. *Current Topics in Membranes*, v. 38, pp. 113-154.

Hoffman, EP; Brown Jr., RH & Kunkel, LM. (1987). Dystrophin: the protein product of the Duchenne Muscular Dystrophy locus. *Cell*, v. 51, pp. 919-928.

Howell, JM; Fletcher, S; Kakulas, BA; O'Hara, M; Lochmuller, H & Kaparti, G. (1997). Use of the dog model for Duchenne muscular dystrophy in gene therapy trials. Neuromuscular disorders, v. 7, n. 5, pp. 325-8.

Howell, JM; Lochmuller, H; O'Hara, A; Fletcher, S; Kakulas, BA; Massie, B; Nalbantoglu, J & Karpati, G.(1998). High-level dystrophin expression after adenovirus-mediated dystrophin minigene transfer to skeletal muscle of dystrophic dogs: prolongation of expression with immunosuppression. *Human Gene Therapy, v.* 9, pp. 629–34.

Huebner, KD; Jassal, DS; Halevy, O; Pines, M & Aanderson, JE. (2008). Functional resolution of fibrosis in *mdx* mouse dystrophic heart and skeletal muscle by halofuginone. *American journal of Physiology. Heart and Circulatory Physiology*, v. 294, pp. 1550-1561.

Jones, BR; Brennan, S; Mooney, CT; Callanan, JJ; Mcallister, H; Guo, LT; Martin, PT; Engvall, E & Shelton, GD. (2004). Muscular dystrophy with truncated dystrophin in a family of Japanese spitz dogs. *Journal of Neurological Science*, v. 217, pp. 143-149.

Kacsor, JJ; Hall, JE; Payne, E & Tarnopolsky, MA. (2007). Low intensity training decreases markers of oxidative stress in skeletal muscle of *mdx* mouse. *Free Radical Biology and Medicine*, v. 43, pp. 145-154.

Kerkis, I; Ambrosio, CE; Kerkis, A; Martins, DS; Zucconi, E; Fonseca, SAS; Cabral, RM; Maranduba, CMC; Gaiad, TP; Morini, AC; Vieira, NM; Brolio, MP; Sant'anna, OA; Miglino, MA & Zatz, M. (2008). Early transplantation of human immature dental pulp stem cells from baby teeth to golden retriever muscular dystrophy (GRMD) dogs: local or systemic? *Journal of Translational Medicine*, v. 6, p. 35, doi:10.1186/1479-5876-6-35.

Kimura, S; Ikesawa, M; Nomura, K; Ito, K; Ozasa, S; Ueno, H; Yoshioka, K; Yano, S; Yamashita, T; Matuskura, M & Miike, T (2006). Immobility reduces muscle fiber necrosis in dystrophin deficient muscular dystrophy. *Brain & Development*, v. 28, n. 7, pp. 473-6.

Koenig, M; Hoffman, EP; Bertelson, CJ; Monaco, AP; Feener, C & Kunkel, LM. (1987). Complete cloning of the Duchenne muscular dystrophy (DMD) cDNA and preliminary genomic organization of the DMD gene in normal and affected individuals. *Cell*, v.50, n. 3, pp.509–517.

Kornegay, JN; Li, J; Bogan, JR; Bogan, DJ; Chen, C; Zheng, H; Wang, B; Qiao, C; Howard Jr, JF & Xiao, X. (2010). Widespread Muscle Expression of an AAV9 Human Mini-dystrophin Vector After Intravenous Injection in Neonatal Dystrophin-deficient Dogs. *Molecular Therapy*, v. 18, n. 8, pp. 1501–1508.

Kornegay, JN; Sharp, NJH; Schueler, RO & Betts, CW. (1994). Tarsal joint contracture in dogs with golden retriever muscular dystrophy. *Laboratory Animal Science*, v. 44, pp. 331-333.

Kornegay, JN; Tuler, SM; Miller, DM & Levesaue, DC. (1988). Muscular dystrophy in a litter of golden retriever dogs. *Muscle nerve*, v. 11, pp. 1056-1064.

Landisch, RM; Kosir, AM; Nelson, SA; Baltgalvis & KA; Lowe, DA. (2008). Adaptative and nonadaptative responses to voluntary wheel running by *mdx* mice. *Muscle Nerve*, v. 38, pp. 1290-1303.

Liu, F; Nishikawa, M; Clemens, PR & Huang, L. (2001). Transfer of full-length Dmd to the diaphragm muscle of Dmd (*mdx/mdx*) mice through systemic administration of plasmid DNA. *Molecular Therapy*, v. 4, pp. 45–51.

Martin, PT; Shelton, GD; Dickinson, PJ; Sturges, BK; Xu, R; LeCouteur, RA; Guo, LT; Grahn, RA; Lo, HP; North, KN; Malik, R; Engvall, E & Lyons, LA. (2008). Muscular dystrophy associated with a-dystroglycan deficiency in Sphynx and Devon Rex cats. *Neuromuscular Disorders*, v. 18, pp. 942–952.

Mathur, S; Vohra, R; Germain, SA; Forbes, S; Bryant, ND; Vandenborne, K & Walter, G.A. (2011). Changes in muscle T2 and tissue damage after downhill running in mdx mice. *Muscle & Nerve*, v. 43, pp. 878-886.

McDonald, CM. (2002). Physical activity, health impairments, and disability in neuromuscular disease. *American Journal of Physical Medicine & Rehabilitation* , v. 81 Suppl 11, pp. 108-20.

Mercuri, E; Mayhew, A; Muntoni, F; Messina, S; Straub, V; Van Ommen, GJ; Voit, T; Bertini, E & Bushby, K. (2008). TREAT-NMD Neuromuscular Network: Towards harmonisation of outcome measures for DMD and SMA within TREAT-NMD. *Neuromuscular Disorders*, v. 18, n. 11, pp. 894-903.

Mokhtarian, A; Lefaucheur, JP; Even, PC & Sebille, A. (1999). Hindlimb immobilization applied to 21-day-old *mdx* mice prevents the occurrence of muscle degeneration. *Journal of Applied Physiology*, v. 86, n. 3, pp. 924-931.

Moxley, RT; Ashwal, S; Pandya, S; Connolly, A; Florence, J; Mathews, K; Baumbach, L; Mcdonald, C; Sussman, M & Wade, C. (2005). Practice Parameter: Corticosteroid treatment of Duchenne dystrophy. *Neurology*, v. 64, pp. 13-20.

Muntoni, F; Fisher, I; Morgan, JE & Abraham, D. (2002). Steroids in Duchenne muscular dystrophy: from clinical trials to genomic research. *Neuromuscular Disorders*, v. 12 (Suppl), pp. 162-165.

Nakamura, A &Takeda, S. (2011). Mammalian models of Duchenne Muscular Dystrophy: Pathological characteristics and therapeutic applications. *Journal of Biomedicine and Biotechnology*, v. 2011, 8p. doi:10.1155/2011/184393

Nguyen, F; Guigand, L; Goubault-Leroux, I; Wyers, M & Cherel, Y. (2005). Microvessel density in muscles of dogs with golden retriever muscular dystrophy. *Neuromuscular Disorders*, v. 15, pp. 154-163.

O'Brien, DP; Johnson, GC; Liu, LA; Guo, LT; Engvall, E; Powell, HC & Shelton, GD. (2001). Laminin alpha 2 (merosin)-deficient muscular dystrophy and demyelinating neuropathy in two cats. *Journal of Neurological Science*, v. 15, v. 189, pp. 37-43.

Ohlendieck, K & Campbell, KP. (1991). Dystrophin-associated proteins are greatly reduced in skeletal muscle from *mdx* mice. *Journal of Cell Biology*, v. 115, pp. 1685–1694.

Paola, JP; Podell, M & Shelton, GD. (1993). Muscular dystrophy in a miniature Schnauzer. *Progress in Veterinary Neurology*, v. 4, pp. 14-18.

Podhorska-Okow, M; Sandri, M; Zampieri, S; Brun, B; Rossini, K & Carraro, U. (1998). Apoptosis of myofibers and satellite cells: exercise-induced damage in skeletal muscle of the mouse. *Neuropathology and Applied Neurobiology*, v. 24, pp. 518-531.

Presthus, J & Nordstoga, K. (1993). Congenital myopathy in a litter of Samoyed dogs. *Progress in Veterinary Neurology*, v. 4, pp. 37-40.

Salvadori, C; Vattemi, G; Lombardo, R; Marini, M; Cantile, C & Shelton, GD. (2009). Muscular Dystrophy with Reduced b-Sarcoglycan. *Journal Compendium of Pathology*, v. 140, pp. 278-282.

Schatzberg, SJ; Olby, NJ; Breen, M; Anderson, LVB; Langford, CF; Dickens, HF; Wilton, SD; Zeiss, CJ; Binns, MM; Kornegay, JN; Morris, GE & Sharp, NJH. (1999). Molecular analysis of a spontaneous dystrophin 'knockout' dog. *Neuromuscular Disorders*, v. 9, pp. 289-295.

Sharp, N; Kornegay, J; Van Camp, SD; Herbstreith, MH; Secore, SL; Kettle, S; Hung, WY; Constantinou, CD; Dykstra, MJ & Roses, AD. (1992). An error in dystrophin mRNA processing in golden retriever muscular dystrophy, an animal homologue of Duchenne muscular dystrophy. *Genomics*, v. 13, pp. 115–121.

Shelton, GD & Engvall, E. (2005). Canine and feline models of human inherited muscle diseases. *Neuromuscular Disorders*, v. 15, n. 2, pp. 127–138.

Shelton, GD. & Engvall, (2002). E. Muscular dystrophies and other inherited myopathies. *Veterinary Clinics of North America - Small Animal Practice*, v. 32, n. 1, pp. 103-124.

Shelton, GD; Liu, LA; Guo, LT; Smith, GK; Christiansen, JS; Thomas, WB; Smith, MO; Kline, KL; March, PA; Flegel, T & Engvall, E. (2001). Muscular dystrophy in female dogs. *Journal Veterinary Internal Medicine*, v. 15, pp. 240-244.

Shelton, GD. (2010). Routine and specialized laboratory testing for the diagnosis of neuromuscular diseases in dogs and cats. *Veterinary Clinical pathology*, v. 39, pp. 278-295.

Shimatsu, Y; Yoshimura, M; Yuasa, K; Urasawa, N; Tomohiro, M; Nakura, M; Tanigawa, M; Nakamura, A; Takeda, S. (2005). Major clinical and histopathological characteristics of canine X-linked muscular dystrophy in Japan, CXMD. *ActaMyologica*, v. 24, n. 2, pp. 145–154.

Sicinski, P; Geng, Y; Ryder-Cook, A; Barnard, E; Darlison, M & Barnard, P. (1989). The molecular basis of muscular dystrophy in the *mdx* mouse: a point mutation. *Science*, v. 244, pp. 1578–1580.

Straub, V; Rafael, JA; Chamberlain, JS & Campbell, KP. (1997). Animal models for muscular dystrophy show different patterns of sarcolemmal disruption. *The Journal of Cell Biology*, v. 139, n. 2, pp. 375–385.

Strober, J.B. (2006). Therapeutics in duchenne muscular dystrophy. *NeuroRx*, v. 3, n. 2, pp. 225-34.

Tegeler, CJ; Grange, RW; Bogan, DJ; Markert, CD; Case, D; Kornegay, JN. & Childers, MK. (2010). Eccentric contractions induce rapid isometric torque drop in dystrophin-deficient dogs. *Muscle & Nerve*, v. 42, pp. 130-132.

Thibaud, JL; Monnet, A; Bertoldi, D; Barthelémy, I; Blot, S & Carlier, PG. (2007). Characterization of dystrophic muscle in golden retriever muscular dystrophy dogs by nuclear magnetic resonance imaging. *Neuromuscular disorders*, v. 17, pp. 575-584.

Uchikawa, K; Liu, M; Hanayama, K; Tsuji, T; Fujiwara, T &Chino, N. (2004). Functional status and muscle strength in people with Duchenne muscular dystrophy living in the community. *Journal of Rehabilitation Medicine*, v. 36, n. 3, pp.124-9.

Vainzof M. Ayub-Guerrieri, D; Onofre, PC; Martins, PC; Lopes, VF; Zilberztajn, D; Maia, LS; Sell, K & Yamamoto, L. (2008). Animal models for genetic neuromuscular disease. *Journal of Molecular Neuroscience*, v. 34, pp. 241-248.

Valentine, BA; Blue, JT; Shelley, SM & Cooper, BJ. (1990a) Increase Serum Alanine Aminotransferase Activity Associated with Muscle Necrosis in the Dog. *Journal of Veterinary Internal Medicine*, v. 4, pp. 140-143.

Valentine, BA; Cooper, BJ; Cummings, JF & Lahunta, AL. (1990b). Canine X-linked muscular dystrophy: morphologic lesions. *Journal of the Neurological Science*, v. 97,p p. 1-23.

Valentine, BA; Cooper, BJ; Delahunta, A; Oquinn, R & Blue, JT. (1988). Canine x-linked muscular-dystrophy - an animal-model of duchenne muscular-dystrophy - clinical-studies. *Journal of the Neurological Sciences*, v. 88, pp. 69-81.

Van ham, LM L; Roels, S . & Hoorens, JK. (1995). Congenital dystrophy like myopathy in a Brittany spaniel puppy. *Progress in Veterinary Neurology*, v. 6, pp. 135-138.

Van Putten, M; de Winter, C; van Roon-Mom, W; van Ommen, G; 't Hoen, PAC & Aartsma-Rus, A. (2010). A 3 months mild functional test regime does not affect disease parameters in young *mdx* mice. *Neuromuscular disorders*, v. 20, pp. 273-280.

Vignos, PJ; Wagner, MB; Karlinchak, B & Kairji, B. (1996). Evaluation of a program for long-term treatment of Duchenne muscular dystrophy. Experience at the University Hospitals of Cleveland. *Journal of Bone & Joint Surgery*, v. 78, n. 12, pp.1844-52.

Wentink, G; Linde-Sipman, JS & Van Der Meijer, AEFH. (1972). Myopathy with a possible recessive X-linked inheritance in a litter of Irish terriers. *Veterinary Pathology*, v. 9, pp. 328-349.

Wieczorek, LA; Garosi, LS & Shelton, GD. (2006). Dystrophin-deficient muscular dystrophy in an Old English sheepdog. *Veterinary Record*, v. 158, pp. 270-273.

Willmann, R; De Luca, A; Benatar, M; Grounds, M; Dubach, J; Raymackers, JM & Nagaraju, K.(2011). Enhancing translation: Guidelines for standard pre-clinical experiments in *mdx* mice. *Neuromuscular Disorders*. Article in Press

Willmann, R; Possekel, S; Dubach-Powell, J; Meier, T & Ruegg, M.A. (2009). Mammalian animal models for Duchenne muscular dystrophy. *Neuromuscular disorders*, v. 19, n. 4, 241-249.

Winand, N; Edwards, M; Pradhan, D; Berian, C & Cooper, B. (1994). Deletion of the dystrophin muscle promoter in feline muscular dystrophy. *Neuromuscular Disorders*, v. 4, pp. 433–445.

Yokota, T; Lu, QL; Partridge, T; Kobayashi, M; Nakamura, A; Takeda, S & Hoffman, E. (2009). Efficacy of systemic morpholino exon-skipping in duchenne dystrophy dogs, *Annals of Neurology*, v. 65, n. 6, pp. 667–676.